Autism and Child Psychopathology Series

Series Editor

Johnny L. Matson, Louisiana State University, Baton Rouge, LA, USA

Brief Overview
The purpose of this series is to advance knowledge in the broad multidisciplinary fields of autism and various forms of psychopathology (e.g., anxiety and depression). Volumes synthesize research on a range of rapidly expanding topics on assessment, treatment, and etiology.

Description
The **Autism and Child Psychopathology Series** explores a wide range of research and professional methods, procedures, and theories used to enhance positive development and outcomes across the lifespan. Developments in education, medicine, psychology, and applied behavior analysis as well as child and adolescent development across home, school, hospital, and community settings are the focus of this series. Series volumes are both authored and edited, and they provide critical reviews of evidence-based methods. As such, these books serve as a critical reference source for researchers and professionals who deal with developmental disorders and disabilities, most notably autism, intellectual disabilities, challenging behaviors, anxiety, depression, ADHD, developmental coordination disorder, communication disorders, and other common childhood problems. The series addresses important mental health and development difficulties that children and youth, their caregivers, and the professionals who treat them must face. Each volume in the series provides an analysis of methods and procedures that may assist in effectively treating these developmental problems.

Johnny L. Matson
Editor

Assessment and Diagnosis in Autism

Springer

Editor
Johnny L. Matson
Louisiana State University
Baton Rouge, LA, USA

ISSN 2192-922X ISSN 2192-9238 (electronic)
Autism and Child Psychopathology Series
ISBN 978-3-032-11801-1 ISBN 978-3-032-11802-8 (eBook)
https://doi.org/10.1007/978-3-032-11802-8

This Springer imprint is published by the registered company Springer Nature Switzerland AG
The registered company address is: Gewerbestrasse 11, 6330 Cham, Switzerland

Contents

Autism Assessment Across the Lifespan: Integrating Research and Clinical Practice

Jessica Emick, Sonia S. Agarwal, and A. J. McConnell

Abstract This chapter provides a detailed overview of the assessment of Autism Spectrum Disorder (ASD) across the lifespan, beginning with a definition of ASD, its core characteristics and symptoms, and the importance of early identification in shaping intervention outcomes. The chapter emphasizes a multidisciplinary team approach to assessment, incorporating expertise from various fields to ensure a comprehensive evaluation. A detailed review of both generalized and autism-specific assessment measures is provided, covering tools used across the lifespan from early childhood through adulthood, as well as adaptive functioning and executive function (EF) measures. Tailoring the assessment process to the individual's needs and profile is highlighted, ensuring the use of appropriate methods for each unique presentation. The chapter also explores differential diagnosis and co-occurring conditions, including developmental, communication, and anxiety disorders, to aid clinicians in distinguishing ASD from other conditions and understanding the broader clinical context. Modern research on racial and ethnic bias in ASD diagnosis is discussed, with an emphasis on addressing disparities and promoting equitable care. The female phenotype of ASD and the barriers to diagnosis faced by women and gender nonconforming individuals are also examined, highlighting the need for increased clinician awareness of diverse presentations. The chapter concludes with case vignettes that illustrate the factors influencing the selection of an appropriate testing battery and provide practical examples of how demographic considerations can inform the design of the diagnostic interview and the interpretation of testing results.

Keywords Autism · Autism Spectrum Disorder (ASD) · Screening tools · Autism diagnostic measures · Neurodevelopmental assessment · Co-occurring conditions · differential diagnosis · Sex differences · Telehealth assessment · Cultural responsiveness

J. Emick (✉)
Fielding Graduate University, Santa Barbara, CA, USA
e-mail: jemick@fielding.edu

S. S. Agarwal · A. J. McConnell
NADD-LC, Alvis Inc., Columbus, OH, USA

J. L. Matson (ed.), *Assessment and Diagnosis in Autism*, Autism and Child Psychopathology Series, https://doi.org/10.1007/978-3-032-11802-8_1

Introduction to Autism Spectrum Disorder (ASD)

Autism Spectrum Disorder (ASD) is a neurodevelopmental disorder characterized by challenges in communication and social interaction, and restricted, repetitive patterns of behavior (American Psychiatric Association (APA), 2022). Recent prevalence data suggests roughly 1 in every 36 children in the United States and 1 in 100 children globally are diagnosed with ASD (Centers for Disease Control & Prevention, 2022; Zeidan et al., 2022). The impact of ASD extends beyond the individual, affecting family dynamics, educational settings, and community support systems. Given the heterogeneity of ASD presentations, accurate assessment is essential to tailor interventions to the unique needs of each individual. Furthermore, early identification and intervention have been shown to significantly improve long-term outcomes, underscoring the importance of comprehensive and timely assessment practices.

This chapter will provide an in-depth exploration of autism assessment across the lifespan. It will examine a range of assessment measures including screening tools, observational assessments, and diagnostic interviews used to identify ASD. Recent trends in assessment, such as the incorporation of technology-based assessments and telehealth services, will be discussed, along with considerations for cultural diversity and linguistic diversity in assessment practices. By incorporating the latest research and evidence-based practices in autism assessment, this chapter aims to equip clinicians and educators with the knowledge and tools necessary to effectively identify and support individuals with ASD across diverse developmental stages and cultural backgrounds.

The authors of this chapter would like to note recent trends in language use within the autism community. Professionals, academics, and caregivers often report preferring person-first language (i.e., person with autism) to emphasize that the diagnosis does not define impacted individuals. Conversely, autistic advocates promote the use of identity-first language (i.e., autistic person) for reasons including de-stigmatization and taking pride in autistic identity (Botha et al., 2023; Kenny et al., 2016). Within the broader autism community, there is poor consensus on most appropriate terminology usage, and the choice to use person-first or identity-first language is made on an individual basis. Within this chapter, the term ASD will be used in discussion of diagnostic characteristics and processes, with person-first and identity-first language used interchangeably in discussion of the experiences of autistic individuals and their families and caregivers.

Definition, Overview, and Key Characteristics and Symptoms

Autism has been a diagnosis recognized by mental health professionals for several decades; however, there is often confusion and inaccurate information about autism found even among mental health professionals. It is important to have an accurate understanding of the diagnostic requirements and history of autism as many individuals and families may have a misunderstanding of autism based on inaccurate information found on the internet and social media. For example, only 27% of the most popular autism videos on Tik Tok contained accurate information with 32% of videos on autism featuring overgeneralized information and 41% containing inaccurate information (Aragon-Guevara et al., 2023). To help better understand the main features of Autism, a brief history is outlined below along with the diagnostic features outlined in the current Diagnostic Statistical Manual of Mental Disorders (DSM; APA, 2022).

In the first two editions of the DSM, autism was initially referred to as Schizophrenic Reaction—Childhood Type. During its early years, Autism often referred to children with very severe symptoms and extensive intellectual deficits. Over the past 45 years, the diagnostic criteria for Autism have become more specified. Beginning with the DSM-III in 1980, a new category was introduced known as Pervasive Developmental Disorders (PDD). This included diagnoses such as Autism, Asperger Disorder, and Pervasive Developmental Disorder—Not Otherwise Specified (PDD-NOS). A diagnosis of Autism from 1980 to 2012 indicated that an individual had persistent deficits in socialization, communication, and restricted interests and repetitive/stereotyped behaviors. A diagnosis of Asperger's Disorder was similar except that deficits in communication were not part of the diagnostic criteria. Lastly, an individual may have received a diagnosis of PDD-NOS if they exhibited some symptoms associated with Autism, Asperger's, or another type of PDD; however, the individual did not meet full diagnostic criteria for any specific disorder in the PDD category.

In 2013, the DSM-5 diagnostic criteria for autism changed significantly. As scientific research has evolved, it was determined that communication deficits alone did not indicate a person met diagnostic criteria for an Autism Spectrum Disorder. Instead, it was the social aspects of communication that were relevant. Furthermore, autism was viewed as a spectrum with some individuals exhibiting substantial deficits in social communication and behavior, whereas, other individuals varied on the severity of their deficits. Therefore, the terminology for the diagnoses of Autism, Asperger's Disorder, and PDD-NOS changed. A diagnosis of Autism Spectrum Disorder is now the appropriate clinical term. Individuals previously diagnosed with Autism, Asperger's Disorder, or PDD-NOS are considered to still meet DSM-5 and DSM-5-TR diagnostic criteria for an Autism Spectrum Disorder. The DSM-5-TR is the current edition of the DSM. The diagnostic criteria for Autism Spectrum Disorder did not substantially change from the DSM-5 to the DSM-5-TR.

There are now two main symptom categories associated with a diagnosis of an Autism Spectrum Disorder: (A) Persistent deficits in social communication and social interaction across multiple contexts, and (B) restricted, repetitive patterns of behavior interests, or activities (see Table 1 below for examples of symptoms commonly exhibited by individuals with ASD).

There are a few additional caveats to consider as part of an ASD diagnostic assessment. First, clinical diagnostic assessments are different from evaluations completed

Table 1 Common symptoms and traits associated with ASD

Autism spectrum disorder in the DSM-5-TR	
Social communication	Examples of Behaviors in Individuals with ASD
Deficits in social-emotional reciprocity	An individual struggles to have a back-and-forth conversation. They may dominate a conversation. They do not pick up on social cues that others are not interested in what they are talking about or that others would like a turn to speak. An individual may also be withdrawn and not ask questions or participate in a back-and-forth exchange A young child does not respond when a parent calls their name An individual does not initiate or respond to social interactions
Deficits in nonverbal communicative behaviors used for social interactions	An individual struggles to establish or maintain Eye Contact An individual does not show a range of facial expressions. They may look emotionless An individual may say something but not look at the person they are speaking to
Deficits in developing, maintaining, and understanding relationships	A child does not engage in make-believe, creative play An individual is blunt and makes comments that offend others An individual has no interest in interacting with others
Restricted, Repetitive Patterns of Behavior, Interests, or Activities	Examples of Behaviors in Individuals with ASD
Stereotyped or repetitive motor movements, use of objects or speech	An individual lines up toys or objects in a line. They become upset if the line is disrupted An individual echoes or repeats what others say to them. Some individuals may script such that they sound like they are quoting from their favorite movie, show, or song when they respond to others An individual repeatedly flaps their hands, makes certain hand gestures, flicks their fingers in front of their eyes, or rocks their body back-and-forth

(continued)

Table 1 (continued)

Autism spectrum disorder in the DSM-5-TR	
Social communication	Examples of Behaviors in Individuals with ASD
Insistence on sameness, inflexible adherence to routines, or ritualized patterns of verbal or nonverbal behavior	An individual wants to eat the same thing for breakfast, lunch, and dinner each day. They refuse to eat if it is not their preferred food items Individuals become extremely upset or distressed at small changes in their daily routine. They may struggle to transition to new activities. At school, they may not respond well to a substitute teacher, fire drill, or changing to a new subject in class An individual is concrete and does not understand sarcasm, jokes, or humor. They struggle to understand the perspective of others
Highly restricted, fixated interests that are abnormal in intensity or focus	A child may have a strong interest in unusual objects such as fire alarms, drain pipes, or parts of an object An individual may perseverate on their interests. A child may be interested in scientific topics, such as dinosaurs, or pop culture topics, such as Minecraft, Pokemon, My Little Pony, etc
Hyper- or hyporeactivity to sensory input or unusual interest in sensory aspects of the environment	An individual has a strong pain tolerance. Children may not tell others that they are not feeling well and parents may not recognize this until the child is seen by a medical professional An individual dislikes certain clothing. They may avoid wearing clothing with tags or other clothing that feels awkward on their skin An individual with severe autism may stare excessively at a ceiling fan and is fascinated by its movement

as part of a special education evaluation (e.g., Evaluation Team Report, Individualized Education Program). Clinical diagnostic evaluations are based on criteria outlined in the current edition of the DSM and often provide treatment recommendations that can be implemented in clinical settings, an individual's home, and/or at school. In contrast, special education evaluations focus primarily on how an individual's functioning is impacting their learning in a school setting. Requirements for a student to be eligible for special education services under an Autism classification vary by state and, therefore, may not always necessitate comprehensive testing to support a diagnosis. This can result in an individual needing a more comprehensive evaluation in the future if they seek services outside of a school setting (e.g., social security benefits, eligibility for government service agencies, etc.). An understanding of differential diagnoses is also important when completing autism assessments. There are several overlapping symptoms that may be better explained by other diagnoses than autism. We discuss differential diagnoses later in this chapter. Another caveat is understanding how autism presents across the lifespan. According to the DSM-5 and DSM-5-TR, autism spectrum disorder may be currently present or historically present in older individuals. Adults that meet diagnostic criteria may not currently exhibit all of the symptoms related to autism but may have done so during their foundational developmental years. In other words, the severity of autism-related symptoms may improve as an individual transitions into adulthood (Bernier et al., 2010).

The Importance of Assessment

Early Identification and Intervention

Research has consistently shown that early detection and intervention significantly improve outcomes in children with autism spectrum disorder (ASD). By identifying the signs of ASD as early as possible, clinicians can initiate appropriate interventions tailored to a child's unique needs, promoting optimal development and functioning (AAP, 2021; Estes et al., 2015). Early interventions typically focus on enhancing communication skills, social interaction, and adaptive behaviors, laying a strong foundation for future learning and independence. Moreover, early identification allows for the early involvement of families in intervention programs, empowering them with knowledge and resources to support their child's development effectively. Through collaborative efforts among psychologists, educators, and healthcare professionals, early identification and intervention play a crucial role in maximizing the potential and quality of life of children with autism.

The ability to accurately diagnose autism has seen significant improvement over the past two decades, particularly in very young children. This progress is attributed to empirical investigations focused on refining the diagnostic criteria outlined in the DSM-5 alongside the development of reliable assessment instruments. The early detection of autism has critical implications for facilitating timely referral to intervention services. While the importance of early identification and subsequent intervention is well established, concerns regarding false positives necessitate investigation of the stability of diagnoses and developmental trajectories of symptoms. Research indicates that symptoms typically emerge between 12 and 18 months of age, with diagnoses made at 18 months of age showing reliability and stability. Studies have demonstrated that diagnoses before the age of three tend to have a relatively low false-positive rate, although false negatives are more common. According to a study by Smith et al. (2015), early diagnoses have been found to have a low false-positive rate, but false negatives remain a significant concern. In fact, 30% of children who were diagnosed before the age of three had false negatives, emphasizing the importance of ongoing monitoring and evaluation (Smith et al., 2015). Late-diagnosed cases present heterogeneity in early outcomes and phenotypes, suggesting the need for expanded screening beyond three years of age (Landa et al., 2022; Yu et al., 2024). Overall, early detection and intervention are pivotal for improving outcomes and maximizing the potential of children with autism, highlighting the importance of collaborative efforts among psychologists, educators, and healthcare professionals.

Understanding Individual Needs and Individual Reasons for Pursuing a Psychological Evaluation

The purpose of psychological and neurodevelopmental assessments varies depending on the individual and context. While some clients and their families seek to determine whether they have Autism Spectrum Disorder (ASD), it is important for clinicians to emphasize the broader value of these assessments. As emphasized by Smith et al. (2015), clinical assessments for ASD not only provide a diagnosis but also offer valuable insights into the individual's strengths and challenges, which can inform the development of personalized treatment plans. Beyond identifying and formulating diagnostic impressions, comprehensive neurodevelopmental evaluations help to understand a client's strengths and weaknesses across key domains. This comprehensive understanding allows the development of individualized evidence-based recommendations and provides a holistic view of the client (Steiner & Gengoux, 2018).

Parents and caregivers might pursue a diagnosis for their child to secure the necessary therapeutic support to enhance their child's development and well-being. For some clients and families, obtaining a diagnostic label is essential to access appropriate services, making the assessment process potentially anxiety-provoking, with long wait times particularly frustrating. For other individuals, the assessment process is intended to increase self-understanding and validation of experiences that may have been confusing or isolating. An official diagnosis can provide a framework for interpreting past difficulties, offer access to tailored support and interventions, and foster a sense of belonging within the autism community. Additionally, some may seek a diagnosis to qualify for educational accommodations or workplace adjustments, enabling them to thrive in environments that are not designed with their needs in mind.

Thus, the motivation behind seeking an autism diagnosis intertwines with the personal, practical, and systemic elements. As a clinician, it is crucial to ask clients and their families why they are seeking an evaluation at this time, and tailor the evaluation to their specific needs and purposes.

Implementing a Multidisciplinary Approach to Assessment

Having a multidisciplinary team of professionals is often recommended for autism diagnostic assessments (Volkmar et al., 2014; Yu et al., 2024). Multidisciplinary team assessments often include a medical, psychological, psychiatric, speech-language, and occupational therapy assessment at minimum. The team is often led by a medical provider, such as a developmental pediatrician, that completes a physical examination and assesses for other medical conditions that may mimic or be associated with ASD. This can include genetic testing, neurological testing, or examination of other potential organic etiologies or conditions the individual may experience. Psychiatrists may also be utilized to provide a more in-depth evaluation of medical components to ASD and provide treatment recommendations to address challenging behaviors that an individual with ASD may engage in across various settings.

Psychologists are also a core component of a multidisciplinary team approach. Psychologists often assist developmental pediatricians in conducting a comprehensive interview assessing an individual's developmental history and behavioral functioning in order to identify if any core social communication and/or restricted, repetitive patterns of behaviors, interests, and activities are present. Psychological testing is also conducted to assess for ASD symptoms, cognitive abilities, adaptive behavior skills, and social-emotional functioning. Psychological testing helps supplement medical testing by providing a description of the individual's strengths and weaknesses to help the team design effective behavioral interventions.

Specialized therapists, such as speech-language therapists, physical therapists, and occupational therapists, also provide important clinical data on an individual's development. Individuals with ASD may be nonverbal or have communication delays; therefore, speech-language testing can provide information on an individual's receptive and expressive vocabulary and social and pragmatic use of language (Volkmar et al., 2014). Furthermore, physical therapy and occupational therapy evaluations include measurements of sensory and/or motor difficulties that are commonly associated with ASD.

The use of collateral sources is also a component to most diagnostic assessments, including the multidisciplinary team approach. Family and caregivers are often interviewed to provide background information on the individual's history, including relevant developmental milestones, mental health, engagement in treatment, maladaptive behaviors, and other relevant factors. Educators can also be part of the process by providing information on how the individual is performing academically, emotionally, socially, and behaviorally within the school setting. Furthermore, educators can provide insight into interventions that have worked or have not worked with individuals so that the multidisciplinary team can collaborate on developing an effective intervention plan that can be used clinically, at home, and/or within the school setting.

Multidisciplinary team assessments for ASD are often completed in one to two appointments. Once each team member completes their part of the evaluation, the team gathers together to discuss the individual's developmental history and testing results. This helps provide diagnostic clarification and assist the team with transitioning to the next stage involving the development of a treatment plan for the individual and family. Feedback is provided to the individual and family along with recommended interventions and next steps. Care coordination is often provided following the conclusion of the assessment. This involves a social worker and/or other professional following up with the family within one month after diagnosis to check-in and evaluate any unaddressed needs of the individual and family. The goal is to assist the family in following up with recommendations from the assessment and link the individual and family with additional resources to help address any gaps in the treatment plan.

There is debate among the effectiveness of the multidisciplinary approach to ASD assessment. Benefits include having a comprehensive evaluation completed and the process being a "one stop for all" so that families have fewer appointments with different professionals. Furthermore, it is believed that having a diverse team of professionals allows the team to collaborate on whether an ASD diagnosis is appropriate, helps reduce clinician bias, and provides family with a targeted intervention plan to address an individual's needs across many domains (Volkmar et al., 2014; Yu et al., 2024). A multidisciplinary team approach is also beneficial for more complicated diagnostic presentations (e.g., Yu et al., 2024) in which an individual presents with various mental health symptoms and developmental concerns that make it more difficult for professionals to ascertain if the individual truly presents with a clinical and behavioral presentation that is consistent with an ASD diagnosis. Multidisciplinary team assessment also typically provides accurate diagnoses given the comprehensiveness of the evaluation (Gerdts et al., 2018). Comprehensive and accurate assessments are vital because brief diagnostic assessments have been found to lead to high rates of inaccurate diagnoses (Bishop & Lord, 2023; Gabrielsen et al., 2015). A multidisciplinary team approach to assessment may also improve service delivery, provide delineated roles and responsibilities for providers, and improve information sharing that may otherwise be complicated by interacting with professionals from other agencies and schools due to privacy laws and other barriers to care coordination.

In contrast, limitations of this approach is that it is not always covered by insurance and third-party payors, not available in all health systems or geographic locations, and not always efficient for simple, uncomplicated cases (Penner et al., 2018, Yu et al., 2024). The multidisciplinary approach also discounts the expertise of solo practitioners that are effective and efficient in identifying and diagnosing ASD in diverse populations. Research has indicated that professionals can provide accurate diagnoses without using a multidisciplinary approach if they have adequate training on ASD assessments (Nowell et al., 2020; Penner et al., 2023). More concerning for families is that many health care systems that utilize the multidisciplinary team approach often have lengthy waitlists and families may have to travel long distances to receive services (Christensen et al., 2018; Nowell et al., 2020); therefore, families are waiting several months to years in order for their child to be evaluated. This prolongs the individual with ASD from being linked to appropriate services and resources, which can be crucial for young children who need services as soon as possible to address their developmental delays.

Tools for Assessing ASD

Best-practice evaluations for assessing autism involve two essential elements: a thorough examination of developmental history and direct observation, including interactions with the individual (Bishop & Lord, 2023; Duvall et al., 2022). Therefore, it is crucial for practitioners conducting assessments to gain a deep understanding of typical and atypical development across domains. Additionally, as ASD has strong genetic links, and understanding the family history of ASD and related conditions can inform the diagnostic process and are an important part of the assessment process. Although assessment tools play a crucial role, the standard is the clinician's comprehensive interpretation of all available information. No single measure or set of measures diagnose ASD; instead, we rely on clinical judgment based on a preponderance of evidence that is ideally gathered during a comprehensive evaluation (Bishop & Lord, 2023; Kaufman, 2022). Therefore, we will review the available tools and their psychometric properties to assist clinicians in selecting the most appropriate measures for each client. *See* Fig. 1 *for a comprehensive diagram of assessment measures organized by type and age.*

Screening vs. Diagnosis

M-CHAT-R: The Modified Checklist for Autism in Toddlers, Revised (M-CHAT-R) is a widely used parent-report screening tool used to identify children who may have ASD at an early age (Robins et al., 2014). The M-CHAT-R is validated for children aged 16 to 30 months and designed to detect early signs of social and communicative deficits associated with ASD. Consisting of 20 yes/no questions administered to a parent or caregiver, the M-CHAT is a simple and brief screener which evaluates behaviors related to social interaction, joint attention, and language development. The simplicity and brief nature of the measure make it a practical tool for a broad range of professionals, with many pediatricians incorporating the screener into routine check-ups.

The M-CHAT-R is scored using an identified cutoff score which categorizes responses into low, medium, or high risk for ASD. The cutoff score is identified as 4 points, with a sensitivity of 0.88 and a specificity of 0.92 (see Robins et al., 2014 for psychometric details). Children who score within the medium or high-risk categories are recommended for further evaluation by a trained clinician. The M-CHAT-R is valuable as a means of early detection of ASD, and can support children in receiving early diagnosis and subsequent early intervention.

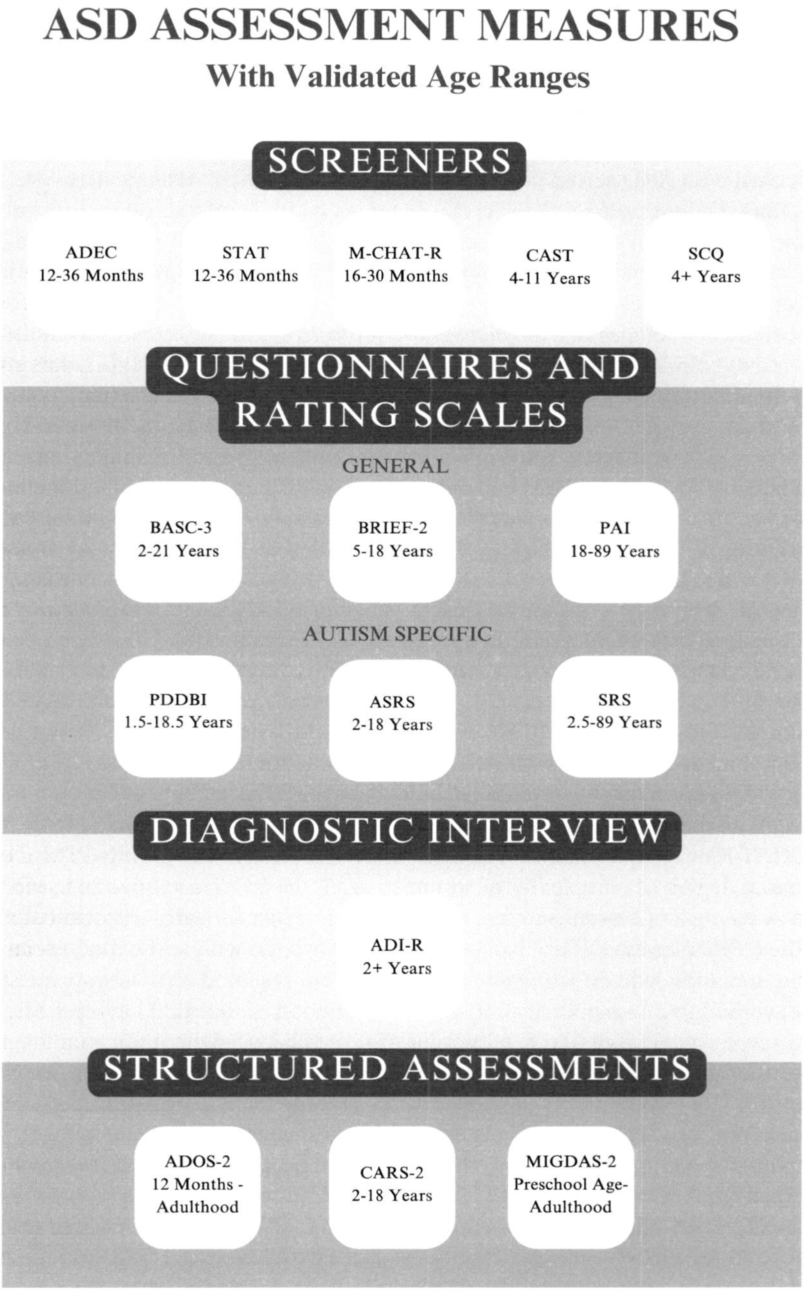

Fig. 1 ASD assessment measures with validated age ranges

***ADEC*:** The Autism Detection in Early Childhood (ADEC) is screening tool designed to identify ASD in children as young as 12 months of age (Young, 2007). The ADEC is unique in its early age range, allowing for early detection and timely intervention which can significantly improve developmental outcomes. The measure consists of 16 items which assess behaviors and developmental deficits commonly associated with ASD across domains of social interaction, communication, and play behaviors. Unlike the M-CHAT-R, the ADEC is administered through direct observation of the child in a naturalistic setting, making the test suitable for young children who may experience distress in more structured assessment formats, thus limiting interpretability of results.

The ADEC includes two distinct versions: the Professional version (administered by a trained clinician), and the Parent version (completed by the child's caregiver). Both versions are used in scoring the test, ensuring a comprehensive understanding of the child's current functioning across contexts and sources. Items are scored based on the presence or absence of specific behaviors, with higher scores indicating greater likelihood of ASD. The ADEC manual includes cutoff scores which identify children who may have ASD, with a cutoff score of at least 11 on the professional version (sensitivity = 0.94, specificity = 0.63; see Hedley et al., 2015 for psychometric details) and at least 14 on the parent version indicating a need for further diagnostic evaluation. The ADEC's focus on early behavioral indicators of ASD make it an effective tool for screening children as young as 12 months old.

***STAT*:** The Screening Tool for Autism in Toddlers and Young Children (STAT) is an interactive screening tool designed to identify possible ASD in children aged 12 to 36 months (Stone et al., 2000). The STAT consists of 12 items which assess key developmental areas associated with ASD, with items administered as a series of structured activities conducted by a trained clinician. The STAT takes place in a controlled setting with the examiner directly observing the child's behaviors, differing from the M-CHAT-R or ADEC which can be administered in naturalistic settings. Despite this increased degree of complexity in administration, the STAT's validation in children aged as young as 12 months makes it a valuable screener for early detection of ASD.

The STAT measures four distinct domains associated with ASD: play, communication, imitation, and directing attention. Each item is scored on a three-point Likert scale, with higher scores indicating greater likelihood of the child having ASD. The Total score ranges from 0 to 4, with a cutoff score of 2 or higher indicating the need for further diagnostic evaluation (sensitivity = 0.83, specificity = 0.86; see Stone et al., 2000 for psychometric details). The STAT's interactive format makes it a valuable tool for identifying early signs of ASD in children who may not exhibit obvious symptoms in naturalistic settings, and can be used by a broad range of professionals to screen for ASD.

***CAST*:** The Childhood Autism Spectrum Test (CAST), formerly referred to as the Childhood Asperger Syndrome Test, is a screening tool designed to identify children aged 4 to 11 years who may have ASD (Scott et al., 2002). The CAST consists of 37 yes/no questions completed by a parent or primary caregiver which focus on symptoms commonly associated with ASD. As a parent-report questionnaire, the

CAST is designed to be straightforward and easy to administer, making it a practical screener for use in clinical, educational, and medical settings.

The CAST covers a range of behaviors associated with ASD including difficulties in social interactions and communication, and the presence of repetitive behaviors and narrow interests. Items are scored dichotomously, with scores of 1 indicating an atypical response indicative of ASD and scores of 0 indicating a typical response. The test yields a Total score which ranges from 0 to 37, with a cutoff score of 15 or higher indicating the need for further diagnostic evaluation (sensitivity = 1.00, specificity = 0.97; see Williams et al., 2005 for psychometric details). The CAST is particularly valuable in its utility for screening ASD in older children who demonstrate developmental delays that were missed by early developmental screeners.

SCQ: Previously referred to as the Autism Screening Questionnaire (ASQ; Berument et al., 1999), the Social Communication Questionnaire (SCQ) is a parent-administered ASD screening measure. Items in the SCQ were derived from the content of the ADI-R, a gold-standard autism diagnostic instrument. The SCQ is a 40-item yes/no behavioral checklist designed to identify the presence of social and communicative behaviors, abnormal language uses, and stereotyped behaviors associated with ASD. The SCQ has been validated for children of at least four years; recent psychometric research examining the utility of the SCQ with children younger than 4 years has yielded promising results (Marvin et al., 2017).

The SCQ is available in two distinct versions: *Lifetime* and *Current*. The *Lifetime* version is interpreted with reference to cutoff points as a screener for potential ASD. Scores above the cutoff of 15 indicate the individual may have ASD and a full diagnostic evaluation is warranted (sensitivity = 0.85, specificity = 0.75; see Berument et al., 1999 for psychometric details). The *Current* version examines the individual's behavior over the last three months and includes three domains of Social Relating, Communication, and Range of interests. SCQ *Current* scores can inform clinical and educational treatment planning and progress tracking.

Questionnaires and Rating Scales

Broad Based Measures

BASC-3: The Behavior Assessment System for Children—3rd edition (BASC-3) is a set of scales and forms designed to measure the behaviors and self-perceptions of children and young adults (Reynolds & Kamphaus, 2015). It is widely used in clinical and educational settings to assess psychological functioning and inform differential diagnosis. The BASC-3 is validated in ages 2 to 21 and covers a broad range of domains including adaptive skills, anxiety, aggression, depression, social skills, and executive functioning, making it particularly useful in assessment of complex behavioral presentations. The BASC-3 also includes a Developmental Social Disorders content scale which measures a child's tendency to display social and communicative deficits commonly associated with developmental disorders, and an Autism Probability Index which indicates the similarity of a child's scores in the domains of social relationships to a sample of children with ASD.

The BASC-3 (Behavior Assessment System for Children, Third Edition) includes a variety of rating forms, such as the Teacher Rating Scales (TRS), Parent Rating Scales (PRS), Self-Report of Personality (SRP), and the Student Observation System (SOS). The TRS consists of 105 to 165 items, depending on the age group being assessed, and the PRS consists of 139–160 items, also varying by age group, with all items scored on a four-point Likert scale. Raw scores are converted into standardized T-scores for interpretation, with scores above the cutoff of 70 indicating clinically significant elevation, and T-scores between 6069 indicative of a child being at-risk. In assessment of ASD, the BASC-3 can be used to elucidate differences in behavioral presentation across settings (by comparing the TRS and PRS) and consider differential diagnosis or potential comorbidity.

BRIEF-2: The Behavior Rating Inventory of Executive Function, Second Edition (BRIEF-2), is a widely used assessment tool designed to evaluate executive functioning in children and adolescents aged 5 to 18 (Gioia et al., 2015). Executive functioning (EF) is a cognitive process that enables goal-directed behavior and includes skills such as planning, organization, working memory, and inhibition. Children with ASD often exhibit significant deficits related to executive functioning, with EF identified as a theoretical construct underpinning ASD symptomatology (Hill, 2004). For this reason, clinicians often administer the BRIEF-2 to investigate a child's current executive functioning.

The BRIEF-2 includes three forms: the Parent Form, the Teacher Form, and a Self-Report Form. These forms assess the child's executive functioning across contexts and perspectives, making it valuable in understanding differences in a child's behavioral presentation across settings. Each form consists of 63 items scored on a three-point Likert scale assessing nine EF scales: Inhibit, Monitor, Shift, Emotional Control, Initiate, Working Memory, Plan/Organize, Organization of Materials, and Self- and Task- Monitor (Gioia et al., 2015). Raw scale scores are converted into standardized T-scores for interpretation, with the test providing three index scores (Behavioral Regulation Index, Emotional Regulation Index, and Cognitive Regulation Index) and a Global Executive Composite score which provides a comprehensive view of the child's executive functioning. T-scores above 65 indicate significant EF difficulties, while scores between 60 and 64 suggest heightened EF concerns. The multidimensional nature of the BRIEF-2 supports its use in assessment of complex presentations of EF deficits as is commonly seen in co-occurring ASD and ADHD. Furthermore, the BRIEF-2's scale and index scores can be used clinically to inform EF support strategies and monitor treatment response over time.

PAI: The Personality Assessment Inventory (PAI) is a comprehensive tool used to broadly assess personality and psychopathology in adults aged 18 to 89 years (Morey, 1991). The PAI consists of 344 items scored on a four-point Likert scale and includes Validity Scales, Clinical Scales, Treatment Consideration Scales, and

Interpersonal Scales. The Validity Scales determine the examinee's approach to the test and identify tendencies towards exaggeration or minimization of symptoms. The Clinical Scales measure psychological constructs such as anxiety, depression, paranoia, schizophrenia, antisocial features, and substance use problems, while the Treatment Scales indicate factors which may influence treatment receptivity such as suicidality, stress, and support. The Interpersonal Scales assess the examinee's interpersonal style, including constructs such as warmth and dominance.

Individual scales within the PAI are interpreted distinctly, with higher Clinical Scale scores generally indicative of significant elevations warranting further clinical investigation. The PAI is commonly used in adult ASD assessments as a generalized measure to provide a broad understanding of an individual's current functioning, personality, and psychopathology. Similar to the BASC-3, the PAI supports differential diagnosis and can be used to identify potential comorbidity.

Autism Specific Measures

SRS-2: The Social Responsiveness Scale—Second Edition (SRS-2) is a rating scale which measures deficits in social behavior related to ASD (Constantino & Gruber, 2012). The measure consists of 65 items scored on a 4-point Likert-type rating scale, with results reported as standardized T-scores. The SRS-2 is distinct from other similar measures as it provides a continuous measure of social ability/impairment instead of a categorical (yes/no) checklist of deficits, allowing for identification of individuals with ASD who demonstrate more subtle social impairment, as well as the identification of social impairment in individuals without ASD.

The SRS-2 is available in four distinct versions spanning three age groups: the Preschool form, the School-Age form, the Adult form, and the Adult form (self-report). The Preschool Form is validated for ages 2.5 to 4.5 years and can be completed by a teacher or a parent. The School-Age form is validated for ages 4 through 18, and can also be completed by a teacher or a parent. The Adult form is validated for ages 19 through 89 years, and can be completed by parents, friends, spouses, and other relatives. There is also a separate Adult form written for self-reporting of social impairment, the Self-Report form, which can be administered directly to the examinee in adult assessments.

The SRS-2 yields a Total score and treatment subscale scores for the domains of Social Awareness, Social Cognition, Social Communication, Social Motivation, and Restricted Interests and Repetitive Behavior. The Total score is calculated using distinct normed references for males and females, and for parents vs. teacher raters (for the Preschool and School-Age forms), and is the most widely utilized score for clinical interpretation. Total T-scores of 76 or higher are indicative of severe deficits in social impairment, while T-scores between 66 and 75 indicate moderate deficits in social impairment and T-scores of 60 to 65 suggest mild to moderate deficits (cutoff of 60 points, sensitivity = 0.92, specificity = 0.92; see Bruni, 2014 for psychometric details). A total T-score of below 60 indicates an individual does not demonstrate social difficulties associated with ASD.

ASRS: The Autism Spectrum Rating Scales (ASRS) are informant rating scales which measure symptoms and behaviors of ASD (Goldstein & Naglieri, 2009). The ASRS are distinct in their versatility, with forms available in both English and Spanish, for screening and evaluation purposes, and covering examinee age ranges of 2 to 5 and 6 to 18 years. Items in the forms are scored on a five-point Likert scale, with results reported as standardized T-scores.

The ASRS are available in English or Spanish, and in two distinct forms: the Parent/Caregiver form and the Teacher/Childcare Provider form. Each of these forms is available in a full-length (70 items for ages 2–5, 71 items for ages 6–18) version or a short-form (15 item) version. The full-length form is used in comprehensive evaluations, while the short-form version may be used to screen children for ASD and identify if further evaluation is needed. Items across the parent and teacher forms are identical except for the inclusion of questions regarding early language development on the Parent/Caregiver form.

The ASRS full-length forms yield the following scores: Total score, DSM-IV-TR Scale, ASRS scales (social/communication; unusual behaviors), and Treatment scales (peer socialization; adult socialization; social/emotional reciprocity; atypical language; stereotypy; behavioral rigidity; sensory sensitivity; attention/self-regulation [for ages 2–5]; attention [for ages 6–18]). The ASRS Total score is the most widely utilized score for clinical decision-making in assessment. Total T-scores of 70 or higher are considered Very Elevated scores indicative of many more ASD-related behavioral concerns than typically reported for children at that age. T-scores between 65 and 69 are Elevated and indicate more ASD-related behavioral concerns than typical, while T-scores between 60 and 64 are Slightly Elevated and indicate mildly more ASD-related behavioral concerns than expected (cutoff of 60 points, sensitivity = 0.92, specificity = 0.91; see Goldstein & Naglieri, 2009 for psychometric details). A T-score of 59 or below indicates the examinee does not demonstrate behavioral concerns related to ASD. The ASRS short-form version yields only one Total T-score, which can be interpreted using the same cutoffs as the full-length forms.

PDDBI: The Pervasive Developmental Disorder Behavior Inventory (PDDBI) is an informant rating scale which measures behaviors associated with ASD which can be used in both assessment and progress tracking (Cohen et al., 2003). Designed to independently assess types of maladaptive and adaptive behavior, the PDDBI contains 10 subscales which can be administered independently or as part of the full inventory. Due to the PDDBI's focus on both adaptive and maladaptive behaviors and its independent subscale design, the measure is commonly used to track intervention responsiveness among children with ASD, making it distinct from other similar measures. Furthermore, the PDDBI is unique in that it can be used to examine children as young as 1.5 years old. The measure is available in two distinct versions: the Teacher form and the Parent form.

The PDDBI Teacher form is validated for ages 1:6 to 18:5 and can be completed by the child's teacher. It consists of 144 items across eight subscales assessing differing aspects of ASD organized as adaptive or maladaptive. The Teacher form assesses four maladaptive subscales (sensory/perceptual approach behaviors; behavior problems; social pragmatic problems; semantic/pragmatic problems) and four adaptive subscales (social approach behaviors; learning, memory, and receptive language; phonological skills; semantic/pragmatic ability). Items are scored on a four-point Likert scale, with results reported as standardized T-scores. The PDDBI Parent form is validated for ages 1:6 to 18:5 and consists of 176 items measuring the eight subscales covered in the Teacher form as well as two additional maladaptive behavior domains of specific fears and arousal problems.

The PDDBI yields a composite Autism score and individual scores for each subscale in the form. The composite Autism score is primarily used for assessment purposes and is calculated from six subscales identified as closely related to DSM-IV autism criteria: sensory/perceptual approach behaviors, social approach behaviors, social pragmatic problems, phonological skills, semantic/pragmatic ability, and semantic/pragmatic problems (Cohen et al., 2003). This composite T-score ranges from 10–100, with scores between 40 and 60 indicating likelihood of ASD (sensitivity = 0.74, specificity = 0.68 for cutoff score of 45; see Reel et al., 2012 and Cohen et al., 2010 for psychometric details). Individual subscale scores can be used in assessment settings to inform evaluators of an examinee's adaptive strengths and weaknesses, and can be used in clinical settings to track intervention responsiveness.

Diagnostic Interview

ADI-R: The Autism Diagnostic Interview-Revised (ADI-R) is a standardized, semi-structured interview designed to assess symptoms associated with ASD and inform diagnosis (Rutter et al., 2003). The ADI-R is conducted with a parent or caregiver and covers the examinee's developmental history and current functioning across three primary domains: Communication, Social Interaction, and Restricted and Repetitive Behaviors. Validated for children and adults with a mental age of two years or older, the ADI-R is a valuable assessment tool for diagnosing ASD across the lifespan. Due to its in-depth and standardized nature, the ADI-R is considered a gold-standard interview in the assessment of ASD and is used internationally in both clinical and research settings.

The ADI-R consists of 93 items scored based on both frequency and severity of behaviors. The test yields domain scores for each of the three primary domains, as well as Algorithm scores which indicate the presence and severity of ASD symptoms. ADI-R Algorithm scores are generated to account for the age and developmental level of the examinee, thus ensuring that the assessment is tailored to the child (see Zander et al., 2017 for psychometric details). Distinct cutoff scores for each domain indicate whether a child meets criteria for ASD diagnosis; examinees must score above the cutoff in the domains of Communication and Social Interaction, and at or above the cutoff for Restricted and Repetitive Behaviors, to meet criteria for ASD. While the ADI-R is widely considered a gold-standard assessment instrument with robust psychometric properties, it is essential for clinicians to administer additional tests as relevant and to draw upon their own clinical judgment in making diagnostic determinations (Kaufman, 2022).

Semi-Structured Assessment

ADOS-2: The Autism Diagnostic Observation Schedule, Second Edition (ADOS-2) is a gold-standard semi-structured assessment measure used in the diagnosis of ASD (Lord et al., 2012). Designed to assess the social behaviors, communication skills, and repetitive behaviors characteristic of ASD, the ADOS-2 provides a standardized opportunity for observation and interaction conducted by a trained clinician. The ADOS-2 includes five modules designed for varying age ranges, developmental levels, and language abilities, allowing for flexibility in administration across heterogeneous examinee presentations. Each module includes a series of activities and social interactions designed to elicit behaviors associated with ASD such as playing with toys, engaging in reciprocal conversation, or participating in a joint activity with the examiner. The clinician observes the examinee's behaviors and responses throughout the testing period, and administers prompts and activities in accordance with the specific instructions outlined in the ADOS-2 manual. Items are scored based on predetermined criteria specific to the module used in assessment, with the test yielding two Domain Scores (Social Affect; Restricted and Repetitive Behaviors) and a Total score, with distinct cut-off thresholds identified for each module. The Modules for the ADOS-2 are as follows:

Toddler Module: designed for children who are pre-verbal or minimally verbal and aged approximately 12 to 30 months, focusing on early social behavior such as joint attention and social referencing.

Module 1: designed for children aged 31 months and older who are pre-verbal or minimally verbal and shares some items with the Toddler Module, assessing early social behaviors such as social referencing and imitation.

Module 2: designed for children aged 31 months and older who use phrases well but are not fluently verbal, and expands upon Module 1 to include assessment of social initiation and response, as well as the presence of restricted and repetitive behaviors and interests.

Module 3: designed for children and adolescents below the age of 16 with fluent speech and an expressive language level of at least 4 years old. This module includes assessment of higher-order social skills such as reciprocal conversation and storytelling, and identifies the presence of restricted and repetitive behaviors and interests.

Module 4: designed for adolescents and adults with fluent speech and typical or above-typical intelligence. This module focuses on assessing social skills and communication across complex social settings reflective of adult life, such as interpreting nonverbal cues and understanding social relationships. Module 4 also identifies the presence of restricted and repetitive behaviors and interests.

Recently, researchers have developed and published initial psychometric information on the Adapted ADOS (A-ADOS), a new module designed to assess autism symptoms in minimally verbal adolescents and adults; see Bal and colleagues' (2020) initial publication for more information.

The ADOS-2 boasts strong psychometric properties, and its standardized structure enables the test to consistently measure characteristics associated with ASD across diverse populations. The test has been translated into 9 languages other than English (Czech, Danish, Dutch, Finnish, French, German, Italian, Norwegian, and Swedish) and is used internationally in ASD research and clinical practice, making it a powerful assessment tool for clinicians who diagnose autism. While recent research with the ADOS-2 indicated minimal bias related to race and sex, evidence of potential underdetection of autism spectrum disorder (ASD) in Black/African American and female children suggested the need for further research (Kalb et al., 2022). See Lord et al. (2000) for English-language psychometric details.

CARS-2: The Childhood Autism Rating Scale, Second Edition (CARS-2) is a clinician-administered rating scale that assesses autism-related behaviors based on direct observation and interaction with the examinee (Schloper et al., 2010). Designed to aid in diagnosis of ASD and in differentiation of ASD from other developmental disorders, the CARS-2 is a widely used neurodevelopmental assessment instrument. It is essential to note that while the original CARS was often clinically misused as a parent questionnaire, both forms of the CARS-2 are intended to be completed by a trained clinician who has directly observed the child. The CARS Standard Form (CARS-ST) is designed for all children between the age of 2–6 years, and children aged above 6 years with IQs of 79 or lower and/or a notable communication impairment. The CARS High Functioning Form (CARS-HF) is designed for children aged 6 years or older with an IQ of 80 or higher and fluent verbal communication.

Both forms of the CARS-2 consist of 15 items which assess behaviors across domains of communication, social interaction, repetitive behaviors, and sensory responses. Items are scored on a four-point Likert scale, with both raw scores and standardized T-scores used for interpretation. Distinct cutoff scores for the two forms identify individuals who are likely to meet criteria for ASD, with higher scores indicating higher levels of autism symptom severity. See Ji et al. (2023) for psychometric details.

MIGDAS-2: The Monteiro Interview Guidelines for Diagnosing the Autism Spectrum, Second Edition (MIGDAS-2) is a qualitative diagnostic tool designed to assess ASD symptoms across the lifespan (Monteiro & Stegall, 2018). The MIGDAS-2 differs from other measures due to its qualitative nature, with the measure structured as an interview framework for gathering qualitative information from multiple sources. The MIGDAS-2 gathers in-depth information on the examinee's behavioral and sensory experiences, and is often used to assess individuals with diverse or subtle presentations which require nuanced diagnostic decision-making.

The MIGDAS-2 consists of three components: the Parent/Caregiver Interview, the Teacher/Professional Interview, and the Sensory-Based Diagnostic Interview, the latter of which is conducted directly with the examinee. Each component gathers specific information about the examinee's developmental history, social interactions, communication skills, and sensory processing patterns. Items are open-ended, encouraging detailed responses which comprise the qualitative data used for analysis. In lieu of quantitative scoring, the MIGDAS-2 manual guides clinicians in synthesizing interview data from multiple sources and creating a comprehensive diagnostic profile of the examinee. The MIGDAS-2 is sensitive to ASD in high-masking individuals who are fluently verbal and have typical intelligence, making it a valuable assessment tool for clinicians diagnosing ASD in adolescents and adults. But more research related to clinical utility is needed (Pagán et al., 2024).

Assessing ASD in adults presents unique challenges and complexities that differ notably from the assessment of children and adolescents. One primary issue is the historical underdiagnosis or misdiagnosis of ASD in adults, particularly those without intellectual disabilities or with high-functioning phenotypes. Many adults may have developed sophisticated coping mechanisms that mask their symptoms, making it difficult to identify ASD through traditional diagnostic criteria. Additionally, the presentation of ASD symptoms can change over time, and adults might not exhibit the same behaviors observed in children. Furthermore, many adults may lack access to comprehensive developmental histories, which are often crucial for accurate diagnosis. These challenges necessitate the use of specialized assessment tools designed specifically for adults, which can accurately capture the nuances of adult ASD presentation and provide a detailed understanding of their social, communication, and sensory processing difficulties.

Other Relevant Assessment Domains

Adaptive Functioning

Adaptive behavior refers to the skills that an individual needs to function independently at an age appropriate level at home, school, and the community. Adaptive behavior measures typically assess communication, socialization, and daily living skills. The Vineland Adaptive Behavior Scales-Third Edition (Vineland-3) and the Adaptive Behavior Assessment System—Third Edition (ABAS-3) are two common measures given to individuals with ASD and other neurodevelopmental disorders. Research on adaptive behavior in individuals with ASD indicate that they typically have deficits in all areas, particularly in social and daily living skills, regardless of their cognitive abilities (McQuaid et al., 2021; Tamm et al., 2022). The use of an adaptive behavior measure is recommended in ASD evaluations as it provides additional data on an individual's strengths and areas needed for growth, which, therefore, can be used to help clinicians identify targets for intervention. There is no conclusive evidence indicating which adaptive behavior measure provides a more efficient and accurate assessment in individuals with ASD (Tamm et al., 2022). Furthermore, there can be discrepancies between input from parents/caregivers and teachers (Stevens et al., 2023). Clinicians may consider completing a behavioral observation of the individual in addition to administering an adaptive behavior measure to provide additional data points that can be used for clinical interpretation, decision-making, and treatment planning.

Vineland-3: The Vineland (Sparrow et al., 2016) was updated in 2016 and has normative data for individuals from birth to 90 years old. Parents, caregivers, teachers, or other informants that know the individual can complete the Vineland-3. There are three main formats of the Vineland-3. There is an interview form that allows clinicians to complete a semi-structured interview with an informant. Next, there is a parent/caregiver form in which the informant answers questions themselves rather than participating in the interview. The focus of the parent/caregiver form is on adaptive behavior within the home, family, and community. A teacher form is also available for individuals between the ages of 3 to 21 years old and provides information on the individual's adaptive behavior abilities within an educational setting. New to the Vineland-3 is a comprehensive version or a brief domain version.

Each version of the Vineland-3 provides an Adaptive Behavior Composite, which gives an overall summary of the individual's abilities. There are four domains that are also measured: communication, daily living skills, and motor skills. The Communication domain focuses on an individual's receptive, expressive, and written communication abilities. The Daily Living Skills domain assesses skills the individual needs to manage their personal well-being, household tasks, and skills needed in the community (e.g., financial skills, travel, safety). The Socialization domain focuses on how an individual relates to others, their play and leisure skills and interests, and ability to use coping skills. The Motor Domain assesses the individual's fine and gross motor skills. Data on motor skills is provided only for individuals up to age 9 years old. The Vineland-3 also has an optional maladaptive behavior scale that examines internalizing and externalizing problem behaviors the individual may engage in. See Pepperdine & McCrimmon, 2018 for psychometric details.

ABAS-3: The ABAS-3 was updated in 2015 (Harrison & Oakland, 2015). It is appropriate for individuals from birth to 89 years old. It provides clinicians with a comprehensive assessment of an individual's adaptive behavior abilities that is norm-referenced. According to the manual, the ABAS-3 requires a sixth-grade reading ability and can be completed by an informant within 20 min. There are five rating forms that allow parents, teachers, and other informants that know the individual to provide information on various domains of adaptive behavior. For each form, a General Adaptive Composite (GAC) score is provided as reference to an individual's overall adaptive behavior abilities. There are also three domains that provide more specific information on an individual's functioning: conceptual, social, and practical. The conceptual domain focuses on adaptive behaviors such as communication abilities, application of knowledge, ability to complete various tasks, and self-direction. The social domain focuses on social skills, social responsibility, and the use of leisure time. The practical domain emphasizes behaviors related to self-care, health and safety, household responsibilities, and skills needed in the community and/or work environment. See Harrison and Oakland (2015) for psychometric details.

Cognitive Functioning

It is beyond the scope of our chapter to cover specific tests and measures utilized by clinicians, researchers, and other professionals to assess cognitive and intellectual functioning in individuals with ASD. However, cognitive and intelligence testing is important in autism assessments as research indicates that low IQ scores is a predictor for an ASD diagnosis, particularly during the early developmental years (Denisova & Lin, 2023). Obtaining a Full Scale IQ and scores on different cognitive domains is important as individuals with ASD may have significant discrepancies in their cognitive abilities. Historically, individuals with ASD have exhibited lower processing speed but perform better on fluid reasoning or visual spatial processing domains (Muth et al., 2014; Oliveras-Rentas et al., 2012). As the ASD spectrum has broadened over time, it is not as common for individuals with ASD to meet criteria for an Intellectual Disability. The number of individuals with co-occurring diagnoses of ASD and ID has decreased from 70 to 30% over the past 50 years (Wolf et al., 2022). The current consensus is that higher intellectual abilities are associated with a better prognosis in many life areas (Wolf et al., 2022).

Executive Functioning

Consideration of neuropsychological batteries that assess social perception, language, attention, and other executive-functioning abilities can also be considered as part of a testing battery for individuals with ASD. Individuals with ASD have been found to have significant deficits in many executive functioning domains, including concept formation/set shifting, cognitive flexibility, fluency, planning, response inhibition, and working memory (Demetriou et al., 2018). Therefore, neuropsychological testing can assist with differential diagnoses, treatment planning, establishing baseline abilities, and track changes in an individual's abilities overtime.

NEPSY-II: The NEPSY-Second Edition (NEPSY-II) allows for the assessment of various cognitive abilities and is appropriate for use in children between the ages of 3 to 16 years old (Korkman, Kirk, & Kemp, 2007). The NEPSY-II includes 19 subtests over six different domains, which include the following: Attention and Executive Functioning, Language, Memory and Learning, Motor Skills, Social Perception, and Visual and Visuoperceptual Processing. Clinicians can select specific subtests and/or domains of the NEPSY-II to administer based on the referral question. The Social Perception battery in particular may be useful for ASD assessments as it is used to evaluate an individual's ability to identify emotions and affect through facial expressions, while also assessing an individual's theory of mind. Typically individuals with ASD show greater deficits in the areas assessed by the social perception battery than individuals that are typically developing or present with other neurodevelopmental difficulties, such as ADHD (Braconnier & Siper, 2021; Korkman et al., 2007). Caution is recommended when utilizing the NEPSY-II as it has not been updated since 2007 and, therefore, normative data may not fully represent abilities in children in our current society. See Brooks et al. (2009) for further psychometric details.

D-KEFS: The Delis-Kaplan Executive Functioning System (D-KEFS; Delis et al., 2001) allows for the comprehensive assessment of executive functioning domains and includes normative data on individuals between the ages of 8 to 89 years old (see Shunk et al., 2006 for psychometric details). The D-KEFS consists of nine subtests that assess cognitive flexibility, inhibition, fluency, problem-solving, verbal and spatial concept formation, planning and reasoning, impulsivity, and abstract thinking. Similar to the NEPSY-II, professionals completing an assessment can select individual subtests to answer a referral question rather than administering the full battery. The D-KEFS can be used as a supplement to the NEPSY-II for children, or it can be used as a stand-alone neuropsychological assessment for individuals in which the NEPSY-II battery is not appropriate (e.g., individuals over the age of 16 years old). Clinicians may be interested in the Verbal Fluency and the Proverb test, which assesses metaphorical thinking and comprehension of abstract thought, as individuals with ASD tend to score lower in these areas compared to other subtests of the D-KEFS (MacDonald et al., 2024; Nyrenius & Billstedt, 2020). Of note, an updated version of the D-KEFS is slated to be available in 2024.

Common Behaviors Observed During the Assessment Process

When testing for ASD, clinicians commonly observe a range of behaviors that reflect the unique challenges and characteristics associated with the condition. These behaviors may include difficulties with sustained attention, which can manifest as fleeting engagement or frequent distractions during assessment tasks, especially in uninteresting tasks, and present challenges, particularly during timed assessments (e.g., attention may wax and wane even within subtests). Additionally, children with ASD often exhibit challenges in social communication, such as limited or inconsistent eye contact, atypical prosody, and deficits in reciprocal conversation skills (e.g., struggle with sustaining age-appropriate back-and-forth conversations). Sensory sensitivities may also influence testing outcomes, with some children demonstrating aversion or heightened responses to certain stimuli in the testing environment (e.g., noises such as the air conditioner turning on or white noise machines may be distracting for a child with ASD). Moreover, rigid adherence to routines, perseverations, or preferences for sameness may affect the client's willingness to engage with novel tasks, instructions, or shifts during assessment sessions (e.g., a child with ASD may have trouble flexibly moving between tasks or incorporating new information into play schemas). Behavioral difficulties, particularly disruptive behaviors under stress, are common (e.g., behavioral dysregulation is common and often out of proportion to the situation). Understanding and accommodating these behaviors is essential for accurate assessment and effective intervention planning in children with ASD.

To effectively accommodate clients with autism during testing, special considerations may be needed, including testing the limits or occasionally breaking test standardization. When this occurs, it is important to thoroughly document the ways in which the standardization administration was not followed (e.g., subtests were administered out of order to maintain the child's focus and attention based on their preferred interests). Other ways to accommodate children with ASD include establishing rapport by engaging in preferred activities or discussing interests to build trust and reduce anxiety. Additionally, it is sometimes necessary to test multiple sessions for a shorter duration. For some clients, it is important to adjust the testing environment to minimize distractions or environmental stimuli that can create sensory overload (e.g., fluorescent lights) and, when appropriate, provide access to sensory tools such as fidget toys or breaks that can enhance focus. For some clients, employing visual schedules that outline the testing session's activities helps clients anticipate tasks and reduce anxiety. Additionally, increasing positive reinforcement with rewards, such as stickers or brief breaks, can motivate and help maintain attention. While brief breaks can be effective for some clients with ASD, for other clients with ASD, the challenges of transitioning back to testing after a brief break can be difficult and result in significant dysregulation. Similarly, it is important for clinicians to be well versed in test administration and able to move fluidly between tasks, as children with ASD often struggle to regulate while waiting. Clinicians should carefully consider the use of technology for test administration. Tablet technology for assessment, in particular, has been successful in enhancing motivation and attention in folks with ASD (Bouck et al., 2014). Finally, clinicians should carefully observe and gather information from multiple sources, such as parents and teachers, to ensure clinical validity when ASD symptoms may impact standardized testing results. Ultimately, clinicians, not instruments, make diagnoses, and it is important to consider information beyond scores to understand the process and context of the scores.

Cultural Considerations in Assessment

Recent events, including the pandemic and heightened awareness of social injustices, have underscored long-standing disparities in our systems and tools. According to the Centers for Disease Control and Prevention (CDC, 2022), the median age at autism diagnosis in the United States is around 4 years, despite the availability of reliable diagnostic tools for children as young as 2 years of age. Racial and ethnic disparities in ASD prevalence have been well documented, with recent findings indicating a similar overall prevalence across groups, but certain disparities persist, particularly among Hispanic and Black children. According to a study by Aylward et al. (2021)the prevalence of ASD among Hispanic and Black children was lower than that among White children, despite no significant differences in socioeconomic status. These findings suggest that other factors, such as cultural and environmental factors, may contribute to the disparities in ASD prevalence.

Various factors contribute to diagnostic disparities in underrepresented communities, including limited access to services, provider shortages, stigma, and diverse cultural interpretations of symptoms. Additionally, the lack of culturally competent healthcare providers and language barriers are also significant contributors to diagnostic disparities in underrepresented communities (Aylward et al., 2021; La Roche et al., 2018). However, a key barrier is the lack of culturally and linguistically sensitive assessment instruments. Many widely used ASD tools were originally developed and validated using homogeneous samples potentially introducing a bias. Some researchers have suggested that using diverse samples in ASD tool development may help to mitigate this bias and improve the accuracy of diagnostic tools (Bishop & Lord, 2023). While some efforts have been made to develop culturally responsive adaptations to improve diversity in standardization samples and enhance the validity of assessment instruments in underrepresented populations, clinicians need to be aware of these limitations and ensure that they use a culturally appropriate strength-based lens during the assessment process.

ASD assessments often operate under a deficit model, spotlighting weaknesses and vulnerabilities while overlooking the strengths inherent in ASD in individuals, families, and communities. However, acknowledging and amplifying these strengths is crucial, particularly in the context of supporting families and individuals with ASD, as it cultivates optimism and facilitates positive adaptation to the challenges of parenting children with ASD. For instance, Hayes et al. (2022) found that fostering resilience in families of children with ASD can lead to improved mental health outcomes and greater overall well-being. Employing a strength-based assessment framework aims to pinpoint and leverage these inherent strengths within the child, family, and broader community, while informing personalized intervention strategies.

To adopt a strength-based approach, clinicians should initially identify strengths across various domains, encompassing the client's unique attributes, family dynamics, and the support systems available within the community and school. For instance, clinicians may highlight how a client's strong attention to detail can serve as a valuable asset in problem-solving endeavors or how individuals with ASD often demonstrate a strong sense of morality, contributing to their understanding of social justice. Regarding family strengths, clinicians may identify the involvement of extended or chosen family members who play significant roles in the client's life as well as identify the family's resilience and coping strategies. For example, highlighting shared activities such as hiking or close relationships with family members can underscore familial strengths. Similarly, identifying school and community support, such as dedicated educators or active involvement in autism advocacy groups, can further bolster the client's network of support. Conducting a strength-based assessment enables clinicians to portray the client in a positive light, nurturing hope, and optimism. By focusing on strengths and emphasizing competence and quality of life rather than solely focusing on symptom reduction, clinicians can instill a sense of empowerment and better reflect the true abilities of individuals with ASD.

Language and Communication Differences

Additional considerations are necessary when conducting assessments with families who speak languages other than English in the home. On average, children who are English language learners (ELLs) are diagnosed later than their monolingual peers (Fahim & Nedwick, 2014). Clinicians who work with ELLs must consider the role of language differences in communication with families, choice of assessment instruments, and evaluation of the child's social and communicative functioning within the context of their language acquisition.

Children who are ELLs often exhibit differences in communication and socialization when compared to their monolingual peers, posing additional challenges to diagnosing ASD in this group. For example, while the absence of joint attention is a common indicator of ASD, typically developing ELLs may similarly display a lack of joint attention within an observation setting due to the cultural value of deference to elders.

For typically developing ELLs, the first language (L1) develops at a similar rate to others who speak that language, with some language confusion and possible language loss in L1 observed as the second language (L2) is introduced. While typically developing ELLs may "echo" L2 words in an attempt to reproduce pronunciation, it is expected that each successive attempt at a word would sound qualitatively different as the child approximates the word with more success. This differs from echolalia observed in ASD, where each repetition of a word is likely to sound qualitatively similar.

While typically developing ELLs demonstrate differences in their nonverbal communication compared to their monolingual peers, their facial expressions and gesture use are often grounded in the culturally bound social rules of their L1. Conversely, ELLs with ASD may display an absence of non-verbal communication behaviors or mismatched non-verbal communications not grounded in either L1 or L2 norms. For this reason, clinicians should be sensitive to differing cultural norms surrounding nonverbal communication to elucidate if a child's nonverbal differences are cultural or indicative of a true developmental delay.

Recent research on ASD presentations among bilingual children has provided valuable information on differentiating between ELL children with and without ASD (Dennison et al., 2019). In addition to the broader cultural considerations reviewed in the above section, the following considerations may support accurate identification and diagnosis among ELL children referred for ASD assessment.

(1) Consider context of impairment: Language and setting
    (a) To what degree is language impairment documented in both the L1 and L2? Particular attention should be given to L1 language development, as delays in L2 development are expected.
    (b) To what degree is the language impairment documented across settings? Particular attention should be given to settings in which L1 is the dominant language, such as home.

(2) Focus on facets of ASD symptomology unrelated to language
   (a) Does the child respond to their name?
   (b) Does the child display sensory sensitivities and/or stereotypy?
   (c) Does the child demonstrate unusual preoccupation with their interests?
(3) Choose culturally and linguistically valid assessment instruments
   (a) What was the normative sample that an instrument was built upon, and did it include individuals of this family's cultural and linguistic background?
   (b) Is there a linguistically adapted version of this assessment?
      (i) The ADI-R and ADOS-2 have available adaptations in Spanish and several other languages; see assessments section for more detail.
   (c) Consider measuring bilingual language ability as supplemental information.
   (d) Consider using nonverbal measures of intelligence if no linguistically-adapted version is available.

Racial and Ethnic Differences

Current research indicates that ASD occurs at a similar rate in all racial, ethnic, and socioeconomic groups (Maenner et al., 2020). However, there is a discrepancy in diagnostic rates between White and racial/ethnic minority individuals, with White children more likely to be diagnosed and more likely to be diagnosed earlier than their racial/ethnic minority peers (Stoll et al., 2021). Cultural differences in the reporting of ASD symptomatology, culturally invalid assessment tools, and language differences contribute to this diagnostic discrepancy.

While the presentation of ASD symptomatology is constant across racial and ethnic groups, the reporting of symptoms by parents and caregivers can be highly influenced by cultural beliefs and norms. Families may have different ideas of ASD and neurodevelopmental disabilities more broadly based on their cultural or religious backgrounds and may come from cultures in which there is no specific label for ASD. This influences the way families report symptoms and how they observe and interpret their child's presentation. These cultural beliefs can also influence attitudes towards seeking help for their child's symptoms, with evidence that white families are more likely to seek professional medical help than racial and ethnic minority groups (Ennis-Cole et al., 2013). In comparison, black families are more likely to turn to their community or church, Latinx families are more likely to seek nontraditional services, and Asian families may avoid seeking help (Bernier et al., 2010). When working with racially and ethnically diverse families, it is important to consider how these factors may influence the clinician-family relationship and the family's reporting of ASD symptoms.

Research on specific cultural groups suggests that Latinx parents may be less likely to report concerns related to their child's communication, social interaction, and areas of RRBIs when compared to White parents and may endorse a lower frequency of

ASD symptomatology than that observed by clinicians (Magana & Smith, 2013). Parents from cultural groups that value deference and respect for authority (e.g., Asian and Hispanic/Latinx groups) may be less likely to engage collaboratively with healthcare providers and assessors, a cultural barrier compounded by the communication barriers often faced by these groups due to language differences. These cultural differences are essential for clinicians to consider in the diagnostic process, especially due to the reliance on parent-reported measures in diagnosing ASD. Clinicians working with diverse families may wish to prioritize clinical observation throughout the diagnostic process to develop an understanding of the child's current functioning.

In working with culturally diverse families, clinicians and practitioners are encouraged to rely on clinical judgment and integrate data from multiple informants on the child's functioning to reduce issues of cultural bias and insensitivity of assessment instruments.

Sex Differences and Female Phenotype

Emerging research indicates a trend of underdiagnosis of autism spectrum disorder (ASD) in females, which poses significant barriers to accessing appropriate support services. Lai and colleagues (2023) highlighted that females with ASD often present with different symptomatology compared to males, which contributes to diagnostic disparity and underscores the need for gender-sensitive assessment tools and diagnostic criteria. This discrepancy is evident in the reported difference between the estimated prevalence of ASD in the general population, where there are three males for every female, and the actual diagnosed cases where there are four males per female (Maenner et al., 2020). The underdiagnosis phenomenon appears to stem from the nuanced presentation of ASD in females compared to the stereotypical male manifestation. According to recent research, girls and women with ASD often present with more social communication impairments and fewer restricted interests than boys and men with ASD, which may contribute to underdiagnosis (Hull et al., 2020). Females may exhibit fewer overtly atypical behaviors and employ compensation strategies such as camouflaging, making their symptoms less conspicuous.

Other challenges include diagnostic instruments, predominantly designed based on male presentations, which may inadequately capture the subtleties of ASD in females, potentially resulting in misinterpretation or oversight of the symptoms. Moreover, biases among clinicians and other observers, influenced by societal norms regarding gendered behavior, may contribute to the under-detection of ASD in females.

Recent empirical studies have highlighted biases in the perception of ASD behaviors, with potential referrers demonstrating a tendency to raise concerns more readily for males than for females exhibiting similar behaviors. For example, educators, when presented with vignettes, were less likely to identify females as autistic than males, indicating a systemic bias in recognizing ASD in females; however, the extent of bias among diagnosticians during assessments remains largely unexplored. Sex-related clinician expectancy bias, wherein ASD is more readily considered for males due to historical prevalence patterns, may perpetuate higher diagnostic rates among males. Additionally, gender expectancy biases may influence the interpretation of behaviors, with those aligning more closely with ASD symptoms in males being more readily recognized as indicative of the disorder.

Addressing these biases and refining diagnostic practices to account for the unique presentation of ASD in females is crucial for ensuring equitable access to support services and accurate diagnosis across sexes. Sex-related clinician expectancy bias refers to the tendency of clinicians to consider or diagnose a condition more frequently in a particular sex or sex based on prevalence rates or perceived alignment with normative behaviors of that sex. In the context of ASD, such bias can manifest in two main ways: first, in clinicians' readiness to consider ASD, and second, in the interpretation of behaviors associated with ASD.

For example, gender expectancy bias may lead clinicians to more readily interpret unusual behaviors as indicative of ASD in males than in females. For instance, social avoidance may be interpreted differently for girls (e.g., shyness, anxiety) than for boys (e.g., aloofness, social disinterest), with the latter being more strongly associated with developmental abnormalities and possibly ASD. Emerging evidence indicates that commonly used screening and diagnostic tools may be less sensitive to autistic traits in females, contributing to systematic under-recognition of ASD in girls and women (de Giambattista et al., 2021). Consistent with this pattern, high-risk male siblings have been found to receive ASD diagnoses at roughly twice the rate of high-risk female siblings, highlighting potential measurement bias and sex-linked differences in clinical presentation (Baby Siblings Research Consortium, 2025).

Clinicians need to consider that females with ASD often show greater social motivation and interest in relationships than male with ASD (Sedgewick et al., 2019); therefore, more variability may be present related to friendship. Females often report having friendships but trouble sustaining friendships (e.g., females may be more likely to have a new best friend each year, but have limited insight into why the friendships end). The Camouflage Hypothesis suggests that females with ASD are more likely to engage in strategies to appear more neurotypical, such as practicing gestures, facial expressions, and eye contact (Hull et al., 2020). The practice of "camouflaging" or "masking" autistic traits, particularly prevalent among females, helps them navigate social situations, but can lead to increased mental health issues such as fatigue and depression. Females who report using masking behaviors also socially situations being very taxing, and sustained engagement is often very difficult. Differences have also been reported in the intensity and frequency of externalizing and internalizing disorders, with males being more likely to display dysregulation and aggression, and females with ASD being more likely to have internalizing disorders such as anxiety (Mandy et al., 2012). Similarly, repetitive behaviors and interests vary according to gender and societal norms. Males tend to display more frequent restricted and repetitive behaviors, which are more predictive of an ASD diagnosis in males than in females (Duvekot et al., 2017). Intense interest in males often focuses on mechanics and mathematics, whereas females are more likely to have socially oriented or normative interests (e.g., unicorns or reading; however, the intensity of the interest is out of proportion (Bargiela et al., 2016).

Addressing Bias in ASD Assessment

Clinicians should adopt a broad perspective on patients' culture, recognizing the diversity within racial and ethnic groups and the intersectionality of those identities. Cultural factors such as socioeconomic status, gender roles, sexual orientation, and disability status should be considered alongside race and ethnicity when working with families with ASD. It is crucial to avoid assumptions and stereotypes based on these identities. For example, clinicians should be aware of using ableist language that promotes discrimination and stigma, such as replacing "at risk for autism" with more neutral terms like "increased likelihood of autism." Additionally, clinicians must continuously examine their biases and privileges and recognize cultural biases in ASD research, assessment, and intervention. Addressing structural biases is essential for ensuring equitable care for individuals with ASD and their families. This may include advocating for more funding for training more diagnosticians who are knowledgeable about ASD within certain underserved locations or considering the impact of other social determinants of health on the diagnostic process and systems. Clinicians should seek specialized training in cultural competence related to working with individuals with ASD and their families and learn more about cultural factors related to neurodivergence and ASD. Clinicians who have received specialized training in cultural competence report higher levels of confidence in their ability to provide effective interventions to individuals with ASD from diverse cultural backgrounds.

When using ASD assessment tools, clinicians should be aware of the standardization sample and exercise caution with instruments that are not validated for use in diverse cultural groups. These tools should be used carefully until they are properly validated. During the assessment process, it is important to recognize that caregivers' concerns about their children may differ from those expressed by clinicians or other professionals. Gathering information from multiple observers is crucial, as interpretations of behaviors can vary based on the cultural backgrounds of both parents, clinicians, and other professionals. For instance, researchers have identified cultural differences in how parents report symptoms on the Modified Checklist for Autism in Toddlers Revised (M-CHAT-R). Items assessing joint attention, social engagement, and language comprehension—such as "points to show," "brings things to show," and "follows your gaze"—tend to be interpreted consistently across cultures as indicative of atypical development. However, cultural variations have been noted in behaviors, such as making eye contact, responding to one's name, and reciprocal smiling (Stevanovic et al., 2022). Cultural variations have also been observed in nonverbal communication, including body language, facial expressions, and gestures. For instance, in some cultures, direct eye contact is considered a sign of respect, whereas in others, it may be seen as a challenge. Similarly, the way people respond to their names can vary cross-culturally, with some cultures valuing formal titles and honorifics, whereas others prioritize first names or no names at all.

Psychoeducation about ASD should be provided in a culturally sensitive manner, considering the patients' knowledge levels and familiarity with the disorder. Questions about client and caregiver understanding of ASD should be answered early and often during the assessment process to facilitate a shared understanding. For example, asking questions about clients' and caregivers' understanding of ASD during the initial consultation can help establish a foundation for a collaborative working relationship. To further reduce bias, it is important to be flexible in the ASD assessment process to support accessibility, which may include offering evening and weekend hours, reserving slots for low-income patients, using telehealth when appropriate, and encouraging extended and kinship family involvement. The consistent use of interpreters is crucial when working with cultural minority families that are not fluent in English. Interpreters should be carefully selected and trained to facilitate communication between the patients and clinicians. Translated materials, including copies of the report, should be offered to ensure clarity. There are many important ways to address bias in ASD assessment, and clinicians should ensure that they actively seek ways to reduce this bias in ASD assessment.

Differential Diagnosis and Co-Occurring Comorbidities

Co-occurring conditions, also referred to as comorbidities, are common among individuals with autism and complicate differential diagnosis. While prevalence rates vary, they range from 70 to 94% of individuals diagnosed with autism have at least one additional psychiatric condition, with over 40% experiencing two or more (Hossain et al., 2020; Simonoff et al., 2008). Specifically, anxiety disorders, affecting approximately 40% of individuals with autism compared to 7.3% of the general population, along with attention-deficit/hyperactivity disorder (ADHD) are among the most prevalent comorbidities (Lai et al., 2019). The assessment of autism is complicated by the presence of co-occurring conditions.

As clinicians, it is important to recognize overlapping features across common conditions (e.g., ASD and social anxiety both may manifest in avoidant behavior; ADHD and ASD may result in social challenges and attentional concerns) as well as transdiagnostic symptoms that may be more subtle associated features and symptoms common across several neurodivergent conditions (e.g., sensory challenges). Additionally, it is important to acknowledge that co-occurring medical, genetic, or psychiatric conditions can overshadow ASD diagnosis, leading to misdiagnosis or delayed diagnosis (Duvall et al., 2022, Pagan et al., 2024). Therefore, it is crucial for healthcare professionals to consider the possibility of co-occurring conditions and conduct a thorough evaluation to ensure accurate diagnosis and timely intervention. Recognizing the inherent clinical challenges related to both differential diagnosis and diagnosis of comorbid conditions, it is necessary for clinicians to ensure an individualized and comprehensive neurodevelopmental evaluation that focuses on key aspects, including evaluating the trajectory of symptom development, including onset, duration, and course. This process often starts with a thorough diagnostic interview to systematically determine the etiology of symptoms in order to accurately diagnose or rule out ASD. For example, if a child has a history of strong social motivation in elementary school with typical friendships and no early developmental history concerns, but as an adolescent, their parents are currently reporting decreased social motivation and irritability than the timing may suggest depression, as opposed to ASD. One known challenge related to the comorbid diagnosis of internalizing conditions, such as anxiety and depression, relies heavily on self-reported internal experiences, which can be particularly challenging for autistic individuals, especially those with intellectual disabilities and limited language skills (Mazefsky et al., 2011). Given the significant complexities of untangling comorbid conditions, some important assessment strategies may be necessary, including slowing down the assessment process to allow an anxious client more time to become familiar and to build rapport, considering incidental observations (e.g., how the client and their family function in the waiting room), reviewing videos or recordings of the client in other more familiar social situations or settings that they have shared, and recognizing relevant limitations to clinical diagnostic decision-making (e.g., including a statement about diagnostic certainty in reports). In cases where there is low diagnostic certainty, it is important to develop a plan of care and a plan for re-evaluation, if applicable.

Distinguishing ASD from Other Disorders

The broad category of neurodevelopmental categories was first introduced in the DSM-5 that was published in 2013. Previously, ASD was categorized under the PDD category but is now considered one of several disorders that have an onset in the developmental period and are characterized by some level of neurological deficit that causes impairment in adaptive functioning. Thus, it is common for many neurodevelopmental disorders to co-occur with one another (APA, 2022). A challenge for many clinicians completing diagnostic assessments is determining which neurodevelopmental symptoms and behaviors are best categorized as being related to ASD compared to other neurodevelopmental disorders.

Attention-Deficit/Hyperactivity Disorder

ADHD is characterized as a persistent pattern of inattention and hyperactivity/impulsivity that interferes with functioning or development (APA, 2022). Historically, ASD and autism were not dually diagnosed as it was presumed that individuals with ASD exhibited symptoms of inattention and hyperactivity/impulsivity as part of their ASD presentation. Current standards allow clinicians to diagnose an individual with both ASD and ADHD when clinically relevant and, therefore, ADHD is one of the most common co-occurring diagnoses in individuals diagnosed with ASD (American Psychiatric Association, 2022). The rates of ADHD among individuals with ASD range from 2.6% to 70.6% (Eaton et al., 2023; Hossain et al., 2020; Rong et al., 2021). ADHD and ASD have many similarities and are often diagnosed more in males than females (May et al., 2016). Both conditions also involve deficits in executive functioning, social abilities, motor skills, sensory processing, and reward processing (Scheerer et al., 2024); therefore, many features of ADHD and ASD are transdiagnostic. A distinguishing factor between the two diagnoses is the presence of restricted, repetitive patterns of behavior, interests, and activities. Many individuals with ADHD experience social difficulties that are also often observed in individuals with ASD; however, individuals with ADHD will not exhibit the restricted, repetitive patterns of behaviors, interests, or activities to the threshold that is required for a diagnosis of ASD. Recent research on adults also indicated that hyperactivity/impulsivity features tend to be less prevalent in adults diagnosed only with ASD but are more likely to be present in individuals that have co-occurring diagnoses of ASD and ADHD.

Intellectual Developmental Disorder

Intellectual Developmental Disorder is a neurodevelopmental disorder characterized by deficits in intellectual functioning and adaptive behavior with an onset during the developmental period (APA, 2022). Intellectual disability is one of the more frequent co-occurring diagnoses associated with ASD (McKenzie et al., 2023). Distinguishing an intellectual disability from ASD can be difficult in young children as well as individuals with severe to profound deficits in cognitive functioning (Thurm et al., 2019). The DSM-5-TR recommends reassessment of intellectual abilities in individuals with ASD across the lifespan because of the variability and instability of IQ scores in younger individuals with ASD. Individuals with ASD may have a diverse range of cognitive abilities. As we noted earlier in this chapter, individuals with ASD may have superior cognitive abilities in one domain of functioning but average to delayed functioning in other areas. Individuals diagnosed with an intellectual disability and/or ASD may also present with deficits in adaptive behavior, engage in self-injurious behaviors, or engage in repetitive behaviors or show restricted interests. Researchers have noted that a greater frequency of unusual body movements, have strong restricted interests, and sensory seeking or sensory avoidance behaviors tend to be more prevalent in individuals with comorbid ASD and intellectual disability compared to individuals solely diagnosed with an intellectual disability (Duvall et al., 2022).

When evaluating an individual with an ID for a potential ASD diagnosis, it is essential to consider the client's cognitive ability and understand any other factors that may have influenced those scores. Along with measurements of adaptive behavior, this information provides context for the individual's developmental level and any behavioral, motor, or sensory impairments that may contribute to the overall presentation. Given that ASD criteria are related to social communication at the expected level for development, it is critical to consider the client's social communication profile relative to cognitive/developmental functioning and the larger social context. In older clients with suspected ASD and ID, the developmental trajectory may be particularly useful. Clinicians should consider whether social communication delays have always been approximately commensurate with other developmental domains or if they have been an isolated or more significant impairment.

When diagnosing ASD in individuals with severe Intellectual and Developmental Disabilities (IDD), it is crucial to exercise heightened caution due to the limitations of current diagnostic instruments and the risk of misdiagnosis. The interaction between cognitive abilities, developmental levels, and comorbid conditions necessitates a nuanced and individualized diagnostic approach. Individuals with severe IDD often have mental ages lower than the typical developmental milestones for observable ASD traits, such as spoken language. This discrepancy complicates the accurate assessment of certain ASD symptoms, as the cognitive and developmental benchmarks required for these assessments may not be attainable for these individuals. For example, widely used diagnostic instruments like the Autism Diagnostic Interview-Revised (ADI-R) and the Autism Diagnostic Observation Schedule (ADOS) lose specificity below certain mental ages, leading to caution or recommendations against their use in very young children or those with significant cognitive impairments (Christiansz et al., 2016).

There is a complex interrelation between ASD and cognitive impairment, with a high rate of co-occurrence between the two conditions, complicating the diagnostic process due to overlapping symptoms and behaviors. This overlap poses challenges in differential diagnosis since both conditions share common signs related to behavioral, communicative, social, and adaptive functioning. As a result, individuals with both conditions often present with more complex needs and may require distinct approaches to diagnosis, support, and intervention. Understanding and identifying the dual presence of these conditions is crucial for tailored clinical management and for facilitating research aimed at improving outcomes.

Anxiety Disorders

Children and adolescents with ASD) are significantly more likely to develop anxiety disorders than their typically developing peers or those with other developmental disorders. Epidemiological studies and meta-analyses suggest that approximately 40% of youth with ASD have co-occurring anxiety disorders, although reported rates vary widely from 11 to 84% in different samples, generally around 40% (Simonoff et al., 2008; Vasa et al., 2020). This variability may be due to the differences in the populations studied and the sensitivity of the assessment tools. Historically, anxiety in individuals with ASD has often been overlooked or attributed to ASD–a phenomenon known as diagnostic overshadowing. Since changes in the DSM-5 have allowed for comorbid diagnoses, clinicians are increasingly recognizing that individuals with ASD can have anxiety disorders that are distinct and independent of their ASD symptoms, and that co-occurring anxiety disorders can exacerbate the difficulties associated with ASD, leading to increased self-injury, depression, gastrointestinal issues, social skill deficits, family stress, and greater healthcare needs (Chang et al., 2012). Researchers have suggested that anxiety follows a similar developmental trajectory in children with and without ASD, with anxiety symptoms worsening with age, peaking in adolescence and declining in adulthood (Vasa et al., 2020). In younger children with ASD, correlates of anxiety include sensory overresponsivity, sleep disturbance, aggression/defiance, and attention deficit/hyperactivity disorder (Vasa et al., 2020). A family history of psychiatric conditions is a stronger predictor of anxiety in youth with ASD than is a family history of ASD alone (Avni et al., 2018).

Given the high comorbidity, it is necessary to systematically assess anxiety as part of a comprehensive ASD assessment and diagnosis, as appropriate. While anxiety assessment can be performed via a checklist or rating scale, given the potential overlap in symptom presentation between ASD and anxiety (e.g., social withdrawal or avoidance, minimal facial expressions, reduced gestures, and limited or avoidant eye contact), it is important to consider ways to gather additional observations or colloratral information about social communication skills outside the clinical setting, which can be done through review of home videos or observations of social communication with a trusted person. Individuals with anxiety, but not ASD, typically have intact social pragmatics, although their ability to use these skills in daily functioning varies. Additionally, it is critical to gather early developmental history, as individuals with ASD tend to have early developmental markers that differ from anxiety. Finally, it is important to consider the function of anxiety. For example, is anxiety related to sensory experiences as part of ASD for generalized anxiety about the future? A close examination of these behaviors can help to differentiate their sources.

Communication Disorders

Communication disorders in the DSM-5-TR include Language Disorder, Speech Sound Disorder, Childhood-Onset Fluency Disorder (Stuttering), and Social (Pragmatic) Communication Disorder. Communication disorders are common in individuals with ASD (Vogindroukas et al., 2022), and may include varying challenges in semantics, articulation, rhythm, grammar, use of gestures, and pragmatic communication. Clinicians sometimes confuse communication deficits with autism; therefore, it is important to focus on communication deficits that impact social interactions in determining if an individual meets criteria for ASD compared to a communication disorder. Individuals with ASD may use abnormal language skills that are distinct from communication disorders. For example, individuals with ASD may engage in echolalia in which they echo or repeat what they hear. Other individuals with ASD may use stereotyped phrases to the point that they script lines from their favorite television show or movie as a means to socially interact with others. It can also be common for individuals with ASD to speak in a flat, monotonous voice, talk about themselves in the third person, reverse pronouns, or engage in other speech abnormalities that interfere with their ability to interact socially.

A relatively new diagnosis introduced in the DSM-5 is Social (Pragmatic) Communication Disorder, which has many similarities to ASD. A diagnosis of Social (Pragmatic) Communication Disorder is appropriate when assessment results indicate that an individual exhibits many of the social communication deficits found in ASD but does not exhibit any restricted, repetitive patterns of behaviors, interests, or activities that are required for an ASD diagnosis. The distinction between SPCD and ASD remains controversial, as both disorders share pragmatic communication challenges (Mandy et al., 2017). Diagnostically, SPCD should be considered after ruling out ASD as a potential diagnosis. Assessing for pragmatic language skills is not based on a singular formal assessment but based on observations, collateral interviews, completing checklists, or inventories, and using informal situations to observe pragmatic language skills to get a holistic understanding of an individual's pragmatic strengths and weaknesses as no singular test can evaluate the complexity of situational pragmatic skills.

Motor Disorders

Motor disorders in the DSM-5-TR include Developmental Coordination Disorder, Stereotypic Movement Disorder, and Tic Disorders. Up to 83% of individuals with ASD experience some degree of motor impairment (Hilton et al., 2012; Martel et al., 2024). Motor impairments in individuals with ASD may include issues with balance, gait, coordination, or sudden and rapid nonrhythmic motor movements. Symptoms associated with motor disorders may mimic repetitive behaviors that are commonly featured in ASD. A key differential difference between ASD and Tic Disorder is that motor movements in ASD tend to be more rhythmic and involve more than one part of the body; whereas, motor movements in tic disorder tend to be more localized in the eyes, face, head, shoulders, or other parts of the body (Duvall et al., 2022). Motor disorders can also co-occur with ASD; therefore, it is appropriate to diagnose a motor disorder if an individual meets criteria. The DSM-5-TR does specify, however, that stereotypic movement disorder should only be diagnosed in individuals with ASD only in cases in which an individual is engaging in self-injurious behaviors or their stereotypic movements are a focus in treatment (APA, 2022).

Future Directions in Autism Assessment

Emerging Approaches in Diagnosis

Advancements in diagnosing autism spectrum disorder (ASD) have been significantly influenced by integrating telehealth technologies into clinical practices, a trend catalyzed, in part, by the COVID-19 pandemic. However, the adoption of telehealth has posed challenges for comprehensive evaluations, especially for ASD, which relies heavily on nonverbal communication and social interactions (Stavropoulos et al., 2022). Concerns arose regarding the impact of personal protective equipment, such as face masks, on the validity of traditional assessment tools. To address this, modified measures such as the Brief Observation of Symptoms of Autism (BOSA) have been developed, facilitating autism-related evaluations in naturalistic settings without direct clinician contact (Dow et al., 2022).

Prior to the pandemic, two telehealth models, TELE-ASD-PEDS and TEDI, were devised to bridge the gap between research and clinical practice for early ASD diagnosis (Wagner et al., 2023). These tools enable remote observation of caregiver-child interactions and exhibit promising psychometric properties. Similarly, the BOSA demonstrates good validity and reliability across a broad population compared to traditional methods such as the ADOS-2, although it may be less precise for nuanced presentations of ASD, particularly with adolescents (Dow et al., 2022; Corona et al., 2024). Further technological advancements, such as mobile applications and artificial intelligence, offer additional screening and diagnostic capabilities for ASD (Reddy et al., 2024). These technologies leverage caregiver—reported behavioral markers, eye tracking, and machine learning algorithms to enhance early detection of autism, though further validation is warranted. For example, a recent study examined the performance of ChatGPT in evaluating developmental and behavioral pediatrics (DBP) case studies, including those with autism, to assess its diagnostic accuracy and treatment recommendation generation. ChatGPT was tested in 97 cases, and a panel of physicians evaluated its performance. The results showed that the ChatGPT achieved a diagnosis agreement rate of 66.2% with the physician panel. Physicians rated the treatment recommendations as reasonably accurate and comprehensive. ChatGPT also demonstrated an ability to address relevant cultural and ethical considerations in DBP cases (Kim et al, 2024).

Despite these strides, challenges persist in standardizing telehealth protocols, ensuring patient privacy and data security, and addressing disparities in technological access. Future research is imperative to validate the efficacy of telehealth-based assessments across diverse populations and settings, as well as to explore the integration of emerging technologies into telehealth platforms for ASD diagnosis (Stavropoulos et al., 2022). Telehealth presents a novel assessment approach by providing remote access to diagnostic evaluations, thereby overcoming geographical, accessibility, and cost barriers. As clinicians continue to embrace telehealth, it is crucial to screen clients to ensure their appropriateness and adequately prepare them for telehealth assessments, including informing them of the necessary technologies and resources (Gibbs et al., 2021).

Individualized and Dynamic Assessment Approaches

An area for needed growth in ASD assessment is recognizing and better understanding the unique connection between a broader autism phenotype (BAP) and higher levels of gender nonconformity (GNC). While non-binary gender identities are especially common among individuals with autism, current tools for measuring gender experiences in autism are insufficient and there is limited information on the needs and mental health of people with autism (Greene et al., 2024; Kallitsounaki & Williams, 2023). Traditional assessment approaches have often conflated sex and gender or viewed them through a binary lens, overlooking the nuanced experiences of autistic individuals, particularly those who are gender-diverse (Strang et al., 2020). It is theorized that individuals with autism may feel less pressure to conform to societal gender roles, leading to higher expressions of gender diversity. The concept of a "female autism phenotype" highlights differences in the expression of autism between males and females, noting that girls and women with autism may exhibit fewer repetitive behaviors and have stronger social motivations than their male counterparts. For example, Halladay et al. (2015) found that female participants with autism spectrum disorder (ASD) demonstrated more advanced communication skills and fewer restricted interests compared to males with ASD, supporting the concept of a female autism phenotype. These differences are influenced by both biological factors and the greater social expectations of females. Additionally, higher levels of internalizing symptoms were associated with increased gender nonconformity, BAP features, and autistic traits.

As clinicians move towards a more individualized and dynamic assessment process, they should consider the overlap between autistic traits and gender nonconformity when assessing ASD and comorbid mental health issues in young adults (Greene et al., 2024). It is crucial to recognize that both elevated autistic traits and gender nonconformity may contribute to heightened internalizing symptoms. Given the high incidence of ASD among adolescents with GNC, routine screening for gender nonconformity and autistic traits in mental health assessments using validated tools is recommended (Strang et al., 2018). It is important to include and measure sex and gender as separate constructs in assessments, recognizing their multicomponent nature as well as develop new tools to capture both binary and non-binary gender experiences.

If ASD is suspected and the screening clinician is not an ASD specialist, ideally the client should be referred to an ASD specialist for comprehensive evaluation. An ASD diagnosis should not exclude the possibility of GNC or GD diagnosis and appropriate GD-related treatment. Clinicians and parents should avoid dismissing GD as merely an aspect of ASD, or vice versa, as both conditions should be assessed and treated independently. Diagnosing ASD in gender nonconforming youth can be complicated by social awkwardness or withdrawal stemming from their GNC history, while diagnosing GD in adolescents with ASD can be challenging due to ASD-related weaknesses in communication, self-awareness, and executive function. For example, a gender nonconforming youth who is socially withdrawn may be misdiagnosed with ASD when their social withdrawal is actually a result of their GNC identity and the discrimination they face. Similarly, an adolescent with ASD who struggles with communication, self-awareness, and executive function may be overlooked for a GD diagnosis due to diagnostic overshadowing which is the assumption that these difficulties are a standard part of their ASD (Strang et al., 2018).

When assessing co-occurring ASD and GNC/GD, collaboration between gender specialists and autism specialists is essential if no clinician skilled in either area is available. This collaborative approach may extend the diagnostic period and slow clinical decision-making because of the complexity of these cases. Providing training for clinicians on the intersectionality of autism and gender diversity, and educating mental health professionals about the specific needs and challenges of these populations can foster more inclusive and effective care. Integrating these findings and recommendations into clinical practice will better support the mental well-being of individuals navigating both gender and neurodiversity. Further research should focus on the lived experiences of autistic individuals regarding their gender identities and expressions, and policies should be developed to support gender-diverse autistic individuals, recognizing the unique intersectionalities that affect their mental health and well-being.

Diagnostic Versus Strength-Based Assessments

Diagnostic models of autism assessment have traditionally followed a medical model that focuses on the behavioral deficits and symptoms outlined in the current edition of the DSM. This emphasis often identifies specific behaviors that clinicians, educators, and other professionals try to eliminate to reduce the severity of ASD. The traditional diagnostic approach has utility as it has resulted in greater research focus on the etiology of autism and evidence-based practices (Donaldson et al., 2017). Furthermore, the traditional diagnostic assessment approach offers a diagnosis and recommendations for treatment that are often needed for individuals with ASD to be linked with educational, governmental, and clinical services. A critique of this approach is that it often has a negative focus on a person's deficits, with minimal attention placed on the unique strengths of individuals with ASD (Monteiro, 2022).

More recently, professionals working with individuals with ASD have advocated for a strength-based assessment approach. Unlike traditional diagnostic assessment, strength-based assessment uses a positive framework to identify the specific strengths, interests, and skills of the individual (Urbanowicz et al., 2019). This is a culturally competent approach, as it emphasizes professional partnering with individuals to help them achieve their personal goals. It focuses on strengths rather than deficits, acknowledges the individual's personal interests and skills, and offers modifications and accommodations to help individuals achieve success, rather than prescribed treatment interventions that have been criticized as being overly generalized towards common autistic behaviors. Individuals with ASD may not always be aware of their strengths and how to utilize their abilities to achieve success in their environment; however, emerging research indicates that individuals with ASD who have knowledge of their strengths and abilities experience an improvement in well-being, quality of life, and overall mental health (Taylor et al., 2023). Furthermore, a strength-based approach is helpful not only for youth with ASD but also for individuals transitioning to adulthood (Urbanowicz et al., 2019) and is exploring ways to reach their personal goals and contribute to society. There is a debate on whether a strength-based approach should focus on specific autistic abilities in the individual versus a more general assessment of individual strengths (Taylor et al., 2023). In the spirit of an individualized approach to assessments, we recommend that evaluators focus not only on autistic-related strengths (e.g., specific interests and passions, sensory responses that make individuals more attuned to their environment, or advanced knowledge in nuanced subjects/topics), but also on other strengths that are not specifically autism-related (e.g., strong vocabulary, quick and efficient problem-solving, organization, etc.).

Addressing Disparities in Access to Assessment Services

As described earlier in this chapter, there are known disparities in the autism diagnosis process and systems that support the process, which negatively impacts outcomes. One emerging approach to reducing disparities in the diagnostic assessment of ASD is the inclusion of navigation services (Emick & Catanase, 2022). Patient navigators roles were first developed to reduce health disparities in cancer care (Riley & Riley, 2016). There is strong evidence that oncology patient navigation programs effectively reduce barriers to high-quality medical care by improving timely access to medical services and related support (Riley & Riley, 2016). Family Navigation within the field of autism has a relatively brief history, and early models of Autism Family Navigation (AFN) focused on navigation for at-risk children and navigating the diagnostic process (Feinberg et al., 2016). Later, models focused on providing navigation services after a child was diagnosed with ASD (Gordon-Lipkin et al., 2016; Roth et al., 2016).

Research suggests that AFN can help reduce barriers to accessing healthcare services related to ASD diagnosis and treatment. Children who received family navigation services were more likely to complete ASD diagnostic assessments than those who received routine clinical care (Feinberg et al. 2016). Additionally, caregivers of young children with Medicaid and a recent ASD diagnosis were more successful in scheduling and completing appointments and found that AFN services were more useful than caregivers of young children with insurance other than Medicaid (Roth et al., 2016). In a recent study, family navigation services decreased the time to diagnosis and increased the likelihood of diagnostic ascertainment in children from racial/ethnic minorities and low-income families who were identified as being at risk for ASD. Ethnicity appeared to moderate the strength of these findings (Feinberg et al., 2021). Navigation services have increased the number of at-risk toddlers evaluated for ASD from an urban, low-income population, as well as the quality of ASD screening in primary care clinics (DiGuiseppi et al., 2021). Research on the effectiveness of a pre-diagnostic navigation model is encouraging as a possible pathway to decreasing disparities in the diagnosis of autism (Hightshoe et al., 2023).

These findings underscore the importance of AFN programs to address significant systemic racial, ethnic, and socioeconomic inequalities in the early identification and treatment of young children with ASD. Future research should focus on refining the structure of interventions, such as embedding AFNs within clinics, to improve access and acceptance, particularly in environments in which language and immigration status are barriers. Moreover, efforts are needed to understand and address the engagement of low-income families and families of color in family navigation programs. Overall, family navigation shows promise as a vital tool for reducing disparities in ASD identification and treatment.

Case Vignettes

Early Identification with Young Child

Anderson is a 28-month-old African-American male referred for a neurodevelopmental evaluation because of concerns raised by his pediatrician stemming from a failed M-CHAT at his 18 month well check and developmental issues noted in the Ages and Stages Questionnaire. He lives with his parents and older sister and attends full-time day care. Despite achieving gross motor milestones on time, Anderson exhibited delays in social, fine motor, language, and adaptive skills. He had prior hearing concerns but passed a hearing screening at birth, although he does not consistently respond to auditory stimuli. There was no relevant history of hospitalizations, surgeries, or illness. There is an immediate maternal family history of anxiety.

Current concerns from parents and daycare teachers include delayed development, limited interaction with others including inconsistent response to name, minimal use of gestures, inconsistent response to requests for joint attention, stimming behaviors including arm flapping when excited, aggression toward the self and others including biting, and frequent nighttime waking. Anderson communicates primarily through non directed vocalization; he engages in non-functional play and shows narrow food preferences, along with safety concerns, such as mouthing or attempting to eat nonfood items.

To better understand Anderson's strengths, service needs, and diagnosis, a comprehensive multidisciplinary clinic evaluation involving a pediatric psychologist, speech pathologist, and occupational therapist was conducted. The assessments were selected as follows.

- clarify diagnosis (e.g., Autism Spectrum Rating Scales, Childhood Autism Rating Scale–Second Edition, Autism Diagnostic Observation Schedule-2nd edition)
- identify and screen for comorbid conditions/concerns (e.g., BASC-3)
- assesses developmental strengths and weaknesses (e.g., Developmental Assessment of Young Children-Second Edition and Preschool Language Scales Fifth Edition).

Anderson demonstrated strengths in enjoying outdoor activities, having a supportive immediate and extended family, and showing persistence in preferred activities, the results indicated that Anderson met the criteria for Autism Spectrum Disorder (ASD) level 2 in both the social communication criteria and restricted and repetitive behaviors and a global developmental delay. He exhibited significant deficits in social interaction/communication and restricted/stereotyped behaviors, alongside notable adaptive and cognitive vulnerabilities that affect attention, cognition, and executive functioning. Expressive and receptive language skills were significantly delayed, with reduced use of pragmatic behaviors, including limited joint attention, inconsistent social responsiveness, and limited eye contact.

Intensive evidence-based interventions were recommended including Applied Behavioral Analysis (ABA), particularly the Denver Early Start Model was recommended for skill acquisition. Additionally, Autism family navigation services are suggested to aid families in accessing services given the known disparities in treatment delays among African American children (La Roche et al., 2018). In Anderson's case, members of both immediate and extended families were invited to participate in navigation, which resulted in better support for Anderson and his parents. Follow-up with the pediatrician for genetic testing to rule out associated genetic conditions and reassessment at 12 to 18 months for progress monitoring are also recommended, in line with the AAP guidelines (Hyman et al., 2020).

When evaluating Anderson, it was crucial to refer the family for genetic testing because of his global developmental delay and the parents' specific questions about genetic risk for family planning. Although genetic testing cannot diagnose autism, it can reveal its origin and identify co-occurring medical conditions. These tests can lead to specific medical diagnoses (e.g., fragile X, Retts syndrome, Angelman syndrome, etc.), allowing for personalized care plans, appropriate surveillance, and targeted interventions. In addition, such diagnoses provide access to community support and valuable information for family planning. In Anderson's case, genetic testing occurred approximately four months after the initial autism diagnosis and indicated a chromosomal abnormality. By being aware of this genetic condition, his family was able to receive additional support through a state agency, and Anderson was medically monitored by the local children's hospital, as his chromosomal abnormality is known to have cardiac complications. As part of the diagnostic assessment process, it is important to be aware of guidelines related to genetic testing (Hyman et al., 2020).

In approaching Anderson's evaluation, it was important to acknowledge that the ASD diagnostic process was delayed because of a lack of ASD providers in his geographic areas (i.e., Anderson was referred for an ASD evaluation at 18 months, but not evaluated until nearly a year later). This delay in evaluation and subsequent delay in intervention services is a widespread interconnected systematic issue with waitlists ranging from several months to several years, depending on the geographic area and insurance status. To address waitlist issues, there have been a range of solutions focusing on alternative service delivery models, increasing system capacity, and improving intake and assessment processes (Eichstedt et al., 2024). While no single approach appears to be sufficient, clinically, it is important to ensure that efforts to reduce wait times should not compromise the quality of care. Kanne and Bishop (2021) make a strong argument that emphasis should be on increasing the number of expert providers to meet the growing demand for care.

Differential Diagnosis in Middle Childhood

Alex is an 11-year-old European-American child referred for a neurodevelopmental evaluation following concerns raised by the child's fourth grade teacher. Alex was assigned female at birth and recently came out to their family as non-binary, preferring they/them pronouns. Alex lives with their mother, father, and younger sister and attends school full-time. There were no developmental concerns reported in early childhood, with Alex meeting all gross motor milestones on time and speaking their first words at 8 months of age. Their family history is positive for ADHD, anxiety, and tics; Alex was diagnosed with ADHD in preschool and is currently prescribed prozac to address ongoing anxiety, typically arising within the school setting. Alex is also diagnosed with Specific Learning Disorder in Reading (Dyslexia) and attends a private school for children with learning disorders. No relevant medical history was reported.

A primary concern reported by both teachers and parents is immense difficulty forming friendships, with Alex reportedly having no friends. Additional concerns include over-reactivity to sensory stimuli (evinced by strong reactions to noises of other students in the classroom, refusal to wear shoes or socks, restrictive preferences for food textures, and aversion to most smells), difficulty understanding language directed to them, unusual behaviors (e.g., skin-picking, toe-walking, echolalia of sounds from Youtube videos) and a narrow range of intense and unusual interests (e.g., socio-political conflict in the Middle East). Alex's teacher also reports concerns that Alex is below grade level in reading comprehension and often struggles to understand character's feelings or intentions, instead preferring fact-based statements; this is despite Alex's otherwise strong intellectual abilities and their successful use of assistive technology for reading in the classroom. In recent months, Alex ceased completing schoolwork and has instead been conducting research on an unrelated topic of interest. This has caused them to fall further behind in school and led to several disciplinary meetings, with the possibility that Alex will have to repeat fourth grade.

A comprehensive evaluation led by a neuropsychologist was conducted to assess Alex's current functioning. Assessments were selected to:

- Clarify diagnosis (e.g., Autism Diagnostic Interview- Revised, The Monteiro Interview Guidelines for Diagnosing the Autism Spectrum, 2nd Edition).
- Provide comprehensive understanding of current functioning, strengths, and weaknesses (Behavior Assessment System for Children, 3rd Edition, Vineland Adaptive Behavior Scales, 3rd Edition, Delis-Kaplan Executive Functioning System).

Results indicated Alex meets criteria for Autism Spectrum Disorder (ASD)-Level 1. They exhibited significant deficits in social interaction and communication, alongside notably restricted areas of interest and the presence of repetitive behaviors. While Alex presented as a bright and friendly child capable of maintaining brief reciprocal conversation with adults, they faced immense difficulty interacting with children their age and struggled to engage in discussion about non-preferred topics. Alex's high cognitive skills, love for learning, and passion for social justice are valuable and unique strengths which were highlighted in their diagnostic report in line with best practices for neuro-informed assessment. Alex's family were provided referrals for Occupational therapy (for sensory integration), Speech Language therapy (for support building skills necessary to make friends), and a therapist specializing in work with twice-exceptional children.

In approaching Alex's diagnostic evaluation, it was essential to consider their both gender identity and their high cognitive skills. Some assessment tools used to diagnose ASD are normed differently by gender, based on a theoretical assumption that presentations of autism differ significantly on the basis of gender. This assumption fails to account for genderfluid and gender nonconforming (GNC) individuals who do not identify solely or primarily with one binary gender. If using these gender-normed assessment instruments within the trans/GNC population, clinicians should score the test twice using both Male and Female norms, and compare the two scores to identify any important differences in scoring thresholds.

Furthermore, conducting assessments with twice-exceptional children, or children who are cognitively gifted with additional developmental/emotional/learning needs, requires additional attention to the child's full profile of strengths and weaknesses. Alex did not display early language delay, their verbal skills were advanced for their age, and they were capable of maintaining high-level conversations about topics of interest. Alex was additionally able to inhibit their stereotyped behaviors and socially "mask" for brief periods of time, although this took a notable toll on her emotional wellbeing. Children like Alex present with many obvious strengths, and clinicians may wish to take more time to gather a comprehensive understanding of the child's functional abilities across various settings to inform diagnostic decision-making within the twice-exceptional or cognitively gifted population.

Conclusion

Autism Spectrum Disorder (ASD) is a neurodevelopmental condition characterized by social communication challenges and repetitive behaviors, with significant variations in presentation among individuals. Clinicians must remain informed about the latest research, tools, and culturally competent practices to provide accurate and comprehensive ASD assessments. A multidisciplinary, individualized approach that encourages early identification, sensitivity to cultural and gender differences, and a focus on strengths can significantly improve the outcomes of individuals with ASD. Early identification and intervention are crucial for improving outcomes, highlighting the need for clinicians to be proficient in using reliable assessment tools and in recognizing early signs. The use of multidisciplinary teams incorporating professionals such as developmental pediatricians, psychologists, occupational therapists, and speech-language therapists can provide a comprehensive understanding of an individual's strengths and weaknesses. However, accessibility to such teams varies, necessitating well-trained solo practitioners. Culturally and linguistically sensitive assessments, along with a strength-based approach that focuses on an individual's abilities, are essential for an accurate diagnosis and effective intervention planning. Advancements in telehealth have facilitated remote assessments and addressed geographical and accessibility barriers, although ongoing research is needed to validate these methods and clinicians should proceed with appropriate caution. Differential diagnosis is complex due to the high prevalence of comorbid conditions, such as ADHD and anxiety, requiring thorough evaluation and consideration of symptom trajectories. Clinicians should be aware of sex differences in ASD presentations, particularly in females, who may exhibit less overt symptoms. Efforts to reduce disparities in access to diagnostic services such as family navigation programs are vital for equitable care. Overall, a holistic, individualized approach that integrates the latest research and emphasizes strengths can significantly enhance the quality of life for individuals with ASD.

References

American Academy of Pediatrics. (2021). Autism spectrum disorder. https://www.aap.org/en/patient-care/autism

American Psychiatric Association. (2022). *Diagnostic and statistical manual for mental disorders* (5th ed., text rev.). https://doi.org/10.1176/appi.books.9780890425787

Aragon-Guevara, D., Castle, G., Sheridan, E., & Vivanti, G. (2023). The reach and accuracy of information on autism on Tiktok. *Journal of Autism and Developmental Disorders*, 1–6.https://doi.org/10.1007/s10803-023-06084-6

Avni, E., Ben-Itzchak, E., & Zachor, D. A. (2018). The Presence of Comorbid ADHD and Anxiety Symptoms in Autism Spectrum Disorder: Clinical Presentation and Predictors. *Frontiers in Psychiatry*, *9*. https://doi.org/10.3389/fpsyt.2018.00717

Aylward, B. S., Gal-Szabo, D. E., & Taraman, S. (2021). Racial, ethnic, and sociodemographic disparities in diagnosis of children with autism spectrum disorder. *Journal of Developmental and Behavioral Pediatrics, 42*(8), 682. https://doi.org/10.1097/DBP.0000000000000996

Baby Siblings Research Consortium. (2025). Sex-related measurement bias in autism spectrum disorder symptoms in the Baby Siblings Research Consortium. *JAMA Network Open, 8*(8), e2525887. https://doi.org/10.1001/jamanetworkopen.2025.25887

Bal, V. H., Maye, M., Salzman, E., Huerta, M., Pepa, L., Risi, S., & Lord, C. (2020). The adapted ADOS: A new module set for the assessment of minimally verbal adolescents and adults. *Journal of Autism and Developmental Disorders, 50*(3), 719–729. https://doi.org/10.1007/s10803-019-04302-8

Bargiela, S., Steward, R., & Mandy, W. (2016). The experiences of late-diagnosed women with autism spectrum conditions: An investigation of the female autism phenotype. *Journal of Autism and Developmental Disorders, 46*(10), 3281–3294. https://doi.org/10.1007/s10803-016-2872-8

Bernier, R., Mao, A., & Yen, J. (2010). Psychopathology, families, and culture: Autism. *Child and Adolescent Psychiatric Clinics of North America, 19*(4), 855–867. https://doi.org/10.1016/j.chc.2010.07.005

Berument, S. K., Rutter, M., Lord, C., Pickles, A., & Bailey, A. (1999). Autism screening questionnaire: Diagnostic validity. *The British Journal of Psychiatry, 175*, 444–451. https://doi.org/10.1192/bjp.175.5.444

Bishop, S. L., & Lord, C. (2023). Commentary: Best practices and processes for assessment of autism spectrum disorder—the intended role of standardized diagnostic instruments. *Journal of Child Psychology and Psychiatry, 64*(5), 834–838. https://doi.org/10.1111/jcpp.13802

Botha, M., Hanlon, J., & Williams, G. L. (2023). Does language matter? Identity-first versus person-first language use in autism research: A response to Vivanti. *Journal of Autism and Developmental Disorders, 53*(2), 870–878. https://doi.org/10.1007/s10803-020-04858-w

Bouck, E. C., Savage, M., Meyer, N. K., Taber-Doughty, T., & Hunley, M. (2014). High-tech or low-tech? Comparing self-monitoring systems to increase task independence for students with autism. *Focus on Autism and Other Developmental Disabilities, 29*(3), 156–167. https://doi.org/10.1177/1088357614528797

Braconnier, M. L., & Siper, P. M. (2021). Neuropsychological assessment in autism spectrum disorder. *Current Psychiatry Reports, 23*, 1–9.

Brooks, B. L., Sherman, E. M. S., & Strauss, E. (2009). NEPSY-II: A developmental neuropsychological assessment, second edition. *Child Neuropsychology, 16*(1), 80–101.https://doi.org/10.1080/09297040903146966

Bruni, T. P. (2014). Review of social responsiveness scale-second edition (SRS-2). *Journal of Psychoeducational Assessment, 32*(4), 365–369. https://doi.org/10.1177/0734282913517525

Centers for Disease Control and Prevention. (2022). *Data & statistics on autism spectrum disorder*. CDC. https://www.cdc.gov/ncbddd/autism/data.html#print

Chang, Y.-C., Quan, J., & Wood, J. J. (2012). Effects of anxiety disorder severity on social functioning in children with autism spectrum disorders. *Journal of Developmental and Physical Disabilities, 24*(3), 235–245. https://doi.org/10.1007/s10882-012-9268-2

Christiansz, J. A., Gray, K. M., Taffe, J., & Tonge, B. J. (2016). Autism spectrum disorder in the DSM-5: Diagnostic sensitivity and specificity in early childhood. *Journal of Autism and Developmental Disorders, 46*(6), 2054–2063. https://doi.org/10.1007/s10803-016-2734-4

Christensen, D. L., Braun, K. V. N., Baio, J., Bilder, D., Charles, J., Constantino, J. N., Daniels, J., Durkin, M. S., Fitzgerald, R. T., Kurzius-Spencer, M., Lee, L. C., Pettygrove, S., Robinson, C., Schulz, E., Wells, C., Wingate, M. S., Zahorodny, W., & Yeargin-Allsopp, M. (2018). Prevalence and characteristics of autism spectrum disorder among children aged 8 Years—autism and developmental disabilities monitoring network, 11 Sites, United States, 2012. Morbidity and mortality weekly report. *Surveillance Summaries, 65*(13), 1–23. https://doi.org/10.15585/mmwr.ss6513a1

Cohen, I. L., Schmidt-Lackner, S., Romanczyk, R., & Sudhalter, V. (2003). The PDD behavior inventory: A rating scale for assessing response to intervention in children with pervasive developmental disorder. *Journal of Autism and Developmental Disorders, 33*(1), 31–45. https://doi.org/10.1023/a:1022226403878

Cohen, I. L., Gomez, T. R., Gonzalez, M. G., Lennon, E. M., Karmel, B. Z., & Gardner, J. M. (2010). Parent PDD behavior inventory profiles of young children classified according to autism diagnostic observation schedule-generic and autism diagnostic interview-revised criteria. *Journal of Autism and Developmental Disorders, 40*(2), 246–254. https://doi.org/10.1007/s10803-009-0863-8

Constantino, J. N. & Gruber, C. P. (2012). *Social responsiveness scale—second edition (SRS-2).* Western Psychological Services.

Corona, L. L., Wagner, L., Hooper, M., Weitlauf, A., Foster, T. E., Hine, J., Miceli, A., Nicholson, A., Stone, C., Vehorn, A., & Warren, Z. (2024). A randomized trial of the accuracy of novel telehealth instruments for the assessment of autism in toddlers. *Journal of Autism and Developmental Disorders, 54*(6), 2069–2080. https://doi.org/10.1007/s10803-023-05908-9

Dellis, D. C., Kaplan, E., & Kramer, J. H. (2001). Delis-Kaplan executive function system (D-KEFS). APA Psyc Tests. https://doi.org/10.1037/t15082-000

Demetriou, E. A., Lampit, A., Quintana, D. S., Naismith, S. L., Song, Y. J. C., Pye, J. E., & Guastella, A. J. (2018). Autism spectrum disorders: A meta-analysis of executive functioning. *Molecular Psychiatry, 23*(5), 1198–1204.

Denisova, K., & Lin, Z. (2023). The importance of low IQ to early diagnosis of autism. *Autism Research, 16*(1), 122–214.

Dennison, A., Hall, S. P., Leal, J., & Madres, D. A. (2019). ASD or ELL? Distinguishing differences in patterns of communication and behavior. *Contemporary School Psychology, 23*(1), 57–67. https://doi.org/10.1007/s40688-018-0206-x

DiGuiseppi, C., Rosenberg, S. A., Tomcho, M. A., Colborn, K., Hightshoe, K., Gutiérrez-Raghunath, S., Cordova, J. M., Dooling-Litfin, J. K., & Robinson Rosenberg, C. (2021). Family navigation to increase evaluation for autism spectrum disorder in toddlers: Screening and Linkage to Services for Autism (SaLSA) pragmatic randomized trial. *Autism : The International Journal of Research and Practice, 25*(4), 946–957. https://doi.org/10.1177/1362361320974175

Donaldson, A. L., Krejcha, K., & McMillin, A. (2017). A strengths-based approach to autism: Neurodiversity and partnering with the autism community. *Perspectives of the ASHA Special Interest Groups, 2*(1), 56–68.

Dow, D., Holbrook, A., Toolan, C., McDonald, N., Sterrett, K., Rosen, N., Kim, S. H., & Lord, C. (2022). The Brief Observation of Symptoms of Autism (BOSA): Development of a new adapted assessment measure for remote telehealth administration through COVID-19 and beyond. *Journal of Autism and Developmental Disorders, 52*(12), 5383–5394. https://doi.org/10.1007/s10803-021-05395-w

Duvall, S., Armstrong, K., Shahabuddin, A., Grantz, C., Fein, D., & Lord, C. (2022). A road map for identifying autism spectrum disorder: Recognizing and evaluating characteristics that should raise red or "pink" flags to guide accurate differential diagnosis. *The Clinical Neuropsychologist, 36*(5), 1172–1207. https://doi.org/10.1080/13854046.2021.1921276

Duvekot, J., van der Ende, J., Verhulst, F. C., Slappendel, G., van Daalen, E., Maras, A., & Greaves-Lord, K. (2017). Factors influencing the probability of a diagnosis of autism spectrum disorder in girls versus boys. *Autism: The International Journal of Research and Practice*, *21*(6), 646–658. https://doi.org/10.1177/1362361316672178

Eaton, C., Roarty, K., Doval, N., Shetty, S., Goodall, K., & Rhodes, S. M. (2023). The prevalence of attention deficit/hyperactivity disorder symptoms in children and adolescents with autism spectrum disorder without intellectual disability: A systematic review. *Journal of Attention Disorders, 27*(12), 1360–1376.

Eichstedt, J. A., Turcotte, K., Golden, G., Arbuthnott, A. E., Chen, S., Collins, K. A., Mowat, S., & Reid, G. J. (2024). Waitlist management in child and adolescent mental health care: A scoping review. *Children and Youth Services Review, 160*, Article 107529. https://doi.org/10.1016/j.chi ldyouth.2024.107529

Emick, J., & Catanese, K. (2022). Autism Family Navigation: A Novel Solution *Ohio Psychologist* 10–14.

Ennis-Cole, D., Durodoye, B. A., & Harris, H. L. (2013). The impact of culture on autism diagnosis and treatment: Considerations for counselors and other professionals. *The Family Journal, 21*(3), 279–287. https://doi.org/10.1177/1066480713476834

Estes, A., Munson, J., Rogers, S. J., Greenson, J., Winter, J., & Dawson, G. (2015). Long-term outcomes of early intervention in 6-Year-old children with autism spectrum disorder. *Journal of the American Academy of Child & Adolescent Psychiatry, 54*(7), 580–587. https://doi.org/10.1016/j.jaac.2015.04.005

Fahim, D., & Nedwick, K. (2014). Around the world: Supporting young children with ASD who are dual language learners. *Young Exceptional Children, 17*(2), 3–20. https://doi.org/10.1177/1096250613477870

Feinberg, E., Abufhele, M., Sandler, J., Augustyn, M., Cabral, H., Chen, N., Diaz Linhart, Y., Cesar Levesque, Z., Aebi, M., & Silverstein, M. (2016). Reducing disparities in timely autism diagnosis through family navigation: Results from a randomized pilot trial. *Psychiatric Services, 67*(8), 912–915. https://doi.org/10.1176/appi.ps.201500162

Feinberg, E., Augustyn, M., Broder-Fingert, S., Bennett, A., Weitzman, C., Kuhn, J., Hickey, E., Chu, A., Levinson, J., Sandler Eilenberg, J., Silverstein, M., Cabral, H. J., Patts, G., Diaz-Linhart, Y., Fernandez-Pastrana, I., Rosenberg, J., Miller, J. S., Guevara, J. P., Fenick, A. M., & Blum, N. J. (2021). Effect of family navigation on diagnostic ascertainment among children at risk for autism: A randomized clinical trial from DBPNet. *JAMA Pediatrics, 175*(3), 243–250. https://doi.org/10.1001/jamapediatrics.2020.5218

Gabrielsen, T. P., Farley, M., Speer, L., Villalobos, M., Baker, C. N., & Miller, J. (2015). Identifying autism in a brief observation. *Pediatrics, 135*, e330–e338.

Gerdts, J., Mancini, J., Fox, E., Rhoads, C., Ward, T., Easley, E., & Bernier, R. A. (2018). Interdisciplinary team evaluation: An effective method for the diagnostic assessment of autism spectrum disorder. *Journal of Developmental & Behavioral Pediatrics, 39*(4), 271–281. https://doi.org/10.1097/DBP.0000000000000549

Gibbs, V., Cai, R. Y., Aldridge, F., & Wong, M. (2021). Autism assessment via telehealth during the Covid 19 pandemic: Experiences and perspectives of autistic adults, parents/carers and clinicians. *Research in Autism Spectrum Disorders, 88*, Article 101859. https://doi.org/10.1016/j.rasd.2021.101859

Gioia G. A., Isquith P. K., Guy S. C., Kenworthy L. (2015). *Behavior rating inventory of executive function-2 professional manual*. Psychological Assessment Resources.

Goldstein, S., & Naglieri, J.A. (2009). *Autism spectrum rating scales*. Multi-Health Systems Inc.

Goldstein, S., & Ozonoff, S. (2018). *Assessment of autism spectrum disorder*. Guilford Publications.

Gordon-Lipkin, E., Foster, J., & Peacock, G. (2016). Whittling down the wait time: Exploring models to minimize the delay from initial concern to diagnosis and treatment of autism spectrum disorder. *Pediatric Clinics of North America, 63*(5), 851–859. https://doi.org/10.1016/j.pcl.2016.06.007

Greene, R. K., Rutter, T. M., Phelps, R. A., Olsen, E. K., Harmon, R., & Moyer, D. N. (2024). Diagnostic assessment of autism spectrum disorder in transgender and gender diverse youth. *The Clinical Neuropsychologist*, 1–22. Advance online publication. https://doi.org/10.1080/13854046.2024.2331272

Halladay, A. K., Bishop, S., Constantino, J. N., Daniels, A. M., Koenig, K., Palmer, K., Messinger, D., Pelphrey, K., Sanders, S. J., Singer, A. T., Taylor, J. L., & Szatmari, P. (2015). Sex and gender differences in autism spectrum disorder: Summarizing evidence gaps and identifying emerging areas of priority. *Molecular Autism, 6*, 36. https://doi.org/10.1186/s13229-015-0019-y

Harrison, P., & Oakland, T. (2015). *Adaptive behavior assessment system* (3rd Ed). Pearson.

Hayes, K. N., Rossetti, K. G., & Zlomke, K. (2022). Community support, family resilience and mental health among caregivers of youth with autism spectrum disorder. *Child: Care, Health and Development, 49*(2), 307–317. https://doi.org/10.1111/cch.13025

Hedley, D., Nevill, R. E., Monroy-Moreno, Y., Fields, N., Wilkins, J., Butter, E., & Mulick, J. A. (2015). Efficacy of the ADEC in identifying autism spectrum disorder in clinically referred toddlers in the US. *Journal of Autism and Developmental Disorders, 45*(8), 2337–2348. https://doi.org/10.1007/s10803-015-2398-5

Hightshoe, K., Gutiérrez-Raghunath, S., Tomcho, M. M., Robinson Rosenberg, C., Rosenberg, S. A., Dooling-Litfin, J. K., Cordova, J. M., Colborn, K., & DiGuiseppi, C. (2023). Barriers to referral and evaluation and corresponding navigation services for toddlers screening positive for autism spectrum disorder. *Families, Systems, & Health, 41*(3), 342–357. https://doi.org/10.1037/fsh0000786

Hill, E. L. (2004). Executive dysfunction in autism. *Trends in Cognitive Sciences, 8*(1), 26–32. https://doi.org/10.1016/j.tics.2003.11.003

Hilton, C. L., Zhang, Y., Whilte, M. R., Klohr, C. L., & Constantino, J. (2012). Motor impairment in sibling pairs concordant and discordant for autism spectrum disorders. *Autism, 16*(4), 430–441. https://doi.org/10.1177/1362361311423018

Hossain, M. M., Khan, N., Sultana, A., Ma, P., McKyer, E. L. J., Ahmed, H. U., & Purohit, N. (2020). Prevalence of comorbid psychiatric disorders among people with autism spectrum disorder: An umbrella review of systematic reviews and meta-analyses. *Psychiatry Research, 287*, Article 112922.

Hull, L., Petrides, K. V., & Mandy, W. (2020). The female autism phenotype and camouflaging: A narrative review. *Review Journal of Autism and Developmental Disorders, 7*(4), 306–317. https://doi.org/10.1007/s40489-020-00197-9

Hyman, S. L., Levy, S. E., Myers, S. M., & Council on Children with Disabilities, Section on Developmental and Behavioral Pediatrics. (2020). Identification, evaluation, and management of children with autism spectrum disorder. *Pediatrics, 145*(1), e20193447. https://doi.org/10.1542/peds.2019-3447

Ji, S. I., Park, H., Yoon, S. A., & Hong, S. B. (2023). A validation study of the CARS-2 compared with the ADOS-2 in the diagnosis of autism spectrum disorder: A suggestion for cutoff scores. *Journal of the Korean Academy of Child and Adolescent Psychiatry, 34*(1), 45–50. https://doi.org/10.5765/jkacap.220027

Kalb, L. G., Singh, V., Hong, J. S., Holingue, C., Ludwig, N. N., Pfeiffer, D., Reetzke, R., Gross, A. L., & Landa, R. (2022). Analysis of race and sex bias in the Autism Diagnostic Observation Schedule (ADOS-2). *JAMA Network Open, 5*(4), Article e229498. https://doi.org/10.1001/jamanetworkopen.2022.9498

Kallitsounaki, A., & Williams, D. M. (2023). Autism Spectrum Disorder and Gender Dysphoria/Incongruence. A systematic Literature Review and Meta-Analysis. *Journal of Autism and Developmental Disorders, 53*(8), 3103–3117. https://doi.org/10.1007/s10803-022-05517-y

Kanne, S. M., & Bishop, S. L. (2021). Editorial perspective: The autism waitlist crisis and remembering what families need. *Journal of Child Psychology and Psychiatry, 62*(2), 140–142. https://doi.org/10.1111/jcpp.13254

Kaufman, N. K. (2022). Rethinking "gold standards" and "best practices" in the assessment of autism. *Applied Neuropsychology: Child, 11*(3), 529–540. https://doi.org/10.1080/21622965.2020.1809414

Kenny, L., Hattersley, C., Molins, B., Buckley, C., Povey, C., & Pellicano, E. (2016). Which terms should be used to describe autism? Perspectives from the UK autism community. *Autism, 20*(4), 442–462. https://doi.org/10.1177/1362361315588200

Kim, R., Margolis, A., Barile, J., Han, K., Kalash, S., Papaioannou, H., Krevskaya, A., & Milanaik, R. (2024). Challenging the chatbot: An assessment of ChatGPT's diagnoses and recommendations for DBP case studies. *Journal of Developmental and Behavioral Pediatrics, 45*(1), e8–e13. https://doi.org/10.1097/DBP.0000000000001255

Korkman, M., Kirk, U., & Kemp, S. (2007). NEPSY—Second Edition (NEPSY-II). APA Psyc Tests. https://doi.org/10.1037/t15125-000

La Roche, M. J., Bush, H. H., & D'Angelo, E. (2018). The assessment and treatment of autism spectrum disorder: A cultural examination. *Practice Innovations, 3*(2), 107–122. https://doi.org/10.1037/pri0000067

Lai, M.-C., Kassee, C., Besney, R., Bonato, S., Hull, L., Mandy, W., Szatmari, P., & Ameis, S. H. (2019). Prevalence of co-occurring mental health diagnoses in the autism population: A systematic review and meta-analysis. *The Lancet. Psychiatry, 6*(10), 819–829. https://doi.org/10.1016/S2215-0366(19)30289-5

Lai, M.-C., Amestoy, A., Bishop, S., Brown, H. M., Giwa Onaiwu, M., Halladay, A., Harrop, C., Hotez, E., Huerta, M., Kelly, A., Miller, D., Nordahl, C. W., Ratto, A. B., Saulnier, C., Siper, P. M., Sohl, K., Zwaigenbaum, L., & Goldman, S. (2023). Improving autism identification and support for individuals assigned female at birth: Clinical suggestions and research priorities. *The Lancet Child & Adolescent Health, 7*(12), 897–908. https://doi.org/10.1016/S2352-4642(23)00221-3

La Roche, M. J., Bush, H. H., & D'Angelo, E. (2018). The assessment and treatment of autism spectrum disorder: A cultural examination. *Practice Innovations, 3*(2), 107. https://doi.org/10.1037/pri0000067

Landa, R. J., Reetzke, R., Holingue, C. B., Herman, D., & Hess, C. R. (2022). Diagnostic stability and phenotypic differences among school-age children diagnosed with ASD before age 2. *Frontiers in Psychiatry, 13*, Article 805686. https://doi.org/10.3389/fpsyt.2022.805686

Lord C., Rutter M., DiLavore P. C., Risi S., Gotham K., & Bishop S. (2012). *Autism diagnostic observation schedule* (2nd ed.). Western Psychological Services.

Lord, C., Risi, S., Lambrecht, L., Cook, E. H., Jr., Leventhal, B. L., DiLavore, P. C., Pickles, A., & Rutter, M. (2000). The autism diagnostic observation schedule—generic: A standard measure of social and communication deficits associated with the spectrum of autism. *Journal of Autism and Developmental Disorders, 30*(3), 205–223. https://doi.org/10.1023/A:1005592401947

MacDonald, R., Baker-Ericzen, M., Roesch, S., Yeh, M., Dickson, K. S., & Smith, J. (2024). The latent structure of the Delis-Kaplan system for autism. *Autism Research, 17*(4), 728–738.

Maenner, M. J., Shaw, K. A., Baio, J., Washington, A., Patrick, M., DiRienzo, M., Christensen, D. L., Wiggins, L. D., Pettygrove, S., Andrews, J. G., Lopez, M., Hudson, A., Baroud, T., Schwenk, Y., White, T., Rosenberg, C. R., Lee, L. C., Harrington, R. A., Huston, M., Hewitt, A., Esler, A. A., Hall-Lande, J.,… Dietz, P. M. (2020). Prevalence of autism spectrum disorder among children aged 8 years—autism and developmental disabilities monitoring network, 11 sites, United States, 2016. *Morbidity and Mortality Weekly Report: Surveillance Summaries, 69*(4), 1–12. https://doi.org/10.15585/mmwr.ss6904a1

Magaña, S., & Smith, L. E. (2013). The use of the autism diagnostic interview-revised with a Latino population of adolescents and adults with autism. *Journal of Autism and Developmental Disorders, 43*(5), 1098–1105. https://doi.org/10.1007/s10803-012-1652-3

Mandy, W., Chilvers, R., Chowdhury, U., Salter, G., Seigal, A., & Skuse, D. (2012). Sex differences in autism spectrum disorder: Evidence from a large sample of children and adolescents. *Journal of Autism and Developmental Disorders, 42*(7), 1304–1313. https://doi.org/10.1007/s10803-011-1356-0

Mandy, W., Wang, A., Lee, I., & Skuse, D. (2017). Evaluating social (pragmatic) communication disorder. *Journal of Child Psychology and Psychiatry, 58*(10), 1166–1175. https://doi.org/10.1111/jcpp.12785

Martel, M., Finos, L., Bahmad, S., Koun, E., Salemme, R., Sonié, S., Fourneret, P., Schmitz, C., & Roy, A. C. (2024). Motor deficits in autism differ from that of developmental coordination disorder. *Autism, 28*(2), 415–432.

Marvin, A. R., Marvin, D. J., Lipkin, P. H., & Law, J. K. (2017). Analysis of social communication questionnaire (SCQ) screening for children less than age 4. *Current Developmental Disorders Reports, 4*(4), 137–144. https://doi.org/10.1007/s40474-017-0122-1

May, T., Cornish, K., & Rinehart, N. J. (2016). Gender profiles of behavioral attention in children with autism spectrum disorder. *Journal of Attention Disorders, 20*(7), 627–635. https://doi.org/10.1177/1087054712455502

Mazefsky, C. A., Kao, J., & Oswald, D. P. (2011). Preliminary evidence suggesting caution in the use of psychiatric self-report measures with adolescents with high-functioning autism spectrum disorders. *Research in Autism Spectrum Disorders, 5*(1), 164–174. https://doi.org/10.1016/j.rasd.2010.03.006

McQuaid, G. A., Pelphrey, K. A., Bookheimer, S. Y., Dapretto, M., Webb, S. J., Bernier, R. A., McPartland, J. C., Van Horn, J. D., & Wallace, G. L. (2021). The gap between IQ and adaptive functioning in autism spectrum disorder: Disentangling diagnostic and sex differences. *Autism, 25*(6), 1565–1579.

McKenzie, K., Metcalfe, D., & Murray, A. L. (2023). Screening for intellectual disability in autistic people: A brief report. *Research in Autism Spectrum Disorders, 100*, Article 102076. https://doi.org/10.1016/j.rasd.2022.102076

Monteiro, M. J. (2022). Individualizing the autism assessment process: A framework for school psychologists. *Psychology in the Schools, 59*(7), 1377–1389.

Monteiro, M. J. & Stegall, S. (2018). *Monteiro interview guidelines for diagnosing the autism spectrum* (2nd ed.). Western Psychological Services.

Morey, L. C. (1991). *Personality assessment inventory.* Psychological Assessment Resources.

Muth, A., Hönekopp, J., & Falter, C. M. (2014). Visuo-spatial performance in autism: A meta-analysis. *Journal of Autism and Devevlopmental Disorders, 44*, 3245–3263. https://doi.org/10.1007/s10803-014-2188-5

Nowell, K. P., Christopher, K., & Sohl, K. (2020). Equipping community based psychologists to deliver best practice ASD diagnoses using the ECHO autism model. *Children's Health Care, 49*(4), 403–424. https://doi.org/10.1080/02739615.2020.1771564

Nyrenius, J., & Billstedt, E. (2020). The functional impact of cognition in adults with autism spectrum disorders. *Nordic Journal of Psychiatry, 74*(3), 220–225.

Oliveras-Rentas, R. E., Kenworthy, L., Roberson, R. B., Martin, A., & Wallace, G. L. (2012). WISC-IV profile in high-functioning autism spectrum disorders: Impaired processing speed is associated with increased autism communication symptoms and decreased adaptive communication abilities. *Journal of Autism and Developmental Disorders, 42*, 655–664. https://doi.org/10.1007/s10803-011-1289-7

Pagán, A. F., Flint, D. D., & Loveland, K. A. (2024). Diagnosing autism in adults: Clinically focused recommendations. *Journal of Health Service Psychology, 50*(2), 103–111. https://doi.org/10.1007/s42843-024-00108-0

Penner, M., Anagnostou, E., Andoni, L. Y., & Ungar, W. J. (2018). Systematic review of clinical guidance documents for autism spectrum disorder diagnostic assessment in select regions. *Autism, 22*(5), 517–527. https://doi.org/10.1177/1362361316685879

Penner, M., Senman, L., Andoni, L., Dupuis, A., Anagnostou, E., Kao, S., Solish, A., Shouldice, M., Ferguson, G., & Brian, J. (2023). Concordance of diagnosis of autism spectrum disorder made by pediatricians vs a multidisciplinary specialist team. *JAMA Network Open, 6*(1), e2252879. https://doi.org/10.1001/jamanetworkopen.2022.52879

Pepperdine, C. R., & McCrimmon, A. W. (2018). Test review: Vineland adaptive behavior scales, third edition (Vineland-3) by Sparrow, S. S., Cicchetti, D. V., & Saulnier, C. A. *Canadian Journal of School Psychology, 33*(2), 157–163. https://doi.org/10.1177/0829573517733845

Reddy, K., Taksande, A., & Kurian, B. (2024). Harnessing the power of mobile phone technology: Screening and identifying autism spectrum disorder with smartphone apps. *Cureus, 16*(2), e55004. https://doi.org/10.7759/cureus.55004

Reel, K. H., Lecavalier, L., Butter, E., & Mulick, J. A. (2012). Diagnostic utility of the pervasive developmental disorder behavior inventory. *Research in Autism Spectrum Disorders, 6*(1), 458–465. https://doi.org/10.1016/j.rasd.2011.07.006

Reynolds, C. R., & Kamphaus, R. W. (2015). *Behavior assessment system for children* (3rd ed.). Pearson.

Riley, S., & Riley, C. (2016). The role of patient navigation in improving the value of oncology care. *Journal of Clinical Pathways, 2*(1), 41–47.

Robins, D. L., Casagrande, K., Barton, M., Chen, C. M., Dumont-Mathieu, T., & Fein, D. (2014). Validation of the modified checklist for Autism in toddlers, revised with follow-up (M-CHAT-R/F). *Pediatrics, 133*(1), 37–45. https://doi.org/10.1542/peds.2013-1813

Rong, Y., Yang, C. J., Jin, Y., & Wang, Y. (2021). Prevalence of attention-deficit/hyperactivity disorder in individuals with autism spectrum disorder: A meta-analysis. *Research in Autism Spectrum Disorders, 83*, Article 101759.

Roth, B. M., Kralovic, S., Roizen, N. J., Spannagel, S. C., Minich, N., & Knapp, J. (2016). Impact of autism navigator on access to services. *Journal of Developmental and Behavioral Pediatrics, 37*(3), 188–195. https://doi.org/10.1097/DBP.0000000000000261

Rutter, M., Lecouteur, A., & Lord, C. (2003). *Autism diagnostic interview, revised*. Pearson.

Sappok, T., Heinrich, M., & Underwood, L. (2015). Screening tools for autism spectrum disorders. *Advances in Autism, 1*(1), 12–29. https://doi.org/10.1108/AIA-03-2015-0001

Scheerer, N. E., Pourtousi, A., Yang, C., Ding, Z., Stojanoski, B., Anagnostou, E., Nicolson, R., Kelley, E., Georgiades, S., Crosbie, J., Schachar, R., Ayub, M., & Stevenson, R. A. (2024). Transdiagnostic patterns of sensory processing in autism and ADHD. *Journal of autism and developmental disorders, 54*(1), 280–292.

Schopler, E., Van Bourgondien, M. E., Wellman, G. J., & Love, S.R. (2010). *Childhood autism rating scale* (2nd ed.). Western Psychological Services.

Scott, F. J., Baron-Cohen, S., Bolton, P., & Brayne, C. (2002). The CAST (Childhood Asperger Syndrome Test): Preliminary development of a UK screen for mainstream primary-school-age children. *Autism, 6*(1), 9–31. https://doi.org/10.1177/1362361302006001003

Sedgewick, F., Hill, V., & Pellicano, E. (2019). "It's different for girls": Gender differences in the friendships and conflict of autistic and neurotypical adolescents. *Autism: The International Journal of Research and Practice, 23*(5), 1119–1132. https://doi.org/10.1177/1362361318794930

Simonoff, E., Pickles, A., Charman, T., Chandler, S., Loucas, T., & Baird, G. (2008). Psychiatric disorders in children with autism spectrum disorders: Prevalence, comorbidity, and associated factors in a population-derived sample. *Journal of the American Academy of Child and Adolescent Psychiatry, 47*(8), 921–929. https://doi.org/10.1097/CHI.0b013e318179964f

Shunk, A. W., Davis, A. S., & Dean, R. S. (2006). Test review: Delis Kaplan Executive Function System (D-KEFS). *Applied Neuropsychology, 13*(4), 275–327. https://doi.org/10.1207/s15324826an1304_9

Smith, I. C., Reichow, B., & Volkmar, F. R. (2015). The effects of DSM-5 criteria on number of individuals diagnosed with autism spectrum disorder: A systematic review. *Journal of Autism and Developmental Disorders, 45*(8), 2541–2552. https://doi.org/10.1007/s10803-015-2423-8

Sparrow, S. S., Cicchetti, D. V., & Saulnier, C. A. (2016). *Vineland Adaptive Behavior Scales* (3rd ed.). Pearson.

Stavropoulos, K.K.-M., Bolourian, Y., & Blacher, J. (2022). A scoping review of telehealth diagnosis of autism spectrum disorder. *PLoS One, 17*(2), Article e0263062. https://doi.org/10.1371/journal.pone.0263062

Steiner, A. M., & Gengoux, G. W. (2018). Strength-Based Approaches to Working with Families of Children with ASD. In M. Siller & L. Morgan (Eds.), *Handbook of Parent-Implemented Interventions for Very Young Children with Autism* (pp. 155–168). Springer International Publishing. https://doi.org/10.1007/978-3-319-90994-3_10

Stevanovic, D., Robins, D. L., Costanzo, F., Fucà, E., Valeri, G., Vicari, S., Erkuran, H. O., Yaylaci, F., Albores-Gallo, L., Gatica-Bahamonde, G., Gabunia, M., Zirakashvili, M., Charman, T., Samadi, S. A., Toh, T.-H., Gayle, W., Brennan, L., Zorcec, T., Auza, A., de Jonge, M. V., Shoqirat, N., Robins, D. L., Knez, R. (2022). Cross-cultural similarities and differences in reporting autistic symptoms in toddlers: A study synthesizing M-CHAT(-R) data from ten countries. *Research in Autism Spectrum Disorders, 95*, 101984. https://doi.org/10.1016/j.rasd.2022.101984

Stevens, M. A., Selders, K. J., Jeckel, O., Brownfield, V., & Nowell, K. P. (2023). An evaluation of parent and teacher discrepancies on an adaptive behavior measure for youth with autism spectrum disorder, intellectual disability, and global developmental delay. *Journal of Autism and Developmental Disorders, 53*(7), 2818–2834.

Stoll, M. M., Bergamo, N., & Rossetti, K. G. (2021). Analyzing modes of assessment for children with autism spectrum disorder (ASD) using a culturally sensitive lens. *Advances in Neurodevelopmental Disorders, 5*(3), 233–244. https://doi.org/10.1007/s41252-021-00210-0

Stone, W. L., Coonrod, E. E., & Ousley, O. Y. (2000). Brief report: Screening tool for autism in two-year-olds (STAT): Development and preliminary data. *Journal of Autism and Developmental Disorders, 30*(6), 607–612. https://doi.org/10.1023/a:1005647629002

Strang, J. F., Meagher, H., Kenworthy, L., de Vries, A. L. C., Menvielle, E., Leibowitz, S., Janssen, A., Cohen-Kettenis, P., Shumer, D. E., Edwards-Leeper, L., Pleak, R. R., Spack, N., Karasic, D. H., Schreier, H., Balleur, A., Tishelman, A., Ehrensaft, D., Rodnan, L., Kuschner, E. S., Mandel, F., Caretto, A., Lewis, H. C., Anthony, L. G. (2018). Initial clinical guidelines for co-occurring autism spectrum disorder and gender dysphoria or incongruence in adolescence. *Journal of Clinical Child and Adolescent Psychology, 47*(1), 105–115.https://doi.org/10.1080/15374416.2016.1228462

Strang, J. F., van der Miesen, A. I., Caplan, R., Hughes, C., daVanport, S., & Lai, M.-C. (2020). Both sex- and gender-related factors should be considered in autism research and clinical practice. *Autism, 24*(3), 539–543. https://doi.org/10.1177/1362361320913192

Tamm, L., Day, H. A., & Duncan, A. (2022). Comparison of adaptive functioning measures in adolescents with autism spectrum disorder without intellectual disability. *Journal of Autism and Developmental Disorders, 52*(3), 1247–1256.

Taylor, E. C., Livingston, L. A., Clutterbuck, R. A., Callan, M. J., & Shah, P. (2023). Psychological strengths and well-being: Strengths use predicts quality of life, well-being and mental health in autism. *Autism, 27*(6), 1826–1839.

Thurm, A., Farmer, C., Salzman, E., Lord, C., & Bishop, S. (2019). State of the field: Differentiating intellectual disability from autism spectrum disorder. *Frontiers in Psychiatry, 10*. https://doi.org/10.3389/fpsyt.2019.00526

Urbanowicz, A., Nicolaidis, C., Houting, J. D., Shore, S. M., Gaudion, K., Girdler, S., & Savarese, R. J. (2019). An expert discussion on strengths-based approaches in autism. *Autism in Adulthood, 1*(2), 82–89.

Van Wijngaarden-Carlisle, J. M., & Ciesla, J. A. (2021). Sex differences in autism: Diagnostic, neurobiological, and behavioral features. *Frontiers in Psychiatry, 12*, 539835. https://doi.org/10.3389/fpsyt.2021.539835

Vasa, R. A., Keefer, A., McDonald, R. G., Hunsche, M. C., & Kerns, C. M. (2020). A scoping review of anxiety in young children with autism spectrum disorder. *Autism Research, 13*(12), 2038–2057. https://doi.org/10.1002/aur.2395

Vogindroukas, I., Stankova, M., Chelas, E. N., & Proedrou, A. (2022). Language and speech characteristics in autism. *Neuropsychiatric Disease and Treatment*, 2367–2377.

Volkmar, F. R., Reichow, B., & McPartland, J. C. (Eds.). (2014). *Adolescents and adults with autism spectrum disorders*. Springer Science + Business Media. https://doi.org/10.1007/978-1-4939-0506-5

Wagner, L., Vehorn, A., Weitlauf, A. S., Lavanderos, A. M., Wade, J., Corona, L., & Warren, Z. (2023). Development of a novel telemedicine tool to reduce disparities related to the identification of preschool children with autism. *Journal of Autism and Developmental Disorders, 10*. Advance online publication. https://doi.org/10.1007/s10803-023-06176-3

Williams, J., Scott, F., Stott, C., Allison, C., Bolton, P., Baron-Cohen, S., & Brayne, C. (2005). The CAST (Childhood Asperger Syndrome Test): Test accuracy. *Autism, 9*(1), 45–68. https://doi.org/10.1177/1362361305049029

Wolff, N., Stroth, S., Kamp-Becker, I., Roepke, S., & Roessner, V. (2022). Autism spectrum disorder and IQ–A complex interplay. *Frontiers in Psychiatry, 13*, Article 856084.

Young, R. L. (2007). *Autism detection in early childhood: ADEC*. Australian Council of Educational Research.

Yu, Y., Ozonoff, S., & Miller, M. (2024). Assessment of autism spectrum disorder. *Assessment, 31*(1), 24–41. https://doi.org/10.1177/10731911231173089

Zander, E., Willfors, C., Berggren, S., Coco, C., Holm, A., Jifält, I., Kosieradzki, R., Linder, J., Nordin, V., Olafsdottir, K., & Bölte, S. (2017). The interrater reliability of the autism diagnostic interview-revised (ADI-R) in clinical settings. *Psychopathology, 50*(3), 219–227. https://doi.org/10.1159/000474949

Zeidan, J., Fombonne, E., Scorah, J., Ibrahim, A., Durkin, M. S., Saxena, S., Yusuf, A., Shih, A., & Elsabbagh, M. (2022). Global prevalence of autism: A systematic review update. *Autism Research, 15*(5), 778–790. https://doi.org/10.1002/aur.2696

Reference to the book

Emick, J., Agarwal, S. S., & McConnell, A. J (2025). Autism assessment across the lifespan: Integrating research and clinical practice. In J. Matson (Ed.), *Handbook of assessment and diagnosis of autism spectrum disorder* (2nd ed.). Springer International Publishing.

Monitoring Progress in Autism

Valsamma Eapen, Katrina Williams, Nicole Rinehart, Emily Wall, Charmaine Bernie, David Moseley, and Jane McGillivray

Keywords Monitoring progress · Autism scale · Diagnostic progress · Autism · Assessment · Behaviour

Overview

Most professionals agree that autism is a lifelong condition, but abilities, associated problems, functioning, and management needs can change over time. Thus, while identification and accurate diagnosis constitute a first step, ongoing monitoring is essential to help individuals with autism to reach their potential and manage developmental challenges and transitional periods that arise throughout their lives. This chapter will highlight the key issues in the process of monitoring, including current opportunities and potential pitfalls.

V. Eapen (✉)
Discipline of Psychiatry and Mental Health, School of Clinical Medicine, University of New South Wales, Sydney, NSW, Australia
e-mail: v.eapen@unsw.edu.au

Academic Unit of Child Psychiatry, South West Sydney (AUCS), South-Western Sydney Local Health District & Ingham Institute, L1, Liverpool Hospital, Liverpool, Sydney, NSW, Australia

K. Williams
Department of Paediatrics, Monash University, Clayton, VIC, Australia
e-mail: Katrina.Williams@rch.org.au

Developmental Paediatrics, Monash Children's Hospital, Clayton, VIC, Australia

Murdoch Childrens Research Institute, Parkville, VIC, Australia

J. L. Matson (ed.), *Assessment and Diagnosis in Autism*, Autism and Child Psychopathology Series, https://doi.org/10.1007/978-3-032-11802-8_2

Context

Heterogeneity and Complexity

Each individual diagnosed with autism varies in their unique strengths and difficulties across behavioural, social and cognitive dimensions, and each individual's behaviours or interests may vary. Also unique to each individual are their circumstances and values. These key factors come together to influence their unique needs and goals. Autism can also co-occur with physical and mental health conditions such as epilepsy, intellectual disability, as well as ADHD, and anxiety (Al-Beltagi, 2021; Rosen et al., 2018; Simonoff et al., 2008). If there is a co-occurring condition, that may need to be prioritized as the focus of interventions or strategies to improve well-being, function, participation, and quality of (Maskey et al., 2013), will require modifications to monitoring over time, in keeping with their priorities for management, support, and intervention. Adding the unique strengths, difficulties, circumstances, and values that each individual and their family bring, it becomes clear that the goals of each person—and therefore what should be monitored—will vary as much as they align. Due to this variation, measuring changes and monitoring progress is complex, but also crucial to improving the lives of each individual with autism and their families.

N. Rinehart · D. Moseley
School of Psychological Sciences, Faculty of Medicine, Nursing, and Health Sciences, Monash University, Clayton, VIC, Australia
e-mail: nicole.rinehart@monash.edu

D. Moseley
e-mail: david.moseley@monash.edu

E. Wall
Academic Unit of Infant Child and Adolescent Psychiatry (AUCS), University of New South Wales, Sydney, NSW, Australia
e-mail: emily.wall@unsw.edu.au

C. Bernie
Early Years Research Lab, Southern Cross University, Lismore, NSW, Australia
e-mail: Charmaine.Bernie@scu.edu.au

Department of Paediatrics, Monash University, Melbourne, VIC, Australia

J. McGillivray
School of Psychology, Faculty of Health, Deakin University, Burwood, NSW, Australia
e-mail: jane.mcgillivray@deakin.edu.au

International Classification of Functioning, Disability, and Health

The development of The International Classification of Impairments, Disabilities, and Handicaps (World Health Organization, 1980), now The International Classification of Functioning, Disability, and Health (World Health Organization, 2001), provides a useful structure for assessing or monitoring individuals with autism and other disabilities, with a focus on function and participation, in addition to impairments, and within a framework of children's rights. This approach has several advantages including that disability is understood as one of impairment to activity and participation which also interacts with the health condition, the environment, and personal factors and having a distinct impact on human experiences at the levels of body, person, and society. In addition, by differentiating these terms conceptually and semantically, it is emphasized that disability is not unidimensional but rather manifests at different levels of human functioning in the form of impairments, performance limitations that impact activity and participation, and the experience of disadvantage (environmental and personal factors). It also provides a taxonomy with numeric codes that can be used to document the elements unique to each of the three levels, with applicability for clinical and administrative purposes (Bölte, 2023; Simeonsson et al., 2003).

The ICF allows the classification of functioning as universal human experiences involving "body function and body structures" which can be conceptualized as well-being, "personal activities and performance" such as mobility and self-care that can be conceptualized as function, and "participation in community" such as school, work, and civic life. Since the barriers and facilitators within the environment at each of these three levels can also be recognized through the "environmental factors qualifiers" option, this classification offers a distinct advantage in terms of assessing eligibility and prioritization of interventions as well as in monitoring progress. However, one limitation is the application to, and coverage of child characteristics and hence additional considerations are required during the early developmental years. For example for children with limited cognitive and language abilities there is a reliance on parental and caregiver giver reports (Hus & Segal, 2021; Rivard et al., 2021). It would be important to include wherever possible, reports of children through interview, play or other direct observations. Further, it is important to recognize that the disability may arise from the lack of supports and adaptations that the society provides for the individual and in this regard social change may help reduce the disability.

Initial Identification

Monitoring for early signs and symptoms of autism can assist timely identification and opportunities for early intervention. Studies based on the siblings of children with an affected older sibling have indicated delay or differences in early attentional control, emotion regulation, social orienting/approach, and communication development (Brian et al., 2015). Another study has found developmental differences as early as 2 months including lack of eye contact, lack of smiling, reciprocal cooing, and babbling (Sallows & Graupner, 2005; Zwaigenbaum et al., 2013). Although some autistic symptoms may be evident from as early as the first year of life, ongoing surveillance is needed to assess their developmental course and ensure accurate diagnosis. Some of the main domains of autism that are relevant to monitoring for early identification are described below. However, it is worth noting that while it is important to monitor for early symptoms if there are concerns about emerging autism, no clinical or behavioural features or assessment would provide 100% sensitivity or specificity.

Evaluating Interventions

Although it is outside the scope of this chapter to discuss the various behavioural and developmental interventions available, some background is necessary for an understanding of how the success of such interventions and management strategies may be measured. Further, systematic reviews have identified that some of the outcomes that and individuals and families value are not necessarily monitored or measured. For example, in preschool children the highest ranked outcomes by parents were those that impacted their daily life and functioning including anxiety, distress, hypersensitivity, sleep problems, happiness, relationships with siblings, and parent stress (McConachie et al., 2018). This calls for the need to have a consensus between parents/caregivers, professionals, and researchers to agree on a core set of evaluation outcomes for use in research.

Typically, in efficacy studies, each individual's developmental skills, abilities, and behaviours that challenge or are unwanted will be assessed at the start and the end of intervention. The selected monitoring tools, also called outcome measures in this context, will also reflect the form of intervention chosen. For example, if a child is undergoing a Comprehensive Treatment Model (CTM) which is designed to elicit a broad developmental response, progress may be monitored across autism severity and developmental milestones using treatment specific tools as well as other assessment tools for autism specific symptoms. The domains that assist early identification may also be appropriate targets for early intervention, supports, and management based on identified needs and goals, with a tailored approach based on personalized care plan that allows progress towards achieving goals over time to be monitored (Whitehouse et al., 2018, 2019).

When establishing intervention goals in practice domains as described above, along with overall development, it is important to include other aspects of functioning, participation, and quality of life, for the individual with autism and their family.

Validity, Utility, and Appropriateness of Tools

There are significant challenges in monitoring the impact of management, supports, and interventions in the context of autism (Eldevik et al., 2009; Howlin et al., 2009; Levin et al., 2021). Recent reviews of assessment tools have identified problems with validity and utility, including their appropriateness for measuring change over time and the need for measures of health-related quality of life to allow evaluation of economic impacts of management and supports (Levin et al., 2021; McConachie & Fletcher-Watson, 2014; Payakachat et al., 2012). As a result, evaluators have resorted to using measures that are primarily diagnostic instruments but typically these are not sensitive to change. Further, most longitudinal studies have focused on overall developmental trajectories using standardized developmental instruments. These measures have substantial limitations as they are primarily developed in general population cohorts and therefore only report variation in relation to population norms. A major additional concern is that these measures only monitor abilities and behaviours against developmental norms, while individuals with neurodivergence or disability, including autism, and their families value different outcomes (Allard et al., 2014). Although there are some exceptions, most of these instruments do not allow measurements spanning the age range from preschool to adolescence and adulthood.

Individualized Planning (IP)

Good practice dictates that intervention, support, and management should be person and family centred with shared decision making, also known as individualized care plannings (Fuentes et al., 2021; Hume et al., 2021; Trembath et al., 2022). For autism the care plan must be tailored to the individual's needs and goals, have research evidence supporting their effectiveness, and that goals must be measurable, continuously monitored, and frequently revised (National Institute for Health and Care Excellence, 2013; Prior et al., 2011; Trembath et al., 2022). As young children with autism mature into adolescents and young adults, delivery of best-practice becomes more challenging as the context and circumstances of individuals diverge (Hume et al., 2021; National Institute for Health and Care Excellence, 2012). Individual care plans should incorporate as much input from the individual with autism as possible and include all of those involved with their care, including their family, physicians, therapists, and educators in a collaborative process. Although the specifics of the IP processes must necessarily change as each individual develops across educational, employment and other settings, the main guiding principles of an effective individual plan remain the same. These principles are seen as best-practice and they also align with recommendations from different developed nations such as the United States (Individuals with Disabilities Education Improvement Act 2004), the United Kingdom (Children and Families Act 2014), and Australia (Trembath et al., 2022). Accordingly, the individual plan should be re-evaluated at least every six months and

Table 1 Key items for consideration in an individualized plan (IP) for children with autism

Overarching long-term goal(s) for the person with autism incorporating planning for life transitions (e.g., starting school or finishing education and starting work)
A thorough assessment of current strengths and difficulties in key developmental and academic/employment/adaptive skills areas
Measurable goals for health outcomes for each specified period three monthly during the initial period following diagnosis, six monthly for younger children, and later at 12 monthly interval or if changes warrant earlier review)
A strategy for measuring overall progress across different domains including health, education, societal participation, and quality of life and an outline of when periodic progress reports will be provided
Assessment of resources and consideration of which services and educational strategies are to be provided by whom, in order to reach, monitor, and assess the goals
A process for the collaborative review and revision of the IP is critical using case conferences or other inter-disciplinary reviews

there should be accurate and objective measurement of progress in accordance with the set goals that address individual strengths and needs as detailed in Table 1.

Empowering individuals with autism to express their thoughts, feelings, and experiences provides crucial insights into their unique needs and goals. This self-advocacy allows for a more personalized approach to intervention, support, and management, ensuring that the needs and goals align with their preferences and aspirations. By prioritizing the autistic person's voice, greater autonomy is fostered and also a more inclusive environment where progress is measured not just by external standards, but by the individual's own sense of growth and fulfillment (Mullally et al., 2024).

Goal Setting as a Core Element of Monitoring Progress and Transitions

Intervention, support, and management vary over time, as do needs and goals and the tools used to measure whether these goals have been achieved. A number of tools and processes are available to help individuals and families establish goals, as well as measure their attainment following selected time intervals. Some tools, such as the Canadian Occupational Performance Measure (Law, 2022) and Goal Attainment Scaling (Ottenbacher & Cusick, 1990) are widely adopted in intervention and rehabilitation settings. Others, such as the Family and Adolescent/Adult Goal Setting Tool (Ashburner et al., 2023) are specific to the autism population. Goal selection and monitoring is a key component of rehabilitation and disability support services worldwide (Pritchard-Wiart et al., 2019; Souza et al., 2021), allowing for defined service-related targets, reflection opportunities, and measurement of progress with one or more intervention.

Key Ages and Stages

Four main stages in life can be identified during which there are changes to a person's environment, their abilities, and the priorities of individuals and families that are likely to lead to different needs and goals over time. The first is the preschool years, the second the primary years, the third the secondary school years, and the fourth the adult years.

As the individual goes through the different stages in the lifecycle, the needs and goals will also vary with different priorities, such as learning and educational goals early in life may shift to participation in employment, or civic life-related goals in adulthood. Some guidelines advise focusing on improvements in the core autism characteristics, especially social interaction and reciprocal communication, by including techniques to expand the child or young person's communication, interactive play and social routines, and working with parents', carers', teachers', or peers' to facilitate greater understanding of, and responsiveness to, the child or young person's patterns of communication and interaction (National Institute for Health and Care Excellence, 2013; Trembath et al., 2022). For the preschool age group some recommended techniques include the integration of play-based strategies with parents, carers, and teachers with therapist modelling and video-interaction feedback to increase joint attention and engagement (Vyshedskiy & Khokhlovich, 2022). Additionally, clinicians, educators, and carers may employ techniques such as pivotal response training (Ona et al., 2020), prompting, reinforcement, and discrete trial teaching (Odom et al., 2003) over a short period of time to enact a change in a specific behaviour or to develop a targeted skill.

Time points for assessments would also deserve special attention in the monitoring process. Times of transitions are identified as times of additional stress for individuals and their families. Issues relating to life skills, personal, social, and sexual relationships, driving and independent living as well as mental health also deserve due consideration. Further, any other major life event in the life of individuals with autism will create additional needs for themselves and their families, over and above those experienced by the general population. Since it will be difficult to initiate contact with services and agencies for the first time during such times of crisis, specific attention to how families and individuals could easily connect with appropriate agencies at these times needs to be built into the monitoring framework.

Further, monitoring information should always cause professionals to pause and reflect on what could be creating the patterns that are being observed, and how that information would assist in decision making based on needs and goals guiding intervention, support, and management in the ongoing care plan. Things that might need modification could include the nature, frequency, or setting of interventions, the professionals involved, the way the treatment plan is being coordinated and provided, or the environment, community supports, or other aspects of care. Ongoing monitoring and assessing progress are central to intervention, education, and social programmes in autism, and fundamental to all programs that include goals.

A Fit-for-Purpose Model for Monitoring

An approach that can add value to what we know about appropriate monitoring for different ages and stages of children with autism is consideration of the purpose of monitoring. In this approach, monitoring can be to identify autism, to assess autism interventions, to identify strengths, and difficulties early, or to ensure that ongoing management is maximizing opportunities for an individual with autism and their family. Monitoring also provides the opportunity to acknowledge advances in an individual's abilities and celebrate this progress. Embedding the ICF with this approach ensures monitoring that includes information about wellbeing, function, and participation, as well as changes in impairments, personal factors and environmental factors, as relevant. Considering biopsychosocial or social models of disability ensures that the environment is not ignored in relation to its impact on the individual's participation and wellbeing, and consideration of quality of life allows an understanding of how important factors that could be changed are influencing wellbeing of each individual. Here, we will use the framework of the ICF to describe tools, opportunities and processes for monitoring that can support individuals with autism and their care providers across the lifespan. Table 2 includes some tools relevant to each ICF domain as example, but is not intended to be a comprehensive list.

Health Condition

The ICF as a framework describes all other constructs or factors as influencing one's health condition. In relation to autism, there are a number of tools and processes that allow for monitoring of an individual's presentation of overall autism characteristics.

Autism Diagnostic Tools

Autism Diagnostic Observation Schedule (ADOS)

The *Autism Diagnostic Observation Schedule (*ADOS; Lord et al., 2000) is a standardized tool for the direct observation and measurement of autistic symptomatology. The ADOS consists of a series of investigator-led processes designed to elicit naturalistic social and communicative behaviours from the child. The investigator thus builds a profile of the child's social communication, social relatedness, play and imagination, and restricted and/or repetitive behaviours. Despite its reputation as the "gold standard" measure of autistic severity (Janvier et al., 2022), the ADOS was designed as a diagnostic tool to measure relatively stable traits in autism which are not anticipated to vary greatly over a lifetime. Longitudinal studies have demonstrated the stability of these standardized scores throughout childhood (Chawarska et al., 2007; Gotham et al., 2009; Hedvall et al., 2014). Indeed, even when children

Table 2 Commonly used assessment tools for monitoring progress throughout life

ICF domain	Subcategory	Measures	Supporting features	Potential challenges
Health condition	Global autism measures	Autism Diagnostic Observation Schedule (ADOS)	• Direct observation of a person's responses to a series of investigator-led procedures designed to elicit naturalistic social and communicative behaviours • Widespread utility • Diagnostic tool	• In person assessment • Takes 1–2 h to administer and score • Bias reported in some populations • Mental age of 12 months or more required • Not designed to measure change over time
		CARS	Can be completed by multiple informants	Responsiveness and test–retest reliability not reported at high levels to date
		AIM	Designed to evaluates outcomes, brief scoring system	Potentially prone to recall bias
		ATEC	Evaluates outcomes, scored online, multiple informants	Large number of items to complete
	Quality of life	PEDSQL	Widespread use, use across childhood	No specific module for autism
		QoLA	Measures overall QoL and those specific to autistic features; parent and self-report version available	Can be lengthy to complete
Participation	Participation in childhood through to early adulthood	YC-PEM PEM-CY Y-PEM	Strong psychometric properties, various tools across lifespan	Some measures still new and not yet adopted widely
		CAPE	Widely used participation measure	Social communication challenges may impact on interpretation of results

(continued)

Table 2 (continued)

ICF domain	Subcategory	Measures	Supporting features	Potential challenges
		CASP	Wide age range, used across clinical populations	Some psychometric properties not well established as yet
	School participation	TRSSA	Measures school adjustment and participation. Short Form TRSSA demonstrates acceptable internal consistency and stability as repeated measure	Full version lengthy to complete; some psychometric properties yet to be investigated
Activity	Adaptive behaviour	VABS-3	Widespread use across the lifespan, strong psychometric properties, multiple informants	Length of time to complete and expertise required to score
		ABAS 3	Easy administration, Widespread use across the lifespan, strong psychometric properties, multiple informants	Less detailed than other adaptive functioning measures
		BASC	Good coverage of range of clinical and adaptive domains. Commonly used in practice	Long questionnaire for parents & teachers to complete (134–160 items)
		CGAS	Good general clinician rated measure. Able to support tracking of changes in functioning over time. Helpful as additional measure alongside other measures	Broad measure that cannot give specific information about the type or context of changes observed
	Educational activities	PEP 3	Informs educational programming, multiple informants	Length of time to complete
	Self-care activities	CSHQ	Comprehensive and valid parent report measure around sleep; CSHQ Autism version available	Autism version relatively new, with recently-published cut-off scores; not yet widely adopted
		Sleep diary	Flexible tool to record sleep patterns	Non-standardized tool to be populated over time

(continued)

Table 2 (continued)

ICF domain	Subcategory	Measures	Supporting features	Potential challenges
		Self-care inventory	Emerging high quality tool for self-care assessment in adults	New tool, not widely adopted as yet
		Aut-eat questionnaire (AEQ)	Parent report of eating patterns	Limited age range (3–8 years)
	Leisure/play	Test of playfulness (TOP)	Established play assessment	Limited uptake in clinical applications
		Child initiated pretend play assessment 2	Comprehensive play assessment used to assess play in children with autism and other clinical presentations. Recent update; improved psychometric properties	Revised version uptake and utility studies limited due to recency of version
		Leisure satisfaction scale	Established scale for assessment of leisure satisfaction	Subjective measure
Body functions and structures	Communication	CCC	Quick to administer Different versions of tool according to age	Originally a screening tool so limited depth of communication skill assessment available
		CELF-P and CELF 5	Robust, well-adopted clinical assessment tool with comprehensive receptive and expressive language subtests	In-clinic assessment, with specific expertise required for evaluation
		CSBS-DP	Combination assessment of parent report and clinical assessment, includes social and direct communication evaluation	Length of time to complete
		MacArthur-Bates CDI	Parent-report based clinical assessment, continuing to be revised and adapted	Narrow age range for children in early stages of language development

(continued)

Table 2 (continued)

ICF domain	Subcategory	Measures	Supporting features	Potential challenges
		Reynell	Direct assessment of child based on language sample	Lacking comprehensive psychometric data, specific expertise required for evaluation
		PLS	Well-adopted clinical assessment tool with comprehensive receptive and expressive language subtests for preschool children	Some questions raised regarding psychometric properties, specific expertise required for evaluation
		PPV	Speed of administration, not reliant on expressive skills for assessment	Training in administration required
		PPECSC	Interviews with primary caregiver that can be scored across a number of age ranges from childhood through to adulthood	Pragmatics focus only
	Social communication	SCQ	Based on ADI-R questions. Easy for parents to complete, 40 questions	Not a diagnostic instrument, needs to be considered alongside clinician assessment
		SRS	Can be used to track severity of ASD symptoms	Does not include clinician report
		ESCS	Good clinician-rated measure with use of direct and video observation	Clinician expertise required for evaluation
	Motor skills	PDMSII	Comprehensive motor skill assessment for below school-age children	Lengthy to administer, in clinic assessment
		BOTMP MABC	Wide age range, clinically assesses gross and fine motor skills	Lengthy to administer, clinical assessment requires specific expertise for evaluation

(continued)

Table 2 (continued)

ICF domain	Subcategory	Measures	Supporting features	Potential challenges
	Sensory processing	Sensory profile	Established tool across different age groups, multiple informants	Lengthy to administer, some psychometric properties under question
		Sensory processing measure	Speed of administration, multiple informants and age groups	Responsiveness and use in populations outside of the United States of America requires further evaluation
Environmental factors	Parental support	PSOC-R	Strong psychometric properties. Measures clinically interesting domains of parent's view of parenting. Recently updated	Self-reported and parents may under or over-report and also impacted by other factors
		PSI	Used widely. Short form has 36 items	Many be impacted by other general issues and may not be specific to the child's issues
		PEARR	Covers useful domains for practice. Designed for supporting families experiencing vulnerability	May trigger trauma symptoms
	Family quality of life	FQOL	Good measure of family supports. Useful for treatment planning. Has five subscales: family interaction, parenting, emotional well-being, physical/material well-being, and disability-related support	Subjective and variable
	Quality of environment	APERS	Tool that explores educational programming	New tool, psychometric properties under investigation, not widely adopted
		Autism ASPECTSS design index	Tool that explores environmental design	New tool, psychometric properties under investigation, not widely adopted

(continued)

Table 2 (continued)

ICF domain	Subcategory	Measures	Supporting features	Potential challenges
Personal factors	Behaviour	DBC	Designed for people with developmental and intellectual disability. Covers broad range of domains	Takes long time to complete with 96 items
		ABC	Can measure change over time	Established in 1985
		RBS-R	Parent rated. Good sensitivity to change	44 items for one domain of repetitive behaviours
		CBCL	Broad measure of emotional and behavioural symptoms for typically developing children	Length of time to complete 113 items
		ASR/ABCL	Self-report and carer versions, for adults	Length of time to complete
	Mood and emotional regulation	DASS	Widely used. 42 item and 21 items versions	Developed initially for adults
		SDQ	Good screening measure. Very widely used in clinical practice and research. Good for tracking change over time	Not able to provide comprehensive data
		ASC-ASD	Specifically designed for children aged 8–16 with autism	Challenges with inter-rater reliability between self and parent reported versions
	Overall developmental/ intellectual abilities	Bayley scales	Good measure across broad range of developmental domains	Complex administration and requiring specialized training
		MSEL	Covers relevant developmental domains	Normative sample from 1995
		Griffiths	Comprehensive developmental measure birth-6 years	Length of time and expertise to complete
		Ages and stages	Widely used a screening measure for general development and social-emotional development	Not a robust or detailed assessment
		WPPSI	Gold standard measure of intelligence for ages 2–7 years	Length of time and expertise to complete

(continued)

Table 2 (continued)

ICF domain	Subcategory	Measures	Supporting features	Potential challenges
		WISC	Gold standard measure of intelligence for ages 6–16 years	Length of time and expertise to complete
		SB5	Widely used measure of intelligence	Norms are not available for all populations

demonstrate vast gains in other domains such as expressive and receptive language and adaptive behaviours as a result of an autism-specific intervention, their ADOS scores did not significantly improve (Dawson et al., 2010; Vivanti et al., 2014). While improvements in such measures would undoubtedly indicate robust changes to behaviour, a lack of improvement may indicate insensitivity to subtle improvements and treatment effects, especially when the aim of an intervention does not broadly target autism, but rather a specific behaviour or outcome. Hence, while the ADOS may help assess the progress of a CTM with limited sensitivity, it is unlikely to accurately reflect progress relating to specific tasks or behaviours. However, it can be useful if such progress results in the child no longer reaching a diagnostic status on the repeat ADOS assessment. It is worth noting that some diagnostic items in the ADOS-2 demonstrate bias for African-American children and female children compared to white children and male children. This bias may lead to an under detection of autism in these populations (Kalb et al., 2022). Calibrated severity scores have demonstrated strong test–retest reliability on review (Janvier et al., 2022).

Childhood Autism Rating Scale (CARS)

The Childhood Autism Rating Scale (Schopler et al., 1986) and the revised version, CARS2 (Schopler et al., 2010) can be completed by a parent, teacher, or a clinician, based on subjective observations of the child's behaviours. Based on the findings of a bimodal distribution among these scores, the scale includes criteria to differentiate between those with mild to moderate autism and those with severe autism (Schopler et al., 1980). Responsiveness and sensitivity to change is not widely established, and test–retest reliability has been questioned (Breidbord & Croudace, 2013).

Autism Monitoring Tools

Autism Treatment Evaluation Checklist (ATEC)

The Autism Treatment Evaluation Checklist (ATEC) (Rimland & Edelson, 1999) is a tool that can be used by clinicians and parents to evaluate treatment outcomes and to monitor progress in autism. The ATEC can be accessed and scored online by parents, teachers, and/or other primary carers. The scale covers 77 items in the areas of communication, sociability, sensory, and cognitive awareness and health and physical behaviour, and also provides a total score.

Autism Impact Measure (AIM)

The Autism Impact Measure (AIM; Kanne et al., 2014) is a 25-item questionnaire that has been specifically designed to have greater sensitivity detecting changes in core autism symptoms (Mazurek et al., 2020). It asks respondents to recall a 2-week period with items rated on two corresponding 5-point scales of frequency and impact of core autism symptoms. Using exploratory factor analysis, four factors were found namely (1) repetitive behaviours, (2) odd/atypical behaviours, (3) communication/

language, and (4) social/emotional reciprocity, and these were observed to concur with the reports of symptom severity/impact.

Participation

Across the lifespan, participation has received increasing attention in relation to measuring and monitoring. Participation is stated to be more than just attendance, but rather, attendance and engagement (Adair et al., 2018). Frequency and quality of attendance and engagement require consideration in relation to assessment and monitoring. With regard to participation in community activities, available evidence from the literature suggests that children with autism participate in activities less frequently and with less variety compared to children with other developmental disabilities as well as those without developmental challenges (LaVesser & Berg, 2011). Participation contexts also change across the lifespan, alongside standardized and non-standardized measures of attendance and engagement that are appropriate for a particular age and stage (Lami et al., 2018).

Early Childhood

Participation in self-care routines, learning, play and social activities, as well as engagement across contexts including home, early education settings, and community contexts such as playgrounds, are all notable considerations when monitoring young children with autism. In addition to the individual, the caregiver and family's confidence with, and ability to attend and engage in activities such as home routines, work, and community outings and is also of paramount importance in relation to the child's wellbeing. Goal setting measures outlined above can help to capture participation areas that are important for the child and family, and can be monitored over time. In addition, there are standardized measures that consider a young child's participation across settings.

Young Children's Participation and Environment Measure

The Young Children's Participation and Environment Measure (YC-PEM) has been modelled of the pre-existing school-age measure described below (Khetani, 2015). It assesses participation across home, early education and community settings. It has demonstrated test–retest reliability and is an appropriate measure for young children with developmental delays or disabilities.

School Years

For all children the crudest measure of participation in school is attendance. Attendance includes participation in the academic curriculum, that can be achieved at a school campus or in the home environment. Unfortunately, today many children with autism do not participate in the school curriculum either because they have been excluded from it or because they refuse to go to school. The former indicates problems with ability to manage the types of problems that can occur in children and young people with autism and the latter a failure in addressing issues or concerns to minimise the risk of refusal.

Participation in the social curriculum (sometimes called the "hidden curriculum") is also important. Attendance at a school campus is not sufficient to ensure participation in the social curriculum, nor is it a measure for individuals who participate in home-schooling. For children who are attending school monitoring of participation should include information from the classroom and outside the classroom. Monitoring should be linked to specific program goals designed to enable the student to participate in non-academic aspects of school life. There are also a number of measures for this age group that can help quantify and monitor participation across home, school, and community contexts.

Participation and Environment Measure for Children and Youth

The Participation and Environment Measure for Children and Youth (PEMCY; (Coster et al., 2011), is a measure for children aged 5–17 years, exploring attendance and engagement across home, school and community settings. It has moderate to good test–retest reliability and continues to be used in clinical and research settings for children with autism in this age group (Lamash et al., 2020).

Children's Assessment of Participation and Enjoyment (CAPE)

The Children's Assessment of Participation and Enjoyment (CAPE) is a widely used assessment of participation across settings (King et al., 2000). It has been translated into several different languages and helps to evaluate participation across various dimensions and contexts. While some psychometric properties are well established, less is known about the measure's responsiveness and construct validity (Abid et al., 2023). Children with autism may find this difficult to undertake and assessors may find it difficult to interpret responses due to a child's limited social-communication abilities in some instances.

Child and Adolescent Scale of Participation

The Child and Adolescent Scale of Participation (CASP; Bedell, 2004) is a tool that has been designed, adapted and explored across a wide age range and numerous clinical populations, including autism (Yee et al., 2017). Despite widely reported use of the measure (Adair et al., 2018) psychometric properties require further investigation in the autism population.

Later Adolescence and Adulthood

Post-school participation is typically conceptualized along three dimensions: employment, independent living, and participation in post-secondary education. For a student with autism, the high school years and IP should be catered to maximizing these outcomes and their educational focus shift from aiming to fill in missing gaps in the student's developmental profile to optimize their post-school lifestyle and opportunities preparation for independence. In the United States, for example, students with disabilities are generally required to develop a transition plan as the driving force of their IP at age 14. Hence, while progress in autism may still be measured broadly in regard to cognition and adaptive functioning at this stage in life, there will also be a greater emphasis on the attainment of specific practical skills. Overall, in terms of assessment and monitoring of progress, instead of continuing to assess what the student cannot do and working towards improvements in those areas, the IP must be based on student interests, preferences, strengths, work habits, and describe the supports and modifications necessary for their future success.

At this stage, evaluation of ability should comprise both formal assessment tools as well as more of the auxiliary methods previously described such as structured observations and grading and feedback of work samples. It should include assessment of interests and preferences, career awareness, cognitive development, academic achievement, adaptive behaviour, self-determination, interpersonal relationship and social skills, communication skills, emotional development and mental health, employment and community skills and community participation, and independent living skills. In this regard, age appropriate, specific, and measurable goals as detailed in Table 3 must be set relevant to school and post-school participation in education, employment, and independent living skills.

Youth and Young Adult Participation and Environment Measure

The Youth and Young Adult Participation and Environment Measure (Y-PEM) is a new measure developed for this key transition and early adulthood lifestage (Shahin et al., 2023). It is demonstrating strong psychometric properties though has yet to be taken up widely in research and clinical applications.

Other measures may also be applicable here, including the Participation in childhood Occupations Questionnaire (PICO–Q; Bar-Shalita et al., 2009) or in specific contexts such as the Child Routines Inventory (Sytsma et al., 2001); Children Helping Out: Responsibilities, Expectations, and Supports, (CHORES; Dunn, 2004). Yet, valid general measures of activity participation for specific use with the autism population are lacking. In a recent study, Little et al. (2014), investigated the use of Home and Community Activities Scale (HCAS; adapted from Dunst et al., 2000) in a large cohort of 713 children with autism and found that activity participation of school-age children fell into six dimensions namely Parent–Child Household Activities, Community Activities, Routine Errands, Neighborhood–Social Activities, Outdoor Activities, and Faith-Based Activities (Little et al., 2014).

Table 3 Examples of target goals, measurement of such goals and relevant interventions in Autism

Skill area	Targeted behaviour	Measurement	Intervention	Reference
Academics	Essay writing—total words written and function essay elements included	Number of words and elements	Video modelling and self-monitoring	Delano (2007a)
	Essay writing—total words written, number of unique verbs, adverbs and adjectives	Number of target elements	Instruction, modelling, practice, and feedback	Delano (2007b)
Adaptive skills	Setting the table and putting away groceries	Percentage of tasks performed correctly	Task analysis and video prompting	Cannella-Malone et al. (2006)
	Packing and unpacking bag, brushing teeth	Percentage of tasks performed correctly	Task analysis and video prompting	Rayner (2010)
	Washing dishes	Percentage of tasks performed correctly	Task analysis and video prompting	Sigafoos et al. (2007)
Challenging behaviour	Disruptions, physical and verbal aggression, and straightening (obsessive) behaviour	Behaviour per minute and percentage of items straightened	Functional communication training with extinction	Kuhn et al. (2009)
	Physical aggression and destructive behaviour	Frequency of aggressive behaviour	Mindfulness exercise	Singh et al. (2011)
Social skills	Conversational basics; providing positive feedback to a speaker and answering open-ended questions	Percentage of steps performed correctly	Group instruction, modelling, roleplay, and feedback	Dotson et al. (2010)
	Initiation to peers and responses to peers	Frequency of behaviour	Script and prompting	Krantz and McClannahan (1993)

(continued)

Table 3 (continued)

Skill area	Targeted behaviour	Measurement	Intervention	Reference
Vocational skills	Prepare folders with advertising material, prepare folders and information notebooks	Percentage of tasks completed successfully and independently	Simulation training: most-to-least prompting and task instruction	Lattimore et al. (2008)
	Cleaning of sinks and mirrors in a company bathroom, and washing up in the break room	Percentage of tasks completed successfully and independently	Simulation training: most-to-least prompting and task instruction	Lattimore et al. (2008)

Quality of Life

Quality of life is another important construct in relation to participation and well-being. Quality of life measures are used extensively in clinical practice and research, across cultures, ages, and contexts (Eapen et al., 2023).

Paediatric Quality of Life Inventory

The Paediatric Quality of Life Inventory (PedsQL; Varni et al., 1999) follows a modular approach to measuring health-related quality of life (HRQOL) in healthy children and adolescents and those with acute and chronic health conditions. The PedsQL Measurement Model integrates seamlessly both generic core scales and disease-specific modules into one measurement system and different developmentally appropriate (Ages 2–18; Child Self-Report Ages 5–7, 8–12, 13–18; Parent Proxy-Report Ages 2–4, 5–7, 8–12, 13–18) forms are available. While disease specific modules are available for some of the chronic health conditions, there is no specific module for autism.

The Quality of Life in Autism

The Quality of Life in Autism (QoLA) contains two subscales to be completed by the parent or carer: Part A, with questions pertaining to overall quality of life, and Part B, with questions asking parents to rate the impact of autism-specific symptoms of their child on parental daily activities. A preliminary study showed good psychometric properties with strong internal consistency and convergent validity (Eapen et al., 2014, 2023) and self-report version is also available as well as Family Quality of Life.

Activity

Activity is a broad term encapsulating how children and adults carry out tasks that they want, need or are expected to do. While reduction in autism characteristics has been extensively studied, the improvement in functioning at the level of activity has not been sufficiently addressed in autism.

While some characteristics may be persistent, pervasive or occur frequently but have limited impact on day-to-day functioning, others although infrequent may have a more profound functional impact. Also, it has been suggested that functional impairment may be independent of the presence and frequency of the characteristics as is the case with psychiatric disorders, where the course and outcomes are different based on the presence or not of functional impairment (Bird et al., 1996). Evidence has indicated that the relationship between autism characteristics and function is not straightforward (Szatmari et al., 2015). Further there are issues pertaining to inconsistencies with the operational definition as well as the measurement of functional impairment (Canino et al., 1999). Measures such as the AIM hold promise in this regard by linking the frequency, impact and interference of each symptom with overall functioning that would have significant advantage in assisting with treatment planning and outcome assessment (Kanne et al., 2014).

A number of measures perform at an activity level, determining frequency and duration of activity performance. Common measures with the potential to monitor progress for individuals with autism are discussed herein under the titles of broad adaptive functioning, self-care (including sleeping and mealtimes), work or productivity, and leisure.

Broad Adaptive Functioning

Adaptive functioning refers to how well a person is able to perform the activities of daily living including conceptual, social and practical skills and how independently they can do this compared to those of similar age and background. There is some evidence to suggest that there is a cognitive advantage over adaptive functioning in children with autism and similar results have been found in a recent study in an older sample (Matthews et al., 2015). Compared to communication and socialization skills, adults with autism showed relative strength in daily living skills although this was not true for adolescents. However, all standard scores were well below average, regardless of their level of cognitive functioning which suggests the need for interventions that target adaptive functioning across the lifespan.

Vineland Adaptive Behaviour Scales

One critical indicator of an individual's functioning and progress is their ability to translate their theoretical intelligence to practical intelligence, or their cognitive potential into real-life skills, hereafter defined as adaptive behaviour. The Vineland Adaptive Behaviour Scales, now in its third edition (Sparrow et al., 2016) assesses social, communication, motor, and daily living skills reflective of an individual's ability to navigate life in the community. It is administered by parent interview and provides both age-equivalent and standardized scores. VABS is used for both baseline assessment and for monitoring progress, and maps comprehensively onto the ICF core sets for autism (Bölte et al., 2014; Hayden-Evans et al., 2022). There is the parent-report version and the interview version completed by the professional and there can be differences in the outcomes between parent versus professional observations, and also variations in observations between settings and assessors.

Adaptive Behaviour Assessment System Third Edition (ABAS-3)

The Adaptive Behaviour Assessment System Third Edition (ABAS-3) is a similar measure of adaptive functioning across a number of subscales (Harrison, 2015). It maps comprehensively on to the ICF core sets for autism (Hayden-Evans et al., 2022) and is broadly applicable due to its wide age range and flexible utility. Its psychometric properties are rated as excellent for school-age children with autism.

Behaviour Assessment System for Children

The Behaviour Assessment System for Children (3rd ed) can be used to measure adaptive functioning across core domains including adaptive/functional skill development and to monitor change (Reynolds et al., 2015). The assessment focuses on the measurement of adaptive and maladaptive behaviour, which are important outcomes for intervention programs. It is standardized (valid and reliable) for age range 2–21 years. For those in the 2–5 year age range, the 134–160 items cover the key areas of activities of daily living, adaptability, aggression, anxiety, attention problems, depression, functional communication, hyperactivity, social skills, somatization, and withdrawal. There is a parent rating form and a teacher form (except activities of daily living scale) and the parent and teacher observation forms can be used to measure change following an intervention program or over time.

Children's Global Assessment Scale

Children's Global Assessment Scale (Shaffer et al., 1983) is a comprehensive tool that can be used to assess function and predict outcomes in adulthood when undertaken with adolescents (Lundh et al., 2016).

Paediatric Evaluation of Disability Inventory–Computer Adaptive Test

Paediatric Evaluation of Disability Inventory-Computer Adaptive Test (PEDI-CAT) is a broad measure of functioning that is delivered electronically to assess children and teenagers up to 21 years of age (Haley et al., 2019). It has been used broadly and has a specific version developed for young people with autism (PEDI-CAT ASD). It has excellent test–retest reliability and adequate responsiveness for school-age children with autism (Hayden-Evans et al., 2022).

Self-Care Activities: Sleep

Sleep disturbances can have significant impact on a child's cognition, academic functioning, behaviour, and mental health. Although sleep problems in children with autism are similar to those of the general population, they occur at markedly higher rates. Approximately 73–86% of children with autism experience problems with sleep onset and maintenance (e.g., long sleep onset latency, short sleep duration, early morning waking Liu et al., 2006; Polimeni et al., 2005). May et al. recently found that 78% of children with autism had parent-reported sleep problems compared to 29% of typically developing controls, with 65% of children with autism having persistent sleep problems one-year later ($n = 84$; 5–12 years) (May et al., 2013). This study also showed that children with autism who were poor sleepers were more aggressive, hyperactive, and experienced greater social problems. Papadopoulos et al. (2015) showed that a brief, behaviourally focused intervention delivered to parents resulted in significantly improved sleep problems and behavioural problems for children with autism. In addition, parents reported improvements in their own mental health after participating in this program. This is an important finding given sleep problems in children with autism have a pervasive impact on the family, including elevated risk for parental stress and poor mental health (Doo & Wing, 2006).

Children's Sleep Habits Questionnaire

A useful tool for monitoring sleep in children with autism is the Children's Sleep Habits Questionnaire (CSHQ; Owens et al. (2000). The CSHQ is 33-item, behaviour parent-reported validated measure of disorders of initiating and maintaining sleep that can distinguish clinical from community samples. Eight subscale scores reflect major behavioural sleep disorders (bedtime resistance, sleep onset delay, sleep duration, sleep anxiety, night wakings, parasomnias, sleep disordered breathing, daytime sleepiness).

Paediatric Sleep Practices Questionnaire

The Paediatric Sleep Practices Questionnaire (PSPQ) measures sleep timing, duration, routines, technology use, and sleep environment and has moderate to strong psychometric properties, being relevant, useful, and comprehensive (Meltzer et al., 2021).

Sleep Diary

Sleep diaries are also commonly used to monitor sleep disturbances in children with autism. Sleep diaries typically involve parents recording the time their child gets into bed at night, falls asleep, any awakenings, and morning wake time, permitting the calculation of sleep duration, sleep onset latency, and number and duration of night wakings.

Self-Care Activities: Mealtimes

\Children with autism have been described to have atypical eating behaviours and food selectivity is the most frequent of these problems (Lee et al., 2024)The everyday management of mealtime behaviours among children with autism can have a negative impact on family routines and become a significant stressor for families. Postorino et al. (2015) investigated the clinical and behavioural features in individuals with autism with the aim of identifying distinctive clinical profiles in children with and without food selectivity. These authors observed that, while there was no statistically significant difference on gastrointestinal symptoms and growth adequacy between those with and without food sensitivity, parents of those with food sensitivity reported significantly higher levels of parental stress and attributed a larger degree of their children's behavioural problems to this. These findings suggest that early identification and appropriate intervention coupled with ongoing monitoring of distinctive clinical and behavioural patterns linked to food sensitivity should be an important consideration in children with autism.

Aut-Eat Questionnaire

The Aut-Eat Questionnaire (AEQ) is a parent report questionnaire that measures eating patterns and problematic eating behaviours of children with ASD aged 3–8 years (Gal et al., 2022). The questionnaire includes demographics, developmental information, and a food list regarding the child with ASD. Six categories of eating problems are measured including: chewing and swallowing problems, eating avoidance, eating selectivity, eating sameness and rituals, over-eating, and problem behaviour during mealtimes.

Self-Care Activities: Other

Dressing, hygiene, and grooming activities can all be challenging areas in need of support and monitoring for individuals with autism. Expectations in this area change greatly over time, across different ages and stages. Some tools, such as the adaptive functioning tools described above, or rehabilitation measures such as the Functional Independence Measure for children (WEE-FIM; McCabe & Granger, 1990) and adults (FIM; Keith et al., 1987), allow for reliable repeated monitoring of self-care independence in these domains, within a specific self-care or activities of daily living subtests. Other tools, such as the newly developed Self-Care Inventory for adults (Luciani et al., 2022), focus specifically on self-care as a construct for assessment and review.

Work, Schoolwork, or Productivity

Work, school, and productivity-related endeavours are of importance to individuals with and without autism. Of these, academic programming and progress monitoring is particularly complex in this context as many core aspects of an individualized plan may not align to a prescribed curriculum and may focus instead on non-academic skills. For example, skills such as communication, socialization, and independence which underpin success in all areas of learning and are associated with positive outcomes, are intrinsically difficult to measure and incorporate into a curriculum. Individualized plans must include measurable academic and functional goals that are not merely restatements of curriculum, standards, or expectations, but are observable, relevant, and assessable objectives intended to facilitate specific gains in academic standards and life skills.

The usual approach to measuring achievement in school is standardized testing. Administering a standardised test to a child with autism can be difficult, and the results somewhat misleading. Students with autism may demonstrate challenging behaviour during the assessment, and research shows that test scores may improve significantly if specialized procedures are implemented to increase the student's engagement in the assessment task (Koegel et al., 1997). Further, although criterion-based or observation-based assessments often provide valuable complementary information, numerous studies have shown that contextual variables such as the amount of attention given to the student prior to the assessment (McComas et al., 2003; Roantree & Kennedy, 2006), the environment (Lang et al., 2009), the person implementing the assessment (Ringdahl & Sellers, 2000) and the motivation of the person with autism and interest in the test materials can all affect the outcome.

It is important to consider what data will need to be collected to document student progress towards IP goals, which tools will be used to generate the data, and how frequently and who will collect data and report progress. Popular methods employed by educators include: direct methods, indirect methods, and authentic methods. As has been discussed, each of these approaches in isolation may not be effective in assessing the child with autism. Direct methods include behaviour observation, such as frequency, duration and interval recording, and curriculum-based assessment. Indirect methods are often auxiliary and include rubrics, which describe performance in qualitative or quantitative terms, attainment scaling, in which the educator rates the student responses on a best-to-worst scale, and student self-monitoring. Authentic methods such as anecdotal notes of informal interviews with students and portfolios of student work involving relevant skills as appropriate for the age.

A number of tools and methods of monitoring can be incorporated to ensure this activity area is optimal for the individual.

The Psycho Educational Profile 3

The Psycho Educational Profile 3 (PEP3;Schopler et al. (2005) is designed to provide information to inform educational programming (IEP) by evaluating uneven learning strengths and weaknesses that characterise autism, and provide information on developmental skill levels. The test also provides a measure of severity, establishes developmental/adaptive levels, and serves as a research tool in outcome research and learning. This is particularly useful for program development and targets social communication and adaptive behaviour. It can be administered by competent and experienced staff and is norm referenced, and provides a measure across core domains of communication, motor and adaptive/maladaptive behaviour, and collects information from a variety of sources; parents, teachers, and direct observation (enabling triangulation of data).

Teacher Rating Scale of School Adjustment

The Teacher Rating Scale of School Adjustment (TRSSA; Betts & Rotenberg, 2007) has been demonstrated to have acceptable internal consistency and stability and can be used to evaluate school adjustment and participation across different time points. An exploratory factor analysis of the TRSSA has yielded three associated factors namely On-Task Classroom Involvement, Positive Orientation, and Maturity.

Leisure and Play

Leisure and play activities are also of critical importance to individuals with and without autism. For children and adults with social communication and behavioural challenges, leisure or play engagement can be reduced, with associated impacts on physical, emotional, and cognitive areas of wellbeing (Manente et al., 2022; Roscoe et al., 2024). Monitoring of leisure and play pursuits is an important area of focus when determining one's progress in childhood and adulthood.

A range of measures are available exploring play and leisure in children and adults with and without autism. In children, tools such as the Test of Playfulness (ToP; Bundy, 1998) and the Child Initiated Pretend Play Assessment 2 (Stagnitti & Unsworth, 2004) are available to assess and monitor play skills in relevant settings. In adolescence and adulthood, exploration of leisure for individuals with autism is receiving increasing attention (Song et al., 2023; Stacey et al., 2018),, with studies using existing measures to understand leisure pursuits in this group, including the Leisure Satisfaction Scale (Beard & Ragheb, 1980).

Body Functions and Structures

This section will focus on autism characteristics and associated areas of deficit relating to specific physical, cognitive, communication, and social abilities, which allows any specific needs to be identified while also setting goals and celebrating strengths, efforts, and achievements. Detailed below are some examples of tools that could be used to monitor progress in these areas, although this is not a comprehensive or exhaustive list. Each has strengths and weaknesses and hence careful selection of the measure based on the target outcome is important.

Social Communication (SC)

It has been suggested that early low-level deficits in recognition and orientation towards social stimuli which then cascades to lack of social engagement with primary caregivers during infancy and resulting in decreased exposure to the reciprocal social interactions critical for development of typical social behaviour. There is substantial evidence to support the presence of these types of differences and it would be a potential target for monitoring which in turn could also help determine the need for intervention, support, and management as development of early social engagement and reciprocity can minimize divergence from a typical developmental trajectory (Webb et al., 2014). Emerging evidence indicates that interventions that address early deficits in joint attention and social reciprocity using strategies that involve interpersonal exchange and positive affect, shared engagement with real-life materials, and activities, sensitivity to child cues and adult responsivity facilitate the development of age-appropriate socio-communicative behaviours.

Social Responsiveness Scale (SRS)

The Social Responsiveness Scale (Constantino & Gruber, 2005) is a brief quantitative measure of autism severity in children and teenagers. It focuses on the degree of impairment in the core autism domains of social awareness, social information processing, reciprocal social communication, social anxiety/avoidance, and stereotypic behaviour/restricted interests. The SRS compares favourably with the ADI-R (Constantino et al., 2003), however is scored based on the observations of parents or teachers, and hence has the limitation of lacking clinician input. Test–retest reliability has been demonstrated in preschool and school-aged versions (Patti et al., 2024).

Early Social Communication Scales (ESCS)

The Early Social Communication Scales (Mundy et al., 2003) is used to measure social behaviour and joint attention skills in a structured setting. During the ESCS, the child is seated at a table while an experimenter presents a range of standardized probes assessing social responsiveness and communication skills, including initiation and response to joint attention, as reflected in frequencies of child alternating gaze, showing, and pointing to share. The ESCS has shown good reliability and validity and has been used in studies of children with autism, including treatment studies (Kasari et al., 2006; Remington et al., 2007; Salt et al., 2002).

Social Communication Questionnaire (SCQ)

The Social Communication Questionnaire (SCQ; Berument et al., 1999), formerly known as Autism Screening Questionnaire is based on a well-validated parent interview, the original Autism Diagnostic Interview (ADI; Rutter et al., 2003). The SCQ covers the areas of communication, reciprocal social interaction, and restricted and repetitive behaviours and interests, which are core diagnostic criteria for autism. There are two versions: a "current" version designed for children under 5 years and a 'lifetime" version designed for children ≥5yrs. The current version is helpful for treatment/planning in that it indicates the type and severity of the characteristics of autism in individual children. The items can be used for setting treatment goals for example, if the child has no ability to take turns in a conversation, conversational turn taking can be targeted in the intervention program. The SCQ can be used for monitoring purposes as it can measure change over time (Eapen et al., 2013a, 2013b).

Sensory Over or Under-Responsiveness

Research has demonstrated that there are distinct sensory profiles in autism relating to behaviours associated with sensory reactivity (the intensity of the response to a sensory stimulus) and multisensory integration (combining information from multiple sensory stimuli) which links with specific patterns of behaviours (Lane et al., 2014). This would suggest that specific intervention strategies matching the sensory difficulties in those affected would be beneficial.

Sensory Processing Measures

The Sensory Profile (Dunn, 2014) and Sensory Processing Measure (Miller-Kuhaneck et al., 2007) are two common tools used to evaluate sensory processing in children with and without autism. They can be completed by caregivers, inclusive of parents and teachers, as well as individuals themselves in the adolescent and adult versions typically. Sufficient responsiveness of these tools in relation to change detection has yet to be established (Brown et al., 2024; Licciardi & Brown, 2023).

Communication

Autism is unique in that essentially the development of communication may not be directly linked to the development of language. More than in any other condition, in autism, language development may occur separately from communication development (Jordan & Jones, 2012). Very young children with autism usually show divergent communication development with differences in the development of joint attention and early engagement with others (Charman & Stone, 2008; Toth et al., 2006). Also, young children with autism are less interested in people than in objects (Kasari et al., 2006) and primarily as a result of paying less attention to other people in their environment, have poor early social communication development (Mo et al., 2019). This extends to the development of language; for example, at the most basic level the learning of the names for things is highly dependent on joint attention and interaction with primary caregivers. Assessment of communication in autism needs to be broad and address all aspects of communication including language development and the structure and function of language and communication. For preverbal, nonverbal, and verbal individuals with autism, assessment of communication as well as of language development is essential. Accurate assessment of receptive and expressive communication are also important because unlike other conditions, in autism receptive language is often more impaired than expressive language (Hudry et al., 2010). This can be misleading when those around the child or adult with autism assume, not unreasonably, that they understand at the same level at which they speak. Children with autism appear to learn language primarily through a process of rote learning chunks of language, which they associate with particular internal and external contexts. Speech often gives a stereotyped impression and echolalia is common. It is important to assess exactly what the child understands and what cues they follow. They may be expert at interpreting visual cues and contextual information while understanding very little of what is actually being said to them.

Children's Communication Checklist (CCC)

Children's Communication Checklist (CCC-2; Bishop (2003) is a 70 item questionnaire completed by a caregiver and screens for communication problems in children aged 4–16 years. The test evaluates a broad range of language skills such as recalling and formulating sentences, word classes, word definition, understanding spoken paragraphs, semantic relationships. There is also a version for older adolescents and adults.

Clinical Evaluation of Language Fundamentals (CELF)

There are preschool and 5–22 years version of this assessment (CELF-P; Wiig et al., 2004), for pre-school to early school age children. Subtests include basic concepts, sentence and word structure, formulating labels, recalling meaning, and linguistic concepts. CELF-5 (Wiig et al., 2013) is a quick and accurate assessment for ages 5 to 22 years to assess for a language disorder. The test evaluates a broad range of language skills such as recalling and formulating sentences, word classes, word definition, understanding spoken paragraphs, semantic relationships. The current battery of tests provides a comprehensive language assessment including a robust assessment of pragmatics using observations and interactive activities.

Communication and Symbolic Behaviour Scales Developmental Profile

Communication and Symbolic Behaviour Scales Developmental Profile (CSBS-DP; 6 months—6 years (Wetherby & Prizant, 2002). This assessment is a combination of parent report and face-to-face evaluation of the child. The assessment measures 7 language predictors: emotion and eye gaze, communication, gestures, sounds, words, understanding, and object use and is sensitive to early delays in social communication, expressive speech/language, and symbolic functioning.

MacArthur-Bates Communication Development Inventories

The MacArthur-Bates Communication Development Inventories (Fenson et al., 2007) (1–3), 3–37 months. The assessment consists of three inventories using parent report to probe use of gestures, words, and sentence.

Reynell Developmental Language Scales

The New Reynell Developmental Language Scales (NRDLS; Edwards et al. (2011). This is a direct assessment of the child designed to identify speech and language delays and impairments in very young children, from 2 to 7 years 6 months.

Peabody Picture Vocabulary

The Peabody Picture Vocabulary Test 4 (PPVT-4; Dunn & Dunn, 2012). Measures listening comprehension of vocabulary in standard English from 2.5 years.

Pragmatics Profile of Everyday Communication Skills in Children

The Pragmatics Profile of Everyday Communication Skills in Children (Dewart & Summers, 1996). Version for preschool aged children 0–4 years, school aged children 5–10 years and adolescents/adults. The assessments are structured interviews with a primary carer designed to assess child communicative functions, response to communication, interaction, and conversation and contextual variation.

Preschool Language Scale

The Preschool Language Scale 5thed (PLS5; Zimmerman et al., 2011). Birth-7 years. This is a direct assessment of the child designed to evaluate maturational lags, strengths, and deficiencies by testing auditory comprehension and verbal ability.

Movement Skills

While not a core area of deficit in children and adults with autism, challenges in the areas of movement and motor skill development are widely reported (Lim et al., 2021; Mohd Nordin et al., 2021), and notably linked to established core challenges in this population (Wang et al., 2022). While motor skill assessments such as the Peabody Developmental Motor Scales II (Folio & Fewell, 2000) Bruininks-Oseretsky Test of Motor Proficiency (Bruininks, 1978) and the Movement ABC (Henderson & Sugden, 1992) are well-utilized in studies exploring motor skill development in children with autism, movement competence, and engagement in motor-based activities across the lifespan has only recently received comparable attention (Tomaszewski et al., 2021). Nonetheless, movement skills, sense of motor competence, and engagement in physical activity presents as important areas for monitoring in relation to individuals with autism of all ages.

Environmental Factors

Families: Parents, Carers, and Siblings

Families of children with autism face unique challenges, and as a result autism families experience higher levels of stress (Hoffman et al., 2009) which can have a significant impact on their quality of life. Siblings can also experience significant challenges and a number of factors may affect the dynamic of the relationship, continually evolving and changing across the course of life (Orsmond & Seltzer, 2007). Monitoring progress in autism would therefore need to include family adjustment and quality of life, stress and coping as well as parental satisfaction, competence, and confidence to manage their child as well as parental perception of their capacity to participate in their community.

The interactions between brothers and sisters provide them with opportunity to experience sharing, companionship, rivalry, and other outcomes. Researchers who study autism do not have a clear understanding of why some sibling pairs experience warm, supportive relationships, whereas others experience conflict and isolation (Rivers & Stoneman, 2003). Many individuals with autism have behaviour repertoires that might be expected to affect sibling relationships and the social, behavioural, and psychological adjustment of their typically developing siblings. Findings regarding the effects of having a sibling with autism have been mixed and inconsistent (Macks & Reeve, 2007; Mascha & Boucher, 2006; Verté et al., 2003). Some researchers (e.g., Hastings, 2003b; Ross & Cuskelly, 2006) have reported negative outcomes (e.g., loneliness, behavioural difficulties, depression) for the typically developing siblings, whereas other researchers (e.g., Jones et al., 2020; Kaminsky & Dewey, 2001; Mascha & Boucher, 2006; Zucker et al., 2022) have found positive outcomes (e.g., less conflict within the relationship, high self-esteem and self-concept) or no evidence of negative effects (Hastings, 2003a; Orsmond & Seltzer, 2007). Orsmond and Seltzer investigated adult siblings of individuals with autism and DS and found that typically developing adult siblings of individuals with autism reported significantly less contact and less positive effect in the relationship with their sibling with autism than did the DS group. Pilowsky et al. (2004) reported that most siblings of individuals with autism were well-adjusted, but emphasized that the stress of having a sibling with autism cannot be overlooked.

Comprehensive monitoring of outcomes should include the well-being of parents, siblings and carers involved in the life of a young person with autism. Thus for the overall improvement, independent living outcomes, maladaptive behaviours as well as general well-being, family stress, coping and quality of life, other relevant measures are indicated. Examples include Autism Treatment Evaluation Checklist (ATEC: Rimland & Edelson, 1999), Parent Stress Index (PSI: Abidin, 1990a), and Quality of Life in Autism (QoLA: Eapen et al., 2014).

The Parenting Sense of Competence Scale (Revised)

The Parenting Sense of Competence Scale (PSOC; Johnston & Mash, 1989) has recently been revised and includes 16 items designed to measure parental self-efficacy (Gilmore & Cuskelly, 2024). Based on the factor structure found in Australian populations (Rogers & Matthews, 2004), the scale generates scores on three subscales: Satisfaction, Efficacy, and Interest, with higher scores indicative of higher levels of parental satisfaction and self-efficacy. The PSOC has been found to have strong psychometric properties (Rogers & Matthews, 2004).

Parenting Stress Index

Parenting Stress Index Short Form (PSI-SF) (Abidin, 1990b): The PSI Short Form (PSI/SF) has 36 items written at a 5th-grade reading level, for parents of children

12 years and younger. The PSI/SF yields a Total Stress score from three scales: Parental Distress, Parent–Child Dysfunctional Interaction, and Difficult Child.

The Parental Empowerment Through Awareness, Relationships, and Resources

The Parental Empowerment through Awareness, Relationships, and Resources (PEARR) (Figueroa et al., 2020). This is a 21-item scale designed to measure three subdimensions of empowerment including resource empowerment, critical awareness, and relational empowerment.

Bullying and Victimization

Bullying and victimization are more prevalent among youth with autism than in the general population, a recent meta-analysis revealing the victimisation in 44% of individuals with autism (Trundle et al., 2023). The role of anxiety in these situations is complex, it appears that parenting stress moderates the association between bullying victimization and anxiety (Weiss et al., 2015). This study also found that when mothers reported high levels of stress, the severity of anxiety was most strongly associated with bullying victimization which has implications for the management of both child anxiety and parental stress in addressing bullying and victimization.

Bullying Measures

Questionnaires measuring a range of child experiences may contain items that capture bullying experiences. Examples include the item "gets teased a lot" from the Child Behaviour Checklist (CBCL; Achenbach & Rescorla, 2001), and selected questions from the Strengths and Difficulties Questionnaire (SDQ; Goodman, 1997) such as "has at least one good friend," "often fights with other children or bullies them," and "picked on by other children." The Self-report of Peer Victimization scale is a 12-item scale measuring overt and indirect peer victimization, including verbal, relational, and physical bullying experiences (Adams et al., 2014).

Physical Environments and Access

Physical environments and access issues for individuals with autism have been receiving increasing attention across studies in recent years. Measures such as the Autism Programme Environmental Rating Scale (APERS; Odom et al., 2018) and the Autism ASPECTSS Design Index are changing the focus of assessment away from the individual with autism, to the features of the environment that can support individuals over time (Mostafa, 2020). This is a relatively novel area in relation to monitoring for individuals with autism, but in line with the ICF and social models of disability, a focus worthy of further consideration for this group.

Personal Factors

Early Development and General Abilities

In infants and toddlers, the symptoms of an autism may only be starting to become apparent, and any differences between an affected child and their peers may not seem too extreme. However, this is one of the greatest opportunities for an early intervention, as it provides intensive support for young children to make more early gains, potentially before their developmental trajectories uncouple from those of their peers. To focus on improving developmental outcomes in young children it is essential to accurately monitor and measure progress in the five developmental domains of early childhood: physical, social, emotional, language, and cognitive skills. A child with autism may experience general or specific impairments in any or all of these domains and associated sub-domains, from a particular sensory processing abnormality to pervasive intellectual impairment.

Moreover, it is important to take into consideration a child's motor profile in their overall management plan. In a study by Papadopoulos et al. (2011) of fifty-three 7–12-year-old children with autism, a significant positive correlation between impairments in motor proficiency (in particular ball skills and balance) and DBC measures of emotional/behavioural disturbance, autistic symptoms, and communication disturbance was reported. These authors suggest that adjunct motor measures (in particular balance) may be a useful objective measure to help monitor the overall developmental profile of a child with autism over time (Papadopoulos et al., 2011). For children with autism who have significant motor impairment that might range from problems with clumsiness, difficulty with motor planning, hand writing difficulties and dystonia's, there is a need for clinical planning around whether motor symptoms should be directly addressed, for example, through intensive occupational therapy, or whether these difficulties should be "monitored" over time. This is particularly relevant in the primary school years. Given that motor impairment is associated with reduced physical activity and participation, there are health as well as psychological benefits for ongoing monitoring of a child's motor development. By monitoring a child's functioning in relation to their individual motor profile and potential limitations, a holistic management approach can be put in place that includes the optimization of activity and participation (Emck et al., 2009).

The Mullen Scales of Early Learning

The Mullen Scales of Early Learning (MSEL; Mullen, 1995) is a standardized, normed developmental assessment for children aged birth through 68 months. It provides an overall index of ability, the Early Learning Composite, and subscale scores of Receptive Language, Expressive Language, Visual Reception, and Fine Motor skill.

Ages and Stages Questionnaire

The Ages and Stages Questionnaire (ASQ; Squires et al., 2009): Parents or caregivers can use the ASQ questionnaires to check a child's general development and the ASQ:SE (socio-emotional) questionnaire to check a child's social emotional development.

The Bayley Scales of Infant Development

Bayley (1993): The Bayley Scales of Infant Development (BSID-III is the current version) is a standard series of measurements used to assess the motor (fine and gross), language (receptive and expressive), and cognitive development of children aged 0–3 years.

Griffiths Mental Developmental Scales

Griffiths Mental Developmental Scale (3rd edition; Griffiths, 2006) The six subscales include Locomotor (Gross motor skills including the ability to balance and to co-ordinate and control movements); Personal-Social (Proficiency in the activities of daily living, level of independence and interaction with other children); Language (Receptive and expressive language); Eye and Hand Co-ordination (Fine motor skills, manual dexterity, and visual monitoring skills); Performance (Visuospatial skills including speed of working and precision) and Practical Reasoning (ability to solve practical problems, understanding of basic mathematical concepts and understanding of moral issues).

General Intellectual Abilities

There is considerable variability in levels of cognition in individuals with autism and therefore accurate intelligence assessment is important in treatment planning.

Weschler Scales (WISC/WPPSI)

Wechsler Pre-school and Primary Scale of Intelligence (WPPSI-IV; Wechsler, 1989, 2002) or the Wechsler Intelligence Scale for Children (WISC–V; Wechsler, 2003) are commonly used tests of intelligence for children. The WISC provides a score that represents a child's overall intellectual ability (FSIQ), and index scores that measure verbal comprehension, visual spatial abilities fluid reasoning, working memory, and processing speed. Scores for quantitative reasoning, auditory working memory, nonverbal ability, general ability, and cognitive proficiency are also available. Although it was originally thought that most people with autism also had co-occurring intellectual disability (ID; i.e., IQ < 70), more recent estimates have reduced this co-occurrence to approximately one-third to one-half of cases (Shenouda et al., 2023). Additionally, epidemiological studies indicate that more than a quarter of participants with autism have average or above average intelligence (i.e., IQ > 85) (Charman et al., 2011).

Stanford-Binet Intelligence Scales: Fifth Edition

The Stanford-Binet Intelligence Scales: Fifth Edition (SB5; Roid, 2003) is a widely used standardized intelligence scale which assesses multiple components of intelligence. It includes ten subtests, five verbal and five nonverbal, which can be used to determine verbal intelligence (VIQ), nonverbal intelligence, and full-scale or abbreviated intelligence.

Behaviour

The presence of co-occurring behavioural difficulties in young people with autism can significantly limit engagement in treatment programs, as well as compromise future educational and vocational opportunities (Fulton et al., 2014). Therefore, understanding and supporting behaviour is a critical focus for interventions and subsequent monitoring. Several authors have suggested that there is a relationship between inability to communicate and the prevalence of behavioural difficulties (Dominick et al., 2007) and self-injurious behaviours (Vismara & Rogers, 2010). Both internalized behaviours (e.g., self-injurious behaviour) and externalised behaviour (e.g., aggression to others) may also be a response to environmental stress (Bartak et al., 2006). Supporting behaviour and ongoing monitoring have significant implications for integration in educational settings and for the overall functioning of the person with autism. Contemporary positive behaviour support approaches have increasing emphasis on culturally responsiveness, trauma-informed principles, and person-centred planning, assessment, and intervention (Schall & Irwin, 2024).

Restricted and Repetitive Behaviours

As repetitive and restrictive behaviours (RRBs) are a core symptom of autism and can be a significant cause of impairment affecting multiple facets of life, it is important to monitor these features for early identification. In addition, these specific behaviours are frequent targets for intervention, support, and management programmes. However, while other social communication symptoms are strongly related to general developmental level and correlate with cognition and IQ, RRBs such as insistence on sameness does not share this relationship with these variables (Bishop et al., 2006; Richler et al., 2010). Further, RBBs are not unique to autism but can also occur in other psychiatric and neurological disorders such as Obsessive Compulsive Disorder (OCD) and Tourette Syndrome (Eapen & Usherwood, 2022) and hence ongoing monitoring to differentiate from, and to identify any co-occurrence of other conditions is needed. In this regard, while monitoring for tics and stereotypes, the points to note would be that tics are brief rapid movements whereas stereotypies are rhythmic, coordinated, and purposeful. Moreover, tics predominately occur in the head and neck region whereas, stereotypies usually involve the limbs or entire body. Further, stereotypies remain much the same with little variation, but tics can follow a waxing and waning course, often reducing with age. In OCD on the other hand, this is driven by a need to relieve anxiety and intrusive thoughts, while in Tourette Syndrome this follows a need to relieve a premonitory urge, and in autism these behaviours are characterized largely by an insistence on sameness and unwavering rigidity in routine. Some studies have shown that despite being a major target for therapy, restricted repetitive behaviours and interests (RRBs) appear to persist in severity over time, even when children show progress in other areas of their symptomatology (Dawson et al., 2010; Vivanti et al., 2014). However, other studies have shown that RRBs improve with age (Zhang et al., 2022).

Repetitive Behaviour Scale-Revised (RBS-R)

The Repetitive Behaviour Scale-Revised is a parent-completed questionnaire which characterizes the severity of repetitive behaviours across six subdomains: stereotyped behaviour, self-injurious behaviour, compulsive behaviour, ritualistic behaviour, sameness behaviour, and restricted behaviour (Bodfish et al., 2000). The tool's adequate sensitivity to change has been established (Scahill et al., 2015).

Tics

Available evidence from the literature suggests that tics occur in around 20–40% of individuals with autism, although there is significant variability in the extant research (Valsamma Eapen et al., 2013a, 2013b). Perhaps the largest and best controlled study to date has reported a rate of 6.5% for the occurrence of Tourette Syndrome in autism (Baron-Cohen et al., 1999) with considerably higher rates of up to 50% for tics when individuals with intellectual disability and autism are considered (Eapen et al., 1997). Awareness of tic disorders will allow for tics to be sensitively managed and possible comorbidities anticipated and differentiated from tics, which in turn can lead to the minimum possible disruption to the young person. For example, tics may be mistaken for fidgetiness that can occur with ADHD, and coprolalia may attract negative consequences such as disciplinary action in children and stigma and social embarrassment in adults. Pharmacological treatment for tic disorders may include clonidine, especially when ADHD presents comorbidly, or antipsychotic agents such as risperidone when there are tics and comorbid behavioural problems such as irritability, aggression, and insomnia (Eapen & Gururaj, 2005). Presence of comorbid OCD would need attention and may necessitate treatment with specific serotonin reuptake inhibitors, while co-morbid ADHD would necessitate the use of stimulants (with caution, monitoring for tic exacerbation) or atomoxetine. The risk of drug interactions and side effects may be increased in those with brain damage or epilepsy, and gradual increase in dosage with close monitoring is recommended in these situations (Eapen & Črnčec, 2009). Psychotherapeutic techniques such as cognitive–behaviour therapy for OCD or comprehensive behavioural intervention for tics (CBIT) have established efficacy (Piacentini et al., 2010; Watson & Rees, 2008); however, outcomes may be constrained in individuals where poor cognitive and learning abilities, and hyperactivity, are a factor. Yale Global Tic Severity Rating

Scale (YGTSS; Leckman et al., 1989) can be a useful tool in monitoring progress following intervention for tics.

Developmental Behaviour Checklist

The Developmental Behaviour Checklist (DBC)-Parent/Caregiver or Teacher Version (DBC-P and DBC-T; Einfeld & Tonge, 2002) is a 96-item checklist of behavioural and emotional problems in children aged between 4–18 years old with developmental difficulties.

The DBC provides an excellent measure of emotional and behavioural problems in both children and adolescents with developmental conditions (Einfeld & Tonge, 1992, 1995, 2002). The DBC can be used for children with intellectual disabilities as well as for children who are cognitively able (Brereton et al., 2002; Einfeld & Tonge, 2002). The DBC has 96 items providing quantitative measures of behavioural and emotional disturbance. Each item is scored on a scale ranging from 0—"not true as far as you know" to 3—"often true or very true." The total score of the DBC provides a measure of overall psychopathology. There are five subscales: Disruptive/Antisocial, Self-absorbed, Communication Disturbed, Anxiety, and Social Relating (Dekker et al., 2002). In addition to measuring psychopathology, the DBC can be used as an Autism Screening tool (the DBC-ASA) in children as young as four years of age (Brereton et al., 2002).

The DBC also has screening measures that can identify and monitor individuals at risk of developing comorbidities. One example of use of the DBC is to monitor comorbid ADHD symptomology (see Gargaro et al. 2014). Boys with autism may be particularly at risk for ADHD comorbidity and require further monitoring, than age, IQ, cognitively and academically matched girls with autism (May et al., 2014).

Child Behaviour Checklist

The Child Behaviour Checklist (Achenbach & Rescorla, 2001) version 1.5–5 years (CBCL 1.5-5) or version 6-18 (CBCL 6-18) can be completed by parents and others who see the children in home-like settings. It obtains parents' reports of children's competencies & problems.

The Teachers Report Form 6-18 (TRF 6-18), is completed by teachers and other school staff who have known the child in school settings for at least 2 months. It obtains teachers' ratings of many of the problems rated on the CBCL 6-18, plus additional items appropriate for teachers.

The Youth Self-Report 11-18 (YSR 11-18), is completed by 11–18 year olds to describe their own functioning. It has most of the same competence & problem items as the CBCL 6-18, and open-ended responses to items covering physical problems, concerns, and strengths.

All forms have parallel Internalizing, Externalizing, and Total Problems scales. The TRF also includes Inattention and Hyperactivity-Impulsivity subscales. The following cross-informant syndromes can be derived from the forms: Anxious/Depressed; Withdrawn/Depressed; Somatic Complaints; Social Problem; Thought Problems; Attention Problems; Rule-Breaking Behaviour; Aggressive Behaviour

The Developmental Behaviour Checklist and The Child Behaviour Checklist have emotional scales that also provide robust measures of anxiety and mood symptoms.

Aberrant Behaviour Checklist (ABC)

The Aberrant Behaviour checklist (ABC; Aman et al., 1985). This scale was primarily developed to assess drug and other treatment effects on individuals with significant cognitive impairment. Factor analysis of the 58 item has yielded a five-factors namely (I) Irritability, Agitation, Crying; (II) Lethargy, Social Withdrawal; (III) Stereotypic Behaviour; (IV) Hyperactivity, Noncompliance; and (V) Inappropriate Speech.

Adult Behaviour Checklist (ABCL)

The Adult Self report (ASR/18-59) & Adult Behaviour Checklist (ABCL/18-59); (Achenbach & Rescorla, 2003). The ASR is used to obtain self-reports from adults on aspects of their adaptive functioning and problems. The ABCL on the other hand is used to obtain reports from people who know the adult person with problems well. There are normed scales for adaptive functioning, as well as empirically based syndromes such as Anxious/Depressed; Attention Problems; Withdrawn; Aggressive Behaviour; Somatic Complaints; Rule-Breaking Behaviour; Thought Problems; and Intrusive problems as well as Internalizing and externalizing problems. The profiles also include a Critical Items scale consisting of items of particular concern to clinicians and a total score.

Emotional Regulation Including Mood and Anxiety

High levels of anxiety are observed in around 40% of children with autism (Micai et al., 2023)The most common type of anxiety is specific phobia (30%), followed by Obsessive Compulsive Disorder (OCD; 17%), social anxiety disorder and agoraphobia (17%), generalized anxiety disorder (15%), separation anxiety disorder (9%), and panic disorder (2%; van Steensel et al., 2011). Early identification and appropriate management of anxiety symptoms should form a critical component in the comprehensive management of autism.

Low mood, self-harm, and suicidal behaviours are common in individuals with autism with a recent meta-analysis reporting that suicidal ideation was present in up to 25.2% of individuals with autism and suicide attempts in 8.3% (O'Halloran et al., 2022). However, identifying those at risk may be difficult due to the challenges in obtaining accurate history from individuals with autism and careful informal and formal enquiries with the young person as well as corroborative evidence from parental or care giver reports would be crucial in assessing for depression and suicidal behaviours.

Strengths and Difficulties Questionnaire

The Strengths and Difficulties Questionnaire (SDQ; Goodman, 1997) is a brief 25 item parent report measure to elicit emotional and behavioural attributes of children and adolescents ages 2 through 17 years old. The SCQ has 5 subscales namely emotional problems; conduct problems; hyperactivity/inattention; peer relationship problems; prosocial behaviours and there is also a total difficulties score based on 20 items. It is important to note that behaviours of concern as identified by measures such as SDQ will need to be considered in the context of the environment and monitoring for the overall wellbeing and quality of life with a focus on identifying issues early and empowering families and individuals with autism to address those aspects that might need additional supports.

Anxiety Scale for Children

The Anxiety Scale for Children-ASD (ASC-ASD) is a 24 item self-report anxiety questionnaire (Rodgers et al., 2016). The ASC-ASD has four subscales measuring separation anxiety, uncertainty, performance anxiety, and anxious arousal. The ASC-ASD has been specifically designed for use with children aged 8–16 years with autism.

The Depression Anxiety Stress Scales

The Depression Anxiety Stress Scales (DASS; Lovibond & Lovibond, 1995) is a 21-item self-report measure that assesses negative affect, generating separate scores for the subscales of Depression, Anxiety, and Stress. The Anxiety scale assesses what causes arousal, what situations cause anxiety and what experiences have led to this effect. The Stress scale assesses whether the person has difficulty relaxing, nervous arousal, and being easily upset/agitated, irritable/over-reactive and impatient. Higher scores indicate greater symptomatology. The DASS-21 has been shown to have excellent psychometric properties (Antony et al., 1998; Henry & Crawford, 2005; Lovibond & Lovibond, 1995; Park et al., 2020).

Psychosis and Catatonia

Co-occurrence of psychotic symptoms in patients with autism can be challenging as some of the core features of autism such as deficits in social reciprocity and communication, as well as restricted behaviours and interests, can be mistaken for psychosis. There are also instances of mis-diagnosis or missed diagnosis of psychosis in autism as there is a subset of patients who present with a complex neurodevelopmental disorder with impairments that cross diagnostic categories (Cochran et al., 2013). Further, symptoms of catatonia are being increasingly recognized at a rate of 4–17% in adolescents and adults with autism (Dhossche, 2014). However it is to be noted that behaviours such as repetitive movements, mutism, posturing, and frantic agitation can occur in autism and hence caution should be exercised and a diagnosis of catatonia should not be made unless there is a sharp and sustained increase of these symptoms persisting for several days or weeks. DeJong et al. (2014) in a recent review reported 22 papers that described the treatment of catatonic symptoms in a total of 28 children and adults with autism using Electroconvulsive therapy (ECT), high-dose lorazepam, and behavioural therapy.

Conclusions and Directions for Future Research

Fit-for-purpose monitoring of individuals with autism and their families offers the opportunity to individually tailor interventions, with timely adaptations based on emerging skills and difficulties, identify commonly occurring problems early, with the hope of preventing or minimizing any negative impact, and to ensure that every individual with autism and their family are reaching their potential for optimal functioning and community participation. Along the way we are likely to also discover new information about how to build on the strengths of individuals with autism and how the environment and community can accommodate difference to minimize avoidable disability.

Tools and processes that support effective monitoring of outcomes and progress with supports continue to be evaluated for individuals with autism. More work is needed in this area, particularly around appropriate measures to evaluate participation and function. In addition, studies are needed to better address questions such as with whom and where participation occurs, and changes to levels of functioning and activity participation as individuals with autism transition from preschool to school, and further to post-school options and adult life. Services and providers should continue to value monitoring, which is ideally integrated across different types of services that are accessed by individuals with autism and their families. Seamless monitoring across the lifespan of developmental progress, scholastic achievement and also functional impact and participation in activities and civic life is the exception rather than the rule. A greater understanding of the link between and relative importance of the characteristics of autism and function and participation is also needed, from the perspective of individuals with autism and their families. Only this will ensure that monitoring is fit-for-purpose and relevant.

References

Abid, M., Demers, I., Mercier, C., & Maltais, D. B. (2023). Systematic review of the psychometric properties of cultural adaptations and translations of the Children's Assessment of Participation and Enjoyment (CAPE). *49*(4), 630–644. https://doi.org/10.1111/cch.13086

Abidin, R. R. (1990a). *Parenting stress index (PSI).* Pediatric Psychology Press.

Abidin, R. R. (1990b). *Parenting stress index:(short form).* Pediatric Psychology Press.

Achenbach, T. M., & Rescorla, L. A. (2001). *Manual for the ASEBA School-age Forms & Profiles.* University of Vermont, Research Center for Children, Youth, & Families.

Achenbach, T. M., & Rescorla, L. A. (2003). *Manual for the ASEBA adult forms & profiles.* University of Vermont, Research Center for Children, Youth, & Families.

Adair, B., Ullenhag, A., Rosenbaum, P., Granlund, M., Keen, D., & Imms, C. (2018). Measures used to quantify participation in childhood disability and their alignment with the family of participation-related constructs: A systematic review. *Developmental Medicine and Child Neurology, 60*(11), 1101–1116. https://doi.org/10.1111/dmcn.13959

Adams, R. E., Fredstrom, B. K., Duncan, A. W., Holleb, L. J., & Bishop, S. L. (2014). Using self- and parent-reports to test the association between peer victimization and internalizing symptoms in verbally fluent adolescents with ASD. *Journal of Autism and Developmental Disorders, 44*(4), 861–872. https://doi.org/10.1007/s10803-013-1938-0

Al-Beltagi, M. (2021). Autism medical comorbidities. *World J Clin Pediatr, 10*(3), 15–28. https://doi.org/10.5409/wjcp.v10.i3.15

Allard, A., Fellowes, A., Shilling, V., Janssens, A., Beresford, B., & Morris, C. (2014). Key health outcomes for children and young people with neurodisability: Qualitative research with young people and parents. *British Medical Journal Open, 4*(4), Article e004611.

Aman, M. G., Singh, N. N., Stewart, A. W., & Field, C. J. (1985). The aberrant behavior checklist: a behavior rating scale for the assessment of treatment effects. *American Journal of Mental Deficiency,* (89), 485–491.

Antony, M. M., Bieling, P. J., Cox, B. J., Enns, M. W., & Swinson, R. P. (1998). Psychometric properties of the 42-item and 21-item versions of the depression anxiety stress scales in clinical groups and a community sample. *Psychological Assessment, 10*(2), 176.

Ashburner, J., Tomkins, V., Bobir, N., Jones, J., Smith, D., Hautsalo, J., & Swift, E. (2023). Co-design and co-production of a goal setting tool for autistic adolescents and adults. *Autism Adulthood, 5*(1), 37–50. https://doi.org/10.1089/aut.2021.0067

Bar-Shalita, T., Yochman, A., Shapiro-Rihtman, T., Vatine, J.-J., & Parush, S. (2009). The participation in childhood occupations questionnaire (PICO-Q): A pilot study. *Physical & Occupational Therapy in Pediatrics, 29*(3), 295–310.

Baron-Cohen, S., Scahill, V. L., Izaguirre, J., Hornsey, H., & Robertson, M. (1999). The prevalence of Gilles de la Tourette syndrome in children and adolescents with autism: A large scale study. *Psychological Medicine, 29*(05), 1151–1159.

Bartak, L., Bottroff, V., Zeitz, J. (2006). Therapist insights in working with stress in people with Autism Spectrum Disorder. In: G. Baron, J. Groden, G. Groden, Lipsitt LP (Eds.), *Stress and coping in Autism.* Oxford University Press.

Bayley, N. (1993). *Bayley scales of infant development: Manual.* Psychological Corporation.

Beard, J. G., & Ragheb, M. G. (1980). Measuring leisure satisfaction. *Journal of Leisure Research, 12*(1), 20–33. https://doi.org/10.1080/00222216.1980.11969416

Bedell, G. M. (2004). Developing a follow-up survey focused on participation of children and youth with acquired brain injuries after discharge from inpatient rehabilitation. *NeuroRehabilitation, 19*(3), 191–205.

Berument, S. K., Rutter, M., Lord, C., Pickles, A., & Bailey, A. (1999). Autism screening questionnaire: Diagnostic validity. *The British Journal of Psychiatry, 175*(5), 444–451.

Betts, L. R., & Rotenberg, K. J. (2007). A short form of the teacher rating scale of school adjustment. *Journal of Psychoeducational Assessment, 25*(2), 150–164. https://doi.org/10.1177/0734282906296406

Bird, H. R., Andrews, H., Schwab-Stone, M., Goodman, S., Dulcan, M., Richters, J., Hoven, C., et al. (1996). Global measures of impairment for epidemiologic and clinical use with children and adolescents. *International Journal of Methods in Psychiatric Research.*

Bishop, D. (2003). *Children's communication checklist—Second edition (CCC-2).* The Psychological Corporation.

Bishop, S. L., Richler, J., & Lord, C. (2006). Association between restricted and repetitive behaviors and nonverbal IQ in children with autism spectrum disorders. *Child Neuropsychology, 12*(4–5), 247–267. https://doi.org/10.1080/09297040600630288

Bodfish, J., Symons, F., Parker, D., & Lewis, M. (2000). Varieties of repetitive behavior in autism: Comparisons to mental retardation. *Journal of Autism and Developmental Disorders, 30*(3), 237–243. https://doi.org/10.1023/a:1005596502855

Bölte, S. (2023). A more holistic approach to autism using the International Classification of Functioning: The why, what, and how of functioning. *Autism, 27*(1), 3–6. https://doi.org/10.1177/13623613221136444

Bölte, S., de Schipper, E., Robison, J. E., Wong, V. C., Selb, M., Singhal, N., de Vries, P. J., & Zwaigenbaum, L. (2014). Classification of functioning and impairment: The development of

ICF core sets for autism spectrum disorder. *Autism Research, 7*(1), 167–172. https://doi.org/10.1002/aur.1335
Breidbord, J., & Croudace, T. J. (2013). Reliability generalization for Childhood Autism Rating Scale. *Journal of Autism and Developmental Disorders, 43*(12), 2855–2865. https://doi.org/10.1007/s10803-013-1832-9
Brereton, A. V., Tonge, B. J., Mackinnon, A. J., & Einfeld, S. L. (2002). Screening young people for autism with the developmental behavior checklist. *Journal of the American Academy of Child & Adolescent Psychiatry, 41*(11), 1369–1375. https://doi.org/10.1097/00004583-200211000-00019
Brian, J. A., Bryson, S. E., & Zwaigenbaum, L. (2015). Autism spectrum disorder in infancy: Developmental considerations in treatment targets. *Current Opinion in Neurology, 28*(2), 117–123.
Brown, T., Almiento, L., Yu, M. L., & Bhopti, A. (2024). The sensory processing measure—Second Edition: A critical review and appraisal. *Occupational Therapy in Health Care, 38*(3), 842–875. https://doi.org/10.1080/07380577.2023.2280216
Bruininks, R. (1978). *Bruininks-Oseretsky test of motor proficiency*. American Guidance Service.
Bundy, A. (1998). *Test of playfulness (ToP) manual*. Colorado State University.
Canino, G., Costello, E. J., & Angold, A. (1999). Assessing functional impairment and social adaptation for child mental health services research: A review of measures. *Mental Health Services Research, 1*(2), 93–108. https://doi.org/10.1023/A:1022334303731
Cannella-Malone, H., Sigafoos, J., O'Reilly, M., Cruz, B. d. l., Edrisinha, C., & Lancioni, G. E. (2006). Comparing video prompting to video modeling for teaching daily living skills to six adults with developmental disabilities. *Education and Training in Developmental Disabilities, 41*(4), 344–356. https://doi.org/10.2307/23879661
Charman, T., Pickles, A., Simonoff, E., Chandler, S., Loucas, T., & Baird, G. (2011). IQ in children with autism spectrum disorders: data from the Special Needs and Autism Project (SNAP). *Psychological Medicine, 41*(03), 619–627. https://doi.org/10.1017/S0033291710000991
Charman, T., & Stone, W. (2008). *Social and communication development in autism spectrum disorders: Early identification, diagnosis, and intervention*. Guilford Press.
Chawarska, K., Klin, A., Paul, R., & Volkmar, F. (2007). Autism spectrum disorder in the second year: Stability and change in syndrome expression. *Journal of Child Psychology and Psychiatry, 48*(2), 128–138. https://doi.org/10.1111/j.1469-7610.2006.01685.x
Cochran, D. M., Dvir, Y., & Frazier, J. A. (2013). "Autism-plus" spectrum disorders: Intersection with psychosis and the schizophrenia spectrum. *Child and Adolescent Psychiatric Clinics of North America, 22*(4), 609–627. https://doi.org/10.1016/j.chc.2013.04.005
Constantino, J. N., Davis, S. A., Todd, R. D., Schindler, M. K., Gross, M. M., Brophy, S. L., Metzger, L. M., Shoushtari, C. S., Splinter, R., & Reich, W. (2003). Validation of a brief quantitative measure of autistic traits: Comparison of the social responsiveness scale with the autism diagnostic interview-revised. *Journal of Autism and Developmental Disorders, 33*(4), 427–433. https://doi.org/10.1023/a:1025014929212
Constantino, J. N., & Gruber, C. P. (2005). *The social responsiveness scale*. Western Psychological Services.
Coster, W., Bedell, G., Law, M., Khetani, M. A., Teplicky, R., Liljenquist, K., Kao, Y.-C., et al. (2011). Psychometric evaluation of the participation and environment measure for children and youth. *Developmental Medicine and Child Neurology, 53*(11), 1030–1037. http://search.proquest.com/docview/901822581?accountid=12763
Dawson, G., Rogers, S., Munson, J., Smith, M., Winter, J., Greenson, J., Donaldson, A., &Varley, J. (2010). Randomized, controlled trial of an intervention for toddlers with autism: The early start denver model. *Pediatrics, 125*(1), e17–e23. https://doi.org/10.1542/peds.2009-0958
DeJong, H., Bunton, P., & Hare, D. (2014). A systematic review of interventions used to treat catatonic symptoms in people with autistic spectrum disorders. *Journal of Autism and Developmental Disorders, 44*(9), 2127–2136. https://doi.org/10.1007/s10803-014-2085-y

Dekker, M., Nunn, R., & Koot, H. (2002). Psychometric properties of the revised developmental behaviour checklist scales in Dutch children with intellectual disability. *Journal of Intellectual Disability Research, 46*(1), 61–75.

Delano, M. E. (2007a). Improving written language performance of adolescents with Asperger syndrome. *Journal of Applied Behavior Analysis, 40*(2), 345–351. https://doi.org/10.1901/jaba.2007.50-06

Delano, M. E. (2007b). Use of strategy instruction to improve the story writing skills of a student with Asperger syndrome. *Focus on Autism and Other Developmental Disabilities, 22*(4), 252–258. https://doi.org/10.1177/10883576070220040701

Dewart, H., & Summers, S. (1996). *The pragmatics profile of everyday communication skills in children*. NFER Nelson.

Dhossche, D. M. (2014). Decalogue of catatonia in autism spectrum disorders. *Frontiers in Psychiatry, 5*, 157. https://doi.org/10.3389/fpsyt.2014.00157

Dominick, K. C., Davis, N. O., Lainhart, J., Tager-Flusberg, H., & Folstein, S. (2007). Atypical behaviors in children with autism and children with a history of language impairment [Research Support, N.I.H., Extramural]. *Research in Developmental Disabilities, 28*(2), 145–162. https://doi.org/10.1016/j.ridd.2006.02.003

Doo, S., & Wing, Y. K. (2006). Sleep problems of children with pervasive developmental disorders: Correlation with parental stress. *Developmental Medicine & Child Neurology, 48*(8), 650–655. https://doi.org/10.1111/j.1469-8749.2006.tb01334.x

Dotson, W. H., Leaf, J. B., Sheldon, J. B., & Sherman, J. A. (2010). Group teaching of conversational skills to adolescents on the autism spectrum. *Research in Autism Spectrum Disorders, 4*(2), 199–209.

Dunn, L. (2004). Validation of the CHORES: A measure of school-aged children's participation in household tasks. *Scandinavian Journal of Occupational Therapy, 11*(4), 179–190.

Dunn, L. M., & Dunn, D. M. (2012). *Peabody picture vocabulary test, (PPVT-4)*. Pearson Education Inc.

Dunn, W. (2014). *The sensory profile 2 manual*. Pearson.

Dunst, C. J., Hamby, D., Trivette, C. M., Raab, M., & Bruder, M. B. (2000). Everyday family and community life and children's naturally occurring learning opportunities. *Journal of Early Intervention, 23*(3), 151–164.

Eapen, V., Crncec, R., Walter, A., & Tay, K. P. (2014). Conceptualisation and development of a quality of life measure for parents of children with autism spectrum disorder. *Autism Research and Treatment, 2014*(11), Article 160783. https://doi.org/10.1155/2014/160783

Eapen, V., & Črnčec, R. (2009). Tourette syndrome in children and adolescents: Special considerations. *Journal of Psychosomatic Research, 67*(6), 525–532. https://doi.org/10.1016/j.jpsychores.2009.08.003

Eapen, V., Črnčec, R., McPherson, S., & Snedden, C. (2013a). Tic disorders and learning disability: Clinical characteristics, cognitive performance and comorbidity. *Australasian Journal of Special Education, 37*(02), 162–172.

Eapen, V., Črnčec, R., & Walter, A. (2013). Clinical outcomes of an early intervention program for preschool children with Autism Spectrum Disorder in a community group setting [Comparative Study Research Support, Non-U.S. Gov't]. *BMC Pediatrics, 13*(1), 3. https://doi.org/10.1186/1471-2431-13-3

Eapen, V., & Gururaj, A. K. (2005). Risperidone treatment in 12 children with developmental disorders and attention-deficit/hyperactivity disorder. *Primary Care Companion to The Journal of Clinical Psychiatry, 7*(5), 221–224. http://www.ncbi.nlm.nih.gov/pmc/articles/PMC1257406/

Eapen, V., Karlov, L., John, J. R., Beneytez, C., Grimes, P. Z., Kang, Y. Q., Mardare, I., Minca, D.G., & Volgyesi-Molnar, M. (2023). Quality of life in parents of autistic children: A transcultural perspective. *Frontiers in Psychology, 14*, 1022094. https://doi.org/10.3389/fpsyg.2023.1022094

Eapen, V., Robertson, M. M., Zeitlin, H., & Kurlan, R. (1997). Gilles de la Tourette's syndrome in special education schools: A United Kingdom study. *Journal of Neurology, 244*(6), 378–382.

Eapen, V., & Usherwood, T. (2022). Assessing tics in children. *BMJ, 376*, Article e069346. https://doi.org/10.1136/bmj-2021-069346
Edwards, S., Letts, C., & Sinka, I. (2011). *The new reynell developmental language scales*. GL Assessment Limited.
Einfeld, S. L., & Tonge, B. J. (1992). *Manual for the developmental behaviour checklist primary carer version (DBC-P)* (Vol. 40). School of Psychiatry, University of NSW and Center for Developmental Psychiatry, Monash University.
Einfeld, S. L., & Tonge, B. J. (1995). The developmental behavior checklist: The development and validation of an instrument to assess behavioral and emotional disturbance in children and adolescents with mental retardation. *Journal of Autism and Developmental Disorders, 25*(2), 81–104. https://doi.org/10.1007/bf02178498
Einfeld, S. L., & Tonge, B. J. (2002). *Manual for the developmental behaviour checklist: Primary carer version and teacher version* (2nd ed.). University of NSW and Center for Developmental Psychiatry, Monash University.
Eldevik, S., Hastings, R. P., Hughes, J. C., Jahr, E., Eikeseth, S., & Cross, S. (2009). Meta-analysis of early intensive behavioral intervention for children with autism. *Journal of Clinical Child & Adolescent Psychology, 38*(3), 439–450. https://doi.org/10.1080/15374410902851739
Emck, C., Bosscher, R., Beek, P., & Doreleijers, T. (2009). Gross motor performance and self-perceived motor competence in children with emotional, behavioural, and pervasive developmental disorders: A review. *Developmental Medicine & Child Neurology, 51*(7), 501–517. https://doi.org/10.1111/j.1469-8749.2009.03337.x
Fenson, L., Marchman, V. A., Thal, D. J., Dale, P. S., Reznick, J. S., & Bates, E. (2007). *MacArthur-Bates communicative development inventories*. Paul H Brookes.
Figueroa, R., Gago, C. M., Beckerman-Hsu, J., Aftosmes-Tobio, A., Yu, X., Davison, K. K., & Jurkowski, J. J. (2020). Development and validation of a parental health-related empowerment scale with low income parents. *International Journal of Environmental Research and Public Health, 17*(22). https://doi.org/10.3390/ijerph17228645
Folio, M., & Fewell, R. (2000). *Peabody developmental motor scales II*. DLM Teaching Resources.
Fuentes, J., Hervás, A., & Howlin, P. (2021). ESCAP practice guidance for autism: a summary of evidence-based recommendations for diagnosis and treatment. *European Child & Adolescent Psychiatry, 30*(6), 961–984. https://doi.org/10.1007/s00787-020-01587-4
Fulton, E., Eapen, V., Črnčec, R., Walter, A., & Rogers, S. (2014). Reducing maladaptive behaviors in preschool-aged children with autism spectrum disorder using the early start denver model. *Frontiers in Pediatrics, 2*, 40. https://doi.org/10.3389/fped.2014.00040
Gal, E., Gal-Mishael, R., Enten Vissoker, R., Hedley, D., Bury, S., & Stolar, O. (2022). Eating challenges in children with autism spectrum disorder: Development and validation of the "Aut-Eat" questionnaire (AEQ). *Journal of Autism and Developmental Disorders, 52*. https://doi.org/10.1007/s10803-021-04978-x
Gargaro, B. A., May, T., Tonge, B. J., Sheppard, D. M., Bradshaw, J. L., & Rinehart, N. J. (2014). Using the DBC-P hyperactivity Index to screen for ADHD in young people with autism and ADHD: A pilot study. *Research in Autism Spectrum Disorders, 8*(9), 1008–1015. https://doi.org/10.1016/j.rasd.2014.05.004
Gilmore, L., & Cuskelly, M. (2024). The Parenting Sense of Competence scale: Updating a classic. *Child: Care, Health and Development, 50*(1), e13173. https://doi.org/10.1111/cch.13173
Goodman, R. (1997). The strengths and difficulties questionnaire: A research note. *Journal of Child Psychology and Psychiatry, 38*(5), 581–586. https://doi.org/10.1111/j.1469-7610.1997.tb01545.x
Gotham, K., Pickles, A., & Lord, C. (2009). Standardizing ADOS scores for a measure of severity in autism spectrum disorders. *Journal of Autism and Developmental Disorders, 39*(5), 693–705. https://doi.org/10.1007/s10803-008-0674-3
Griffiths, R. (2006). *Griffiths mental development scales*. Hogrefe Ltd.

Haley, S. M., Coster, W., Dumas, H., Fragala-Pinkham, M., Moed, R., Kramer, J., Ni, P., Feng, T., Kao, Y. C., Ludlow, L. H. (2019). *Pediatric evaluation of disability inventory: development, standardisation and aministration manual*. Boston University.

Harrison, P. L. (2015). *ABAS-3*.

Hastings, R. P. (2003a). Behavioral adjustment of siblings of children with autism engaged in applied behavior analysis early intervention programs: The moderating role of social support. *Journal of Autism and Developmental Disorders, 33*(2), 141–150.

Hastings, R. P. (2003b). Brief report: Behavioral adjustment of siblings of children with autism. *Journal of Autism and Developmental Disorders, 33*(1), 99–104.

Hayden-Evans, M., Milbourn, B., D'Arcy, E., Chamberlain, A., Afsharnejad, B., Evans, K., Whitehouse, A. J. O., Bölte, S., & Girdler, S. (2022). An evaluation of the overall utility of measures of functioning suitable for school-aged children on the autism spectrum: A scoping review. *nternational Journal of Environmental Research and Public Health, 19*(21). https://doi.org/10.3390/ijerph192114114

Hedvall, A., Westerlund, J., Fernell, E., Holm, A., Gillberg, C., & Billstedt, E. (2014). Autism and developmental profiles in preschoolers: Stability and change over time [Research Support, Non-U.S. Gov't]. *Acta Paediatrica, 103*(2), 174–181. https://doi.org/10.1111/apa.12455

Henderson, S., & Sugden, D. (1992). *Movement assessment battery for children*. The Psychological Corporation.

Henry, J. D., & Crawford, J. R. (2005). The short-form version of the Depression Anxiety Stress Scales (DASS-21): Construct validity and normative data in a large non-clinical sample. *British Journal of Clinical Psychology, 44*(2), 227–239.

Hoffman, C. D., Sweeney, D. P., Hodge, D., Lopez-Wagner, M. C., & Looney, L. (2009). Parenting stress and closeness mothers of typically developing children and mothers of children with autism. *Focus on Autism and Other Developmental Disabilities, 24*(3), 178–187.

Howlin, P., Magiati, I., & Charman, T. (2009). Systematic review of early intensive behavioral interventions for children with autism. *Journal Information, 114*(1).

http://primoa.library.unsw.edu.au/openurl/61UNSW_INST/UNSW_SERVICES_PAGE?url_ver=Z39.88-2004&rft_val_fmt=info:ofi/fmt:kev:mtx:journal&genre=article&sid=ProQ:ProQ%3Ahealthcompleteshell&atitle=Psychometric+evaluation+of+the+Participation+and+Environment+Measure+for+Children+and+Youth&title=Developmental+Medicine+and+Child+Neurology&issn=00121622&date=2011-11-01&volume=53&issue=11&spage=1030&au=Coster%2C+Wendy%3BBedell%2C+Gary%3BLaw%2C+Mary%3BKhetani%2C+Mary+Alunkal%3BTeplicky%2C+Rachel%3BLiljenquist%2C+Kendra%3BGleason%2C+Kara%3BKao%2C+Ying-chia&isbn=&jtitle=Developmental+Medicine+and+Child+Neurology&btitle=&rft_id=info:eric/&rft_id=info:doi/

http://primoa.library.unsw.edu.au/openurl/61UNSW_INST/UNSW_SERVICES_PAGE?url_ver=Z39.88-2004&rft_val_fmt=info:ofi/fmt:kev:mtx:journal&genre=unknown&sid=ProQ:ProQ%3Aabiglobal&atitle=A+PARADOXICAL+EFFECT+OF+PRESESSION+ATTENTION+ON+STEREOTYPY%3A+ANTECEDENT+ATTENTION+AS+AN+ESTABLISHING%2C+NOT+AN+ABOLISHING%2C+OPERATION&title=Journal+of+Applied+Behavior+Analysis&issn=00218855&date=2006-10-01&volume=39&issue=3&spage=381&au=Roantree%2C+Christina+F%3BKennedy%2C+Craig+H&isbn=&jtitle=Journal+of+Applied+Behavior+Analysis&btitle=&rft_id=info:eric/&rft_id=info:doi/

Hudry, K., Leadbitter, K., Temple, K., Slonims, V., McConachie, H., Aldred, C., Charman, T., et al. (2010). Preschoolers with autism show greater impairment in receptive compared with expressive language abilities. *International Journal of Language & Communication Disorders, 45*(6), 681–690.

Hume, K., Steinbrenner, J. R., Odom, S. L., Morin, K. L., Nowell, S. W., Tomaszewski, B., Savage, M. N., et al. (2021). Evidence-based practices for children, youth, and young adults with autism: Third generation review. *Journal of Autism and Developmental Disorders, 51*(11), 4013–4032. https://doi.org/10.1007/s10803-020-04844-2

Hus, Y., & Segal, O. (2021). Challenges surrounding the diagnosis of autism in children. *Neuropsychiatric Disease and Treatment, 17*, 3509–3529. https://doi.org/10.2147/ndt.S282569
Individuals with Disabilities Education Improvement Act of 2004, Pub. L. No. 108-446, §611-619, (2004).
Janvier, D., Choi, Y. B., Klein, C., Lord, C., & Kim, S. H. (2022). Brief Report: Examining test-retest reliability of the autism diagnostic observation schedule (ADOS-2) calibrated severity scores (CSS). *Journal of Autism and Developmental Disorders, 52*(3), 1388–1394. https://doi.org/10.1007/s10803-021-04952-7
Johnston, C., & Mash, E. J. (1989). A measure of parenting satisfaction and efficacy. *Journal of Clinical Child Psychology, 18*(2), 167–175. https://doi.org/10.1207/s15374424jccp1802_8
Jones, E. A., Fiani, T., Stewart, J. L., Neil, N., McHugh, S., & Fienup, D. M. (2020). Randomized controlled trial of a sibling support group: Mental health outcomes for siblings of children with autism. *Autism, 24*(6), 1468–1481. https://doi.org/10.1177/1362361320908979
Jordan, R., & Jones, G. (2012). *Meeting the needs of children with autistic spectrum disorders*. Routledge.
Kalb, L. G., Singh, V., Hong, J. S., Holingue, C., Ludwig, N. N., Pfeiffer, D., Landa, R. et al. (2022). Analysis of race and sex bias in the autism diagnostic observation schedule (ADOS-2). *JAMA Netw Open, 5*(4), e229498. https://doi.org/10.1001/jamanetworkopen.2022.9498
Kaminsky, L., & Dewey, D. (2001). Siblings relationships of children with autism. *Journal of Autism and Developmental Disorders, 31*(4), 399–410.
Kanne, S. M., Mazurek, M. O., Sikora, D., Bellando, J., Branum-Martin, L., Handen, B., Warren, Z., et al. (2014). The Autism Impact Measure (AIM): Initial development of a new tool for treatment outcome measurement [Research Support, Non-U.S. Gov't Research Support, U.S. Gov't, P.H.S.]. *J Autism Dev Disord, 44*(1), 168–179. https://doi.org/10.1007/s10803-013-1862-3
Kasari, C., Freeman, S., & Paparella, T. (2006). Joint attention and symbolic play in young children with autism: A randomized controlled intervention study. *Journal of Child Psychology and Psychiatry, 47*(6), 611–620. https://doi.org/10.1111/j.1469-7610.2005.01567.x
Keith, R. A., Granger, C. V., Hamilton, B. B., & Sherwin, F. S. (1987). The functional independence measure: A new tool for rehabilitation. *Advances in Clinical Rehabilitation, 1*, 6–18.
Khetani, M. (2015). Psychometric Evaluation of the Young Children's Participation and Environment Measure (YC–PEM). *The American Journal of Occupational Therapy, 69*(Supplement_1), 6911500184p6911500181–6911500184p6911500181. https://doi.org/10.5014/ajot.2015.69S1-RP301D
King, G. A., Law, M., King, S., Hurley, P., Hanna, S., Kertoy, M., Young, N., et al. (2000). *Children's assessment of participation and enjoyment (CAPE) and preferences for activities of children (PAC)*. PsychCorp.
Koegel, L. K., Koegel, R. L., & Smith, A. (1997). Variables related to differences in standardized test outcomes for children with autism. *Journal of Autism and Developmental Disorders, 27*(3), 233–243. https://doi.org/10.1023/a:1025894213424
Krantz, P. J., & McClannahan, L. E. (1993). Teaching children with autism to initiate to peers: Effects of a script-fading procedure. *Journal of Applied Behavior Analysis, 26*(1), 121–132. https://doi.org/10.1901/jaba.1993.26-121
Kuhn, D. E., Hardesty, S. L., & Sweeney, N. M. (2009). Assessment and treatment of excessive straightening and destructive behavior in an adolescent diagnosed with autism. *Journal of Applied Behavior Analysis, 42*(2), 355–360.
Lamash, L., Bedell, G., & Josman, N. (2020). Participation patterns of adolescents with autism spectrum disorder compared to their peers: Parents' perspectives. *The British Journal of Occupational Therapy, 83*(2), 78–87. https://doi.org/10.1177/0308022619853518
Lami, F., Egberts, K., Ure, A., Conroy, R., & Williams, K. (2018). Measurement properties of instruments that assess participation in young people with autism spectrum disorder: A systematic review. *Developmental Medicine and Child Neurology, 60*(3), 230–243. https://doi.org/10.1111/dmcn.13631

Lane, A. E., Molloy, C. A., & Bishop, S. L. (2014). Classification of children with autism spectrum disorder by sensory subtype: A case for sensory-based phenotypes. *Autism Research, 7*(3), 322–333.

Lang, R., O'Reilly, M., Lancioni, G., Rispoli, M., Machalicek, W., Chan, J. M., Langthorne, P., & Franco, J. (2009). Discrepancy in functional analysis results across two settings: implications for intervention design. *Journal of Applied Behavior Analysis, 42*(2), 393–397. https://doi.org/10.1901/jaba.2009.42-393

Lattimore, L. P., Parsons, M. B., & Reid, D. H. (2008). Simulation training of community job skills for adults with autism: A further analysis. *Behavior Analysis in Practice, 1*(1), 24–29. http://www.ncbi.nlm.nih.gov/pmc/articles/PMC2848532/

LaVesser, P., & Berg, C. (2011). Participation patterns in preschool children with an autism spectrum disorder. *OTJR: Occupation, Participation and Health, 31*(1), 33–39. https://doi.org/10.3928/15394492-20100823-01

Law, M. (2022). *COPM Canadian occupational performance measure: Revised*. Schulz-Kirchner Verlag GmbH.

Leckman, J. F., Riddle, M. A., Hardin, M. T., Ort, S. I., Swartz, K. L., Stevenson, J., & Cohen, D. J. (1989). The yale global tic severity scale: Initial testing of a clinician-rated scale of tic severity. *Journal of the American Academy of Child & Adolescent Psychiatry, 28*(4), 566–573.

Lee, M., Lee, S., Sohn, J. W., Kim, K. W., & Choi, H. J. (2024). Assessment methods for problematic eating behaviors in children and adolescents with autism spectrum disorder. *Soa Chongsonyon Chongsin Uihak, 35*(1), 57–65. https://doi.org/10.5765/jkacap.230065

Levin, A. R., Baumer, N., Amaral, J., Sargado, S., Pawlowski, K., Chiujdea, M., Bridgemohan, C. et al. (2021). Autism spectrum disorder parent report for outcome monitoring: A preliminary report of development and clinical utility. *Journal of Developmental & Behavioral Pediatrics, 42*(4), 272–282. https://doi.org/10.1097/dbp.0000000000000895

Licciardi, L., & Brown, T. (2023). An overview & critical review of the Sensory Profile—second edition. *Scandinavian Journal of Occupational Therapy, 30*(6), 758–770. https://doi.org/10.1080/11038128.2021.1930148

Lim, Y. H., Licari, M., Spittle, A. J., Watkins, R. E., Zwicker, J. G., Downs, J., & Finlay-Jones, A. (2021). Early motor function of children with autism spectrum disorder: A systematic review. *Pediatrics, 147*(2). https://doi.org/10.1542/peds.2020-011270

Little, L. M., Sideris, J., Ausderau, K., & Baranek, G. T. (2014). Activity participation among children with autism spectrum disorder. *The American Journal of Occupational Therapy, 68*(2), 177.

Liu, X., Hubbard, J., Fabes, R., & Adam, J. (2006). Sleep disturbances and correlates of children with autism spectrum disorders. *Child Psychiatry and Human Development, 37*(2), 179–191. https://doi.org/10.1007/s10578-006-0028-3

Lord, C., Risi, S., Lambrecht, L., Cook, E. H., Jr., Leventhal, B. L., DiLavore, P. C., Pickles, A., & Rutter, M. (2000). The autism diagnostic observation schedule-generic: a standard measure of social and communication deficits associated with the spectrum of autism. *Journal of Autism and Developmental Disorders, 30*(3), 205–223. http://www.ncbi.nlm.nih.gov/pubmed/11055457

Lovibond, S., & Lovibond, P. F. (1995). *Manual for the depression anxiety stress scales*. Psychology Foundation of Australia.

Luciani, M., De Maria, M., Page, S. D., Barbaranelli, C., Ausili, D., & Riegel, B. (2022). Measuring self-care in the general adult population: Development and psychometric testing of the self-care inventory. *BMC Public Health, 22*(1), 598. https://doi.org/10.1186/s12889-022-12913-7

Lundh, A., Forsman, M., Serlachius, E., Långström, N., Lichtenstein, P., & Landén, M. (2016). Psychosocial functioning in adolescent patients assessed with Children's Global Assessment Scale (CGAS) predicts negative outcomes from age 18: A cohort study. *Psychiatry Research, 242*, 295–301. https://doi.org/10.1016/j.psychres.2016.04.050

Macks, R., & Reeve, R. (2007). The adjustment of non-disabled siblings of children with autism. *Journal of Autism and Developmental Disorders, 37*(6), 1060–1067. https://doi.org/10.1007/s10803-006-0249-0

Manente, C. J., LaRue, R. H., Maraventano, J. C., Butler, C., Budge, J., Scarpa, C., & Kahng, S. (2022). Leisure and adaptive behavior for individuals with autism. In *Handbook of quality of life for individuals with autism spectrum disorder* (pp. 333–356). Springer.

Mascha, K., & Boucher, J. (2006). Preliminary investigation of a qualitative method of examining siblings' experiences of living with a child with ASD. *The British Journal of Development Disabilities, 52*(102), 19–28.

Maskey, M., Warnell, F., Parr, J., Le Couteur, A., & McConachie, H. (2013). Emotional and behavioural problems in children with autism spectrum disorder. *Journal of Autism and Developmental Disorders, 43*(4), 851–859. https://doi.org/10.1007/s10803-012-1622-9

Matthews, N., Smith, C., Pollard, E., Ober-Reynolds, S., Kirwan, J., & Malligo, A. (2015). Adaptive functioning in autism spectrum disorder during the transition to adulthood. *Journal of Autism and Developmental Disorders,* 1–12. https://doi.org/10.1007/s10803-015-2400-2

May, T., Cornish, K., Conduit, R., Rajaratnam, S. M. W., & Rinehart, N. J. (2013). Sleep in high-functioning children with autism: Longitudinal developmental change and associations with behavior problems. *Behavioral Sleep Medicine, 13*(1), 2–18. https://doi.org/10.1080/15402002.2013.829064

May, T., Cornish, K., & Rinehart, N. (2014). Does gender matter? A one year follow-up of autistic, attention and anxiety symptoms in high-functioning children with autism spectrum disorder. *Journal of Autism and Developmental Disorders, 44*(5), 1077–1086. https://doi.org/10.1007/s10803-013-1964-y

Mazurek, M. O., Carlson, C., Baker-Ericzén, M., Butter, E., Norris, M., Barr, C., & Kanne, S. (2020). The autism impact measure (AIM): Examination of sensitivity to change. *Autism Research, 13*(11), 1867–1879. https://doi.org/10.1002/aur.2397

McCabe, M. A., & Granger, C. V. (1990). Content validity of a pediatric functional independence measure. *Applied Nursing Research, 3*(3), 120–122. https://doi.org/10.1016/s0897-1897(05)80128-4

McComas, J. J., Thompson, A., & Johnson, L. (2003). The effects of presession attention on problem behavior maintained by different reinforcers. *Journal of Applied Behavior Analysis, 36*(3), 297–307. https://doi.org/10.1901/jaba.2003.36-297

McConachie, H., & Fletcher-Watson, S. (2014). Building capacity for rigorous controlled trials in autism: the importance of measuring treatment adherence. *Child: Care, Health and Development.*

McConachie, H., Livingstone, N., Morris, C., Beresford, B., Le Couteur, A., Gringras, P., Parr, J. R., et al. (2018). Parents suggest which indicators of progress and outcomes should be measured in young children with autism spectrum disorder. *Journal of Autism and Developmental Disorders, 48*(4), 1041–1051. https://doi.org/10.1007/s10803-017-3282-2

Meltzer, L. J., Forrest, C. B., de la Motte, A., Mindell, J. A., & Bevans, K. B. (2021). Development and validation of the pediatric sleep practices questionnaire: A self-report measure for youth ages 8–17 years. *Behavioral Sleep Medicine, 19*(1), 126–143. https://doi.org/10.1080/15402002.2020.1714625

Micai, M., Fatta, L. M., Gila, L., Caruso, A., Salvitti, T., Fulceri, F., Scattoni, M. L., et al. (2023). Prevalence of co-occurring conditions in children and adults with autism spectrum disorder: A systematic review and meta-analysis. *Neuroscience and BioBehavioral Reviews, 155*, 105436. https://doi.org/10.1016/j.neubiorev.2023.105436

Miller-Kuhaneck, H., Henry, D. A., Glennon, T. J., & Mu, K. (2007). Development of the sensory processing measure–School: Initial studies of reliability and validity. *The American Journal of Occupational Therapy, 61*(2), 170–175.

Mo, S., Liang, L., Bardikoff, N., & Sabbagh, M. A. (2019). Shifting visual attention to social and non-social stimuli in autism spectrum disorders. *Research in Autism Spectrum Disorders, 65*, 56–64. https://doi.org/10.1016/j.rasd.2019.05.006

Mohd Nordin, A., Ismail, J., & Kamal Nor, N. (2021). Motor development in children with autism spectrum disorder. *Frontiers in Pediatrics, 9*, Article 598276. https://doi.org/10.3389/fped.2021.598276

Mostafa, M. (2020). Chapter 23—Architecture for autism: Built environment performance in accordance to the autism ASPECTSS design index. In U. Das, N. Papaneophytou, & T. El-Kour (Eds.), *Autism 360* (pp. 479–500). Academic Press. https://doi.org/10.1016/B978-0-12-818466-0.00023-X

Mullally, S. L., Wood, A. E., Edwards, C. C., Connolly, S. E., Constable, H., Watson, S., King, N. et al. (2024). Autistic voice: Sharing autistic children's experiences and insights. *medRxiv*. https://doi.org/10.1101/2024.07.22.24310796

Mullen, E. (1995). *Mullen scales of early learning (AGS ed.)*. American Guidance Service Inc.

Mundy, P., Delgado, C., Block, J., Venezia, M., Hogan, A., & Seibert, J. (2003). *Early social communication scales (ESCS)*. University of Miami.

National Institute for Health and Care Excellence. (2012). *Autism: recognition, referral, diagnosis and management of adults on the autism spectrum* (NICE clinical guidelines). Issue.

National Institute for Health and Care Excellence. (2013). *Autism: The management and support of children and young people on the autism spectrum* (NICE clinical guidelines). Issue.

O'Halloran, L., Coey, P., & Wilson, C. (2022). Suicidality in autistic youth: A systematic review and meta-analysis. *Clinical Psychology Review, 93*, Article 102144. https://doi.org/10.1016/j.cpr.2022.102144

Odom, S. L., Brown, W. H., Frey, T., Karasu, N., Lee Smith-Canter, L., & Strain, P. S. (2003). Evidence-based practices for young children with autism: Contributions for single-subject design research. *Focus on Autism and Other Developmental Disabilities, 18*(3), 166–175. https://doi.org/10.1177/10883576030180030401

Odom, S. L., Cox, A., Sideris, J., Hume, K. A., Hedges, S., Kucharczyk, S., Shaw, E., Boyd, B. A., Reszka, S., &Neitzel, J. (2018). Assessing quality of program environments for children and youth with autism: Autism program environment rating scale (APERS). *Journal of Autism and Developmental Disorders, 48*(3), 913–924. https://doi.org/10.1007/s10803-017-3379-7

Ona, H. N., Larsen, K., Nordheim, L., Brurberg, K. G. (2020). Effects of Pivotal Response Treatment (PRT) for children with Autism Spectrum Disorders (ASD): A systematic review. *Review Journal of Autism and Developmental Disorders 7*(3), https://doi.org/10.1007/s40489-019-00180-z

Orsmond, G. I., & Seltzer, M. M. (2007). Siblings of individuals with autism spectrum disorders across the life course. *Mental Retardation and Developmental Disabilities Research Reviews, 13*(4), 313–320.

Ottenbacher, K. J., & Cusick, A. (1990). Goal attainment scaling as a method of clinical service evaluation. *American Journal of Occupational Therapy, 44*(6), 519–525. https://doi.org/10.5014/ajot.44.6.519

Owens, J. A., Spirito, A., & McGuinn, M. (2000). The children's sleep habits questionnaire (CSHQ): Psychometric properties of a survey instrument for school-aged children. *Sleep-New York, 23*(8), 1043–1052.

Papadopoulos, N., McGinley, J., Tonge, B., Bradshaw, J., Saunders, K., Murphy, A., & Rinehart, N. (2011). Motor proficiency and emotional/behavioural disturbance in autism and Asperger's disorder: Another piece of the neurological puzzle? *Autism*. https://doi.org/10.1177/1362361311418692

Papadopoulos, N., Sciberras, E., Hiscock, H., Mulraney, M., McGillivray, J., & Rinehart, N. (2015). The efficacy of a brief behavioral sleep intervention in school-aged children with ADHD and comorbid autism spectrum disorder. *Journal of Attention Disorders*. https://doi.org/10.1177/1087054714568565

Park, S. H., Song, Y. J. C., Demetriou, E. A., Pepper, K. L., Thomas, E. E., Hickie, I. B., & Guastella, A. J. (2020). Validation of the 21-item depression, anxiety, and stress scales (DASS-21) in individuals with autism spectrum disorder. *Psychiatry Research, 291*, 113300. https://doi.org/10.1016/j.psychres.2020.113300

Patti, M. A., Croen, L. A., Dickerson, A. S., Joseph, R. M., Ames, J. L., Ladd-Acosta, C., Lyall, K., et al. (2024). Reproducibility between preschool and school-age Social Responsiveness Scale forms in the Environmental influences on Child Health Outcomes program. *Autism Res, 17*(6), 1187–1204. https://doi.org/10.1002/aur.3147

Payakachat, N., Tilford, J. M., Kovacs, E., & Kuhlthau, K. (2012). Autism spectrum disorders: A review of measures for clinical, health services and cost-effectiveness applications.
Piacentini, J., Woods, D. W., Scahill, L., et al. (2010). Behavior therapy for children with tourette disorder: A randomized controlled trial. *JAMA, 303*(19), 1929–1937. https://doi.org/10.1001/jama.2010.607
Pilowsky, T., Yirmiya, N., Doppelt, O., Gross-Tsur, V., & Shalev, R. S. (2004). Social and emotional adjustment of siblings of children with autism. *Journal of Child Psychology and Psychiatry, 45*(4), 855–865.
Polimeni, M. A., Richdale, A. L., & Francis, A. J. P. (2005). A survey of sleep problems in autism, Asperger's disorder and typically developing children. *Journal of Intellectual Disability Research, 49*(4), 260–268. https://doi.org/10.1111/j.1365-2788.2005.00642.x
Postorino, V., Sanges, V., Giovagnoli, G., Fatta, L. M., De Peppo, L., Armando, M., Mazzone, L., et al. (2015). Clinical differences in children with autism spectrum disorder with and without food selectivity. *Appetite*. https://doi.org/10.1016/j.appet.2015.05.016
Prior, M., Roberts, J., Rodger, S., Williams, K., & Sutherland, R. (2011). A review of the research to identify the most effective models of practice in early intervention for children with autism spectrum disorders. *Australian Government Department of Families, Housing, Community Services and Indigenous Affairs, Australia*. Retrieved May 11, 2012.
Pritchard-Wiart, L., Thompson-Hodgetts, S., & McKillop, A. B. (2019). A review of goal setting theories relevant to goal setting in paediatric rehabilitation. *Clinical Rehabilitation, 33*(9), 1515–1526. https://doi.org/10.1177/0269215519846220
Rayner, C. S. (2010). Video-modelling to improve task completion in a child with autism. *Developmental Neurorehabilitation, 13*(3), 225–230. https://doi.org/10.3109/17518421003801489
Remington, B., Hastings, R. P., Kovshoff, H., Espinosa, F. d., Jahr, E., Brown, T., Ward, N., et al. (2007). Early intensive behavioral intervention: Outcomes for children with autism and their parents after two years. *American Journal on Mental Retardation, 112*(6), 418–438. https://doi.org/10.1352/0895-8017(2007)112[418:EIBIOF]2.0.CO;2
Reynolds, C. R., Kamphaus, R. W., & Vannest, K. J. (2015). *BASC3: Behavior assessment system for children*. PscyhCorp.
Richler, J., Huerta, M., Bishop, S. L., & Lord, C. (2010). Developmental trajectories of restricted and repetitive behaviors and interests in children with autism spectrum disorders. *Development and Psychopathology, 22*(1), 55–69. https://doi.org/10.1017/s0954579409990265
Rimland, B., & Edelson, M. (1999). *Autism treatment evaluation checklist*. Autism Research Institute.
Ringdahl, J. E., & Sellers, J. A. (2000). The effects of different adults as therapists during functional analyses. *Journal of Applied Behavior Analysis, 33*(2), 247–250. https://doi.org/10.1901/jaba.2000.33-247
Rivard, M., Patrick, C., Mello, C., Morin, D., & Morin, M. (2021). The diagnostic trajectory in autism and intellectual disability in Quebec: Pathways and parents' perspective. *BMC Pediatrics, 21*(1), 393. https://doi.org/10.1186/s12887-021-02864-0
Rivers, J., & Stoneman, Z. (2003). Sibling relationships when a child has autism: Marital stress and support coping. *Journal of Autism and Developmental Disorders, 33*(4), 383–394. https://doi.org/10.1023/A:1025006727395
Roantree, C. F., & Kennedy, C. H. (2006). A paradoxical effect of presession attention on stereotypy: antecedent attention as an establishing, not an abolishing, operation. *Journal of Applied Behavior Analysis, 39*(3), 381–384. http://search.proquest.com/docview/225047198?accountid=12763
Rodgers, J., Wigham, S., McConachie, H., Freeston, M., Honey, E., & Parr, J. R. (2016). Development of the anxiety scale for children with autism spectrum disorder (ASC-ASD). *Autism Research, 9*(11), 1205–1215. https://doi.org/10.1002/aur.1603
Rogers, H., & Matthews, J. (2004). The parenting sense of competence scale: Investigation of the factor structure, reliability, and validity for an Australian sample. *Australian Psychologist, 39*(1), 88–96. https://doi.org/10.1080/00050060410001660380

Roid, G. (2003). Stanford-Binet Intelligence Scales (SB5). *Rolling Meadows, IL: Riverside.*

Roscoe, E. M., Hall, V. A., McVarish, A. E., & Cornaglia, R. B. (2024). Increasing leisure-item engagement in individuals with autism. *39*(1), e1981. https://doi.org/10.1002/bin.1981

Rosen, T. E., Mazefsky, C. A., Vasa, R. A., & Lerner, M. D. (2018). Co-occurring psychiatric conditions in autism spectrum disorder. *International Review of Psychiatry, 30*(1), 40–61. https://doi.org/10.1080/09540261.2018.1450229

Ross, P., & Cuskelly, M. (2006). Adjustment, sibling problems and coping strategies of brothers and sisters of children with autistic spectrum disorder. *Journal of Intellectual and Developmental Disability, 31*(2), 77–86.

Rutter, M., Le Couteur, A., & Lord, C. (2003). *Autism diagnostic interview—revised*. Western Psychological Services.

Sallows, G. O., & Graupner, T. D. (2005). Intensive behavioral treatment for children with autism: Four-year outcome and predictors. *American Journal of Mental Retardation, 110*(6), 417–438. https://doi.org/10.1352/0895-8017(2005)110[417:Ibtfcw]2.0.Co;2

Salt, J., Shemilt, J., Sellars, V., Boyd, S., Coulson, T., & Mc Cool, S. (2002). The Scottish Centre for Autism Preschool Treatment Programme: II: The results of a controlled treatment outcome study. *Autism, 6*(1), 33–46. https://doi.org/10.1177/1362361302006001004

Scahill, L., Aman, M. G., Lecavalier, L., Halladay, A. K., Bishop, S. L., Bodfish, J. W., Dawson, G., et al. (2015). Measuring repetitive behaviors as a treatment endpoint in youth with autism spectrum disorder. *Autism, 19*(1), 38–52. https://doi.org/10.1177/1362361313510069

Schall, C., & Irwin, D. J. (2024). Positive behavior interventions and supports for students with intellectual disability: Ensuring culturally responsive, trauma-informed, person-centered supports. In *Handbook of research-based practices for educating students with intellectual disability* (pp. 236–257).

Schopler, E., Bourgondien, M. E., Wellman, G. J., & Love, S. R. (2010). *Childhood autism rating scale, second edition (CARS2)*. Western Psychological Services.

Schopler, E., Lansing, M. D., Reichler, R. J., & Marcus, L. M. (2005). *Psychoeducational Profile, Third Edition (PEP-3)*. Pro-ed Incorporation.

Schopler, E., Reichler, R. J., DeVellis, R. F., & Daly, K. (1980). Toward objective classification of childhood autism: Childhood Autism Rating Scale (CARS). *Journal of Autism and Developmental Disorders, 10*(1), 91–103. https://doi.org/10.1007/bf02408436

Schopler, E., Reichler, R. J., & Renner, B. R. (1986). *The childhood autism rating scale (CARS)*.

Shaffer, D., Gould, M. S., Brasic, J., Ambrosini, P., Fisher, P., Bird, H., & Aluwahlia, S. (1983). A children's global assessment scale (CGAS). *Archives of General Psychiatry, 40*(11), 1228–1231.

Shahin, S., DiRezze, B., Ahmed, S., & Anaby, D. (2023). Development and content validity of the youth and young-adult participation and environment measure (Y-PEM). *Disability and Rehabilitation, 45*(3), 549–561. https://doi.org/10.1080/09638288.2022.2030809

Shenouda, J., Barrett, E., Davidow, A. L., Sidwell, K., Lescott, C., Halperin, W., Zahorodny, W. et al. (2023). Prevalence and disparities in the detection of autism without intellectual disability. *Pediatrics, 151*(2). https://doi.org/10.1542/peds.2022-056594

Sigafoos, J., O'Reilly, M., Cannella, H., Edrisinha, C., de la Cruz, B., Upadhyaya, M., Young, D., et al. (2007). Evaluation of a video prompting and fading procedure for teaching dish washing skills to adults with developmental disabilities. *Journal of Behavioral Education, 16*(2), 93–109. https://doi.org/10.1007/s10864-006-9004-z

Simeonsson, R. J., Leonardi, M., Lollar, D., Bjorck-Akesson, E., Hollenweger, J., & Martinuzzi, A. (2003). Applying the international classification of functioning, disability and health (ICF) to measure childhood disability. *Disability and Rehabilitation, 25*(11–12), 602–610. https://doi.org/10.1080/0963828031000137117

Simonoff, E., Pickles, A., Charman, T., Chandler, S., Loucas, T., & Baird, G. (2008). Psychiatric disorders in children with autism spectrum disorders: Prevalence, comorbidity, and associated factors in a population-derived sample. *Journal of the American Academy of Child & Adolescent Psychiatry, 47*(8), 921–929. https://doi.org/10.1097/CHI.0b013e318179964f

Singh, N. N., Lancioni, G. E., Manikam, R., Winton, A. S., Singh, A. N., Singh, J., & Singh, A. D. (2011). A mindfulness-based strategy for self-management of aggressive behavior in adolescents with autism. *Research in Autism Spectrum Disorders, 5*(3), 1153–1158.
Song, W., Zheng, L., Tichá, R., Abery, B., & Nguyen-Feng, V. N. (2023). Leisure participation of autistic adults: An ecological momentary assessment feasibility study. *American Journal on Intellectual and Developmental Disabilities, 128*(4), 319–333. https://doi.org/10.1352/1944-7558-128.4.319
Souza, F., Duff, G., & Swait, J. (2021). "Whose plan is it?" understanding how the goal pursuit of consumers and carers influence choices in the australian disability sector. *Journal of Choice Modelling,* 100300. https://doi.org/10.1016/j.jocm.2021.100300
Sparrow, S., Cicchetti, D. V., & Saulnier, C. A. (2016). *Vineland adaptive behavior scales, (Vineland-3).* Psychological Corporation.
Squires, J., Bricker, D., & Twombly, E. (2009). Ages & stages questionnaires. *Baltimore, Maryland,* 257–182.
Stacey, T.-L., Froude, E. H., Trollor, J., & Foley, K.-R. (2018). Leisure participation and satisfaction in autistic adults and neurotypical adults. *Autism, 23*(4), 993–1004. https://doi.org/10.1177/1362361318791275
Stagnitti, K., & Unsworth, C. (2004). The test-retest reliability of the child-initiated pretend play assessment. *American Journal of Occupational Therapy, 58*(1), 93–99. https://doi.org/10.5014/ajot.58.1.93
Sytsma, S. E., Kelley, M. L., & Wymer, J. H. (2001). Development and initial validation of the Child Routines Inventory. *Journal of Psychopathology and Behavioral Assessment, 23*(4), 241–251.
Szatmari, P., Georgiades, S., Duku, E., Bennett, T. A., Bryson, S., Fombonne, E., Vaillancourt, T., et al. (2015). Developmental trajectories of symptom severity and adaptive functioning in an inception cohort of preschool children with autism spectrum disorder. *JAMA psychiatry, 72*(3), 276–283.
Tomaszewski, B., Savage, M. N., & Hume, K. (2021). Examining physical activity and quality of life in adults with autism spectrum disorder and intellectual disability. *Journal of Intellectual Disabilities, 26*(4), 1075–1088. https://doi.org/10.1177/17446295211033467
Toth, K., Munson, J., Meltzoff, A. N., & Dawson, G. (2006). Early predictors of communication development in young children with autism spectrum disorder: Joint attention, imitation, and toy play. *Journal of Autism and Developmental Disorders, 36*(8), 993–1005.
Trembath, D., Varcin, K., Waddington, H., Sulek, R., Pillar, S., Allen, G., Goodall, E., et al. (2022). *National guideline for supporting the learning, participation, and wellbeing of autistic children and their families in Australia.* Autism CRC.
Trundle, G., Jones, K. A., Ropar, D., & Egan, V. (2023). Prevalence of victimisation in autistic individuals: A systematic review and meta-analysis. *Trauma, Violence & Abuse, 24*(4), 2282–2296. https://doi.org/10.1177/15248380221093689
van Steensel, F. J., Bögels, S. M., & Perrin, S. (2011). Anxiety disorders in children and adolescents with autistic spectrum disorders: A meta-analysis. *Clinical Child and Family Psychology Review, 14*(3), 302–317.
Varni, J. W., Seid, M., & Rode, C. A. (1999). The PedsQL™: Measurement model for the pediatric quality of life inventory. *Medical Care, 37*(2), 126–139.
Verté, S., Roeyers, H., & Buysse, A. (2003). Behavioural problems, social competence and self-concept in siblings of children with autism. *Child: Care, Health and Development, 29*(3), 193–205. https://doi.org/10.1046/j.1365-2214.2003.00331.x
Vismara, L. A., & Rogers, S. J. (2010). Behavioral treatments in autism spectrum disorder: What Do We Know? *Annual Review of Clinical Psychology, 6*(1), 447–468. https://doi.org/10.1146/annurev.clinpsy.121208.131151
Vivanti, G., Paynter, J., Duncan, E., Fothergill, H., Dissanayake, C., & Rogers, S. (2014). Effectiveness and feasibility of the early start Denver model implemented in a group-based community childcare setting. *Journal of Autism and Developmental Disorders, 44*(12), 3140–3153. https://doi.org/10.1007/s10803-014-2168-9

Vyshedskiy, A., & Khokhlovich, E. (2022). Pretend play predicts receptive and expressive language trajectories in young children with autism. *medRxiv*. https://doi.org/10.1101/2022.04.04.22273397

Wang, L. A. L., Petrulla, V., Zampella, C. J., Waller, R., & Schultz, R. T. (2022). Gross motor impairment and its relation to social skills in autism spectrum disorder: A systematic review and two meta-analyses. *Psychological Bulletin, 148*(3–4), 273–300. https://doi.org/10.1037/bul0000358

Watson, H. J., & Rees, C. S. (2008). Meta-analysis of randomized, controlled treatment trials for pediatric obsessive-compulsive disorder. *Journal of Child Psychology and Psychiatry, 49*(5), 489–498. https://doi.org/10.1111/j.1469-7610.2007.01875.x

Webb, S. J., Jones, E. J. H., Kelly, J., & Dawson, G. (2014). The motivation for very early intervention for infants at high risk for autism spectrum disorders. *International Journal of Speech-Language Pathology, 16*(1), 36–42. https://doi.org/10.3109/17549507.2013.861018

Wechsler, D. (1989). *Wechsler preschool and primary intelligence scale-revised*. Psychological Corporation.

Wechsler, D. (2002). *The Wechsler primary and preschool scale of intelligence—Third Edition*. The Psychological Corporation.

Wechsler, D. (2003). *Wechsler intelligence scale for children–Fourth Edition*. The Psychological Corporation.

Weiss, J. A., Cappadocia, M. C., Tint, A., & Pepler, D. (2015). Bullying victimization, parenting stress, and anxiety among adolescents and young adults with autism spectrum disorder. *Autism Research*, n/a-n/a. https://doi.org/10.1002/aur.1488

Wetherby, A. M., & Prizant, B. M. (2002). *Communication and symbolic behavior scales: Developmental profile*. Paul H Brookes Publishing.

Whitehouse, A., Evans, K., Eapen, V., & Wray, J. (2018). *A National guideline for the assessment and diagnosis of autism spectrum disorder in Australia*. Cooperative Research Centre for Living with Autism.

Whitehouse, A. J., Varcin, K. J., Alvares, G. A., Barbaro, J., Bent, C., Boutrus, M., Davidson, E., et al. (2019). Pre-emptive intervention versus treatment as usual for infants showing early behavioural risk signs of autism spectrum disorder: A single-blind, randomised controlled trial. *Lancet Child Adolesc Health, 3*(9), 605–615. https://doi.org/10.1016/S2352-4642(19)30184-1

Wiig, E. H., Secord, W., & Semel, E. M. (2004). *CELF preschool 2: Clinical evaluation of language fundamentals preschool*. Pearson/PsychCorp.

Wiig, E. H., Semel, E., & Secord, W. A. (2013). *Clinical evaluation of language fundamentals®—Fifth Edition (CELF®-5)*. Pearson.

World Health Organization. (1980). *International classification of impairments, disabilities, and handicaps: a manual of classification relating to the consequences of disease, published in accordance with resolution WHA29. 35 of the Twenty-ninth World Health Assembly, May 1976*. World Heath Organization.

World Health Organization. (2001). *International Classification of functioning, disability, and health*. World Health Organization.

Yee, T., Magill-Evans, J., Zwaigenbaum, L., Sacrey, L.-A.R., Askari, S., & Anaby, D. (2017). Participation measures for preschool children with autism spectrum disorder: A scoping review. *Review Journal of Autism and Developmental Disorders, 4*(2), 132–141. https://doi.org/10.1007/s40489-017-0102-8

Zhang, A., Liu, L., Chang, S., Shi, L., Li, P., Shi, J., Liu, J., et al. (2022). Connectivity-based brain network supports restricted and repetitive behaviors in autism spectrum disorder across development. *Front Psychiatry, 13*, 874090. https://doi.org/10.3389/fpsyt.2022.874090

Zimmerman, I. L., Steiner, V. G., & Evatt Pond, R. (2011). *Preschool language scales—Fifth edition (PLS-5)*. Pearson.

Zucker, A., Chang, Y., Maharaj, R., Wang, W., Fiani, T., McHugh, S., Jones, E. A., et al. (2022). Quality of the sibling relationship when one sibling has autism spectrum disorder: A randomized controlled trial of a sibling support group. *Autism, 26*(5), 1137–1152. https://doi.org/10.1177/13623613211042135

Zwaigenbaum, L., Bryson, S., & Garon, N. (2013). Early identification of autism spectrum disorders. *Behavioural Brain Research, 251*, 133–146. https://doi.org/10.1016/j.bbr.2013.04.004

Machine Learning in Autism Assessments

Selda Ozdemir, Isik Akin-Bulbul, and Ibrahim Kok

Abstract Artificial intelligence (AI) is the science and engineering of creating intelligent systems that imitate human abilities to think, learn, and solve problems. One of the most significant subfields of AI is machine learning (Pramod et al., 2021). Over the past two decades, there has been rapid development in machine learning models across various research fields, including autism (Ozdemir et al., 2022; Wan et al., 2019; Zhao et al., 2021). Machine learning involves algorithms and methods that perform complex tasks such as analysis, prediction, classification, and decision-making by automatically learning from large datasets (Yildirim et al., 2024).

Keywords Artificial intelligence · Autism research · Autism · Clinical · Machine learning

Introduction to Machine Learning in Clinical Assessments

Artificial intelligence (AI) is the science and engineering of creating intelligent systems that imitate human abilities to think, learn, and solve problems. One of the most significant subfields of AI is machine learning (Pramod et al., 2021). Over the past two decades, there has been rapid development in machine learning models across various research fields, including autism (Ozdemir et al., 2022; Wan et al., 2019; Zhao et al., 2021). Machine learning involves algorithms and methods that perform complex tasks such as analysis, prediction, classification, and decision-making by automatically learning from large datasets (Yildirim et al., 2024). It has emerged as a transformative methodology in clinical studies, providing innovative solutions to long-standing challenges in clinical autism assessments (Ozdemir

S. Ozdemir (✉) · I. Akin-Bulbul
Education Faculty, Department of Special Education, Hacettepe University, Ankara, Turkey
e-mail: seldaozdemir@hacettepe.edu.tr

I. Kok
Engineering Faculty, Department of Artificial Intelligence and Data Engineering, Ankara University, Ankara, Turkey

J. L. Matson (ed.), *Assessment and Diagnosis in Autism*, Autism and Child Psychopathology Series, https://doi.org/10.1007/978-3-032-11802-8_3

et al., 2022). By analyzing large datasets and utilizing advanced algorithms, machine learning facilitates the development of predictive models that assist clinicians in identifying at-risk children, diagnosing autism, detecting risk factors, and personalizing intervention plans.

One primary reason machine learning revolutionizes clinical practices is its ability to process and analyze complex, multidimensional datasets beyond human capabilities (Kok & Ozdemir, 2022). Traditional methods often struggle with vast amounts of data generated by behavioral and developmental observations, electronic health records, imaging modalities, eye tracking, and genomic studies. Machine learning algorithms, on the other hand, can uncover hidden patterns and relationships within these datasets, providing valuable insights for early risk assessment and diagnosis (Thabtah & Peebles, 2020). For example, machine learning-powered systems have shown remarkable accuracy in detecting autism in very young children, helping to reduce the time required for diagnosis and enhancing precision.

Machine learning algorithms vary significantly in their capabilities and applications. Simple models, such as Linear Regression, Decision Trees, and Naive Bayes, are often preferred for their ease of interpretation and straightforward application in solving basic classification or regression problems. However, to achieve high accuracy in complex tasks, more advanced models like deep learning, Random Forests, and Gradient Boosting are favored due to their ability to analyze intricate patterns in large datasets effectively. Two primary objectives guide the design and application of machine learning models: (I) achieving high accuracy and (II) ensuring interpretability to prevent the model from being perceived as a black-box (Yildirim et al., 2024). However, a trade-off often exists between these objectives. As machine learning models become more complex to enhance accuracy, their interpretability tends to decrease. This trade-off is particularly noticeable in advanced models such as deep learning, random forests, and gradient-boosting methods, surpassing simpler models like linear regression, decision trees, and Naive Bayes regarding predictive accuracy (Yildirim et al., 2024). Despite their power, these complex models lack transparency, preventing users from understanding how decisions are made and leaving them unaware of the specific factors influencing the model's predictions (ElShawi et al., 2021). For example, in clinical studies, decision-support models require accurate predictions and explanations for the decisions made. These professionals must provide accurate and transparent reasons for diagnosing young children, often necessitating detailed explanations such as "symptom lists" for diagnostic decisions.

Interpretable Machine Learning (IML) has emerged as a solution to address black-box models' challenges (Adadi et al., 2018; Yildirim et al., 2024). It facilitates explanations and illustrates the behavior of machine learning models, offering clearer insights into how these models make predictions. Interpretable Machine Learning models are broadly categorized into intrinsic and agnostic models. Intrinsic models, such as Decision Trees and Lasso are inherently interpretable due to their design. In contrast, agnostic methods, such as SHAPley Additive exPlanations (SHAP) (Nohara et al., 2022), Local Interpretable Model-agnostic Explanations (LIME) (Man & Chan, 2021; Zhu et al., 2022), Explain Like I'm 5 (ELI5) (Gurbuz et al., 2023), and Type-2 Fuzzy Regression (T2FR) (Zare et al., 2022) are designed to explain the decisions of any machine learning model regardless of its complexity. By bridging the gap between performance and interpretability, Interpretable Machine Learning methods enable users to trust and better understand machine learning models, making them particularly valuable in domains like clinical assessments where decision transparency is crucial (ElShawi et al., 2021).

Overall, despite its potential, the integration of machine learning into clinical practices still presents significant challenges. Model transparency, data quality, and accessibility remain critical issues, as autism data is often undefined, unrelated to autism symptoms, incomplete, or inconsistent across many studies. Additionally, methodological concerns such as algorithmic bias and decision validity must be addressed to ensure fair and transparent decision-making. However, these challenges also create opportunities for collaboration among researchers, clinicians, data scientists, and policymakers to develop robust frameworks that facilitate the responsible use of machine learning in clinical autism assessments. As machine learning continues to evolve, its applications in clinical assessments are expected to expand, driving innovations in autism risk assessments, diagnostic assessments, and individualized interventions. By addressing current challenges and leveraging its transformative potential, machine learning continues to provide the evolving potential to redefine the future of clinical practices, making autism clinical assessments faster, more efficient, precise, and centered around the needs of children.

This chapter explores the transformative role of machine learning in clinical autism assessments, beginning with an introduction to its fundamental concepts and its impact on improving autism risk assessments, diagnostic accuracy, and individualized interventions. The distinctions between machine learning and deep learning algorithms are critically analyzed. Furthermore, the discussion addresses the primary machine learning paradigms, supervised, unsupervised, semi-supervised, and reinforcement learning, highlighting their specific applications in diagnosis, clustering, anomaly detection, and optimizing intervention strategies. The chapter outlines the workflow of developing machine learning models for clinical use, including data collection, preprocessing, feature engineering, training, and validation, while also emphasizing the importance of performance metrics such as accuracy, sensitivity, specificity, and F1 score in evaluating model reliability. Challenges associated with research data, such as missing information and unqualified data, are addressed to overcome these issues. A section on explainability and interpretability explores methodologies such as SHAP (Nohara et al., 2022), LIME (Man & Chan, 2021; Zhu et al., 2022), ELI5 (Gurbuz et al., 2023), and T2FR (Zare et al., 2022) aimed at ensuring the transparency and trustworthiness of machine learning models employed in clinical autism applications. Moreover, real-world examples, such as autism detection and risk identification research, show the practical impact of machine learning in the clinical domain. Lastly, this chapter explores future trends such as federated learning, multimodal machine learning systems, the Internet of Things (IoT), and the integration of Natural Language Processing (NLP), providing valuable insights into the evolving body of literature regarding the application of machine learning in clinical practice. The chapter concludes with a discussion on the ongoing potential of these technologies to revolutionize the assessment of autism practices.

Machine Learning and Deep Learning

Developing effective machine learning models remains an evolving research domain, along with AI models that involve deep learning. An important method of machine learning is deep learning. Deep learning is a subfield of machine learning that employs multilayer artificial neural networks to reveal hidden relationships in complex and high-dimensional datasets that may be imperceptible to human capacity (Bzdok & Meyer-Lindenberg, 2018; Jordan & Mitchell, 2015). Both methods show significant potential in clinical studies for identifying complex health conditions without a single cause and/or symptom profile that cannot be diagnosed through definitive medical tests. In recent years, machine learning and deep learning have been increasingly applied in autism research to design highly precise and predictable decision support systems while reducing human involvement in large data. These studies, in general, aim to create fast and accurate diagnostic decision support systems and shorten the duration of the diagnostic process.

The primary difference between the machine learning and deep learning models lies in the complexity of the model and data requirements. Machine learning models are simpler, faster to train, and more effective with smaller datasets. In contrast, deep learning models require large datasets and significant computational resources but can analyze complex and unstructured data to identify unseen patterns. Machine learning might be preferred for tasks using small behavioral datasets, whereas deep learning would be ideal for analyzing high-dimensional data like videos or imaging in research studies. Support Vector Machines (SVM), Decision Trees, and Random Forests are the most commonly used machine learning algorithms in autism studies (Ozdemir et al., 2022). On the other hand, deep learning is a specialized subset of machine learning that uses neural networks with multiple layers to extract features from raw data automatically. Unlike traditional machine learning, deep learning models learn hierarchies of features directly from large data, eliminating the need for manual feature engineering. Specifically, deep learning models can analyze raw research data or images to identify feature patterns associated with autism diagnosis, learning from the data itself without predefined inputs. Techniques like Convolutional Neural Networks (CNNs) are particularly effective for these tasks. In summary, while machine learning and deep learning aim to identify patterns and make predictions, machine learning depends on feature engineering and simpler models. In contrast, deep learning leverages advanced neural networks to learn directly from raw data, providing powerful tools for complex problems.

The Machine Learning Workflow in Clinical Studies

Machine learning models are computational systems designed to learn patterns from data and make predictions or decisions, adapting their performance based on the input they process (Arrieta et al., 2020). Unlike traditional algorithms that rely on predefined rules, machine learning models generalize from examples, enabling them to analyze complex problems across various domains. Developing a machine learning model involves a systematic workflow to ensure accuracy and interpretability. It begins with data collection, where relevant raw data is gathered pertaining to the problem. Next, data preprocessing is applied to clean the dataset by handling missing values, normalizing feature scales, and removing outliers. Dimensionality reduction techniques may also be used during this phase to simplify the dataset while preserving essential information. This structured process forms the foundation for implementing effective and interpretable machine learning models.

Feature selection is carried out to identify the most relevant variables using techniques like Recursive Feature Elimination (RFE) or LASSO regression, enhancing model interpretability and reducing complexity. The model selection phase involves choosing an appropriate algorithm, such as Random Forest, Support Vector Machines (SVM), or Gradient Boosting, based on the problem type (e.g., classification, regression) and data characteristics (Han et al., 2012). Once the model is selected, training and validation follow, where the dataset is split into training and validation sets or subjected to k-fold cross-validation. This step involves iterative parameter tuning and performance assessment using metrics such as accuracy and precision. In the testing phase, the model is evaluated on unseen data to determine its generalization capabilities, ensuring robustness against overfitting. An important step in machine learning models is interpretability, where methods like SHAP or LIME are applied to explain how individual features contribute to predictions, making the model's decisions transparent. Finally, the model deployment phase integrates the trained and validated model into practical systems for real-world clinical applications. The process ensures a comprehensive workflow adaptable to various clinical uses, extending beyond decision support systems into broader machine learning applications.

Types of Machine Learning and Their Clinical Applications

Machine learning involves four primary types of learning paradigms, supervised, unsupervised, semi-supervised, and reinforcement learning, each designed for specific data structures and problem domains (Shalev-Shwartz & Ben-David, 2014). Supervised learning is widely used in problems where labeled data is available, making it ideal for classification (e.g., autism diagnosis) and regression (e.g., predicting developmental scores based on behavioral features). In this approach, the model is trained on data that includes both input features (e.g., behavioral or developmental scale scores) and their corresponding labels (e.g., "autism" or "non-autism"). The goal is to learn a mapping between inputs and outputs, enabling accurate predictions for new, unseen data. For example, a supervised model can be trained on eye-tracking data labeled as "autism" or "non-autism" to classify new samples. Supervised learning techniques, such as Support Vector Machines (SVM) or Decision Trees, are especially effective for classification tasks and can achieve high accuracy when a sufficient amount of labeled data is available (Han et al., 2012).

Unsupervised learning is implemented when labeled data is unavailable, focusing instead on discovering hidden patterns or structures within the data. This approach seeks to uncover hidden patterns or structures in unlabeled data, such as clustering children into subgroups based on similar behavioral, physiological, or developmental features (Sun et al., 2024). For instance, an unsupervised model can identify clusters of children with similar eye movement patterns, potentially revealing subgroups among children with autism and non-autism. Techniques related to clustering or dimensionality reduction assist in revealing relationships that may not be immediately evident, providing new insights into the data.

Semi-supervised learning bridges the gap between labeled and unlabeled data by leveraging a small amount of labeled data alongside a larger set of unlabeled data. This approach is especially useful in clinical assessments, where labeling can be costly or time-consuming. It represents a hybrid machine learning strategy that employs both labeled and unlabeled data for training, typically with a small amount of labeled data and a large amount of unlabeled data. This method leverages the labeled data to guide the model while using the structure or distribution of the unlabeled data to improve generalization and performance. By reducing the dependence on costly labeled datasets, semi-supervised learning is particularly valuable in applications such as medical imaging, speech recognition, and text classification, where obtaining labeled data is expensive or time-intensive.

Finally, reinforcement learning is a dynamic decision-making system in which an agent learns optimal actions through a reward-based mechanism, such as the optimization of individualized intervention plans over time (Shalev-Shwartz & Ben-David, 2014). Reinforcement learning represents a fundamentally different paradigm in which an agent learns to make decisions by interacting with an environment and receiving feedback through rewards or penalties (Kok & Ozdemir, 2022). In the context of autism research, reinforcement learning can be used to develop individualized intervention systems. For instance, a virtual agent might engage with children in a controlled environment, adjusting its behavior to maximize engagement or promote social interactions. Over time, the agent learns an optimal strategy based on the feedback, providing a dynamic and adaptive approach to problem-solving. AI programs like ChatGPT and GEMINI exemplify reinforcement learning. These paradigms collectively address various challenges within machine learning workflows, enabling researchers and practitioners to develop advanced solutions based on data availability and desired outcomes of the model.

When developing a decision support system model using machine learning, selecting the appropriate learning paradigm is critical and typically determined early in the process. The decision depends on the nature of the data and the problem to solve. Supervised learning is applied from the model selection stage, as the labeled data guides the training, validation, and testing of predictive models. In contrast, during feature selection or data preprocessing, unsupervised learning can be utilized earlier in the process to identify hidden patterns, reduce dimensionality, or cluster data into meaningful groups. Semi-supervised learning integrates labeled and unlabeled data, making it suitable for training and validation, especially in clinical assessments where acquiring labeled data is expensive or time-consuming. While less common in clinical decision support systems, reinforcement learning may be employed in dynamic environments, such as optimizing intervention strategies based on evolving intervention data, and is typically introduced after the model selection phase. These learning paradigms are strategically incorporated into different stages of the machine learning workflow to ensure the system's accuracy, interpretability, and practicality for real-world applications.

Performance Metrics for Machine Learning Models

In machine learning research, performance metrics such as accuracy, sensitivity, specificity, and F1 score are commonly employed to evaluate the effectiveness of classification models, particularly in applications like identifying children with autism from non-autistic children (Ozdemir et al., 2022). Accuracy reflects the overall proportion of correct predictions involving autism and non-autistic classifications. It is calculated as the sum of true positives (TP) and true negatives (TN) divided by the total number of samples. However, while accuracy provides a general measure of machine learning performance, it can be misleading in class imbalance cases where one category (e.g., non-autistic) is overrepresented. To address this limitation, sensitivity and specificity offer more detailed insights into model performance. Sensitivity, or the true positive rate, measures the ability of the model to identify individuals with autism correctly, calculated as the proportion of true positives among all actual autism cases (TP/(TP + FN)). This metric is critical in contexts where failing to identify children with autism (false negatives) could delay crucial early interventions. In contrast, specificity, or the true negative rate, quantifies the model's ability to correctly classify non-autistic children, defined as the proportion of true negatives among all actual non-autistic cases (TN/(TN + FP)). High specificity is essential to minimize false positives, which can lead to further testing and misallocated resources.

Lastly, the F1 score is a performance metric used in machine learning to evaluate the accuracy of a classification model, particularly in cases where the dataset is imbalanced (e.g., one class significantly outnumbers another). It balances precision and recall, making it a helpful metric when false positives and negatives must be minimized. The F1 score is calculated as the harmonic mean of precision (the proportion of true positives among predicted positives) and recall (the proportion of true positives among actual positives). The precision is the proportion of true positive predictions out of all positive predictions made by the model, and recall (also called

Table 1 *A sample scenario for a machine learning model applied to 100 children with autism spectrum disorder (ASD) and non-ASD children*

True Class	Predicted: ASD	Predicted: Non-ASD
ASD	30 (TP)	10 (FN)
Non-ASD	5 (FP)	55 (TN)

sensitivity) is the proportion of true positives identified out of all actual positive cases.

In a sample scenario (As shown in Table 1), one can consider a machine learning model applied to a dataset of 100 children, including 40 children with autism and 60 non-autistic children. If the model correctly identifies 30 children with autism (TP) while misclassifying 10 (false negatives) and correctly classifies 55 non-autistic children (TN) with 5 false positives (FP), the resulting metrics would include an accuracy of 85%, a sensitivity of 75%, a specificity of 91.67%, and a F1 score of 79.9%. These metrics indicate the balance between identifying true children with autism and avoiding misclassification of non-autistic children, indicating the importance of sensitivity and specificity in assessing the practical utility of machine learning models in autism screening. Overall, an 85% accuracy score indicates the overall performance of the machine learning model, but it doesn't distinguish between children with autism and non-autistic classification quality. The 75% sensitivity score reveals that 75% of children with autism were correctly identified, but 25% of children (FN) were missed. Additionally, the 91.67% specificity score shows that the model is very effective at identifying non-ASD children, with only a small proportion misclassified as autism. Finally, the F1 score of 79.9% reflects that the model achieves a good balance, as it can effectively identify true positives while keeping misclassifications relatively low. Thus, in machine learning research, particularly in classification tasks like identifying children with autism versus non-autistic children, metrics like accuracy, sensitivity, specificity, and F1 score are crucial for evaluating the model's performance.

Explainability and Interpretability of Machine Learning Models in Clinical Applications

In recent years, machine learning and deep learning studies for supporting early autism diagnosis have increased significantly. Specifically, an analysis of research trends indicates that traditional machine learning methods were more common in the past, while studies employing deep learning models have increased lately. These studies show promise for early autism diagnosis by enhancing risk assessment accuracy and specificity. However, the "black box" nature of certain machine learning and deep learning models complicates understanding how and why these models make decisions (Arrieta et al., 2020). This lack of transparency in the models' decision-making processes presents significant challenges to trust and acceptance, particularly in clinical settings. This issue diminishes confidence in the model's outputs, exposes inherent biases, and ultimately impedes the integration of machine learning applications into critical fields.

This lack of transparency poses a critical problem in fields like autism assessments, where understanding the outcomes and the decision-making process behind them is essential. When diagnosing a young child with autism, both professionals and parents need clarity on which factors contributed to the autism diagnosis to make informed intervention decisions. Without such insights, misdiagnoses or ineffective interventions can lead to severe consequences and ethical problems. The increasing dimensionality of datasets and the growing number of features in machine learning problems have also led to the prominence of Feature Selection methods (Li et al., 2017). Feature Selection preprocesses data to reduce the number of features, thereby improving interpretability to some extent. However, this reduction often comes at the cost of data loss, which may decrease the overall accuracy of the machine learning model (Chandrashekar et., 2014).

Interpretable Machine Learning has emerged as a solution to address this issue, enhancing the transparency of complex machine learning models while maintaining their performance (Arrieta et al., 2020). Interpretable Machine Learning techniques enable users to understand and trust machine learning models by providing local interpretability (understanding individual predictions) and global interpretability (understanding the model as a whole). They offer insights into how decisions are reached, increasing transparency, trust, and validity in applications in clinical decision-making (Yildirim-Okay et al., 2021). Unlike Feature Selection techniques, which focus on reducing the dimensionality of data before training to enhance interpretability (often at the cost of accuracy), Interpretable Machine Learning methods focus on explaining model behavior during or after training. This enables a deeper understanding of how features influence the outcomes.

Interpretable Machine Learning methods can be categorized into intrinsic and agnostic models (Yildirim-Okay et al., 2021). Intrinsic methods, such as Decision Trees and Lasso, are inherently interpretable due to their structure, while agnostic methods, including SHAP, LIME, and ELI5 and are designed to explain the behavior of any model regardless of its complexity. Agnostic Interpretable Machine Learning methods are particularly valuable as they allow post-hoc interpretability without compromising the model's performance.

More specifically, Explainable Artificial Intelligence models, such as SHAP and LIME, have become essential tools for addressing the lack of transparency in complex machine learning models like Random Forest (RF) and Gradient Boosting (GB) (Yildirim et al., 2024). These methods are particularly important in clinical studies, where understanding the reasoning behind predictions is critical for building trust and ensuring informed decision-making. SHAP quantifies the contribution of each feature to a model's prediction, enabling users to pinpoint which factors were most influential. Similarly, LIME creates interpretable local surrogate models around individual predictions, simplifying the decision-making process for specific cases. For example, in an autism diagnosis study, these methods can clarify which clinical variables played a decisive role in the diagnosis. SHAP can rank these factors by importance, while LIME provides a localized explanation for a particular prediction. This information helps clinicians verify the model's reasoning and ensures that patients understand the basis for their diagnosis and intervention plan. By bridging the gap between model performance and interpretability, SHAP and LIME make complex algorithms more transparent and reliable, ultimately enhancing the adoption of machine learning in high-stakes domains like healthcare.

Overall, in domains like autism assessments, where decisions significantly impact human life, the opacity of a model's decision is a critical concern. For example, clinicians using machine learning models for risk assessments or intervention planning require clear explanations of how the model arrived at its conclusions. In the context of clinical assessments, Explainable Artificial Intelligence enable both local and global interpretability, empowering clinicians to understand individual predictions and broader model behaviors (As shown in Fig. 1). These methods foster trust, reliability, and transparency, ensuring that machine learning-based decisions align with ethical standards. Thus, a promising line of research as mentioned before, has started to accumulate regarding the application of Explainable Artificial Intelligence methods.

A study by Garg et al. (2022) suggested that autism classification was achieved by integrating the deep learning model with Explainable Artificial Intelligence methods. Initially, the researchers developed a four-layer DL model and applied it to the autism screening dataset for classification purposes. Subsequently, the SHAP method was used to identify the most effective features in this classification process. The system's performance was evaluated through case studies using various datasets, achieving a maximum classification accuracy of 98%. When using only the features identified as effective by SHAP, an accuracy of 79% was attained. The presented hybrid model significantly contributed to the early detection of autism. Magboo et al. (2022) also implemented machine learning models to classify children with autism. Nine different machine learning models were utilized in the application. Among these models, Logistic Regression (LR), Support Vector Machine (SVM), and AdaBoost achieved accuracy rates ranging from 99% to 100%. An analysis using LIME facilitated the identification of both relevant and irrelevant features, demonstrating that Explainable Artificial Intelligence contributes to the reliability of autism detection. In addition, Torres et al. (2023) used a pre-trained CNN model to identify key clinical features for ASD diagnosis. EEG data were converted into 2D images as input for deep learning. The ROAR method assessed the reliability of Explainable Artificial Intelligence techniques in detecting EEG features related to facial emotion classification in TD and autistic individuals. Feature importance was estimated using LRP, PatternNet, and Smooth-Grad Squared. Furthermore, Atlam et al. (2024) developed an Explainable Artificial Intelligence-based deep learning model for early autism detection. Tested on an autism dataset, the model achieved 98% accuracy. SHAP analysis highlighted key features influencing predictions and enhancing interpretability. This approach improved both autism detection accuracy and decision transparency.

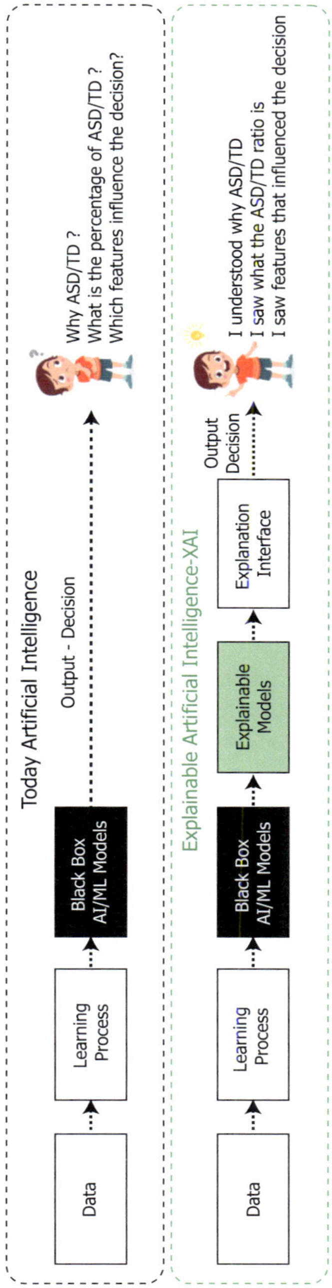

Fig. 1 Figure depicting difference between the Artificial Intelligence and Explainable Artificial Intelligence-XAI models

Moreover, beyond the high performance of algorithms and models, Explainable Artificial Intelligence research provides insights into which features or data significantly impact predictions in decision-making. In autism research, for example, Bargagna et al. (2024) developed an explainable deep learning framework that merges a Bayesian Neural Network (BNN) with an Explainable Artificial Intelligence methodology to classify participants with autism using resting-state functional magnetic resonance imaging (rs-fMRI) data. Their proposed framework leveraged the BNN's capabilities to make predictions and provide insights into model reliability. Biswas et al. (2021) sought to clarify the importance of features in model decisions through correlation and hierarchical visualization, applying Interpretable Machine Learning methods to a support vector machine (SVM) model for early autism diagnosis in children. The researchers highlighted the significance of transparency and explainability in fostering clinicians' trust in AI models and ensuring the ethical and responsible deployment of AI in clinical assessments. In another study, Hilal et al. (2022) introduced an Interpretable Machine Learning-based autism diagnosis model (IML-ASD) that utilized Bacterial Foraging Optimization (BFO) to select optimal feature subsets and a Deep Belief Network (DBN) enhanced with the Whale Optimization Algorithm (WOA) for classification. Similarly, Jeon et al. (2024) developed various models including Random Forest (RF), SVM, Gradient Boosting Machine (GBM), XGBoost, C5.0, neural networks (NNET), k-nearest neighbors (k-NN), and logistic regression (LR)-for pediatric autism diagnosis using the "Autism Spectrum Disorder-ASD Child Characteristics" dataset, which involves a wide range of behavioral and demographic features. To enhance the transparency of models and their clinical interpretability, the researchers utilized Interpretable Machine Learning methodologies, including permutation feature importance (PFI), LIME, and SHAP, to elucidate the most effective models identified as Gradient Boosting Machines (GBM), XGBoost, and others NNET.

The accuracy of machine learning is highly dependent on the features used to construct the dataset. Therefore, feature selection is critical in improving the accuracy of machine learning models. Numerous studies within the existing literature, including studies by Garg et al. (2022) and Atlam et al. (2024), use behavioral data to classify autism in real-world contexts. In contrast, other studies, such as Sujana et al. (2023), focus on behavioral data that require specialized clinical training for the early diagnosis of autism indicators. The Autism Diagnostic Observation Schedule (ADOS) and the Autism Diagnostic Interview-Revised (ADI-R) are complex, time-intensive assessment tools that can only be administered by clinical experts who have received specialized training and possess the necessary materials. However, the utility of autism classification based on data obtained through these specialized assessments may diminish if families do not have access to these evaluations in a timely manner. Despite recent AI and machine learning advancements for autism assessment, challenges persist in developing effective and interpretable machine learning methodologies for detecting autism. Conventional machine learning models often depend on manual feature selection, which limits the discovery of new biomarkers and reduces diagnostic effectiveness. Additionally, many machine learning models function as "black boxes," offering limited transparency regarding their decision-making processes, which poses significant challenges in the healthcare sector. Overall, understanding the reasoning behind a diagnostic decision is crucial for the clinical application of these methodologies as valid and reliable tools.

Despite the advancements, studies on Explainable Artificial Intelligence in autism research remain limited and primarily focus on data such as surveys, medical records, and genetic information. Moreover, a significant gap exists in applying Explainable Artificial Intelligence techniques to early autism assessment studies. Therefore, further research on Explainable Artificial Intelligence is crucial to enhancing trust and transparency in machine learning and deep learning research regarding clinical autism assessments.

Applications of Machine Learning Models and Data-Related Problems in Autism Research

Machine learning plays a significant role in autism risk assessment and treatment, helping researchers and clinicians categorize young children based on the severity of autism symptoms or co-occurring disorders. These models can prioritize cases by analyzing easily obtainable data, such as physiological, behavioral, developmental, and parent-reported data or early developmental milestones. Machine learning-based decision support systems can process large datasets to detect subtle signs of autism earlier than traditional diagnostic methods, facilitating timely interventions that are critical in early childhood. Indeed, a growing number of studies have been published on autism classification and prediction (Akin-Bulbul et al., 2024; Ozdemir et al., 2022; Stahl et al., 2012; Zhou et al., 2024). A review by Hyde et al. (2019) highlighted the extensive use of supervised machine learning algorithms, particularly Support Vector Machines (SVM) and Decision Trees, across 45 studies. Furthermore, a study by Monarca et al. (2023) discussed that the quality and quantity of data are vital when developing diagnostic support systems. Given that training machine learning models requires substantial amounts of data, one might assume that the performance of the proposed models may initially be less than ideal due to limited initial datasets. Monarca focused on evaluating limited data (from 122 children with autism and non-autistic children) from a research experiment on participants' interactions with screens and demonstrated that significant results could be achieved in autism classification.

Even though machine learning holds significant potential for improving autism assessment methodologies, substantial data-related challenges limit its effectiveness. A major concern is the lack of detailed and comprehensive developmental and behavioral data in studies involving individuals diagnosed with autism. Critical information, such as autism symptom severity, cognitive or language functioning, and comorbid psychiatric conditions, is often missing or not adequately addressed in datasets. Another significant limitation is the wide age range of participants in studies. Data collected from individuals aged from toddlerhood to adult years encompasses a broad developmental spectrum, making it difficult to draw consistent conclusions about the neurodevelopmental nature of autism. Moreover, early childhood represents a critical period for the identification of early signs of autism, as timely diagnosis and intervention possess the greatest potential to enhance outcomes. Additionally, a significant challenge concerning datasets is their heavy reliance on parent-reported observations and survey responses, which, while valuable, are inherently subjective and susceptible to bias. This issue may result in inconsistencies within study findings and undermine the reliability of machine learning models. In fact, a recent review conducted by Jordan and Mitchell (2015) systematically evaluated artificial intelligence methods and datasets employed in autism research. The researchers indicated that the majority of studies have not concentrated on physiological or behavioral data, but rather on questionnaire-based datasets such as the Modified Checklist for Autism in Toddlers (M-CHAT).

Furthermore, the data used in some studies may focus on specific tasks or measures, such as motor activities, that are neither symptomatically nor theoretically connected to autism diagnosis. Consequently, these datasets do not effectively capture the essential developmental and behavioral characteristics needed for accurately identifying or understanding autism. For example, Crippa et al. (2015) proposed a machine learning framework to classify low-functioning children with autism based on kinematic analysis of a simple reach-to-drop task. Although motor coordination issues can relate to various neurodevelopmental disorders, including autism, one may question the study's results if the researchers included participants with only motor development disorders. Thus, oversimplified data that are not directly related to autism symptoms, along with insufficient information about data properties and participant characteristics, contribute to skeptical views on the application of machine learning models in the autism field.

It is important to note that a large majority of studies published in the engineering field aim to develop effective machine learning models. A critical concern regarding these studies, which has dominated the machine learning field for many years, involves their purely methodological nature that seeks to evolve machine learning algorithms and design more efficient decision support systems. Much of this research line primarily uses open-access data, often overlooking data properties and participant characteristics. On the other hand, many machine learning studies have focused to explore novel physiological and behavioral data to identify autism markers. For instance, Sarabadani et al. (2020) examined autonomic responses in children with autism using physiological measurements, while Babu et al. (2021) analyzed facial expressions of toddlers with autism and typically developing (TD) controls, identifying significant differences in participant responses. Furthermore, Varsha and Maheswari (2024) utilized facial images to classify autism by implementing a deep learning-based model. Initially, the VGG19, Densenet121, and InceptionV3 CNN models were employed for feature extraction. The data containing these extracted features were subsequently classified using a Deep Neural Network (DNN) model. Densenet121 achieved the highest accuracy score of 96.66% among the tested models. The study's findings emphasized the importance of facial features in detecting autism. Similarly, Kang et al. (2023) developed a deep learning model for autism classification using facial images, emphasizing explainability. Utilizing the Autism-Image-Data dataset (comprising 2940 images), the researchers applied MobileNet, Xception, EfficientNet, and an Ensemble Model. Grad-CAM was employed to highlight image regions that influence predictions, thus enhancing interpretability. The Ensemble Model achieved the highest accuracy of 89%, demonstrating the effectiveness of facial feature extraction for autism detection with Explainable Machine Learning. Despite the reported high accuracy rates, the use of facial images or physiological data for autism classification lacks theoretical support and rationale within the field of autism research.

Some researchers argue that machine learning models need to optimize resources in clinical and research settings, ensuring that young children with the most urgent needs receive attention promptly (Abbas et al., 2018; Kosmicki et al., 2015). This is particularly relevant in contexts where access to diagnostic tools, such as the ADOS, is limited by cost or availability of trained specialists. For example, Kosmicki et al. (2015) utilized data sets obtained from the ADOS Module 2 and Module 3, a clinical observation tool considered the gold standard for autism assessment. They identified 9 and 12 distinguishing items from Modules 2 and 3, respectively, and applied Alternating Decision Trees (DT), Logistic Model Trees, SVM, Naïve Bayes, and Random Forest algorithms to train the dataset. Their findings demonstrated that the sensitivity of these algorithms in distinguishing autism ranged between 96% and 98%, while specificity varied between 87% and 98%. Similarly, in another study, Duda et al. (2014) used machine learning to train a classifier that can reduce 72% in length in the ADOS-G test with 97% accuracy. Abbas et al. (2018) focused on a different type of data rather than eye-tracking and applied machine learning to data collected through the ADI-R, which is completed based on clinical interviews with parents. In their study, 20 features were selected from a total of 155, and the Random Forest algorithm was applied for autism assessment. Using area under the curve (AUC), recall (sensitivity), and precision (specificity) as evaluation metrics, the researchers reported performance rates of 95%, 98%, and 64%, respectively.

Moreover, a recent study by Sujana and Augustine (2023) reported an autism accuracy rate of 91.37% for their machine learning-based autism diagnosis model. The study examined the design of an Interpretable Machine Learning model to provide reliable symptom information for predicting the model's outcomes. The researchers utilized the ABIDE-1 dataset, which included 1114 records of autistic and non-autistic children. Various test scores were analyzed in the study, such as the ADI-R and the ADOS results, along with the children's performance IQ, verbal IQ, and full IQ scores. Similarly, using the ABIDE-1 dataset, Sujana and Augustine (2023) proposed an interpretable Deep Neural Network (DNN) model for classifying autism. The model achieved an accuracy rate of 93.27% in autism classification. Post-hoc explainability methods, including LIME, SHAP, and Anchors, were utilized to clarify the impact of specific features, enhancing the model's interpretability. Given that the ADI and the ADOS instruments are extensively acknowledged as the gold standards for the assessment of autism, it is anticipated that they yield high accuracy rates due to their high sensitivity to early symptoms of autism. In fact, Karuppasamy et al. (2022) conducted an examination of the efficacy of a Convolutional Neural Network (CNN) model in diagnosing autism utilizing the ABIDE dataset, subsequently reporting an accuracy score of 95%.

In conclusion, although machine learning models trained on the ADOS data often report impressive performance metrics, the practical utility of these studies is limited. The application of the ADOS requires trained experts, significant time, and financial resources, making it inaccessible to many children and their parents. Furthermore, using a reduced number of the ADOS items requires scientific evidence and rationale to explain the autism symptomatology in the early years. To address these issues, it is crucial for future research to prioritize the inclusion of objective, symptomatically relevant data and to focus on creating cost-effective data solutions that bridge gaps in access to specialized diagnostic tools.

Eye-Tracking Research in Machine Learning

One of the most important aspects of developing effective machine learning models is the data required to train and support the models. One novel technology providing real-time physiological data is eye-tracking technology. Due to its non-invasive and user-friendly nature, this technology has gained popularity in various research fields, including autism (Akin-Bulbul et al., 2023; 2024; Jones et al., 2013; Ozdemir et al., 2022, 2024). Eye-tracking technology allows researchers to observe young children's visual attention from an early age, providing detailed sensory information about one of the primary symptoms of autism, reduced social visual attention (Jones et al., 2013; Ozdemir et al., 2024; Ozturk et al., 2024). Indeed, visual attention has been a key symptom domain of autism since Kanner's (1943) original definition, and at-risk children are assessed clinically for their reduced social visual attention. However, because eye movement data is highly complex and multidimensional, analyzing this intricate data with traditional statistical methods can be quite challenging. As eye-tracking technology provides more than 30 types of eye movement data, researchers must select only a limited number of data types for analysis using traditional statistical methods. Conversely, the data used to train and support machine learning algorithms is critically important, and eye-tracking data contributes to the development of artificial intelligence models by providing large, multidimensional data sets. Thus, the application of machine learning in studies using eye-tracking data is recognized as a promising pathway for addressing autism risk assessment problems in young children.

Most researchers used machine learning and/or deep learning algorithms to design decision-support models for autism diagnosis. Within the most current studies, research conducted with toddlers with autism provides critically important findings. For example,

in a recent study, Ozdemir et al. (2022) developed a visual attention-based decision support system and analyzed the usability of various machine learning models, including Decision Trees, Naïve Bayes, Random Forests, and Support Vector Machines. The researchers employed a passive viewing paradigm with stimuli consisting of social interaction scenes on one side of the screen and dynamic animations or toys with light and sound on the other side. The study results indicated an 87% accuracy rate in identifying toddlers with autism. The findings suggest the potential of visual attention and eye movement data in classifying toddlers with autism, which significantly enhances machine learning-based decision support systems in this field.

Furthermore, Chanyoung et al. (2022) examined the effects of toddlers' joint attention difficulties in autism classification. The study used video recordings of toddlers' joint attention behavior as model input data. The developed neural network model architecture was built on two main algorithms, LSTM and CNN. The CNN extracted features from each frame in the videos and fed the LSTM. The LSTM performed a classification using the features provided by the CNN model and distinguished whether children have autism or not. Consistent with the previous evidence (Ozdemir et al., 2024), joint attention stimuli and the machine learning model yielded 94.5% accuracy, providing evidence for using joint attention visual stimuli to detect early autism. In another recent machine learning study, Akin-Bulbul et al. (2024) explored the predictive power of machine learning on eye-tracking data of toddlers with autism and TD toddlers (a total of 124 participants aged 18 months and 36 months). Using video stimuli that reflect emotions, the researchers reported that the KNN classification algorithm demonstrated the highest classification success when applied to videos depicting a neutral emotional state. The KNN algorithm achieved a classification success rate of 81.45% for toddlers with autism.

Moreover, Fernandez-Lanvin et al. (2024) investigated the feasibility of a machine learning-based autism screening prototype for toddlers under 24 months of age. The researchers created various videos to assess toddlers' social information gaze exchanges and gaze following. After developing the screening model, at-risk participants viewed short movies, and infants classified as positive for autism using the random forest algorithm were referred to early intervention services. Random Forests had the highest mean area under curve (AUC), the lowest standard deviation, and statistically outperformed most of the algorithms. Children's diagnoses were confirmed when they were typically around three years of age. This machine learning-supported, eye-tracking-based early screening method demonstrated significant progress in detecting early autism by AUC results exceeding 95%. In another eye-tracking study, Alarifi et al. (2023) investigated atypical visual attention patterns of participants with autism (a total of 130 participants with age range between 22 months and 22 years) when watching human and animal faces and eye visuals in joint attention tasks. Study findings showed that the Random Forest algorithms effectively identified participants with autism.

The existing literature includes studies on eye-tracking and machine learning that involve mixed-age groups of participants. Franco et al. (2023) explored the usability of Random Forest algorithms within Artificial Neural Networks using visual attention models and reported the strong performance of Random Forest algorithms over traditional machine learning methods for classifying individuals with autism and non-autistic individuals (a total of 77 participants aged between 3 and 16 years). Wan et al. (2019) identified ten different Areas of Interests (AOIs) based on eye-tracking data, including the background, hair, eyes, and mouth regions. Using a support vector machine (SVM) algorithm with five-fold cross-validation, they analyzed the impact of fixation duration in distinguishing children with autism from TD children, applying sensitivity, specificity, and accuracy metrics. Their findings indicated that fixation duration achieved a sensitivity of 81%, a specificity of 80%, and an accuracy of 82% in differentiating children with autism from TD children.

Several eye-tracking and machine learning studies in the literature have been conducted with adults diagnosed with autism. In a recent study, Khalaji et al. (2023) collected eye-tracking data from adult participants while they completed web-based tasks. The researchers explored how the data measurement process and data quality influence the performance of machine learning algorithms. Their proposed model demonstrated that data quality was crucial for classification performance when identifying autism using cleaned data. Similarly, Yaneva et al. (2018, 2020) examined differences in eye movements among adults participants with autism engaged in web-based search tasks (browsing and searching on web pages) using Random Forest classifiers, revealing eye-tracking parameters for autism classification. Overall, even though the above studies highlighted the development of machine learning models in classifying participants with autism with high accuracy using eye-tracking data, participants' ages should be considered cautiously as they do not reflect early diagnostic years.

Additionally, recent studies systematically explore the best algorithms for distinguishing children with autism from their typically developing peers, focusing on achieving the highest classification performance. Zhao et al. (2021) examined the classification performance of eye-tracking data collected during face-to-face interactions in distinguishing children with autism from TD children. The researchers applied advanced feature selection techniques to optimize classification accuracy and determine the most relevant features, utilizing SVM, Linear Discriminant Analysis (LDA), Decision Tree (DT), and Random Forest algorithms. Their results demonstrated that combining features related to visual fixation and session duration using the SVM classifier led to a classification accuracy of 92.31%. Other studies, such as Akter et al. (2021), have evaluated various machine learning algorithms on scan path images, revealing that the Multilayer Perceptron exhibited the highest accuracy at 87%. However, these studies often lacked information on the experimental stimuli that influenced children with autism and non-autistic children's eye movement patterns.

In eye-tracking and machine learning-focused research, some researchers have examined the role of avoiding direct eye contact in videos, similar to real-life observations, or focusing visual attention on specific facial regions in distinguishing autism. In this context, Wan et al. (2019) investigated the fixation duration of participants aged 4–6 years while watching a 10-second video featuring a female model speaking. Their findings revealed significant differences in fixation duration between children with autism and typically developing (TD) children across six predefined areas of interest. Additionally, discriminant analysis demonstrated that fixation durations on the mouth and body significantly distinguished children with autism from their TD peers, achieving an evaluation accuracy of 85.1%, sensitivity of 86.5%, and specificity of 83.8%. The researchers suggested that the visual attention data obtained from a short video clip could provide sufficient information to differentiate children with autism from TD children.

Some researchers studying machine learning and autism classification have also investigated classification accuracy using either eye-tracking data combined with behavioral data or behavioral data alone. For instance, in a study incorporating both eye-tracking and motor movement-based data, Vabalas et al. (2020) attempted to distinguish 22 adults with autism from 22 adults without an autism diagnosis. Prior to the classification process, the researchers tested feature selection techniques such as SVM-Recursive Feature Elimination (RFE), t-tests, minimum redundancy maximum relevance, and ReliefF. Additionally, they applied a nested validation approach to develop their model and evaluated the results on an independent sample. The developed models yielded an accuracy rate of 73% using movement-based features, 70% using eye-tracking features, and 78% when both data types were combined.

Furthermore, eye scan paths provide significant insights into the visual attention patterns and preferences of individuals with autism in social contexts. For example, Kanhirakadavath et al. (2022) conducted a study utilizing adaptive eye-tracking data derived from machine learning models for the purpose of early autism screening in children, employing eye-tracking scan path images. Both machine learning and deep learning models have been used in autism classification. Similarly, Benabderrahmane et al. (2024) introduced a multimodal machine learning model to assist with autism classification model using eye-tracking data. To achieve a higher accuracy in autism classification, the proposed model examined individual eye scanning paths throughout the presented screen-based images, sequences of distances in eye movements, and durations of each fixation. Furthermore, Alsaidi et al. (2024) developed a Convolutional Deep Neural Network (T-CNN-ASD) to predict autism diagnosis by analyzing eye-tracking data. The T-CNN-ASD model was trained and validated on eye-tracking data collected from 59 children in the study. Results showed that the proposed model outperformed traditional machine learning algorithms. In another study, Zhou et al. (2024) analyzed scan paths capturing eye movement dynamics during social interactions of children with autism. Implementing machine learning and deep learning models, the researchers examined how children attended to both facial expressions and other social cues. Study results revealed that the participants with autism displayed more distinctive visual patterns than the non-autistic participants, suggesting more individual image representations. This study reported that path-based digital phenotyping provides qualitative and quantitative value for autism classification.

In addition, deep learning models have significantly contributed, particularly by using eye-tracking data as visual classification problems. In a recent study, Mehmood et al. (2024) utilized the potential of machine learning with gaze-tracking data to cost-effectively facilitate the early diagnosis of autism for children with limited access to healthcare resources, enhancing the results using both machine learning and deep learning models. In a previous study, Cilia et al. (2021) examined the visual attention patterns of individuals with autism using eye-tracking data and conducted autism diagnoses with a Convolutional Neural Network (CNN) model, demonstrating that these models show great promise. Lastly, Li et al. (2021) examined the role of computer vision in identifying neurodevelopmental disorders, noting that eye-tracking data provides the most valuable insights for classifying autism. In this study, the researchers reviewed techniques that apply deep learning methods on eye-tracking data to identify and profile attention impairments in individuals with autism.

Moreover, Liu et al. (2016) proposed a data-driven model to identify children with autism based on atypical eye movements during face scanning. The study utilized a data-driven feature extraction method, a "leave-one-out" cross-validation strategy, and Support Vector Machine algorithms to analyze eye movement data collected during face recognition tasks. Study findings suggested the machine learning model was high in accuracy (85.51%), specificity (86.21%), and sensitivity (93.10%) in classifying children with autism using eye-tracking data. The researchers showed that eye movements in facial areas were the most discriminative areas in classifying and predicting autism diagnosis. Participants with autism exhibited reduced visual attention in the facial areas compared to TD children, consistent with previous literature (Ozdemir et al., 2024; Ozturk et al., 2024).

In summary, a review of the existing literature reveals that researchers generally aim to test the effectiveness of machine learning models on different data types or to examine the consistency of machine learning-based eye-tracking results with observational data. These recent studies suggest that integrating eye-tracking data with machine learning and deep learning models can effectively identify potential autism markers, such as eye movements and visual attention patterns. On the other hand, reviewed studies have been conducted across various age groups (children, adults) using different eye-tracking stimuli (human faces, objects, animations, static, and dynamic images), distinct experimental paradigms (passive viewing, participant-driven selection of stimuli, task-based viewing), and a range of machine learning algorithms (Support Vector Machines, Decision Trees, Bayesian Classifiers). Additionally, participants were matched based on different criteria (e.g., cognitive age, chronological age). Despite variations in methodologies and datasets, the findings from the machine learning studies consistently report relatively high classification accuracy rates, further highlighting the potential of these models in autism research. Nevertheless, existing literature provides valuable insights into the effectiveness of machine learning algorithms, particularly in eye movement analysis, offering a foundation for future studies in early autism detection.

Social Interaction and Cognitive Processes in Machine Learning and Autism Research

Eye-tracking technologies serve as valuable tools for examining social interactions and the perception of social cues in individuals with autism, showing the areas of attention and the elements that attract children's attention within social contexts (Akin-Bulbul & Ozdemir, 2023; Akin-Bulbul et al., 2024; Ozdemir et al., 2024; Ozturk et al., 2024). Indeed, many machine learning studies have investigated how individuals with autism perceive social stimuli and interact with social cues, including eye contact and facial expressions (Jones et al., 2013; Ozdemir et al., 2024). For instance, Król and Król (2019) analyzed spatial and temporal variations in gaze paths by assessing eye movement data from individuals with autism and those who are not autistic. While existing methodologies predominantly focus on raw gaze data and spatial information, the researchers, for the first time, implemented dimensionality reduction techniques via t-SNE on gaze path similarity matrices and performed statistical analysis to compare differences between the groups. The study's findings revealed statistical significance in the classification outcomes associated with the LightGBM algorithm, suggesting that gaze patterns markedly differ between face-to-face interactions of individuals with and without autism in both spatial and temporal dimensions. In another study, Ruan et al. (2021) investigated the visual perception variations among individuals with autism utilizing deep learning-based Deep Neural Network (DNN) and Convolutional Neural Network (CNN) models. This study revealed that individuals with autism demonstrate atypical visual attention toward social stimuli, suggesting the effectiveness of deep learning methodologies in exploring atypical visual attention in individuals with autism. The results highlight the pivotal role of eye-tracking data in augmenting our comprehension of atypical visual attention during social interactions. Similarly, He et al. (2021) utilized Support Vector Machine (SVM) and Logistic Regression (LR) models to assess how children with autism respond to social and non-social stimuli, demonstrating the influence of machine learning models.

Alcañiz et al. (2022) evaluated the efficacy of eye movements as potential biomarkers using static and dynamic stimuli within a VR environment to assess children's performance in realistic simulated settings. The researchers reported differences in visual attention based on gaze durations as distinguishing measures for autism diagnosis (86% accuracy). Children with autism displayed greater visual attention toward adults than children depicted in the VR compared to the control group. Similarly, Artiran et al. (2024) demonstrated variations in interactions with the social environment among individuals with autism by analyzing attention distribution during a VR-based job interview simulation. Participants with autism gazed at and mirrored the virtual interviewer less frequently than their non-autistic counterparts. De Belen et al. (2024) employed a data-driven approach to analyze the dynamic visual attention of young children with autism and their non-autistic peers while watching videos to extract autism classification and predict symptom severity. The study used machine learning and deep learning techniques to examine eye-tracking data and video features, facilitating the identification of spatiotemporal patterns and dynamic visual attention metrics that predict autism diagnosis and symptom severity. In summary, the results of the studies indicated that machine learning models offer insights into a deeper understanding of the difficulties encountered by individuals with autism within social contexts. The authors emphasized that machine learning models facilitate an objective framework for analyzing individual responses to social stimuli.

Furthermore, recognizing how autism influences cognitive functions like attention and learning is essential for designing effective intervention programs. Research in this field examines the distinctions in cognitive processes between individuals with autism and non-autistic peers, utilizing machine learning and deep learning algorithms that analyze eye-tracking data and webcam inputs from various attention assessments. In a recent study, Varghese et al. (2024) developed an attention assessment model using real-time virtual attention tasks. Researchers employed deep learning for head pose and gaze parameters and machine learning models for attention quantification. They proposed the usability of their attention level assessment model with children with autism. In a similar study involving virtual attention tasks, Banire et al. (2024) introduced a machine learning model to assess the attention of children with autism and a control group by analyzing webcam and eye-tracking data. The researchers proposed three distinct learning models: face-based, gaze-based, and hybrid (face-gaze) models to classify participants as attentive or inattentive, using six different classification algorithms (SVM, CART, LOR, RF, GBC, KNN). The study's findings indicated that the gaze-based model performed best in classifying children with autism and their non-autistic peers as either attentive or inattentive.

Conclusion

Machine learning offers advanced techniques that develop automated classifiers, which can be utilized by both users and experts to significantly enhance sensitivity, specificity, efficiency, and accuracy in diagnostic decision-making processes (Thabtah & Peebles, 2020). Machine learning is expected to be increasingly applied as an evolving methodology and tool to improve the accuracy of autism risk assessment and early risk detection. While each study provides valuable opportunities for acquiring new knowledge, expanding the existing body of research, or facilitating the next phase of future investigation, a critical limitation lies in the inability to translate these developed tools into practical applications.

Advancements in machine learning research indicate that machine learning methods offer promising results in distinguishing children with autism from their TD peers. However, despite the growing number of studies applying machine learning to children and adults with autism, existing research still faces numerous methodological limitations. For instance, many studies conducted in engineering disciplines often lack detailed information about the cognitive and developmental characteristics of autistic participants, treating the autism diagnostic group as a homogeneous entity without considering individual differences in symptom severity. On the other hand, some studies that define the participant characteristics tend to have limited sample sizes due to the difficulties associated with conducting detailed assessments. For example, while Alcaniz et al. (2022) reported participant characteristics using tools such as the ADOS, their eye-tracking and machine learning study was conducted with only 35 children with autism and 20 TD children. Additionally, many studies have been conducted with adults with autism (e.g., Vabalas et al., 2020, with 22 autistic and 22 non-autistic adults). Yet, the reported findings can not be generalized to early childhood populations. Another notable limitation of the existing machine learning literature is the use of data features that are not directly related to autism symptomatology. For example, Crippa et al. (2015) classified 15 preschool-aged children severely affected by autism and 15 TD peers based on hand and arm movements. A significant limitation of this study was that the motor task used, grasping a 10 cm ball with fine motor movements using both hands and placing it into a hole, could also pose challenges for children with developmental delays who do not have autism.

Finally, while machine learning studies based on data types that are difficult for families to access provide valuable scientific insights, their practical application for real-life autism classification remains limited. For instance, Moradi et al. (2017) analyzed cortical thickness data from MRI scans using support vector regression and an elastic net (ENet) penalized linear regression model to predict autism severity in 156 individuals aged 8–40 years. Similarly, Zhang et al. (2018) conducted an MRI-based study involving 70 children with autism and 79 TD children, reporting a classification accuracy of 78.33%. Additionally, some studies investigated early structural and functional connectivity differences in the brain, reporting varying levels of classification accuracy (Zwaigenbaum & Penner, 2018). In summary, while the scientific knowledge gained from these studies is highly valuable, the accessibility of assessment applications remains a significant challenge. The difficulties associated with applying imaging techniques such as EEG and MRI to children with autism, the limited accessibility of these technologies for larger populations, and the complexity of behavioral assessments, which often require highly specialized training (e.g., the ADOS, the ADI-R administration) make the fast and objective evaluation of early autism risks challenging.

Nevertheless, researchers from various countries continue to emphasize the urgent need for screening tools that enable the swift and objective assessment of autism risk (Bolte et al., 2016; Elsabbagh & Johnson, 2016). Although parental concerns related to autism become evident by the time children reach their second birthday (Zwaigenbaum et al., 2009) and the importance of early diagnosis and intervention in mitigating autism's effects is consistently emphasized (Dawson et al., 2010), access to early intervention services remains a major challenge for children with autism and their families. This is largely due to the limited availability of qualified specialists and the lack of valid, reliable, and objective assessment tools for evaluating autism risks. Therefore, the development of rapid and objective assessment methods for identifying early autism risk in children has become a critical necessity.

In the era of big data and the promising advancements of machine learning applications, an increasing number of studies are incorporating machine learning techniques, which has drawn significant attention. While traditional machine learning methods have reported high classification accuracy in distinguishing autism, the difficulty of drawing meaningful inferences from these models poses a major challenge. Moreover, traditional machine learning methods do not offer interpretable information regarding why, how, or under what conditions a specific decision or classification was made. Thus, recent years have seen a rise in innovative research focused on Explainable Artificial Intelligence or Interpretable Machine Learning to address this issue. By leveraging these methods, it becomes possible to identify the specific features that contribute to autism classification, which is not achievable with traditional machine learning models. Consequently, Explainable Artificial Intelligence approaches can provide clear, understandable, and individualized insights into a child's likelihood of being on the autism spectrum, offering more transparent and interpretable assessments tailored to each child's unique profile.

Developing machine learning models in clinical research, particularly in autism assessments, necessitates addressing critical regulatory and ethical considerations to ensure its reliable, valid, and effective implementation. Establishing robust standards and guidelines is essential for integrating machine learning models into clinical autism assessments. These frameworks must define acceptable accuracy, sensitivity, and interpretability levels of model decisions to foster trust among researchers, clinicians, individuals with autism, and caregivers.

Moreover, ensuring reliability and transparency in machine learning models is critical for their adoption in sensitive clinical applications. Transparent models allow clinicians and caregivers to understand how decisions are made in machine learning models. Methods such as SHAP or LIME, can provide insights into the model's behavior, ensuring that decisions align with clinical reasoning. Furthermore, reliability mechanisms must be established to address errors or adverse outcomes, ensuring that machine learning systems operate under ethical responsibility. In conclusion, addressing methodological and ethical challenges is a cornerstone for successfully integrating machine learning into clinical autism assessments. By developing clear standards, addressing biases, and ensuring transparency and reliability, machine learning systems can be effectively implemented in clinical assessments while maintaining reliability and validity.

Lastly, machine learning contributes to individualized intervention plans by integrating diverse data sources, including behavioral, physiological, and genetic information. By analyzing these multidimensional datasets, machine learning models can predict which interventions are most likely to benefit a specific child. Clustering techniques can group children with similar behavioral patterns, aiding in understanding how different autism phenotypes respond to specific interventions. This individualized approach not only improves treatment outcomes but also reduces the trial-and-error process often involved in interventions in autism. In summary, these applications highlight the transformative potential of machine learning in autism assessment, addressing critical gaps in early risk detection, diagnosis, and intervention while advancing the field toward more efficient, data-driven solutions.

Future Research Implications

The future of machine learning in autism clinical studies is poised to be shaped by emerging advancements such as federated learning, multimodal machine learning systems, the integration of the Internet of Things (IoT), and Natural Language Processing (NLP). Federated learning addresses one of the clinical study challenges: maintaining children's privacy while leveraging diverse, large-scale datasets. By enabling collaborative model training across multiple institutions without sharing sensitive data, federated learning preserves data locality while creating globally robust models. This approach facilitates the development of high-performing machine learning systems and fosters cross-institutional collaborations, unlocking the potential to address rare diseases and underrepresented populations more effectively.

Similarly, multimodal machine learning systems are revolutionizing clinical studies by integrating heterogeneous data types such as behavioral and observational data, medical imaging, electronic health records, developmental test results, eye-tracking data, and textual clinical notes. These systems enable a comprehensive analysis of a child's disorder, capturing the complexity of a child's neurodevelopment that single-modality models often miss. For example, combining eye-tracking data with developmental test scores and observational data can improve the accuracy of autism diagnosis. Multimodal machine learning offers the ability to unify disparate data sources, delivering more nuanced insights and facilitating individualized assessments.

The integration of IoT technologies further extends the reach of machine learning into continuous and real-time clinical assessments. IoT devices, such as wearable sensors, speech record devices, and remote monitoring tools, allow for continuous tracking of early symptoms, physical and speech activity, and other parameters outside clinical settings. Wearable devices are becoming vital tools for early autism risk assessment, and advanced sensors and machine learning are being used to monitor behavioral and physiological markers of autism. Devices like smartwatches and wristbands track movement, voice recorders, sleep, and physiological responses, while EEG headbands and eye-tracking glasses capture neural activity and visual attention. Motion sensors and biosensor patches detect motor delays and stress-related markers, and wearable cameras provide objective insights into social interactions. For example, tools like the LENA (Language Environment Analysis) system analyze the child's speech environment by recording the number of words spoken, conversational turns, and caregiver responses. Microphone-equipped wearables, integrated into smart clothing or accessories, can capture speech patterns, vocalizations, and babbling, offering insights into developmental milestones and early detection of speech delays. These tools enable continuous, naturalistic monitoring, supporting traditional diagnostic methods. However, data accuracy, comfort, and ethical compliance must be addressed. Advances in sensor technology and machine learning promise to improve their reliability, making wearable devices a valuable resource for early autism diagnosis and intervention. For example, wearable devices monitoring speech complexity and frequency can alert professionals to early signs of autism, enabling early interventions. Thus, IoT integration generates vast amounts of real-time data, which can uncover patterns and trends to inform decision-making when paired with advanced machine learning techniques.

Natural Language Processing (NLP) plays an increasingly important role in the early detection of autism by analyzing linguistic and speech patterns that may indicate developmental differences. Children with autism often exhibit atypical language development, including delayed speech onset, limited vocabulary, repetitive speech, or differences in prosody and tone. NLP techniques can process and analyze these features by extracting and quantifying linguistic markers from audio recordings, transcripts, or caregiver-child interactions. For instance, NLP algorithms can evaluate sentence complexity, word repetition, speech rhythm, or conversation pauses to identify early signs of autism. Additionally, sentiment analysis and semantic modeling can assess emotional expressions and pragmatic language use, where children with autism may show difficulties. By integrating NLP techniques with other clinical assessments, such as behavioral and physiological data, researchers can develop robust models to improve the accuracy and timeliness of autism diagnosis. Furthermore, NLP-powered mobile apps or digital platforms can provide parents and clinicians access to monitor a child's language development, enabling earlier interventions and better outcomes. As NLP techniques evolve, their potential to uncover nuanced linguistic patterns offers new opportunities for advancing early autism detection.

In summary, as these technologies converge, machine learning models hold immense potential to transform clinical assessments and early intervention services by fostering more collaborative, data-driven, and child-centered autism assessment and intervention systems. The combination of federated learning, multimodal machine learning, IoT, and NLP creates a pathway toward reliable, valid, and accurate machine learning models that address critical gaps in clinical standards. These trends are expected to drive significant innovation in autism assessment research, enabling efficient solutions tailored to children's individual needs.

Machine learning has shown to be a transformative force in autism studies, offering innovative solutions to challenges in clinical assessments, particularly in the early detection and diagnosis of autism. This chapter has highlighted machine learning applications, the challenges associated with data quality, interpretability, and methodological problems in literature, and the importance of integrating diverse methodologies like wearable devices, multimodal machine learning systems, IoT, and NLP. While machine learning continues to evolve, its development in autism assessments depends on overcoming current limitations. Furthermore, advancements in machine learning models must be balanced with transparency, reliability, and ethical considerations to maintain trust and validity. Ultimately, the integration of machine learning into clinical practice holds great promise, but realizing its full potential will require collaboration between clinicians, researchers, and caregivers, ensuring that machine learning models are valid, reliable, and interpretable.

Acknowledgments This book chapter was supported by the Scientific and Technological Research Council of Turkey with grant #123R050.

References

Abbas, H., Garberson, F., Glover, E., & Wall, D. P. (2018). Machine learning approach for early detection of autism by combining questionnaire and home video screening. *Journal of the American Medical Informatics Association, 25*(8), 1000–1007. https://doi.org/10.1093/jamia/ocy039

Adadi, A., & Berrada, M. (2018). Peeking inside the black-box: A survey on explainable artificial intelligence (XAI). *IEEE Access, 6*, 52138–52160. https://doi.org/10.1109/ACCESS.2018.2870052

Akin-Bulbul, I., & Ozdemir, S. (2023). Imitation performance in children with autism and the role of visual attention in imitation. *Journal of Autism and Developmental Disorders, 53*(12), 4604–4617. https://doi.org/10.1007/s10803-022-05726-5

Akin-Bulbul, I., & Ozdemir, S. (2024). Evaluation of the social attention hypothesis: Do children with autism prefer to see objects rather than people? *Journal of Autism and Developmental Disorders*. https://doi.org/10.1007/s10803-024-06596-9

Akin-Bulbul, I., Kok, I., & Ozdemir, S. (2024). Machine learning in classification of autism spectrum disorder: Visual attention directed to the emotional states. *Turkish Journal of Psychology, 39*, 103–129. https://doi.org/10.31828/turkpsikoloji.1537964

Akter, T., Ali, M. H., Khan, M. I., Satu, M. S., & Moni, M. A. (2021). Machine learning model to predict autism investigating eye-tracking dataset. In *2nd international conference on robotics, electrical and signal processing techniques (ICREST)* (pp. 383–387). https://doi.org/10.1109/icrest51555.2021.9331152

Alarifi, H., Aldhalaan, H., Hadjikhani, N., Johnels, J. Å., Alarifi, J., Ascenso, G., & Alabdulaziz, R. (2023). Machine learning for distinguishing Saudi children with and without autism via eye-tracking data. *Child and Adolescent Psychiatry and Mental Health, 17*(1) https://doi.org/ARTN10.1186/s13034-023-00662-3

Alcañiz, M., Chicchi-Giglioli, I. A., Carrasco-Ribelles, L. A., Marín-Morales, J., Minissi, M. E., Teruel-Garcia, G., Sirera, M., & Abad, L. (2022). Eye gaze as a biomarker in the recognition of autism spectrum disorder using virtual reality and machine learning: A proof of concept for diagnosis. *Autism Research, 15*(1), 131–145. https://doi.org/10.1002/aur.2636

Alsaidi, M., Obeid, N., Al-Madi, N., Hiary, H., & Aljarah, I. (2024). A convolutional deep neural network approach to predict autism spectrum disorder based on eye-tracking scan paths. *Information, 15*(3). https://doi.org/10.3390/info15030133

Arrieta, A. B., Díaz-Rodríguez, N., Del Ser, J., Bennetot, A., Tabik, S., Barbado, A., ... & Herrera, F. (2020). Explainable Artificial Intelligence (XAI): Concepts taxonomies opportunities and challenges toward responsible. *AI Information Fusion, 58*, 82–115. https://doi.org/10.1016/j.inffus.2019.12.012

Artiran, S., Bedmutha, P. S., & Cosman, P. (2024). Analysis of gaze, head orientation, and joint attention in autism with triadic VR interviews. *IEEE Transactions on Neural Systems and Rehabilitation Engineering, 32*, 759–769. https://doi.org/10.1109/Tnsre.2024.3363728

Atlam, E. S., Masud, M., Rokaya, M., Meshref, H., Gad, I., & Almars, A. M. (2024). EASDM: Explainable autism spectrum disorder model based on deep learning. *Journal of Disability Research, 3*(1), 20240003. https://doi.org/10.57197/JDR-2024-0003

Babu, P. R. K., Di Martino, J. M., Chang, Z., Perochon, S., Carpenter, K. L. H., Compton, S., ... & Sapiro, G. (2021). Exploring complexity of facial dynamics in autism spectrum disorder. *IEEE Transactions on Affective Computing, 14*(2), 919–930. https://doi.org/10.1109/TAFFC.2021.3113876

Banire, B., Al Thani, D., & Qaraqe, M. (2024). One size does not fit all: Detecting attention in children with autism using machine learning. *User Modeling and User-Adapted Interaction, 34*(2), 259–291. https://doi.org/10.1007/s11257-023-09371-0

Bargagna, F., De Santi, L. A., Santarelli, M. F., Positano, V., & Vanello, N. (2024). Bayesian XAI methods towards a robustness-centric approach to deep learning: An ABIDE I study. *2022 IEEE International Symposium on Medical Measurements and Applications (MeMeA)*, 1–5. https://doi.org/10.1109/memea60663.2024.10596826

de Belen, R. A. J., Eapen, V., Bednarz, T., & Sowmya, A. (2024). Using visual attention estimation on videos for automated prediction of autism spectrum disorder and symptom severity in preschool children. *PLoS One, 19*(2), e0282818. https://doi.org/10.1371/journal.pone.0282818

Benabderrahmane, B., Gharzouli, M., & Benlecheb, A. (2024). A novel multi-modal model to assist the diagnosis of autism spectrum disorder using eye-tracking data. *Health Information Science and Systems, 12*(1). https://doi.org/10.1007/s13755-024-00299-2

Biswas, M., Kaiser, M. S., Mahmud, M., Al Mamun, S., Hossain, M. S., & Rahman, M. A. (2021). An XAI based autism detection: The context behind the detection. *Brain Informatics, 12960*, 448–459. https://doi.org/10.1007/978-3-030-86993-9_40

Bolte, S., Bartl-Pokorny, K. D., Jonsson, U., Berggren, S., Zhang, D., Kostrzewa, E., Falck-Ytter, T., Einspieler, C., Pokorny, F. B., Jones, E. J. H., Roeyers, H., Charman, T., & Marschik, P. B. (2016). How can clinicians detect and treat autism early? Methodological trends of technology use in research. *Acta Pediatrica, 105*(2), 137–144. https://doi.org/10.1136/bmj.k1674

Bzdok, D., & Meyer-Lindenberg, A. (2018). Machine learning for precision psychiatry: Opportunities and challenges. *Biological Psychiatry: Cognitive Neuroscience and Neuroimaging, 3*(3), 223–230. https://doi.org/10.1016/j.bpsc.2017.11.007

Chandrashekar, G., & Sahin, F. (2014). A survey on feature selection methods. *Computers and Electrical Engineering, 40*(1), 16–28. https://doi.org/10.1016/j.compeleceng.2013.11.024

Chanyoung, K., Soyeon, K., Rang, P. Y., Soon-Beom, H., Mindong, S., Lim, J., & Bongkyung, J. (2022, November). AI-assisted initiation to joint attention evaluation for autism spectrum disorder detection. In *In 2022 IEEE 3rd international conference on human-machine systems (ICHMS)* (pp. 1–6). IEEE. https://doi.org/10.1109/ICHMS56717.2022.9980778

Cilia, F., Carette, R., Elbattah, M., Dequen, G., Guérin, J. L., Bosche, J., Vandromme, L., & Le Driant, B. (2021). Computer-aided screening of autism spectrum disorder: Eye-tracking study using data visualization and deep learning. *JMIR Human Factors, 8*(4). https://doi.org/10.2196/27706

Crippa, A., Salvatore, C., Perego, P., Forti, S., Nobile, M., Molteni, M., & Castiglioni, I. (2015). Use of machine learning to identify children with autism and their motor abnormalities. *Journal of Autism and Developmental Disorders, 45*(7), 2146–2156. https://doi.org/10.1007/s10803-015-2379-8

Dawson, G., Rogers, S., Munson, J., Smith, M., Winter, J., Greenson, J., Donaldson, A., & Varley, J. (2010). Randomized, controlled trial of an intervention for toddlers with autism: The early start Denver model. *Pediatrics, 125*(1), e17–e23. https://doi.org/10.1542/peds.2009-0958

Duda, M., Kosmicki, J. A., & Wall, D. P. (2014). Testing the accuracy of an observation-based classifier for rapid detection of autism risk. *Translational Psychiatry, 4*(8), 424–424. https://doi.org/10.1038/tp.2014.65

Elsabbagh, M., & Johnson, M. H. (2016). Autism and the social brain: The first-year puzzle. *Biological Psychiatry, 80*(2), 94–99. https://doi.org/10.1016/j.biopsych.2016.02.019

ElShawi, R., Sherif, Y., Al-Mallah, M., & Sakr, S. (2021). Interpretability in healthcare: A comparative study of local machine learning interpretability techniques. *Computational Intelligence, 37*(4), 1633–1650. https://doi.org/10.1111/coin.12410

Fernandez-Lanvin, D., Gonzalez-Rodriguez, M., De-Andres, J., & Camero, R. (2024). Towards an automatic early screening system for autism spectrum disorder in toddlers based on eye-tracking. *Multimedia Tools and Applications, 83*(18), 55319–55350. https://doi.org/10.1007/s11042-023-17694-8

Franco, F. O., Oliveira, J. S., Portolese, J., Sumiya, F. M., Silva, A. F., Machado-Lima, A., Nunes, F. L. S., & Brentani, H. (2023). Computer-aided autism diagnosis using visual attention models and eye-tracking: Replication and improvement proposal. *BMC Medical Informatics and Decision Making, 23*(1). https://doi.org/10.1186/s12911-023-02389-9

Garg, A., Parashar, A., Barman, D., Jain, S., Singhal, D., Masud, M., & Abouhawwash, M. (2022). Autism spectrum disorder prediction by an explainable deep learning approach. *Computers, Materials and Continua, 71*(1), 1459–1471. https://doi.org/10.32604/cmc.2022.022170

Gurbuz, E., Turgut, O., & Kok, I. (2023, July). Explainable AI-based malicious traffic detection and monitoring system in next-gen IoT healthcare. *IEEE International Conference on Smart Applications, Communications and Networking (SmartNets)*, 1–6. https://doi.org/10.1109/SmartNets58706.2023.10215896

Han, J., Kamber, M., & Pei, J. (2012). *Data mining: Concepts and techniques.* Morgan Kaufmann Publishers.

He, Q., Wang, Q. D., Wu, Y. X., Yi, L., & Wei, K. L. (2021). Automatic classification of children with autism spectrum disorder by using a computerized visual-orienting task. *PsyCh Journal, 10*(4), 550–565. https://doi.org/10.1002/pchj.447

Hilal, A. M., Issaoui, I., Obayya, M., Al-Wesabi, F. N., Nemri, N., Hamza, M. A., Al Duhayyim, M., & Zamani, A. (2022). Modeling of explainable artificial intelligence for biomedical mental disorder diagnosis. *Cmc-Computers Materials and Continua, 71*(2), 3853–3867. https://doi.org/10.32604/cmc.2022.022663

Hyde, K. K., Novack, M. N., LaHaye, N., Parlett-Pelleriti, C., Anden, R., Dixon, D. R., & Linstead, E. (2019). Applications of supervised machine learning in autism spectrum disorder research: A review. *Review Journal of Autism and Developmental Disorders, 6*, 128–146. https://doi.org/10.1007/s40489-019-00158-x

Jeon, I., Kim, M., So, D., Kim, E. Y., Nam, Y., Kim, S., Shim, S., Kim, J., & Moon, J. (2024). Reliable autism spectrum disorder diagnosis for pediatrics using machine learning and explainable AI. *Diagnostics, 14*(22). https://doi.org/10.3390/diagnostics14222504

Jones, W., & Klin, A. (2013). Attention to eyes is present but in decline in 2–6-month-old infants later diagnosed with autism. *Nature, 504*(7480), 427–431. https://doi.org/10.1038/nature12715

Jordan, M. I., & Mitchell, T. M. (2015). Machine learning: Trends, perspectives, and prospects. *Science, 349*(6245), 255–260. https://doi.org/10.1126/science.aaa8415

Kang, H., Yang, M., Kim, G. H., Lee, T. S., & Park, S. (2023, July). DeepASD: Facial image analysis for autism spectrum diagnosis via explainable artificial intelligence. In *Fourteenth international conference on ubiquitous and future networks (ICUFN)* (pp. 625–630). IEEE. https://doi.org/10.1109/ICUFN57995.2023.10200203

Kanhirakadavath, M. R., & Chandran, M. S. M. (2022). Investigation of eye-tracking scan path as a biomarker for autism screening using machine learning algorithms. *Diagnostics, 12*(2). https://doi.org/10.3390/diagnostics12020518

Kanner, L. (1943). Autistic disturbances of affective contact. *Nervous Child, 2*, 217–250.

Karuppasamy, S. G., Muralitharan, D., Gowr, S., Arumugam, S. R., Devi, E. A., & Maharajan, K. (2022, April). Prediction of autism spectrum disorder using convolution neural network. In *2022 6th international conference on trends in electronics and informatics (ICOEI)* (pp. 1096–1100). IEEE. https://doi.org/10.1109/ICOEI53556.2022.9776657

Khalaji, E., Eraslan, S., Yesilada, Y., & Yaneva, V. (2023). Effects of data preprocessing on detecting autism in adults using web-based eye-tracking data. *Behaviour and Information Technology, 42*(14), 2476–2484. https://doi.org/10.1080/0144929x.2022.2127376

Kok, I., & Ozdemir, S. (2022). Content-centric data and computation offloading in AI-supported fog networks for next generation IoT. *Pervasive and Mobile Computing, 85*, 101654. https://doi.org/10.1016/j.pmcj.2022.101654

Kosmicki, J. A., Sochat, V., Duda, M., & Wall, D. P. (2015). Searching for a minimal set of behaviors for autism detection through feature selection-based machine learning. *Translational Psychiatry, 5*, e514. https://doi.org/10.1038/tp.2015.7

Król, M., & Król, M. E. (2019). A novel eye movement data transformation technique that preserves temporal information: A demonstration in a face processing task. *Sensors, 19*(10). https://doi.org/10.3390/s19102377

Li, J., Cheng, K., Wang, S., Morstatter, F., Trevino, R. P., Tang, J., & Liu, H. (2017). Feature selection: A data perspective. *ACM Computing Surveys (CSUR), 50*(6), 1–45. https://doi.org/10.1145/3136625

Li, X. T., Fan, F. F., Chen, X. J., Li, J., Ning, L., Lin, K. G., Chen, Z., Qin, Z. Y., Yeung, A. S., Li, X. J., Wang, L. P., & So, K. F. (2021). Computer vision for brain disorders based primarily on ocular responses. *Frontiers in Neurology, 12*. https://doi.org/10.3389/fneur.2021.584270

Liu, W. B., Li, M., & Yi, L. (2016). Identifying children with autism spectrum disorder based on their face processing abnormality: A machine learning framework. *Autism Research, 9*(8), 888–898. https://doi.org/10.1002/aur.1615

Magboo, M. S. A., & Magboo, V. P. C. (2022). Explainable AI for autism classification in children. In *Smart innovation, systems and technologies* (pp. 195–205). https://doi.org/10.1007/978-981-19-3359-2_17

Man, X., & Chan, E. (2021). The best way to select features? Comparing MDA, LIME, and SHAP. *The Journal of Financial Data Science Winter, 3*(1), 127–139. https://doi.org/10.3905/jfds.2020.1.047

Mehmood, M., Amin, H. U., & Chen, P. L. (2024). Pre-diagnosis for autism spectrum disorder using eye-tracking and machine learning techniques. *Advances in Brain Inspired Cognitive Systems, 14374*, 239–250. https://doi.org/10.1007/978-981-97-1417-9_23

Monarca, I., Cibrian, F. L., Chavez, E., & Tentori, M. (2023). Using a small dataset to classify strength-interactions with an elastic display: A case study for the screening of autism spectrum disorder. *International Journal of Machine Learning and Cybernetics, 14*(1), 151–169. https://doi.org/10.1007/s13042-022-01554-2

Moradi, E., Khundrakpam, B., Lewis, J. D., Evans, A. C., & Tohka, J. (2017). Predicting symptom severity in autism spectrum disorder based on cortical thickness measures in agglomerative data. *NeuroImage, 144*, 128–141. https://doi.org/10.1016/j.neuroimage.2016.09.049

Nohara, Y., Matsumoto, K., Soejima, H., & Nakashima, N. (2022). Explanation of machine learning models using shapley additive explanation and application for real data in hospital. *Computer Methods and Programs in Biomedicine, 214*, 106584. https://doi.org/10.1016/j.cmpb.2021.106584

Ozdemir, S., Akin-Bulbul, I., Kok, I., & Ozdemir, S. (2022). Development of a visual attention based decision support system for autism spectrum disorder screening. *International Journal of Psychophysiology, 173*, 69–81. https://doi.org/10.1016/j.ijpsycho.2022.01.004

Ozdemir, S., Akin-Bulbul, I., & Yildiz, E. (2024). Visual attention in joint attention bids: A comparison between toddlers with autism spectrum disorder and typically developing toddlers. *Journal of Autism and Developmental Disorders, 55*, 408–427. https://doi.org/10.1007/s10803-023-06224-y

Ozturk, D., Aydoğan, S., Kok, İ., Akın Bulbul, I., Ozdemir, S., Ozdemir, S., & Akay, D. (2024). Linguistic summarization of visual attention and developmental functioning of young children with autism spectrum disorder. *Health Information Science and Systems, 12*(1), 39. https://doi.org/10.1007/s13755-024-00297-4

Pramod, A., Naicker, H. S., & Tyagi, A. K. (2021). Machine learning and deep learning: Open issues and future research directions for the next 10 years. *Computational Analysis and Deep Learning for Medical Care: Principles, Methods, and Applications, 463-490.* https://doi.org/10.1002/9781119785750.ch18

Ruan, M. D., Webster, P. J., Li, X., & Wang, S. (2021). Deep neural network reveals the world of autism from a first-person perspective. *Autism Research, 14*(2), 333–342. https://doi.org/10.1002/aur.2376

Sarabadani, S., Schudlo, L. C., Samadani, A. A., & Kushski, A. (2020). Physiological detection of affective states in children with autism spectrum disorder. *IEEE Transactions on Affective Computing, 11*(4), 588–600. https://doi.org/10.1109/TAFFC.2018.2820049

Shalev-Shwartz, S., & Ben-David, S. (2014). *Understanding machine learning: From theory to algorithms.* Cambridge University Press.

Stahl, D., Pickles, A., Elsabbagh, M., Johnson, M. H., & BASIS Team. (2012). Novel machine learning methods for ERP analysis: A validation from research on infants at risk for autism. *Developmental Neuropsychology, 37*(3), 274–298. https://doi.org/10.1080/87565641.2011.650808

Sujana, D. S., & Augustine, D. P. (2023, December). Explaining autism diagnosis model through local interpretability techniques-a post-hoc approach. In *International conference on data science, agents & artificial intelligence (ICDSAAI)* (pp. 1–5). IEEE. https://doi.org/10.1109/ICDSAAI59313.2023.10452575

Sun, K., Roy, A., & Tobin, J. M. (2024). Artificial intelligence and machine learning: Definition of terms and current concepts in critical care research. *Journal of Critical Care, 82*, 154792. https://doi.org/10.1016/j.jcrc.2024.154792

Thabtah, F., & Peebles, D. (2020). A new machine learning model based on induction of rules for autism detection. *Health Informatics Journal, 26*(1), 264–286. https://doi.org/10.1177/1460458218824711

Torres, J. M. M., Medina-DeVilliers, S., Clarkson, T., Lerner, M. D., & Riccardi, G. (2023). Evaluation of interpretability for deep learning algorithms in EEG emotion recognition: A case study in autism. *Artificial Intelligence in Medicine, 143*, 102545. https://doi.org/10.1016/j.artmed.2023.102545

Vabalas, A., Gowen, E., Poliakoff, E., & Casson, A. J. (2020). Applying machine learning to kinematic and eye movement features of a movement imitation task to predict autism diagnosis. *Scientific Reports, 10*(1), 1–13. https://doi.org/10.1038/s41598-020-65384-4

Varghese, E. B., Qaraqe, M., & Al-Thani, D. (2024). Attention level evaluation in children with autism: Leveraging head pose and gaze parameters from videos for educational intervention. *IEEE Transactions on Learning Technologies, 17*, 1777–1793. https://doi.org/10.1109/Tlt.2024.3409702

Varsha, P., & Maheswari, U. (2024). Identification of autism spectrum disorder in children from facial features using deep learning. In *2024 Fourth International Conference on Advances in Electrical, Computing, Communication and Sustainable Technologies (ICAECT)* (pp. 1–6). https://doi.org/10.1109/ICAECT60202.2024.10469379

Wan, G., Kong, X., Sun, B., Yu, S., Tu, Y., Park, J., Lang, C., Koh, M., Wei, Z., Feng, Z., Lin, Y., & Kong, J. (2019). Applying eye tracking to identify autism spectrum disorder in children. *Journal of Autism and Developmental Disorders, 49*, 209–215. https://doi.org/10.1007/s10803-018-3690-y

Yaneva, V., Ha, L. A., Eraslan, S., Yesilada, Y., & Mitkov, R. (2018). Detecting autism based on eye-tracking data from web searching tasks. 15th International Web for All Conference (W4a) 2018. doi:https://doi.org/10.1145/3192714.3192819

Yaneva, V., Ha, L. A., Eraslan, S., Yesilada, Y., & Mitkov, R. (2020). Detecting high-functioning autism in adults using eye tracking and machine learning. *IEEE Transactions on Neural Systems and Rehabilitation Engineering, 28*(6), 1254–1261. https://doi.org/10.1109/Tnsre.2020.2991675

Yildirim, M., Yildirim-Okay, F. Y., & Ozdemir, S. (2024). A comparative analysis on the reliability of interpretable machine learning. *Pamukkale University Journal of Engineering Sciences, 30*(4), 494–508. https://doi.org/10.5505/pajes.2023.49473

Yildirim-Okay, F., Yildirim, M., & Ozdemir, S. (2021, October). Interpretable machine learning: A case study of healthcare. *IEEE International Symposium on Networks, Computers and Communications (ISNCC)*, 1–6. https://doi.org/10.1109/ISNCC52172.2021.9615727

Zare, A., Shoeibi, A., Bajestani, N. S., Moridian, P., Alizadehsani, R., Hallaji, M., & Khosravi, A. (2022). Accurate prediction using triangular type-2 fuzzy linear regression: Simplifying complex T2F calculations. *IEEE Systems, Man, and Cybernetics Magazine, 8*(3), 51–60. https://doi.org/10.1109/MSMC.2022.3148569

Zhang, F., Savadjiev, P., Cai, W., Song, Y., Rathi, Y., Tunç, B., Parker, D., Kapur, T., Schultz, R. T., Makris, N., & Verma, R. (2018). Whole brain white matter connectivity analysis using machine learning: An application to autism. *NeuroImage, 172*, 826–837. https://doi.org/10.1016/j.neuroimage.2017.10.029

Zhao, Z., Tang, H., Zhang, X., Qu, X., Hu, X., & Lu, J. (2021). Classification of children with autism and typical development using eye-tracking data from face-to-face conversations: Machine learning model development and performance evaluation. *Journal of Medical Internet Research, 23*(8), e29328. https://doi.org/10.2196/29328

Zhou, W., Yang, M. Q., Tang, J. S., Wang, J., & Hu, B. (2024). Gaze patterns in children with autism spectrum disorder to emotional faces: Scanpath and similarity. *IEEE Transactions on Neural*

Systems and Rehabilitation Engineering, 32, 865–874. https://doi.org/10.1109/Tnsre.2024.3361935

Zhu, M., Zang, B., Ding, L., Lei, T., Feng, Z., & Fan, J. (2022). LIME-based data selection method for SAR images generation using GAN. *Remote Sensing, 14*(1), 204. https://doi.org/10.3390/rs14010204

Zwaigenbaum, L., Bryson, S., Lord, C., Rogers, S., Carter, A., Carver, L., Chawarska, K., Constantino, J., Dawson, G., Dobkins, K., & Fein, D. (2009). Clinical assessment and management of toddlers with suspected autism spectrum disorder: Insights from studies of high-risk infants. *Pediatrics, 123*(5), 1383–1391. https://doi.org/10.1542/peds.2008-1606

Zwaigenbaum, L., & Penner, M. (2018). Autism spectrum disorder: Advances in diagnosis and evaluation. *BMJ, k1674*. https://doi.org/10.1136/bmj.k1674

Stress and Satisfaction in the Diagnostic Process

James Lynch, Ebony L. Holliday, Hillary C. Stanley, Jill C. Fodstad, and Noha F. Minshawi

Abstract Receiving an autism spectrum disorder (autism) diagnosis is a pivotal moment for families, but the diagnostic process can be lengthy, stressful, and inconsistent. This chapter explores the pathways to diagnosis, highlighting the factors influencing parental stress and satisfaction, including wait times, age of diagnosis, symptom severity, and professional interactions. Parents frequently report delays in obtaining an autism diagnosis, which can stem from prolonged wait times, multiple professional referrals, and systemic barriers such as limited access to qualified providers. These delays are exacerbated by disparities related to race, ethnicity, socioeconomic status, and geographic location, creating inequitable diagnostic experiences. Additionally, symptom severity and developmental presentation influence the timing and complexity of diagnosis, with children exhibiting milder or more subtle symptoms often being diagnosed later. This chapter highlights the importance of empathetic, clear, and supportive communication between professionals and families. Parents express greater satisfaction when professionals provide honest feedback, discuss strengths alongside challenges, and offer practical, individualized recommendations for post-diagnostic care. The emerging telehealth technologies are also explored as a promising avenue for increasing diagnostic accessibility, particularly for underserved populations. While current research provides valuable insights, methodological inconsistencies in measuring parental stress and satisfaction remain a limitation. Future research should focus on refining these constructs and identifying evidence-based strategies to improve diagnostic experiences.

Keywords Parent stress · Parent satisfaction · Diagnostic process · Autism · Assessment · Diagnosis

---

J. Lynch · J. C. Fodstad · N. F. Minshawi (✉)
Department of Psychiatry, Indiana University School of Medicine, Riley Hospital for Children at Indiana University Health, Indianapolis, IN, USA
e-mail: nminshaw@iu.edu

E. L. Holliday
Center for Autism Services, Science and Innovation, Kennedy Krieger Institute, Baltimore, MD, USA

H. C. Stanley
Woodview Psychological Group, Indianapolis, IN, USA

J. L. Matson (ed.), *Assessment and Diagnosis in Autism*, Autism and Child Psychopathology Series, https://doi.org/10.1007/978-3-032-11802-8_4

Autism spectrum disorder (autism) is a neurodevelopmental disability characterized by impairment in social-communication skills and the presence of restricted or repetitive behaviors (American Psychiatric Association, 2013). According to the Centers for Disease Control and Prevention (CDC), autism affects approximately 1 out of 36 children in the United States (Maenner et al., 2023). Even more, the global prevalence of autism has increased nearly 20–30 times since the 1960s (CDC, 2014) and is currently estimated at approximately 1 out of 100 children (Zeidan et al., 2022). These rising rates of autism combined with the importance of early intervention (Boyd et al., 2010; Hyman et al., 2020) have led to increased efforts to maximize awareness, screening, and surveillance (Daniels et al., 2014; Hyman et al., 2020; Zwaigenbaum et al., 2019), though there is still substantial room for growth (Carbone et al., 2020). In those cases where formal assessment is pursued, the diagnostic process for autism can be a complex and challenging experience for both professionals and families. Professionals experience a number of challenges related to expertise and experience, limited resources, communication with parents, and systemic barriers (Hamp et al., 2023; Morris et al., 2019). Most importantly, parents and the individuals being assessed may be confused by the assessment process, overwhelmed by amount of information available to them, or unsure of what their next steps should be. Therefore, it is crucial to explore the experiences and perspectives of families who are at the center of the diagnostic process.

The examination of patient satisfaction has been a focus of health care systems for several decades. This concept, which reflects the type and quality of services as well as overall experience, is often considered a global indicator of health care quality and a significant factor in improving service delivery (e.g., Gonzalez, 2005; Turris, 2005). Given that autism diagnosis and service provision occurs predominantly in childhood, research has primarily examined parent satisfaction, as they are the gatekeepers of patient service use. One particular area of focus in assessing parent satisfaction in autism is in the diagnostic process specifically. In 1994, Smith and colleagues launched a comprehensive evaluation to assess whether the diagnostic process for autism had improved during the previous decade for families. Participants included 127 families of children aged 19 years and younger with autism diagnoses. Outcomes of their investigation yielded a lack of significant progress in diagnosis, support, and early intervention among those families surveyed (Smith et al., 1994). In the 30 years since, research has continued to investigate parental and individual/adult perspectives of the diagnostic process. Although several consistencies have been identified in the literature, numerous discrepancies still exist. Overall, the quality of the research in this area is still emerging. Rich information has been gained from qualitative studies, which have identified meaningful themes that aid in understanding the parent and/or professional experience through the diagnostic process. However, due to methodological limitations including inconsistency in measurement and a lack of rigorous quantitative studies, the ability to generalize on a larger-scale is limited. This is especially significant given the heterogeneity of autism, and the likely impact upon the diversity of parent perspectives.

The focus of this chapter is to explore the reactions and perspectives of parents, and in some cases the individuals themselves, regarding the diagnostic process for autism. First, the most common pathways to diagnosis will be presented, integrated with the factors that can impact stress and satisfaction among families. Within these common steps of the diagnostic process, current research will be discussed in order to highlight strengths and areas that require continued focus. Next, the chapter will outline best practices for working efficiently and effectively with families during the assessment and diagnostic process. Finally, future directions for research will be discussed.

Diagnostic Pathway

Development of Parental Concerns

Developmental milestones are important indicators for parents that their child is progressing as expected. When parents begin noticing that their child is not engaging in typical behaviors expected for his or her age, worry, or anxiety may develop. Among children with autism, most parents' concerns regarding development occur before age 3, with some parents reporting concerns as early as age 12 months (Becerra-Culqui et al., 2018; Crane et al., 2016; Herlihy et al., 2015; Matheis et al., 2017; Mackenzie et al., 2023; Richards et al., 2016; Zablotsky et al., 2017; Zuckerman et al., 2015). Several studies have examined the types of early concerns identified by parents or caregivers. Results consistently indicate that the majority of parents first recognize delays or abnormalities in language development (Becerra-Culqui et al., 2018; Crane et al., 2015; Mitroulaki et al., 2020; Richards et al., 2016) and/or social skills (Crane et al., 2015; Richards et al., 2016). Additional concerns include behavioral disturbances (Crane et al., 2015; Mitroulaki et al., 2020), limited imaginative play (Moh & Magiati, 2012), restricted/repetitive behaviors (Chamak et al., 2011; Moh & Magiati, 2012), sleep or feeding difficulties, (Chamak et al., 2011; Molteni & Maggiolini, 2014), and general delays in motor development (McConkey et al., 2009).

Previous research has highlighted slight differences in these early concerning symptoms based upon autism subtype/severity. For example, Mitroulaki et al. (2020) examined differences in initial parent concerns across different autism spectrum presentations (DSM-IV, DSM-IV-TR, DSM-5, ICD-10) in a sample of 128 children with DSM-IV-TR diagnoses of Autistic disorder (72.7%), Asperger syndrome (18.8), and other developmental diagnoses (e.g., Pervasive Developmental Disorder, Not Otherwise Specified; 8.6%). Speech and language challenges were reported as first concerns significantly more often in the Autistic disorder group, while behavior problems and educational difficulties were significantly more often reported in the Asperger syndrome group (Mitroulaki et al., 2020). Importantly, age of diagnosis also differed across groups, with children with Asperger syndrome diagnosed at significantly later ages than children with Autistic disorder. Sheldrick et al. (2017) also observed a similar pattern of results, finding that across two national children's health surveys, reported age of diagnosis decreased as reported symptom severity increased ("mild", "moderate" "severe"; Sheldrick et al., 2017). These findings suggest that individuals with autism who have higher cognitive and language abilities initially may exhibit more subtle symptoms that are not identified until later years.

Research has also suggested that initial parent concerns may also differ across racial/ethnic identity groups. A recent study by Azad et al. (2022) using a large sample ($n = 489$) children comprising different racial/ethnic identities (White, Hispanic/Latinx, Black/African American, Asian, multiracial) observed significant group differences in the frequency of reported parent concerns across multiple domains including cognition, emotion/behavior, social/communication, and restricted/repetitive behaviors. For example, compared to White children, rates of autism-specific restricted/repetitive behaviors were lower for Asian, Hispanic/Latinx, and Black/African American children, while rates of communication concerns were higher for all three groups, as well as for multiracial children. Additionally, rates of emotional/behavioral concerns were lower for Asian and Black/African American children compared to White children and both Black/African American and multiracial children had lower frequencies of reported cognitive concerns (Azad et al., 2022). Interestingly, other studies have largely not observed significant differences between racial/ethnic groups across these domains (e.g., Donahue et al., 2017; Issarraras et al., 2019), though some differences appear to be more robust, specifically differences in social concerns (Donahue et al., 2017, Issarraras et al., 2018) and cognitive concerns (Zeleke et al., 2019).

Encounters with Professionals

It is not uncommon for a lag time to exist between the period that initial concerns are identified and the point at which families pursue further assessment. Mackenzie et al. (2023) reported an average delay of 5 months. Prior studies have indicated that parents wait between 7 and 8 months prior to scheduling an initial appointment with a professional (Daley, 2004; Howlin & Moore, 1997). It is possible that these delays occur due to familial beliefs that the symptoms will subside over time. Alternately, families or individuals may be uncertain if their concerns are valid. During this pre-diagnostic period, worry and anxiety may continue to develop in the family as decisions are eventually made to pursue further evaluation.

Initial Visit. There are a variety of professionals who serve as the initial point of contact for families to discuss their concerns. These individuals include pediatricians, psychiatrists, psychologists, educators, and other medical or mental health providers. However, the first consultation is often with the primary care provider or general practitioner/pediatrician (Johnson & Myers, 2007). A variety of outcomes can result from this initial consultation. Families may either receive a formal autism diagnosis, a diagnosis of a different condition (e.g., language delay, intellectual disability, behavioral problems), referral for additional assessment, or assurance that there is no cause for concern.

The extent to which general medical providers are attentive and proactive with early warning signs varies, and the issue is complex. Some health and mental health professionals may be insufficiently trained in autism to accurately identify subtle symptoms or various presentations of behaviors (Morris et al., 2019). In some cases, parents lack confidence in their general medical provider's skills to identify autism (Carbone et al., 2010; Harrington et al., 2006). Many times, families simply wait until additional or more significant concerns develop in their child. In an investigation by Carbone and colleagues (2013), 144 parents of children with autism completed a questionnaire assessing perceptions of their general medical provider's abilities to address specific needs and conditions related to their children's diagnoses. Additionally, 144 general medical providers (unmatched to family participants) completed a similar questionnaire regarding self-perceptions of their own abilities in the same areas. Participating providers rated their abilities in addressing early behavioral or developmental concerns more favorably (i.e., 78% rated as "good") than parents (i.e., 62% rated as "good"). Additionally, Carbone and colleagues identified that one of the most discrepant areas between parents and general medical providers was in the ability to make appropriate referrals during the diagnostic process. Approximately 80% of providers perceived that they had "good" abilities to make appropriate referrals, compared to only 50% of parents (Carbone et al., 2013). These discrepancies suggest that there may be a gap between professionals and families related to needs and expectations during the initial contact and subsequent rendered services.

Differences in provider responses may also depend on differences in presenting concerns. For instance, Zuckerman et al. (2015) examined the association between later diagnosis and provider response to initial caregiver concerns in a large sample of children diagnosed with autism ($n = 1420$) and children diagnosed with intellectual disability (ID)/developmental delay (DD) ($n = 2098$). Caregivers of children with autism were significantly more likely than children with ID/DD to receive one or more reassuring/passive responses from providers (e.g., "it was too early to tell if anything was wrong") and significantly less likely to receive one or more proactive responses from providers (e.g., "making a referral to a specialist; such as a developmental pediatrician, child psychologist, occupational, or speech therapist"), with reassuring/passive responses associated with longer delays between initial discussion of concerns with the provider and autism diagnosis (Zuckerman et al., 2015).

Research has also found that primary care providers (PCPs) might not feel comfortable or proficient in identifying early warning signs and symptoms of autism within minority children. Zuckerman et al. (2013) evaluated PCPs self-ratings of perceived difficulty in identifying early warning signs and symptoms of autism within minority children. Among 267 PCPs, approximately 60% reported difficulty in identifying autism symptoms and warnings signs in Spanish-speaking Hispanic/Latinx families. Approximately 37% of PCPs reported the same difficulty for African American/Black children. These ratings were found to be significantly different from that of White children (Zuckerman et al., 2013). Further, disparities exist in developmental screening. Children of color are less likely to be screened in primary care settings, and when screened have higher false positivity rates (Carbone et al., 2020; Guthrie et al., 2019). Further compounding this issue is that language can act as a significant barrier. Indeed, Zuckerman et al. (2013) observed that among the 267 PCPs surveyed, a substantially minority offered screening in Spanish, with 17.7% conducting Spanish language general developmental screening, 28.7% conducting Spanish language autism-specific screening, and only 10.3% offering both. Overall, these outcomes reflect the ways in which cultural and language variables can impact the assessment of autism and perhaps the screening and diagnostic experiences of those families.

Parent reactions to this initial contact with professionals can vary. Some parents cite confidence in the consulted professional's assessment abilities and feel respected and valued during evaluation appointments (Hackett et al., 2009). Other families may be told by professionals that there are no significant issues of concern. In these situations, feelings of stress and frustration can develop, especially for parents who believe there are clear abnormalities occurring in their child's behavior or development. In fact, some parents believe that their initial concerns were not taken seriously by professionals, or that they were unable to accurately describe their worries to their PCP or general practitioner (Braiden et al., 2010).

Subsequent Referrals. When parents and professionals are in agreement about initial concerns, research has demonstrated that 50% to 55% of families are then referred to subsequent providers (Howlin & Moore, 1997; Jones et al., 2014; Moh & Magiati, 2012). During this next stage of the diagnostic process, psychiatrists, psychologists, and multidisciplinary teams are common providers of additional specialized assessment. Even after referrals to these specialists, it is not unusual for some families to be further referred to other professionals for additional evaluation. Although identified estimates have varied, families typically visit an average of four to five professionals before receiving a final autism diagnosis (Goin-Kochel et al., 2006; Moh & Magiati, 2012). In fact, research suggests that families often see three or more providers before receiving a final autism diagnosis (Mackenzie et al., 2023; Makino et al., 2021; Wong et al., 2017; Zavaleta-Ramirez et al., 2020). Wait times for these appointments can compound delays in diagnosis. For example, a study of a large-scale national sample of caregivers of children diagnosed with autism found a mean wait time of five months for referral visits, with an average of 3.5 additional referral visits following the initial provider visit (Mackenzie et al., 2023), meaning that families experienced, on average, a diagnostic process of over a year. A factor that contributes greatly to this high number of referrals is that access to quality services (i.e., autism-specific diagnostic centers, specialized professionals) is sometimes limited due to a shortage in providers who are able to or feel comfortable diagnosing autism (Drahota et al., 2020; Mahapatra et al., 2019; Martinez et al., 2018; Morris et al., 2019).

These referrals and multiple appointments can take a toll on a family. Goin-Kochel and colleagues (2006) found a significant inverse relationship between the number of professional encounters and overall satisfaction. Specifically, increased satisfaction was associated with fewer visits to professionals and decreased satisfaction associated with more professional visits (Goin-Kochel et al., 2006). One aspect of receiving multiple referrals that is likely strongly linked to parent satisfaction is receipt of multiple diagnoses. Many parents report their child's diagnosis of ASD being delayed by receiving other developmental, behavioral, and psychiatric diagnoses (Avlund et al., 2021; Brookman-Frazee et al., 2012; Crane et al., 2016; Martinez et al., 2018; Stahmer et al., 2019). In fact, Mackenzie et al. (2023) observed that in their sample of 406 caregivers of children diagnosed with ASD, only 5% received a formal diagnosis of ASD at their initial visit. Receiving multiple diagnoses can certainly be confusing and upsetting to caregivers who are searching for answers and assistance. Different diagnoses come with vast differences in evidence-based interventions, expected longitudinal trajectories, and associated stigmas. Further, mismatches between diagnoses and parents' perceived difficulties for their child may result in parents feeling that their child's needs are not being met or that their concerns are not being heeded, further contributing to stress and frustration.

Variables Impacting Diagnostic Evaluation Process

The length of the diagnostic process may be influenced by several variables including level of severity, race/ethnicity, and socioeconomic status. These variables can introduce complexity to the evaluation process, which potentially may lead to delays in final diagnoses. Taking into consideration the association between age of diagnosis and parental satisfaction (Goin-Kochel et al., 2006; Siklos & Kerns, 2006), it is important to understand how these additional variables impact parental experiences of the diagnostic process.

Clinical presentation and symptom severity can influence age of diagnosis and diagnostic delay. Though subsumed under the single diagnostic category of autism spectrum disorder in DSM-5, research has traditionally used the previous diagnostic classifications of "pervasive developmental disorder—not otherwise specified (PDD-NOS)", "Asperger's syndrome", and "autistic disorder" to denote varying levels of symptoms and functional impairment. In their systematic review and meta-analysis of studies conducted internationally between 2012 and 2019, van't Hof et al. (2021) observed that the median age of diagnosis across studies ranged from 30 to 68.1 months for autistic disorder, 30 to 84 months for Asperger's syndrome, and 61 to 114 months for PDD-NOS. Further, the number of autism-specific symptoms has also been associated with age of diagnosis, with more symptoms resulting in earlier diagnosis (Daniels & Mandell, 2014). Regarding symptom severity, research suggests that milder autism symptom severity and higher cognitive and communication abilities are associated with later ages of diagnosis (Avlund et al., 2021; Mazurek et al., 2014, Mishaal et al., 2014; Sheldrick et al., 2017; Zwaigenbaum et al., 2019), though other studies have not observed significant differences (Moh & Magiati, 2012). Interestingly and somewhat counterintuitively, studies have found that higher levels of restricted, repetitive behaviors are associated with later ages of diagnosis (Mishaal et al., 2014; Zwaigenbaum et al., 2019).

Symptom severity was also found to impact the number of encounters with professionals. For example, Moh and Magiati (2012) found a negative correlation between the degree of autism severity and the number of professional consultations, such that individuals with more severe symptomology visited fewer professionals in order to obtain a diagnosis. This finding is likely due to a clearer presentation of diagnostic criteria. There are also specific deficits or clinical presentations associated with parental stress and satisfaction. Siklos and Kerns (2006) found that families of children with more impaired communication reported lower levels of stress and higher rates of satisfaction during the diagnostic process. Conversely, parents of children with greater externalizing behavioral difficulties report less satisfaction with their diagnostic experiences. Their research suggested that communication deficits may be identified more efficiently by professionals, leading to quicker referrals, evaluation, and access to services (Siklos & Kerns, 2006), perhaps due to greater diagnostic specificity of these symptoms.

Another crucial component of the diagnostic process are the providers themselves. Importantly, providers' own experiences and expertise with autism can influence the diagnostic process and subsequently influence parents' levels of stress and satisfaction. If providers feel ill-equipped, unsure, or frustrated, this may be apparent in their interactions with patients and families and lead to decreased parent satisfaction. In a recent systematic review, Morris et al. (2019) identified 27 quantitative and qualitative studies comprising 6537 health care providers in the USA, Canada, Australia, United Kingdom, India, Nigeria, and Pakistan. Providers, many of whom were family physicians, endorsed feeling that patients with autism were too complex for their scope of practice in terms of medical needs and service/support needs and that they lacked knowledge of the etiology, symptom presentation, and diagnostic criteria of the disorder (Morris et al., 2019). Providers also shared that limited access to education, training, and experience with autism served as a barrier, while prior professional and personal experience with a child with autism was a facilitator (Morris et al., 2019). Importantly, providers endorsed wanting specialized education and training regarding diagnostic criteria, symptom presentation, co-occurring disorders, and interventions (Morris et al., 2019). More recently, Hamp et al. (2023) identified other challenges for providers that parallel those reported by parents. These challenges include frustration with the prolonged and complicated process of obtaining a diagnosis (which sometimes led to providers not making referrals for formal evaluations to spare families their own frustration), feeling obligated to refer patients for specialist evaluations even when cases were straightforward which unnecessarily complicated the diagnostic process, and needing to exert more energy and patience when parents resisted diagnosis (Hamp et al., 2023).

Past researchers (Brogan & Knussen, 2003; Howlin & Moore, 1997) also found that higher parental satisfaction was associated with receiving a definitive rather than tentative diagnosis. Several researchers have made note of participants with diagnoses of "autistic traits, tendencies, or features" (e.g., Brogan & Knussen, 2003; Howlin & Moore, 1997; Siklos & Kerns, 2006; Smith et al., 1994). These descriptors were often defined as tentative diagnoses in the above studies and identified those individuals who did not meet full diagnostic criteria for autism. When professionals provide a tentative diagnosis, it may be due to their caution or hesitancy in assigning a false positive outcome (Zwaigenbaum & Stone, 2006) or later misdiagnosis (Nissenbaum et al., 2002). However, it is important for professionals to be aware that tentative diagnoses have been associated with lower rates of satisfaction from parents and families (Brogan & Knussen, 2003; Howlin & Moore, 1997).

Overall, parental satisfaction with the evaluation process can correlate with a child's diagnostic age. Fortunately, the outcomes from a literature review on age of autism diagnosis by Daniels and Mandell (2014) yielded a consistent trend for children being diagnosed at earlier ages. This may reflect a recent trend toward increased screening and surveillance for autism among younger children leading to further evaluation (Brian et al., 2008; Johnson & Myers, 2007; Nadel & Poss, 2007). Timely diagnosis can allow children access to earlier intervention services (Boyd et al., 2010; Lord & Richler, 2006) which may positively impact upon their long term prognosis (Klintwall et al., 2015; Osborne et al., 2008) and also serve to decrease rates of parental stress (Wong & Kwan, 2010).

Disclosure of Diagnosis

The delivery of a diagnosis has the potential to be a very stress-inducing period in the diagnostic process for both families and professionals. At this delicate juncture, many parents or family members have already personally identified significant concerns in their child's behaviors, met with numerous professionals, and likely have endured long waiting periods. Given all of these factors, families often present to the feedback/disclosure appointment with heightened anxiety and worry and a variety of contradictory emotions about potential diagnostic outcomes (Molteni & Maggiolini, 2014). Research has been consistent regarding parent/family satisfaction with the actual delivery of diagnosis. Some studies have demonstrated that families are largely satisfied with how they were given the autism diagnosis for their child. For example, in an examination of 102 parents of children with autism in Singapore, Moh and Magiati (2012) found that on average, participants reported moderate satisfaction with the manner in which diagnostic information was shared with them. Parents also conveyed satisfaction with providers who gave specific information about their child's diagnosis, collaborated with caregivers in making decisions, and explained the process and reasons for the diagnosis (Moh & Magiati, 2012). Similar results were observed by Mackenzie et al. (2023) in their survey of 406 parents of children in the U.S. diagnosed with autism. A large proportion of parents reported feeling *very satisfied* with the professional manner in which the diagnosis was provided (70%) and with the information provided at the diagnostic appointment (47%), with only a small minority expressing dissatisfaction (either *somewhat dissatisfied* or *very dissatisfied*) with these two components (6% and 9% respectively; Mackenzie et al., 2023).

Researchers have also examined the perspectives of parents related to the positive and negative factors associated with the delivery of diagnosis. In their scoping review of the literature, Makino et al. (2021) identified several factors that have been reported to influence parents' experiences with receiving their child's diagnosis. General themes that emerged related to more positive experiences included parents wanting providers to be empathetic and to utilize a strengths-based approach, having opportunities to ask questions and process information, and discussions related to their child's prognosis and next steps (Makino et al., 2021). Conversely, negative experiences included believing their child's diagnosis was not sufficiently explained, feeling overwhelmed with the amount of information provided at the feedback appointment, and confusion and lower levels of satisfaction associated with tentative diagnoses of autism (Makino et al., 2021). Further, Anderberg and South (2021) found that increased parent certainty that their child would receive an autism diagnosis was predictive of more positive emotional reactions to the diagnosis and greater pre-feedback appointment parent knowledge of autism and resources felt more prepared for next steps post-diagnosis. Increased provider positivity was also an important predictive factor of greater positive emotional reactions and preparedness. Conversely, higher pre-feedback appointment parent anxiety about receiving the diagnosis and lower pre-appointment knowledge of autism were associated with greater levels of negative emotional reactions and confusion (Anderberg & South, 2021).

Researchers have also examined providers' experiences with sharing autism diagnoses with families. In one study, Rogers et al. (2016) surveyed 116 multidisciplinary health care providers from the UK involved in the autism diagnostic process. Choosing from a list of options, providers were asked to rank their top three most challenging aspects of providing an autism diagnosis. The most common challenge was ensuring caregivers understood the diagnosis and why it was given, with 60% of providers ranking it within their top three and 30% ranking it as their number one most challenging aspect (Rogers et al., 2016). Other frequently ranked challenges include providing technical/medical information at the appropriate level for families, managing family and caregiver distress, and the amount of information that needed to be given to families (Rogers et al., 2016). Positively, only a very small minority of providers ranked having enough information to answer questions (5%) and maintaining and empathetic approach (4%) within their top three challenges (Rogers et al., 2016).

Post-diagnosis

The period immediately following the disclosure of a diagnosis is also considered emotionally intense for many individuals and families. Crucially, parents' processing of their child's diagnosis can have lasting impacts on their own mental health (e.g., Da Paz et al., 2018), emphasizing that the diagnostic process does not end with the feedback appointment. Though many parents experience relief following their child's diagnosis (Makino et al., 2021), there are still substantial challenges that families face. Many studies have highlighted the negative experiences of families following their child's autism diagnosis, such as feeling distressed, alone and unsupported, and wanting more direction regarding next steps and interventions (Legg & Tickle, 2019; Makino et al., 2021). For some parents, the shock or stress of receiving a formal autism diagnosis can interfere with their ability to effectively hear and understand post-diagnostic feedback from professionals (Abbott et al., 2013). Many of the participants in Abbott and colleagues' investigation reported feeling overwhelmed by the overall amount of information provided at the disclosure or feedback session. Researchers have also indicated that individuals and family members identified dissatisfaction due to a lack of post-diagnostic support (Jones et al., 2014; Osborne & Reed, 2008; Siklos & Kerns, 2006) or because information was not described as efficiently or effectively as possible (Jones et al., 2014; Legg & Tickle, 2019; Makino et al., 2021). Considering these findings, it appears crucial to enact a careful balance in the type and quantity of information provided at this sensitive stage of the diagnosis process.

In sum, several variables (i.e., number of professional encounters, diagnostic age/wait time, quality of professional relationship) have been associated with levels of stress and satisfaction of families and individuals during the diagnostic period. The identification and assessment of these variables are essential for increasing the knowledge and awareness of professionals who are engaged in service delivery. With greater understanding of family and patient experiences during the diagnostic process, professionals can strive to implement best practice strategies aimed at improving satisfaction and overall experiences.

Length of Diagnostic Process

Given the number of individual stages of the diagnostic process that families must progress through, the journey to receiving an appropriate diagnosis can be remarkably lengthy and challenging. Importantly, this can have a substantial effect on families' levels of stress and satisfaction. The average period of time between age of initial concerns and diagnosis has varied among studies. Researchers have typically cited a length of time between 2 and 4 years for the diagnostic process, with the typical age of diagnosis ranging from 3 to 6 years among children (CDC, 2014; Crane et al., 2016; Daley, 2004; Daniels & Mandell, 2014; Goin-Kochel et al., 2006; Howlin & Moore, 1997; Maenner et al., 2023; Mansell & Morris, 2004; McMorris et al., 2013; Mitroulaki et al., 2020; Moh & Magiati, 2012; Sheldrick et al., 2017; Siklos & Kerns, 2006; van't Hoff et al., 2021; Wiggins et al., 2006; Zavaleta-Ramirez et al., 2020; Zuckerman et al., 2015; Zuckerman et al., 2017). Caregivers have reported the extensive waiting from age of first concern to receiving the diagnosis to being able to take next steps as particularly challenging (Smith-Young et al., 2020) and quantitative research has demonstrated a significant association between time taken to receive a diagnosis and overall parent satisfaction (Crane et al., 2016).

It is noted that results have varied and some investigators found children diagnosed at younger ages and in a more expedited process (e.g., Harrington et al., 2006). This is encouraging given that rates of satisfaction have been found to be higher among parents whose children were diagnosed at younger ages (Goin-Kochel et al., 2006; Siklos & Kerns, 2006). However, even a wait of only a few months can still be considered a prolonged period of uncertainty and stress in the lives of families.

Racial/Ethnic Differences in Experience with the Diagnostic Process

As outlined above, the autism diagnostic process can be complex, with a multitude of factors across multiple stages affecting parents' experiences. Importantly, racial/ethnic disparities exist across each of these stages, which can make the diagnostic process even more arduous and stressful for racially/ethnically minoritized families. A recent systemic review by Fisher et al. (2023) of qualitative studies examining the caregivers' experiences with the diagnostic process identified 15 studies representing 253 Black, Hispanic/Latinx, Chinese, and Korean caregivers. Caregivers reported adverse experiences due to a number of different factors at all stages of the process. Families' experiences were impacted by systems-level factors such as parental custodial issues and financial constraints, as well as provider-level factors including providers minimizing caregivers' concerns or suggesting a "wait and see" approach before taking next steps and making biased assumptions (Fisher et al., 2023). For example, racially/ethnically minoritized families frequently reported experiencing biased assumptions from providers about family socio-demographics or language delays being the result of limited exposure to English. Cultural and non-English language factors also played a role in negatively affecting caregivers' experiences, as caregivers reported difficulties with stigma, cultural perceptions and knowledge of autism, medical jargon, and lack of materials or interpretive services for non-English speaking families (Fisher et al., 2023).

Similar results have also been observed quantitatively. Using data from the 2011 *Survey of Pathways to Diagnosis and Services* (a follow-up to the 2009–2010 *National Survey of Children with Special Health Care Needs*) of children with, Zeleke et al. (2019) examined differences between White and racial/ethnic minoritized families' experiences obtaining an autism diagnosis for their child. Several key differences emerged. Researchers indicated that while there was no significant difference in the age of caregivers first concerns about their child's development, White families were more likely than racially/ethnically minoritized families to speaks with doctors or health care professionals about those concerns (Zeleke et al., 2019). Providers more often told families they were completing a developmental screening and had children completely developmental tasks (e.g., stacking objects, recognizing colors) for White families than for minoritized families, and White families were more likely to report feeling that providers met their child's needs and that they were satisfied with received health care services (Zeleke et al., 2019). Regarding families' perceptions of the disorder, racially/ethnically minoritized families were more likely than White families to endorse viewing autism as a lifelong, mysterious, genetic/heritable condition (Zeleke et al., 2019).

Virtual Diagnostic Evaluations

The widespread adoption of telehealth services has allowed for even greater service utilization, particularly for families living in rural and underserved areas. Within autism research, studies have highlighted the utility and validity of telehealth assessment (Alfuraydan et al., 2020; Liu & Ma, 2022; Stavropoulos et al., 2022). Though studies have been limited by sample size and available psychometrics, results nonetheless shown that the telehealth screening and assessment have good accuracy compared to in-person visits (Alfuraydan et al., 2020; Liu & Ma, 2022; Stavropoulos et al., 2022). Notably, there is a dearth of studies that have examined caregiver satisfaction with the telehealth assessment, but results have been promising. Reese et al. (2013) assessed parent satisfaction with the diagnostic assessment among a sample 10 children with developmental delays and 11 age-matched children with an existing diagnosis of autism, all of whom had completed an in-person evaluation within the previous two years. Participants were then randomly assigned to either an in-person or telehealth evaluation condition. In addition to no significant differences in diagnostic accuracy or clinician ratings on standardized assessments and measures, there were also no differences in parent satisfaction. Parents in both in-person and telehealth conditions reported high levels of satisfaction regarding aspects such as level of comfort talking with clinicians and feeling that the clinicians were competent and caring, as well as overall level of satisfaction (Reese et al., 2013). Additionally, Corona et al. (2021) found that in a sample of 51 children ages 1–3 comprising 35 children with autism, 10 with developmental delays, and six who were typically developing, parents generally had positive perceptions of the telehealth screening and assessment. The majority of parents found it comfortable to play with their child on while video, easy to follow spoken instructions, and felt that the appointment was an appropriate duration (Corona et al., 2021). However, it is important to note that 12% of parents felt that telehealth screening did not elicit the specific behaviors they were most concerned about. While results have been promising, additional research is needed. Researchers should continue to examine how telehealth can be optimized to ensure the best quality of services provided to families while maximizing their reach, particularly to families facing barriers to in-person services.

Improving the Diagnostic Process

As indicated earlier, it may take several years for a child to obtain an autism diagnosis. The child may be placed on waiting lists (Connolly & Gersch, 2013) or referred to multiple providers before he/she receives a diagnosis (Goin-Kochel et al., 2006). Waiting for a diagnosis is anxiety provoking for parents (Osborne & Reed, 2008). When it comes to receiving the diagnosis, parents report wanting empathy and optimism (Makino et al., 2021). As providers, there are a number of things that we can do to help attenuate the stress that parents experience during the evaluation process and thereby hopefully increase their satisfaction with services.

Preparing Families for the Process

Although parents would like the diagnostic process to take less time, this is not always possible for clinics. To reduce parental distress during this time period, parents find it helpful if professionals inform them about the length of the diagnostic process beforehand (Abbott et al., 2013; Connolly & Gersch, 2013). If the child is completing a multidisciplinary assessment, parents prefer being informed that several different professionals will be completing the exam. This information helps parents understand why the diagnostic process takes a significant amount of time and also helps relieve parental frustration (Abbott et al., 2013).

While waiting for an autism diagnosis, parents may experience fear and anxiety because they have either inaccurate or no information about autism. Parents can find an overwhelming amount of information on the internet. Additionally, they may only obtain information about the most severe cases (Connolly & Gersch, 2013). To reduce parental fear and anxiety, professionals should provide parents with information about autism while they are waiting for their diagnostic assessment. Professionals could provide parents with pamphlets and/or handouts on autism, along with a list of reputable websites and books. This information could be provided to the family via a letter in the mail or be posted on the agency's website. When professionals provide this information to the family, they should clearly state that they do not know if the child meets criteria for autism. Professionals should state that they are providing this information because many parents report that receiving accurate information on autism helps alleviate parental anxiety during the diagnostic process. These statements could be provided in a letter to the family and/or verbally when the family schedules the autism evaluation.

The Feedback Session

Consensus among clinical practice guidelines is that feedback should not be delayed and occur shortly after the diagnostic evaluation, though only one set of guidelines, from the National Institute of Care Excellence (2017), provided a specific time frame—six weeks (Pattison et al., 2022). When planning feedback sessions, consideration should be given to the time and setting. Professionals should allocate a sufficient amount of time to the feedback session (Mulligan et al., 2012). Researchers suggested allocating between 75 and 90 min to the feedback session (Pruett, 2013). Feedback should be provided in a private setting, where the professional and family will not be disturbed (Baird et al., 2000). Since receiving diagnostic feedback can be a stressful experience for parents, it should be delivered in a family friendly setting.

It is recommended that professionals have comfortable chairs or tables in their office (Nissenbaum et al., 2002) and the room be arranged in a manner that is conducive to conversation (Shea, 1993). Since parents can have negative emotional reactions to the diagnosis, it is beneficial to have tissues available (Shea, 1993). While potentially sounding minor to providers, a warm and comfortable environment for delivering feedback may reduce some of the external stress experienced by the parents and therefore allow them to more effectively listen to the information being provided. With the expansion of telehealth capability and accessibility since the COVID-19 pandemic, providers are encouraged to utilize telehealth modalities for delivery of assessment feedback. Providing feedback via telehealth is not only efficient, but may also allow additional caregivers the opportunity to attend the feedback session.

Beyond location and duration, another factor to consider is the people present in a feedback session. During an autism evaluation, families may be assessed by several professionals on a multidisciplinary team or one professional (Mulligan et al., 2012). When a multidisciplinary team completes the evaluation, the team should meet prior to the feedback session in order to discuss the data and results. Together, the team should decide who from the team will be present for the feedback session and how information, results of the assessment, and the diagnosis will be disseminated (i.e., who will speak, lead the session, and deliver the diagnosis). Frequently, it is the psychologist on the team who delivers the diagnosis (Nissenbaum et al., 2002). Additionally, the team should designate one main professional for the family to contact with questions (Cottrell & Summers, 1990). However, if a single professional or multidisciplinary team completes the evaluation, the professional who delivers feedback should have a prior relationship with the family. Parents prefer receiving feedback from someone who has interacted with their child and has firsthand knowledge of his/her skills and behavior (Shea, 1993).

In addition to ensuring the appropriate providers are present for feedback, parents have indicated that they do not like being informed of a diagnosis while they were alone and did not have any support. If the child comes from a multi-caregiver home, the providers should inform parents of the diagnosis when they are together when possible (Baird et al., 2000; Poehlmann et al., 2005). If the child comes from a one-parent household, providers should ask the parent if they would like to bring another individual to the feedback session for support (Baird et al., 2000). If other family members (e.g., grandparents, aunts, uncles) also live in the home or are significantly involved in the child's life (e.g., provide childcare), then it may also be beneficial to invite them. Consideration must be given to parents who are divorced or separated. It is best practice to have all interested parties in the room, which includes all parents and stepparents. However, if parents do not live near each other or have a hostile relationship, then it may be best to have two separate feedback sessions (Tharinger et al., 2008). It is important that providers weigh the time required to coordinate parties for feedback sessions with the need for timely feedback. Providers should make themselves available for questions following the feedback session, especially in cases where all caregiving parties may not be able to attend.

Research and clinical practice guidelines are inconsistent regarding if children should be present in the room during feedback (Pattison et al., 2022). Nissenbaum et al. (2002) interviewed parents and asked them if their child was present during feedback. The majority of parents indicated that their child was not in the room during feedback. Parents who preferred having their child out of the room indicated that their child would not have understood the information and/or that they needed time to grieve the diagnosis without their child present. Tharinger et al. (2008) suggests having a second feedback session with the child and his/her parents after the professional has completed a separate feedback with the parents. It is recommended that this session occur days or weeks after the initial parent feedback session to allow parents time to process their initial emotional reactions to the diagnosis. When delivering feedback to children, information should be provided in a developmentally appropriate manner. Children with autism often have poor insight into their psychological self (Williams, 2010). Therefore, they may be unable to recognize their symptoms. It may be beneficial for professionals to give concrete examples of the child's symptoms when informing the child of his/her diagnosis. Professionals could also use visuals and/or social stories to assist the child in understanding his/her symptoms. Additionally, professionals should use simple language that the child will understand.

It is recommended that parents have the opportunity to ask questions throughout the feedback session (Abbott et al., 2013; Mulligan et al., 2012). When parents ask questions, professionals should do their best to answer all of them. Subsequently, many clinical practice guidelines recommend that professionals should provide honest and accurate information and should do so in a way that is understandable to non-clinical individuals (Pattison et al., 2022). Providers should consider the parents' psychosocial background when providing information, using language that is appropriate for the given context (e.g., verbal and written proficiency, education, possible presence of parental characteristics of autism; Fuentes et al., 2021; Pattison et al., 2022).

Structuring the Feedback Session

In addition to thinking about all of the various factors outlined above that influence the nature of a feedback session, clinicians should also give prior consideration to the way that information is being delivered. Feedback sessions should be a structured session that is outlined and planned beforehand (Abbott et al., 2013). At the beginning of the feedback session, it is beneficial for professionals to check in with the parents and assess their feelings about the assessment process (Tharinger et al., 2008). Next, professionals should review the purpose of the evaluation (Groth-Marnat, 2003) and provide an outline for the session (Tharinger et al., 2008). At this point, it is important that professionals emphasize the importance of collaboration during feedback. Parents must be encouraged to offer their opinions, thoughts, and disagreements. Moreover, professionals should encourage parents to ask questions throughout the feedback session. In addition, it is recommended that professionals thank parents for their participation and validate their feelings about the evaluation process. It is also beneficial if professionals acknowledge the time and energy that parents dedicated to the evaluation (Tharinger et al., 2008).

When professionals inform parents of their child's diagnosis, it is recommended that they provide information about autism, the assessment tools used in the evaluation, and the child's assessment results or leveling of functioning (Pattison et al., 2022). After the diagnosis is rendered, professionals should provide information regarding the child's prognosis (Mansell & Morris, 2004; Mulligan et al., 2012; Nissenbaum et al., 2002) and recommendations (Tharinger et al., 2008). With regard to the child's prognosis, professionals should educate parents on the child's future development and the impact of early intervention (Nissenbaum et al., 2002). When reviewing recommendations, it is beneficial if professionals adequately explain treatment options (Mansell & Morris, 2004) and provide information regarding local resources (Mulligan et al., 2012). All recommendations should be specific and individualized to the child.

Overall, feedback should be provided in a manner that is honest (Mulligan et al., 2012; Nissenbaum et al., 2002), clear (Abrams & Goodman, 1998; Baird et al., 2000; Mulligan et al., 2012), and easy to understand (Abbott et al., 2013; Nissenbaum et al., 2002; Shea, 1993; Watermeyer et al., 2012). Professionals should be honest regarding the child's strengths, needs, weaknesses, and future prognosis (Shea, 1993). At times, professionals avoid using labels during feedback sessions (Abrams & Goodman, 1998; Chamak et al., 2011). They may inform parents that the child has communication problems, a developmental delay, or language problems (Chamak et al., 2011). Instead of avoiding diagnostic labels, which can lead to confusion on the part of the parents, professionals should clearly state that the child meets criteria for autism (Abrams & Goodman, 1998).

To assist with comprehension, professionals should repeat information, have visual aids, and use examples when explaining concepts. Professionals should be aware of parental verbal and nonverbal cues that indicate if they understand the information being presented. Research suggests that parents who do not spontaneously ask questions, appear unwilling to engage in the discussion, and provide minimal verbal (e.g., yes, no, okay, uh huh) and nonverbal responses (e.g., head nod) likely do not understand the information or may be confused (Watermeyer et al., 2012).

Professionals should focus on the child's strengths and provide hope for the family during feedback (Abbott et al., 2013; Mulligan et al., 2012; Nissenbaum et al., 2002). Parents report being more satisfied with feedback when professionals discuss positive attributes of their child (Abbott et al., 2013). When professionals focus on the child's strengths, it provides hope for the parents (Mulligan et al., 2012), which in turn provides motivation for parents to handle the child's behavior and other challenging symptoms of autism. It is recommended that professionals discuss the child's strengths at the end of the feedback session so it ends on a "positive note" (Nissenbaum et al., 2002). Research suggests that parents enjoy hearing optimistic statements about their child's future (Abbott et al., 2013; Nissenbaum et al., 2002). Specifically, parents want to hear that there is hope for improvement and that there are effective interventions that could improve the child's deficits (Cottrell & Summers, 1990; Mulligan et al., 2012). Although professionals should offer hope and focus on the strengths of the child, it is important that he/she provides accurate and honest information (Shea, 1993). In other words, professionals should not provide false hope to the family.

Professionals should be supportive, warm, and empathetic during feedback (Baird et al., 2000). Failure to do so may negatively impact parents' abilities to cope with their child's diagnosis. In fact, parents who perceive their medical professional as being insensitive and lacking empathy indicate that these characteristics negatively impacted their emotional response to their child's diagnosis (Poehlmann et al., 2005). Researchers suggest that having a supportive relationship with professionals assists parents in accepting their child's diagnosis (Abbott et al., 2013).

Written Feedback

Due to the large amount of information provided and the emotional nature of feedback sessions, parents may have difficulty retaining and understanding the information presented (Abbott et al., 2013; Mulligan et al., 2012). Thus, written information should be provided to families at the feedback session so they can revisit information discussed (Braiden et al., 2010; Brogan & Knussen, 2003; Mulligan et al., 2012). Specifically, the family should be provided with a written report regarding the diagnostic process (Shea, 1993). Researchers suggest that professionals inform parents at the beginning of the feedback session that they will be receiving a report in order to relieve their anxiety of having to remember all of the information presented (Tharinger et al., 2008). Notably, many clinical practice guidelines recommend that reports not only be provided to the family, but to other professionals as well such as the referring provider, the child's primary care provider, and other relevant or health care providers (Pattison et al., 2022).

In addition to a written psychological report, parents find it beneficial if they receive pamphlets, booklets, and/or websites on autism (Mulligan et al., 2012; Osborne & Reed, 2008), along with a reading list (Braiden et al., 2010; Mansell & Morris, 2004; Mulligan et al., 2012). Written information about local resources and treatment should also be provided to parents (Mansell & Morris, 2004; Nissenbaum et al., 2002). It is helpful if professionals include the phone number and name of the contact person in this information (Baird et al., 2000; Nissenbaum et al., 2002). All written materials provided to parents should be written using simple language; parents must be able to understand the information (Braiden et al., 2010; Nissenbaum et al., 2002).

Summary

In summary, a variety of factors must be considered when providing feedback to parents. Professionals should be knowledgeable about how to prepare for the feedback session, structure the feedback session, deliver feedback, and provide written information. While it can be quite time consuming to do so, research has demonstrated that parents' reaction to receiving an autism diagnosis are impacted by the quality of the assessment and feedback they receive. A summary of the feedback session is provided in Table 1.

Table 1 Strategies for effective feedback sessions

The feedback session
Preparing for the feedback session • Have comfortable chairs and tables • Have tissues available • Arrange chairs in a manner that is conducive to conversation • Schedule the feedback session for 60–75 min • Ask the parent(s) if he/she would like to bring another adult to the interview (i.e., spouse, partner, family member(s), and/or family friend) • Have the parent(s) decide if he/she would like the child present during the feedback session
Structuring the feedback session • Check-in with the parents and evaluate their feelings about the assessment process • Review the purpose of the evaluation • Invite parents to share their thoughts and opinions • Encourage parents to ask questions at any point • Review the diagnostic criteria of autism and state which symptoms the child demonstrates • Clearly state that the child meets criteria for autism • Discuss the child's strengths • Provide information regarding the child's prognosis (i.e., child's future development and the impact of early intervention) • Provide recommendations • Allow additional time at the end of the session for questions
How to deliver feedback • Use language that the parents will understand • Be honest, supportive, warm, and empathetic • Provide hope for the family
Written information provided at feedback • Written psychological report • Pamphlets, booklets, and/or handouts on autism • List of books and websites on autism • The name, telephone number, and/or website for local resources • The name and telephone number for local treatment providers

Parent Experiences Following a Diagnosis

Following the diagnosis, parents may experience either positive or negative emotional reactions. Research indicates that parents experience many different negative reactions to receiving an autism diagnosis such as shock, anger, denial, grief, sadness, and anxiety (Fernandez-Alcantara et al., 2016; Goff et al., 2013; Legg & Tickle, 2019; Makino et al., 2021; Mitchell & Holdt, 2014; Rabba et al., 2019). Following a diagnosis of autism, parents may experience grief that their child will never be "normal" (Cameron et al., 1992; Poehlmann et al., 2005). They may experience a sense of loss, as they have to alter their image of the child (Fernandez-Alcantara et al., 2016; Goff et al., 2013). Additionally, parents may worry about their child's future (Fernandez-Alcantara et al., 2016; Mansell & Morris, 2004). Specifically, parents worry about the amount of care and support their child may need during their life and how to provide this (Mitchell & Holdt, 2014). Though some parents may react negatively to their child's diagnosis, the majority of parents report experiencing a sense of relief (Makino et al., 2021). They feel relieved because their concerns regarding their child's development and/or behavior were validated (Avdi et al., 2000; Mulligan et al., 2012; Watson, 2008). Parents also report experiencing a sense of relief because a diagnosis allows them to obtain services for their child (Osborne & Reed, 2008). It is vital that professionals allow time for parents to express these concerns and provide information to reduce these concerns and correct misbeliefs, especially pertaining to the causes of autism.

Accepting the Child's Diagnosis

Accepting their child's diagnoses may be harder and take more time for some parents than others (Cameron et al., 1992; Mitchell & Holdt, 2014). However, the majority of parents report reaching this stage at some point of time (Mitchell & Holdt, 2014; Poslawsky et al., 2014). Parents may initially be in denial of their child's diagnosis, limiting their ability to accept the diagnosis (Mitchell & Holdt, 2014; Nissenbaum et al., 2002). Parents must process their negative emotional reactions before they are able to accept their child's diagnosis (Mitchell & Holdt, 2014). Some parents indicate that in order to accept their child's diagnosis, they had to alter how they viewed their child. Instead of focusing on how the child "should be", they began thinking about how "the child is" (Avdi et al., 2000).

Poslawsky et al. (2014) examined parental acceptance of their child's autism diagnosis. Parents were defined as adequately adapting and coping with the diagnosis if they were action, thinking, or feeling oriented. Parents who were action oriented took steps to obtain resources for their child and adjust their child's routine to account for the diagnosis. Thinking-oriented parents obtained information about their child's diagnosis in order to assist their understanding of autism. Feeling-oriented parents experienced both positive and negative emotions about their child's diagnosis. Poslawsky and colleagues found that most parents who accepted their child's diagnosis were action oriented. The study indicated that parents who were unable to accept their child's diagnosis were angry, emotionally overwhelmed, depressed, or neutral to their child's diagnosis. The outcomes of Poslawsky and colleagues investigation indicated that it was harder for parents to accept their child's diagnosis if he/she had more severe symptoms of autism.

Support and Resources

Children with autism should receive tailored, developmentally appropriate, and intensive intervention to address core and co-occurring challenges associated with the disorder (Hyman et al., 2020) and researchers have indicated that intervention should begin as early as possible (Hyman et al., 2020; Zwaigenbaum et al., 2015). Systematic reviews have emphasized the importance of families receiving post-diagnostic information and support for accessing intervention services (Makino et al., 2021; McCrimmon & Gray, 2021); however, many families report high levels of stress and struggle in trying to access these services for their children (Corcoran et al., 2015; Makinno et al., 2021). Mulligan et al. (2012) interviewed parents, who had children diagnosed with autism, regarding their service utilization. Parents reported that services were often limited and difficult to obtain. Many services had strict admission criteria, long wait lists, and/or provided few resources. Additionally, professionals did not assist parents in obtaining services for their child. Following the diagnosis, the professional informed the parent of services he/she would need to obtain for the child; however, they did not provide any referrals. In Crane et al.'s (2016) study of caregiver experiences in the UK, 35% of parents did not receive any offers of help from providers during or after the diagnosis process. Frustration and dissatisfaction with the lack of guidance and support received by parents at a time when they are unsure of what to do next has been echoed in other studies (e.g., Carlsson et al., 2016; Corcoran et al., 2015; Ho et al., 2014; Lappe et al., 2018; Legg & Tickle, 2019; Mackenzie et al., 2023; Rabba et al., 2019).

Facing a lack of post-diagnostic support, parents often express needing to play an active role in securing services for their child. Studies have highlighted parents' need to personally advocate for their child to receive needed services (Carlsson et al., 2016; Lappe et al., 2018; Pearson et al., 2020). Parents also experience many social, economic, and emotional challenges when trying to access services for their child, such as managing uncertainty and unanswered questions, devoting extra time and energy to locating services, social and occupational disruptions, and often needing to be an active participant in their child's treatment, all which can result in significant distress (Brookman-Frazee et al., 2012; Carlsson et al., 2016; Ho et al., 2014; Lappe et al., 2014; Lovelace et al., 2018; Rabba et al., 2019; Sansoti et al., 2012; Stahmer et al., 2019). Further, the high economic costs of care, difficulties obtaining insurance coverage for autism-specific services, and disparities in service availability are also significant obstacles during the post-diagnostic period (Carlsson et al., 2016; Pearson et al., 2020; Sansoti et al., 2012; Smith et al., 2020).

There are several ways in which parents can receive greater post-diagnostic support. Parents often report wanting more information about the disorder, intervention services, and their child's prognosis (Andberg & South, 2021; Hannel et al., 2016; Legg & Tickle, 2019), and the opportunity to get support from someone who understands autism and could provide reassurance (Rabba et al., 2019). Providers could support parents by helping manage expectations and encouraging them to focus on the present (Rabba et al., 2019). Respite services for children can be limited, as many are only available once a month or do not accept adolescents (Hall & Graff, 2010). Therefore, many parents have expressed a need for more respite services (Baile & Costantini, 2013; Bromley et al., 2004; Dillenburger et al., 2010; Osborne & Reed, 2008). Parents want more programs for children with autism that they could attend after school, on the weekends, or during school breaks (Siklos & Kerns, 2006). Parents also express a desire to have more training in Applied Behavior Analysis (ABA) or behavioral therapy services in order to learn better strategies to manage their child's interfering behaviors (Bromley et al., 2004; Dillenburger et al., 2010; Osborne & Reed, 2008).

Furthermore, parents suggest that professionals provide them with referrals to individual therapy for themselves to assist them in coping with the diagnosis (Mansell & Morris, 2004). Whole family supports such as group or family therapy are also recommended by parents to assist the family with stressors related to their child's diagnosis (Hall & Graff, 2010; Osborne & Reed, 2008). Additional services parents would like to receive include childcare (Bromley et al., 2004; Hall & Graff, 2010), a case manager to assist with the coordination of services (Mulligan et al., 2012), educational support, support groups, a professional to assess their child on a regular basis (Osborne & Reed, 2008), a family advocate, ABA schools/centers, multidisciplinary support (Dillenburger et al., 2010), and transportation (Bromley et al., 2004).

Parents who have children with autism may experience financial strain. A parent may be unable to work due to the amount of time he/she has to dedicate to obtaining services for the child (Mitchell & Holdt, 2014). Insurance companies may not cover behavioral therapy and/or diagnostic evaluations (Hall & Graff, 2010). Additionally, parents need financial assistance for other treatments (Siklos & Kerns, 2006). Overall, parents want more financial support for their children (Bromley et al., 2004; Hall & Graff, 2010; Renty & Roeyers, 2006). Relatedly, greater efforts are needed to reduce racial and ethnic disparities in available services (Smith et al., 2020). Potential solutions include increasing telehealth options, Medicaid coverage for autism-specific services, and medical transportation services (Fisher et al., 2022).

Many parents experience distress over their child's future (Siklos & Kerns, 2006). Parents worry about their child's ability to financially support themselves when he/she is an adult (Hall & Graff, 2010). Thus, parents need assistance planning for their child's future income. Other future concerns include: medical support, obtaining employment as an adult, and the child's ability to live independently as an adult

(Renty & Roeyers, 2006). Due to these future concerns, parents need services to assist with their child's transition to adulthood.

Limitations of Current Research and Issues Requiring Further Study

In order to continually identify best practice strategies to implement during the diagnostic process, professionals must have an empirically based understanding of the variables that influence parent and caregiver levels of satisfaction and stress. One area of focus within the literature base is the diversity of participants from several different countries. A significant portion of the research is from the United Kingdom followed by the United States, with other investigations based in regions such as Canada, France, Australia, India, Italy, and Singapore. This diversity of participants is desirable because the global experiences of families can be evaluated, potentially leading to large-scale generalizability. However, this regional diversity can also create further discrepancies within a developing research base. Given some of the likely differences in health care systems related to service delivery and overall patient satisfaction (Thomson et al., 2013), the ability to generalize specific results among countries may be somewhat limited.

Although it appears likely that shared experiences (i.e., satisfaction/dissatisfaction with diagnostic process) may occur regardless of country of origin, it is possible that other cultural/regional factors specific to systems of care could have an influence on outcomes. For example, Daley (2004) described that families in India often experience limited access to health care providers who are qualified to diagnose autism. As a result, some individuals seeking evaluations travel several days to receive care (Daley, 2004). Certainly, in the time since this study, greater access to professionals specializing in autism may have occurred. However, the availability and/or quality of specialized services in non-Western countries can be different than those in Western countries. Furthermore, in a review of health care system performance indicators among 14 industrialized countries, United Kingdom citizens had notably more favorable views of their public health system. In contrast, United States citizens had the least favorable views compared to the other assessed countries. Although the association between global perspectives and more specific clinical/health experiences is unknown, it is worthwhile to consider the potential implications regarding the countries who have contributed most readily to the research base. Going forward, research should continue to explore both the global and cultural/regional-specific experiences of individuals navigating the autism diagnostic process. In this pursuit, researchers may need to delve further into the complexities and norms of health care systems within and between countries in order to better understand the variables that could influence diagnostic perceptions. Further evaluation of the extent to which these regional and cultural differences impact upon overall diagnostic experiences could provide greater conceptual clarity.

In addition to some of the previously identified correlates of overall satisfaction (e.g., age at diagnosis, wait time, number of professional encounters, relationship with professionals, etc.), future investigations should also explore the potential impact of additional variables. Numerous studies have examined stress (e.g., Baker-Ericzén et al., 2005; Hayes & Watson, 2013; Ritzema & Sladeczek, 2011; Rivard et al., 2014) and psychological functioning (e.g., Harper et al., 2013; Minnes et al., 2014) in parents of children with autism, and it would be noteworthy to assess the impact of these variables on ratings of overall satisfaction. It is possible that extraneous factors such as family stressors or general parenting stress may impact perceptions of the diagnostic process. Similarly, further study of child-specific variables could better inform practice. Considering that the level of autism severity has been found to be a significant predictor of parental stress (Lyons et al., 2010), future studies could explore the possible moderating impact of disability severity on parental stress and overall satisfaction during the diagnostic process. Further investigation of these parent and child variables may help professionals to better understand, predict, and plan for future diagnostic experiences.

Additionally, many of the core studies in this area have included qualitative, quantitative, and mixed-method research designs. Many qualitative studies have provided rich information that assists in understanding the themes and experiences of parents and families who encounter the autism diagnostic process. Quantitative studies have also explored a range of issues related to satisfaction with the diagnostic process. In the Makino et al. (2021) review, the authors note that parent satisfaction tends to be ill-defined and inconsistently measured, limiting the ability for researchers to conduct quantitative meta-analyses. Overall, it appears important to build upon the methodological rigor of future research both quantitatively and qualitatively. One particular emphasis should be on further development of the constructs of satisfaction and stress for individuals navigating the autism diagnostic process.

As noted, many variables (e.g., age of diagnosis, wait time, professional response to initial concerns, professional relationship, diagnostic severity/subtype, etc.) have been examined related to overall satisfaction. Further, several other variables have been posited as additional correlates of overall satisfaction with the diagnostic process. Assessing the contribution of each of these factors within the overall construct of satisfaction will enhance conceptual and theoretical understanding. Studies (e.g., Anderberg & South, 2021; Da Paz et al., 2018) have explored predictors and correlates of satisfaction through multivariate analysis. Continued exploration and confirmation of findings is necessary to further develop and refine theory.

As the constructs of stress and satisfaction are further explored, implications for the assessment and measurement of related variables are relevant. In the reviewed studies, many investigators created their own questionnaires/surveys to assess perceptions of stress and satisfaction (e.g., Harrington et al., 2006; Jones et al., 2014; Mansell & Morris, 2004; Smith et al., 1994). The measurement of these variables in other studies (e.g., Brogan & Knussen, 2003; Howlin & Asgharian, 1999) was based on different questionnaires used during previous investigations (i.e., Howlin & Moore, 1997; Sloper & Turner, 1993). When a range of questionnaires/surveys are used with limited or no reported psychometric qualities, it is difficult to condense outcomes and determine the reliability of measurement. Additionally, inconsistencies also exist among scales in the way in which overall satisfaction is measured. Some satisfaction scores were derived from a single item, often based upon a 4- or 5-point Likert scale. Other scores were based upon multiple aspects of a questionnaire or responses to several different items. If researchers are acknowledging the multi-dimensionality of stress and satisfaction, it is unknown if single-item questions can accurately reflect the overall experience and construct of these variables. A more comprehensive emphasis on multi-dimensional assessment may be warranted. As a result, future research should explore scale development and refinement with specific measurement tools. Researchers are encouraged to extend beyond the face validity of questionnaires and continue to examine construct and content validity. Enhanced understanding of the variables primarily contributing to the constructs of stress and satisfaction could assist in more efficient and effective identification of best practice strategies for professionals.

Finally, investigations should strive to narrow the research-to-practice gap that can be common in the health and mental health fields. This gap between the identification of empirically based strategies and their use in regular clinical practice has been discussed related to autism intervention research (e.g., Dingfelder & Mandell, 2011; Stahmer, 2007; Stahmer & Aarons, 2009), and it is possible that similar challenges may be present within autism assessment/diagnostic research. Further, there is considerable inconsistency among research-supported clinical practice guidelines (Pattison et al., 2022). The disconnect between researchers and practitioners might occur due to a lack of attention or acknowledgement of systemic issues and contextual factors in different practice settings (Jensen & Foster, 2010). For example, practitioners may attempt to implement best practice strategies, but find themselves burdened by the realities of limited (or absence of) insurance payment for additional feedback appointments. Additionally, spending increased time with some families in attempts to increase satisfaction and reduce stress may inevitably increase the diagnostic wait time for other families, a factor known to increase stress and decrease satisfaction. This dichotomy, in which research-based strategies may be beneficial for one group of individuals but not another, may lead to inconsistent or limited adoption of the recommendation practice.

To improve effectiveness and consistency of practice, researchers should explore the extent to which implementation of the recommended strategies actually affects overall experiences and satisfaction during the diagnostic process. There are numerous variables that may influence an individual's experiences during this time. As a result, it may be helpful to begin isolating specific strategies (e.g., number of feedback sessions, type of information provided during disclosure, etc.) to explore the extent to which implementation impacts ratings of overall stress and satisfaction. This information may be able to better shape the practices of professionals working with families and individuals.

Conclusion

Navigating the diagnostic process for autism can be a highly stressful period for parents and caregivers. Despite some limitations, the growing body of research in this area contributes to a better understanding of the experiences and perspectives of families and individuals. The current literature provides several implications for professionals who are providing health and mental health services to children, families, and/or adults. As research continues to inform practice, professionals should strive to provide high quality services to individuals and families that are efficient, comprehensive, collaborative, and respectful.

References

Abbott, M., Bernard, P., & Forge, J. (2013). Communicating a diagnosis of autism spectrum disorder - A qualitative study of parents' experiences. *Clinical Child Psychology and Psychiatry, 18*(3), 370–382. https://doi.org/10.1177/1359104512455813

Abrams, E. Z., & Goodman, J. F. (1998). Diagnosing developmental problems in children: Parents and professionals negotiate bad news. *Journal of Pediatric Psychology, 23*(2), 87–98.

Alfuraydan, M., Croxall, J., Hurt, L., Kerr, M., & Brophy, S. (2020). Use of telehealth for facilitating the diagnostic assessment of Autism Spectrum Disorder (ASD): A scoping review. *PLoS One, 15*(7), Article e0236415. https://doi.org/10.1371/journal.pone.0236415

American Psychiatric Association. (2013). *Diagnostic and statistical manual of mental disorders* (5th ed.). https://doi.org/10.1176/appi.books.9780890425596

Anderberg, E., & South, M. (2021). Predicting parent reactions at diagnostic disclosure sessions for autism. *Journal of Autism and Developmental Disorders, 51*(10), 3533–3546. https://doi.org/10.1007/s10803-020-04817-5

Avdi, E., Griffin, C., & Brough, S. (2000). Parents' constructions of professional knowledge, expertise and authority during assessment and diagnosis of their child for an autistic spectrum disorder. *British Journal of Medical Psychology, 73*(3), 327–338.

Avlund, S. H., Thomsen, P. H., Schendel, D., Jorgensen, M., Carlsen, A. H., & Clausen, L. (2021). Factors associated with a delayed autism spectrum disorder diagnosis in children previously assessed on suspicion of autism. *Journal of Autism and Developmental Disorders, 51*(11), 3843–3856. https://doi.org/10.1007/s10803-020-04849-x

Azad, G., Holingue, C., Pfeiffer, D., Dillon, E., Reetzke, R., Kalb, L., Menon, D., Hong, J. S., & Landa, R. (2022). The influence of race on parental beliefs and concerns during an autism diagnosis: A mixed-method analysis. *Autism, 26*(5), 1176–1187. https://doi.org/10.1177/13623613211044345

Baile, W. F., & Costantini, A. (2013). Communicating with cancer patients and their families. In T. N. Wise, M. Biondi, & A. Costantini (Eds.), *Psycho-oncology* (pp. 57–90). American Psychiatric Publishing Inc.

Baird, G., McConachie, H., & Scrutton, D. (2000). Parents' perceptions of disclosure of the diagnosis of cerebral palsy. *Archive of Disabled Child, 83*(6), 475–480.

Baker-Ericzén, M. J., Brookman-Frazee, L., & Stahmer, A. (2005). Stress levels and adaptability in parents of toddlers with and without autism spectrum disorders. *Research and Practice for Persons with Severe Disabilities, 30*(4), 194–204.

Becerra-Culqui, T. A., Lynch, F. L., Owen-Smith, A. A., Spitzer, J., & Croen, L. A. (2018). Parental first concerns and timing of autism spectrum disorder diagnosis. *Journal of Autism and Developmental Disorders, 48*(10), 3367–3376. https://doi.org/10.1007/s10803-018-3598-6

Boyd, B. A., Odom, S. L., Humphreys, B. P., & Sam, A. M. (2010). Infants and toddlers with autism spectrum disorder: Early identification and early intervention. *Journal of Early Intervention, 32*(2), 75–98.

Braiden, H.-J., Bothwell, J., & Duffy, J. (2010). Parents' experience of the diagnostic process for autistic spectrum disorders. *Child Care in Practice, 16*(4), 377–389.

Brian, J., Bryson, S. E., Garon, N., Roberts, W., Smith, I. M., Szatmari, P., & Zwaigenbaum, L. (2008). Clinical assessment of autism in high-risk 18-month-olds. *Autism, 12*(5), 433–456.

Brogan, C. A., & Knussen, C. (2003). The disclosure of a diagnosis of an autistic spectrum disorder: Determinants of satisfaction in a sample of Scottish parents. *Autism, 7*(1), 31–46.

Bromley, J., Hare, D. J., Davison, K., & Emerson, E. (2004). Mothers supporting children with autistic spectrum disorders: Social support, mental health status and satisfaction with services. *Autism, 8*(4), 409–423.

Brookman-Frazee, L., Baker-Ericzen, M., Stadnick, N., & Taylor, R. (2012). Parent perspectives on community mental health services for children with autism spectrum disorders. *Journal of Child and Family Studies, 21*(4). https://doi.org/10.1007/s10826-011-9506-8

Carbone, P. S., Behl, D. D., Azor, V., & Murphy, N. A. (2010). The medical home for children with autism spectrum disorders: Parent and pediatrician perspectives. *Journal of Autism and Developmental Disorders, 40*(3), 317–324.

Carbone, P. S., Campbell, K., Wilkes, J., Stoddard, G. J., Huynh, K., Young, P. C., & Gabrielsen, T. P. (2020). Primary care autism screening and later autism diagnosis. *Pediatrics, 146*(2). https://doi.org/10.1542/peds.2019-2314

Carbone, P. S., Murphy, N. A., Norlin, C., Azor, V., Sheng, X., & Young, P. C. (2013). Parent and pediatrician perspectives regarding the primary care of children with autism spectrum disorders. *Journal of Autism and Developmental Disorders, 43*(4), 964–972.

Centers for Disease Control and Prevention. (2014). *Autism spectrum disorder: From numbers to know-how*. https://archive.cdc.gov/www_cdc_gov/grand-rounds/pp/2014/20140422-autism-spectrum.html

Chamak, B., Bonniau, B., Oudaya, L., & Ehrenberg, A. (2011). The autism diagnostic experiences of French parents. *Autism, 15*(1), 83–97.

Connolly, M., & Gersch, I. (2013). A support group for parents of children on a waiting list for an assessment for autism spectrum disorder. *Educational Psychology in Practice, 29*(3), 293–308.

Corona, L. L., Weitlauf, A. S., Hine, J., Berman, A., Miceli, A., Nicholson, A., Stone, C., Broderick, N., Francis, S., Juarez, A. P., Vehorn, A., Wagner, L., & Warren, Z. (2021). Parent perceptions of caregiver-mediated telemedicine tools for assessing autism risk in toddlers. *Journal of Autism and Developmental Disorders, 51*(2), 476–486. https://doi.org/10.1007/s10803-020-04554-9

Cottrell, D. J., & Summers, K. (1990). Communicating an evolutionary diagnosis of disability to parents. *Child: Care, Health and Development, 16*(4), 211–218.

Crane, L., Chester, J. W., Goddard, L., Henry, L. A., & Hill, E. (2016). Experiences of autism diagnosis: A survey of over 1000 parents in the United Kingdom. *Autism, 20*(2), 153–162. https://doi.org/10.1177/1362361315573636

Da Paz, N. S., Siegel, B., Coccia, M. A., & Epel, E. S. (2018). Acceptance or despair? Maternal adjustment to having a child diagnosed with autism. *Journal of Autism and Developmental Disorders, 48*(6), 1971–1981. https://doi.org/10.1007/s10803-017-3450-4

Daley, T. C. (2004). From symptom recognition to diagnosis: Children with autism in urban India. *Social Science and Medicine, 58*(7), 1323–1335.

Daniels, A. M., & Mandell, D. S. (2014). Explaining differences in age at autism spectrum disorder diagnosis: A critical review. *Autism, 18*(5), 583–597.

Dillenburger, K., Keenan, M., Doherty, A., Byrne, T., & Gallagher, S. (2010). Living with children diagnosed with autistic spectrum disorder: Parental and professional views. *British Journal of Special Education, 37*(1), 1–11.

Dingfelder, H. E., & Mandell, D. S. (2011). Bridging the research-to-practice gap in autism intervention: An application of diffusion of innovation theory. *Journal of Autism and Developmental Disorders, 41*(5), 597–609.

Donohue, M. R., Childs, A. W., Richards, M., & Robins, D. L. (2019). Race influences parent report of concerns about symptoms of autism spectrum disorder. *Autism, 23*(1), 100–111. https://doi.org/10.1177/1362361317722030

Drahota, A., Sadler, R., Hippensteel, C., Ingersoll, B., & Bishop, L. (2020). Service deserts and service oases: Utilizing geographic information systems to evaluate service availability for individuals with autism spectrum disorder. *Autism, 24*(8), 2008–2020. https://doi.org/10.1177/1362361320931265

Fisher, A. P., Lynch, J. D., Jacquez, F. M., Mitchell, M. J., Kamimura-Nishimura, K. I., & Wade, S. L. (2023). A systematic review examining caregivers' of color experiences with the diagnostic process of autism spectrum disorder. *Autism, 27*(4), 876–889. https://doi.org/10.1177/13623613221128171

Fuentes, J., Hervas, A., & Howlin, P. (2021). ESCAP practice guidance for autism: A summary of evidence-based recommendations for diagnosis and treatment. *European Child and Adolescent Psychiatry, 30*(6), 961–984. https://doi.org/10.1007/s00787-020-01587-4

Goff, B. S. N., Springer, N., Foote, L. C., Frantz, C., Peak, M., Tracy, C., Veh, T., Bentley, G. E., & Cross, K. A. (2013). Receiving the initial down syndrome diagnosis: A comparison of prenatal and postnatal parent group experiences. *Intellectual and Developmental Disabilities, 51*(6), 446–457.

Goin-Kochel, R. P., Mackintosh, V. H., & Myers, B. J. (2006). How many doctors does it take to make an autism spectrum diagnosis? *Autism, 10*(5), 439–451.

Gonzalez, N., Quintanta, J. M., Biblao, A., Escobar, A., Aizpuru, F., Thompson, A., Esteban, C., Sebastián, J. A. S., & De la Sierra, E. (2005). Development and validation of an in-patient satisfaction questionnaire. *International Journal for Quality in Health Care, 17*(6), 465–472.

Groth-Marnat, G. (2003). *Handbook of psychological assessment* (4th ed.). John Wiley & Sons Inc.

Guthrie, W., Wallis, K., Bennett, A., Brooks, E., Dudley, J., Gerdes, M., Pandey, J., Levy, S. E., Schultz, R. T., & Miller, J. S. (2019). Accuracy of autism screening in a large pediatric network. *Pediatrics, 144*(4). https://doi.org/10.1542/peds.2018-3963

Hackett, L., Shaikh, S., & Theodosiou, L. (2009). Parental perceptions of the assessment of autistic spectrum disorders in a tier three service. *Child and Adolescent Mental Health, 14*(3), 127–132.

Hall, H. R., & Graff, J. C. (2010). Parenting challenges in families of children with autism: A pilot study. *Issues in Comprehensive Pediatric Nursing, 33*(4), 187–204.

Hamp, N., DeHaan, S. L., Cerf, C. M., & Radesky, J. S. (2023). Primary care pediatricians' perspectives on autism care. *Pediatrics, 151*(1). https://doi.org/10.1542/peds.2022-057712

Harper, A., Dyches, T. T., Harper, J., Roper, S. O., & South, M. (2013). Respite care, marital quality, and stress in parents of children with autism spectrum disorders. *Journal of Autism and Developmental Disorders, 43*(11), 2604–2616.

Harrington, J. W., Patrick, P. A., Edwards, K. S., & Brand, D. A. (2006). Parental beliefs about autism: Implications for the treating physician. *Autism, 10*(5), 452–462.

Hayes, S. A., & Watson, S. L. (2013). The impact of parenting stress: A meta-analysis of studies comparing the experience of parenting stress in parents of children with and without autism spectrum disorder. *Journal of Autism and Developmental Disorders, 43*(3), 629–642.

Herlihy, L., Knoch, K., Vibert, B., & Fein, D. (2015). Parents' first concerns about toddlers with autism spectrum disorder: Effect of sibling status. *Autism, 19*(1), 20–28. https://doi.org/10.1177/1362361313509731

Howlin, P., & Asgharian, A. (1999). The diagnosis of autism and Asperger syndrome: Findings from a survey of 770 families. *Developmental Medicine and Child Neurology, 41*(12), 834–839.

Howlin, P., & Moore, A. (1997). Diagnosis in autism: A survey of over 1200 patients in the UK. *Autism, 1*(2), 135–162.

Hyman, S. L., Levy, S. E., & Myers, S. M. (2020). Identification, evaluation, and management of children with autism spectrum disorder. *Pediatrics, 145*(1). https://doi.org/10.1542/peds.2019-3447

Issarraras, A., Matson, J. L., Matheis, M., & Burns, C. O. (2019). Differences in developmental concerns of young children with autism spectrum disorder across racial/ethnic groups.

Developmental Neurorehabilitation, 22(3), 174–179. https://doi.org/10.1080/17518423.2018.1504828

Jensen, P. S., & Foster, M. (2010). Closing the research to practice gap in children's mental health: Structures, solutions, and strategies. *Administration and Policy in Mental Health and Mental Health Services Research, 37*(1–2), 111–119.

Johnson, C. P., & Meyers, S. M. (2007). Identification and evaluation of children with autism spectrum disorders. *Pediatrics, 120*(5), 1183–1215. https://doi.org/10.1542/peds.2007-2361

Jones, L., Goddard, L., Hill, E. L., Henry, L. A., & Crane, L. (2014). Experiences of receiving a diagnosis of autism spectrum disorder: A survey of adults in the United Kingdom. *Journal of Autism and Developmental Disorders, 44*(12), 3033–3044. https://doi.org/10.1007/s10803-014-2161-3

Klintwall, L., Eldevik, S., & Eikeseth, S. (2015). Narrowing the gap: Effects of intervention on developmental trajectories in autism. *Autism, 19*(1), 53–63.

Legg, H., & Tickle, A. (2019). UK parents' experiences of their child receiving a diagnosis of autism spectrum disorder: A systematic review of the qualitative evidence. *Autism, 23*(8), 1897–1910. https://doi.org/10.1177/1362361319841488

Liu, M., & Ma, Z. (2022). A systematic review of telehealth screening, assessment, and diagnosis of autism spectrum disorder. *Child and Adolescent Psychiatry and Mental Health, 16*(1), 79. https://doi.org/10.1186/s13034-022-00514-6

Lord, C., & Richler, J. (2006). Early diagnosis of children with autism spectrum disorders. In T. Charman & W. Stone (Eds.), *Social and communication development in autism spectrum disorders: Early identification, diagnosis, and intervention* (pp. 35–59). Guilford Press.

Lyons, A. M., Leon, S. C., Phelps, C. E. R., & Dunleavy, A. M. (2010). The impact of child symptom severity on stress among parents of children with AUTISM: The moderating role of coping styles. *Journal of Child and Family Studies, 19*(4), 516–524.

MacKenzie, K. T., Mazefsky, C. A., & Eack, S. M. (2023). Obtaining a first diagnosis of autism spectrum disorder: Descriptions of the diagnostic process and correlates of parent satisfaction from a national sample. *Journal of Autism and Developmental Disorders, 53*(10), 3799–3812. https://doi.org/10.1007/s10803-022-05673-1

Maenner, M. J., Warren, Z., Williams, A. R., Amoakohene, E., Bakian, A. V., Bilder, D. A., Durkin, M. S., Fitzgerald, R. T., Furnier, S. M., Hughes, M. M., Ladd-Acosta, C. M., McArthur, D., Pas, E. T., Salinas, A., Vehorn, A., Williams, S., Esler, A., Grzybowski, A., Hall-Lande, J., & Shaw, K. A. (2023). Prevalence and characteristics of autism spectrum disorder among children aged 8 years - autism and developmental disabilities monitoring network, 11 sites, United States, 2020. *MMWR Surveill Summ, 72*(2), 1–14. https://doi.org/10.15585/mmwr.ss7202a1

Mahapatra, P., Pati, S., Sinha, R., Chauhan, A. S., Nanda, R. R., & Nallala, S. (2019). Parental care-seeking pathway and challenges for autistic spectrum disorders children: A mixed method study from Bhubaneswar, Odisha. *Indian Journal of Psychiatry, 61*(1), 37–44. https://doi.org/10.4103/psychiatry.IndianJPsychiatry_257_18

Makino, A., Hartman, L., King, G., Wong, P. Y., & Penner, M. (2021). Parent experiences of autism spectrum disorder diagnosis: A scoping review. *Review Journal of Autism and Developmental Disorders, 8*(3), 267–284. https://doi.org/10.1007/s40489-021-00237-y

Mansell, W., & Morris, K. (2004). A survey of parents' reactions to the diagnosis of an autistic spectrum disorder by a local service: Access to information and use of services. *Autism, 8*(4), 387–407. https://doi.org/10.1177/1362361304045213

Martinez, M., Thomas, K. C., Williams, C. S., Christian, R., Crais, E., Pretzel, R., & Hooper, S. R. (2018). Family experiences with the diagnosis of autism spectrum disorder: System barriers and facilitators of efficient diagnosis. *Journal of Autism and Developmental Disorders, 48*(7), 2368–2378. https://doi.org/10.1007/s10803-018-3493-1

Matheis, M., Matson, J. L., Burns, C. O., Jiang, X., Peters, W. J., Moore, M., de Back, K. A., & Estabillo, J. (2017). Factors related to parental age of first concern in toddlers with autism spectrum disorder. *Developmental Neurorehabilitation, 20*(4), 228–235. https://doi.org/10.1080/17518423.2016.1211186

Mazurek, M. O., Handen, B. L., Wodka, E. L., Nowinski, L., Butter, E., & Engelhardt, C. R. (2014). Age at first autism spectrum disorder diagnosis: The role of birth cohort, demographic factors, and clinical features. *Journal of Developmental & Behavioral Pediatrics, 35*(9), 561–569. https://doi.org/10.1097/DBP.0000000000000097

McConkey, R., Truesdale-Kennedy, M., & Cassidy, A. (2009). Mother's recollection of early features of autism spectrum disorders. *Child and Adolescent Mental Health, 14*(1), 31–36. https://doi.org/10.1111/j.1475-3588.2008.00495.x

McMorris, C. A., Cox, E., Hudson, M., Liu, X., & Bebko, J. M. (2013). The diagnostic process of children with autism spectrum disorder: Implications for early identification and intervention. *Journal on Developmental Disabilities, 19*(2), 42–49.

Minnes, P., Perry, A., & Weiss, J. A. (2014). Predictors of distress and well-being in parents of young children with developmental delays and disabilities: The importance of parent perceptions. *Journal of Intellectual Disability Research.*

Mishaal, R. A., Ben-Itzchak, E., & Zachor, D. A. (2014). Age of autism spectrum disorder diagnosis is associated with child's variables and parental experience. *Research in Autism Spectrum Disorders, 8*(7), 873–880. https://doi.org/10.1016/j.rasd.2014.04.001

Mitchell, C., & Holdt, N. (2014). The search for a timely diagnosis: Parents' experiences of their child being diagnosed with an autistic spectrum disorder. *Journal of Child and Adolescent Mental Health, 26*(1), 49–62.

Mitroulaki, S., Serdari, A., Tripsianis, G., Gundelfinger, R., Arvaniti, A., Vorvolakos, T., & Samakouri, M. (2020). First alarm and time of diagnosis in autism spectrum disorders. *Comprehensive Child and Adolescent Nursing, 45*(1), 75–91. https://doi.org/10.1080/24694193.2020.1834013

Moh, T. A., & Magiati, I. (2012). Factors associated with parental stress and satisfaction during the process of diagnosis of children with autism spectrum disorders. *Research in Autism Spectrum Disorders, 6*(1), 293–303.

Molteni, P., & Maggiolini, S. (2014). Parents' perspectives towards the diagnosis of autism: An italian case study research. *Journal of Child and Family Studies.*

Morris, R., Greenblatt, A., & Saini, M. (2019). Healthcare providers' experiences with autism: A scoping review. *Journal of Autism and Developmental Disorders, 49*(6), 2374–2388. https://doi.org/10.1007/s10803-019-03912-6

Mulligan, J., MacCulloch, R., Good, B., & Nicholas, D. B. (2012). Transparency, hope, and empowerment: A model for partnering with parents of a child with autism spectrum disorder at diagnosis and beyond. *Social Work in Mental Health, 10*(4), 311–330.

Nadel, S., & Poss, J. E. (2007). Early detection of autism spectrum disorders: Screening between 12 and 24 months of age. *Journal of the American Association of Nurse Practitioners, 19*(8), 408–417. https://doi.org/10.1111/j.1745-7599.2007.00244.x

Nissenbaum, M. S., Tollefson, N., & Reese, R. M. (2002). The interpretive conference: Sharing a diagnosis of autism with families. *Focus on Autism and Other Developmental Disabilities, 17*(1), 30–43.

Osborne, L. A., McHugh, L., Saunders, J., & Reed, P. (2008). Parenting stress reduces the effectiveness of early teaching interventions for autistic spectrum disorders. *Journal of Autism and Developmental Disorders, 38*(6), 1092–1103.

Osborne, L. A., & Reed, P. (2008). Parents' perceptions of communication with professionals during the diagnosis of autism. *Autism, 12*(3), 309–324. https://doi.org/10.1177/1362361307089517

Pattison, E., Ure, A., Mittiga, S. R., Williams, K., & Freeman, N. C. (2022). The feedback session of an autism assessment: A scoping review of clinical practice guideline recommendations. *Journal of Autism and Developmental Disorders, 52*(4), 1821–1840. https://doi.org/10.1007/s10803-021-05067-9

Poehlmann, J., Clements, M., Abbeduto, L., & Farsad, V. (2005). Family experiences associated with a child's diagnosis of fragile X or Down syndrome: Evidence for disruption and resilience. *Mental Retardation, 43*(4), 255–267. https://doi.org/10.1352/0047-6765(2005)43[255:FEAWAC]2.0.CO;2

Poslawsky, I. E., Naber, F. B. A., Van Daalen, E., & Van Engeland, H. (2014). Parental reaction to early diagnosis of their children's autism spectrum disorder: An exploratory study. *Child Psychiatry and Human Development, 45*(3), 294–305.

Pruett, K. D. (2013). Feedback which leads forward: Where intervention begins. *Journal of the American Academy of Child and Adolescent Psychiatry, 52*(8), 769–771.

Reese, R. M., Jamison, R., Wendland, M., Fleming, K., Braun, M. J., Schuttler, J. O., & Turek, J. (2013). Evaluating interactive videoconferencing for assessing symptoms of autism. *Telemedicine Journal and E-Health, 19*(9), 671–677. https://doi.org/10.1089/tmj.2012.0312

Renty, J., & Roeyers, H. (2006). Satisfaction with formal support and education for children with autism spectrum disorder: The voices of the parents. *Child: Care, Health and Development, 32*(3), 371–385.

Richards, M., Mossey, J., & Robins, D. L. (2016). Parents' concerns as they relate to their child's development and later diagnosis of autism spectrum disorder. *Journal of Developmental and Behavioral Pediatrics, 37*(7), 532–540. https://doi.org/10.1097/DBP.0000000000000339

Ritzema, A. M., & Sladeczek, I. E. (2011). Stress in parents of children with developmental disabilities over time. *Journal on Developmental Disabilities, 17*(2), 22–34.

Rivard, M., Terroux, A., Parent-Boursier, C., & Mercier, C. (2014). Determinants of stress in parents of children with autism spectrum disorders. *Journal of Autism and Developmental Disorders, 44*(7), 1609–1620.

Rogers, C. L., Goddard, L., Hill, E. L., Henry, L. A., & Crane, L. (2016). Experiences of diagnosing autism spectrum disorder: A survey of professionals in the United Kingdom. *Autism, 20*(7), 820–831. https://doi.org/10.1177/1362361315611109

Shea, V. (1993). Interpreting results to parents of preschool children. In E. Schopler, M. E. Van Bourgondien, & M. M. Bristol (Eds.), *Preschool issues in autism* (pp. 185–198). Plenum Press.

Sheldrick, R. C., Maye, M. P., & Carter, A. S. (2017). Age at first identification of autism spectrum disorder: An analysis of two US surveys. *Journal of the American Academy of Child and Adolescent Psychiatry, 56*(4), 313–320. https://doi.org/10.1016/j.jaac.2017.01.012

Siklos, S., & Kerns, K. A. (2006). Assessing need for social support in parents of children with autism and down syndrome. *Journal of Autism and Developmental Disorders, 36*(7), 921–923.

Siklos, S., & Kerns, K. A. (2007). Assessing the diagnostic experiences of a small sample of parents of children with autism spectrum disorders. *Research in Developmental Disabilities, 28*(1), 9–22. https://doi.org/10.1016/j.ridd.2005.09.003

Sloper, P., & Turner, S. (1993). Determinants of parental satisfaction with disclosure of disability. *Developmental Medicine and Child Neurology, 35*(9), 816–825.

Smith, B., Chung, M. C., & Vostanis, P. (1994). The path to care in autism: Is it better now? *Journal of Autism and Developmental Disorders, 24*(5), 551–563.

Stahmer, A. C. (2007). The basic structure of community early intervention programs for children with autism: Provider descriptions. *Journal of Autism and Developmental Disorders, 37*(7), 1344–1354.

Stahmer, A. C., & Aarons, G. A. (2009). Attitudes toward adoption of evidence-based practices: A comparison of autism early intervention providers and children's mental health providers. *Psychological Services, 6*(3), 223–234.

Stahmer, A. C., Vejnoska, S., Iadarola, S., Straiton, D., Segovia, F. R., Luelmo, P., Morgan, E. H., Lee, H. S., Javed, A., Bronstein, B., Hochheimer, S., Cho, E., Aranbarri, A., Mandell, D., Hassrick, E. M., Smith, T., & Kasari, C. (2019). Caregiver voices: Cross-cultural input on improving access to autism services. *Journal of Racial and Ethnic Health Disparities, 6*(4), 752–773. https://doi.org/10.1007/s40615-019-00575-y

Stavropoulos, K. K., Bolourian, Y., & Blacher, J. (2022). A scoping review of telehealth diagnosis of autism spectrum disorder. *PLoS One, 17*(2), Article e0263062. https://doi.org/10.1371/journal.pone.0263062

Tharinger, D. J., Finn, S. E., Hersh, B., Wilkinson, A., Christopher, G. B., & Tran, A. (2008). Assessment feedback with parents and preadolescent children: A collaborative approach. *Professional Psychology: Research and Practice, 39*(6), 600–609.

Thomson, S., Osborn, R., Squires, D., & Jun, M. (2013). *International profiles of health care systems, 2013.*
Turris, S. A. (2005). Unpacking the concept of patient satisfaction: A feminist analysis. *Journal of Advanced Nursing, 50*(3), 293–298.
van'T Hof, M., Tisseur, C., van Berckelear-Onnes, I., van Nieuwenhuyzen, A., Daniels, A. M., Deen, M., Hoek, H. W., & Ester, W. A. (2021). Age at autism spectrum disorder diagnosis: A systematic review and meta-analysis from 2012 to 2019. *Autism, 25*(4), 862–873. https://doi.org/10.1177/1362361320971107
Watermeyer, J., Kanji, A., & Cohen, A. (2012). Caregiver recall and understanding of paediatric diagnostic information and assessment feedback. *International Journal of Audiology, 51*(12), 864–869.
Watson, S. L. (2008). Something you have to do'—Why do parents of children with developmental disabilities seek a differential diagnosis? *Developmental Disabilities Bulletin, 36*(1–2), 168–198.
Wiggins, L. D., Baio, J., & Rice, C. (2006). Examination of the time between first evaluation and first autism spectrum diagnosis in a population-based sample. *Journal of Developmental and Behavioral Pediatrics, 27*(Suppl2), S79–S87.
Williams, D. (2010). Theory of own mind in autism: Evidence of a specific deficit in self-awareness? *Autism, 14*(5), 474–494. https://doi.org/10.1177/1362361310366314
Wong, V. C. N., & Kwan, Q. K. (2010). Randomized controlled trial for early intervention for autism: A pilot study of the Autism 1-2-3 project. *Journal of Autism and Developmental Disorders, 40*(6), 677–688.
Wong, V., Yu, Y., Keyes, M. L., & McGrew, J. H. (2017). Pre-diagnostic and diagnostic stages of autism spectrum disorder: A parent perspective. *Child Care in Practice, 23*(2), 195–217. https://doi.org/10.1080/13575279.2016.1199537
Zablotsky, B., Colpe, L. J., Pringle, B. A., Kogan, M. D., Rice, C., & Blumberg, S. J. (2017). Age of parental concern, diagnosis, and service initiation among children with autism spectrum disorder. *American Journal on Intellectual and Developmental Disabilities, 122*(1), 49–61. https://doi.org/10.1352/1944-7558-122.1.49
Zavaleta-Ramirez, P., Rosetti, M. F., Albores-Gallo, L., Vargas-Soberanis, M. A., Lopez, O. N., & Medina-Mora, M. E. (2020). Pathways to a diagnosis of autism spectrum disorder. *Psychiatric Services, 71*(11), 1120–1126. https://doi.org/10.1176/appi.ps.201900518
Zeidan, J., Fombonne, E., Scorah, J., Ibrahim, A., Durkin, M. S., Saxena, S., Yusuf, A., Shih, A., & Elsabbagh, M. (2022). Global prevalence of autism: A systematic review update. *Autism Research, 15*(5), 778–790. https://doi.org/10.1002/aur.2696
Zeleke, W. A., Hughes, T. L., & Drozda, N. (2019). Disparities in diagnosis and service access for minority children with ASD in the United States. *Journal of Autism and Developmental Disorders, 49*(10), 4320–4331. https://doi.org/10.1007/s10803-019-04131-9
Zuckerman, K., Lindly, O. J., & Chavez, A. E. (2017). Timeliness of autism spectrum disorder diagnosis and use of services among U.S. elementary school-aged children. *Psychiatric Services, 68*(1), 33–40. https://doi.org/10.1176/appi.ps.201500549
Zuckerman, K. E., Lindly, O. J., & Sinche, B. K. (2015). Parental concerns, provider response, and timeliness of autism spectrum disorder diagnosis. *The Journal of Pediatrics, 166*(6), 1431–1439. https://doi.org/10.1016/j.jpeds.2015.03.007
Zuckerman, K. E., Mattox, K. E., Donelan, K., Batbayar, O., Baghaee, A., & Bethell, C. (2013). Pediatrician identification of Latino children at risk for autism spectrum disorder. *Pediatrics, 132*(3), 445–453.
Zwaigenbaum, L., Brian, J. A., & Ip, A. (2019). Early detection for autism spectrum disorder in young children. *Paediatr Child Health, 24*(7), 424–443. https://doi.org/10.1093/pch/pxz119
Zwaigenbaum, L., & Stone, W. (2006). Early screening for autism spectrum disorders in clinical practice settings. In T. Charman & W. Stone (Eds.), *Social and communication development in autism spectrum disorders: Early identification, diagnosis, and intervention* (pp. 88–113). Guilford Press.

Preschool, Early Childhood, and Adolescence

Steven G. Little and Angeleque Akin-Little

Abstract The prevalence of autism spectrum disorder (ASD) has increased markedly over the past three decades necessitating the screening, evaluating, and diagnosing of children with ASD as early as possible to ensure that children with ASD receive access the services and supports they need as early in development as possible. The period from 3 to 18 years of age represents an important period for detection and diagnosis of ASD. This chapter reviews a number of screening and diagnostic instruments. Also discussed are other instruments, procedures, and issues that are important in the assessment and diagnosis of ASD to ensure the likelihood of efficacious intervention result.

Keywords ASD Assessment · ASD Screening · ASD Diagnosis · Preschool · Adolescents · Early Childhood · Autistic Regression · ASD Intervention

The prevalence of autism spectrum disorder (ASD) has increased markedly over the past three decades, rising from 2 per 10,000 in 1990, to 1 in 68 children in 2014 (Blumberg et al., 2013; Centers for Disease Control and Prevention, 2014), and 1 in 36 in 2020 (Maenner et al., 2023). ASD can usually be reliably diagnosed by age 2 and the earlier ASD is diagnosed, the sooner treatments and services can begin (Sheldrick et al., 2022). Therefore, the screening, evaluating, and diagnosing of children with ASD as early as possible is important for ensuring that these children access the services and supports they need Table 1 (CDC, 2014; Eikeseth et al., 2007; NIMH, 2024; Zwaigenbaum et al., 2015).

Diagnosis occurs when a psychologist or other professional conducts a comprehensive evaluation to determine if a child has ASD based on the criteria in the Diagnostic and Statistical Manual of Mental Disorders (DSM-5, APA, 2013). According to the DSM-5, ASD diagnosis requires (a) persistent deficits in social communication

Chapter in *Handbook of Assessment and Diagnosis of Autism Spectrum Disorder* (2nd ed.)

S. G. Little (✉) · A. Akin-Little
Walden University, Minneapolis, MN, US
e-mail: stevenlittlephd@yahoo.com

J. L. Matson (ed.), *Assessment and Diagnosis in Autism*, Autism and Child Psychopathology Series, https://doi.org/10.1007/978-3-032-11802-8_5

Table 1 Autism rating scales

Title	Age range	Publication date	Author(s)	Purpose	Scales/scores	Publisher
Ages & stages questionnaire (ASQ-3)	1–5–6	2009	Squires et al.	• Screening	• Communication • Gross motor • Fine motor • Problem solving • Personal-social	Western psychological services
Autism diagnostic interview-revised (ADIR)	2–adult	2003	Rutter et al.	• Diagnosis program planning	• Language/ communication • Reciprocal social interactions • Repetitive behaviors/ interests	Western psychological services
Autism diagnostic observation schedule, second edition (ADOS-2)	12 Months–adult	2012	Lord et al.	• Assessment • Diagnosis	• Five modules, selected on the basis of expressive language and age	Western psychological services
Autism Spectrum rating scales (ASRA)	2–18	2010	Goldstein & Naglieri	• Screening • Diagnosis • Progress monitoring	• Total score • Social/ communication • Unusual behaviors • Self-regulation • Short form score	Multi-health systems, Inc. (MHS)
Childhood Autism rating scale (second ed.) (CARS-2)	2+	2010	Schlopler, Van Bourgondien, Wellman, & Love	• Identification • Determine functional capabilities	• Standard version • High-functioning version	Western psychological services

(continued)

Table 1 (continued)

Title	Age range	Publication date	Author(s)	Purpose	Scales/scores	Publisher
Gilliam Autism rating scale (third ed.) (GARS-3)	3–22	2014	Gilliam	• Identification • Symptom severity	• Restrictive and repetitive behaviors • Social interaction • Social communication • Emotional responses • Cognitive style • Maladaptive speech	PRO-ED
Parents' evaluation of developmental status (PEDS)	Birth–8	2013	Glascoe & Robertshaw	• Screening	• Language • Motor • Self-help • Early academic skills • Behavior • Social/emotional/ mental health	Ellsworth & Vandemeer Press, LLC
PDD behavior inventory (PDDBI)	18 months -12–5	2005	Cohen & Sudhalter	• Diagnosis • Assessing response to intervention	• Repetitive, ritualistic, and pragmatic problems • Approach/withdrawal problems (extended form) • Expressive social communication abilities • Receptive/expressive social communication abilities (extended form) • Autism composite	PAR

(continued)

Table 1 (continued)

Title	Age range	Publication date	Author(s)	Purpose	Scales/scores	Publisher
PDD behavior inventory-screening version (PDDBI-SV)	18 months-12–5	2011	Cohen	• Screening	• Social pragmatic problems • Social approach behaviors • Composite score	PAR

and social interaction across multiple contexts and (b) restricted, repetitive patterns of behavior, interests, or activities. Therefore, the focus of assessment is on identifying language delays, social skill deficits, and restricted, repetitive, and stereotyped patterns of behavior. In addition, as there is a great deal of heterogeneity of features in individual children with ASD (Jeste & Geschwind, 2014) which makes observation and behavioral assessment essential in order to link assessment and subsequent intervention (Little & Akin-Little, 2016). Although diagnosis of ASD is possible in children as young as 14 months of age (Johnston et al., 2009), factors such as autistic regression and difficulty in identifying symptoms of ASD in very young children, results in most children with ASD not being diagnosed until later, especially those with average or above-average language and cognitive abilities (Manning et al., 2011). A meta-analysis of published literature by van't Hof et al. (2020), including 55 cohorts from 35 countries ($n = 66{,}966$), found a mean age at diagnosis of 60.48 months with a range of 30.90 to 234.57 months. Thus, the period from 3 to 18 years of age represents an important period for detection and diagnosis of ASD. This chapter covers evidence-based assessments used for this age group.

Diagnosing Autism

To be classified ASD in the *DSM-5,* a child must present with symptoms in early childhood, which cause impaired ability to function in daily life activities. These symptoms may not fully manifest until social demands exceed capacity, for instance in middle school, later adolescent, and young adulthood (Hughes et al., 2023). ASD is characterized by two core domains dealing with significant difficulties in practical verbal and nonverbal social communication and repetitive patterns of behavior interest and activities. The child must present in all three deficits categories in the social communication domain (APA, 2013, p. 50): (a) deficits in social-emotion reciprocity, ranging, for example, from abnormal social approach and failure of normal back and forth conversation to reduced sharing interests, emotions, or affect and to failure to initiate or respond to social interactions; (b) deficits in non-verbal communicative behaviors used for social interaction, ranging, for example, from poorly integrated verbal and nonverbal communication to abnormalities in eye contact and body language or deficits in understanding and use of gestures and to a total lack of facial expressions and nonverbal communication; and (c) deficits in developing, maintaining, and understanding relationships, ranging, for example, from difficulties adjusting behavior to suit various social contexts to difficulties in sharing imaginative play or in making friends and to absence of interest in peers.

In addition, a minimum of two of the four criteria in the restricted and repetitive patterns of behaviors domain are required for an ASD diagnosis (APA, 2013, p. 50): (a) stereotyped or repetitive motor movements, use of objects, or speech (e.g., stereotypies, lining up toys or flipping objects, echolalia, idiosyncratic phrases); (b) insistence on sameness, inflexible adherence to routines, or ritualized patterns of verbal or non-verbal behavior (e.g., extreme distress at small changes, difficulties with transitions, rigid thinking patterns, greeting rituals, need to take same route or eat same food every day); (c) highly restricted, fixated interests that are abnormal in intensity or focus (e.g., strong attachment to or preoccupation with unusual objects, excessively circumscribed or perseverative interests); and (d) hyper- or hypo-reactivity to sensory input or unusual interest in sensory aspects of environment (e.g., apparent indifference to pain, temperature, adverse response to specific sounds or textures, excessive smelling or touching of objects, visual fascination with lights or movement).

Symptoms must also be present in early development, cause clinically significant impairment in current functioning, and are not better explained by intellectual disability or global developmental delay. The *DSM-5* identifies three severity levels, based on support needed within two domains: (a) social communication and (b) restricted repetitive patterns of behavior. Symptom severity is classified as Level 1 (requiring very substantial support), Level 2 (requiring substantial support), or Level 3 (requiring support).

The behaviors associated with ASD vary in range. Some individuals may have verbal capabilities and still be unable to use language in a socially meaningful manner, whereas others may have no verbal ability whatsoever. Some may engage in self-stimulatory behaviors such as rocking or twirling their bodies, and flapping their hands, whereas others diagnosed with an ASD may not. Individuals diagnosed with an ASD typically do not engage in pretend play, although some may engage in some pretend play at some level that is less than that of same-aged typically developing peers (Jorgenson, 2017).

Autism Assessment: Screening and Comprehensive Evaluation

As previously mentioned, early identification of autism is crucial as it enables early intervention. Early identification and intervention of autism in children as young as age 2 has not only been found to be reliable, valid, and stable; it has been found to promote positive long-term outcomes (Conrood & Stone, 2005; Zwaigenbaum et al., 2015). Nevertheless, many children do not receive a definitive diagnosis until much later, which means they miss out on the long-term benefits of early intervention (Conrood & Stone, 2005).

Although autism cannot be detected with any one medical test, Volker and Lopata (2008) discussed various medical evaluations that are components of the overall ASD assessment process. There are tests used to rule out speech and hearing problems, which may account for the symptoms of language problems common in ASD. Neurological tests are used to assess for seizure activity or other brain abnormalities that may occur either in the presence of ASD or as an exclusion. Genetic testing identifies chromosomal abnormalities and other tests assess for allergies and other medical conditions that may be comorbid with an ASD. However, none of these medical procedures can ascertain whether an individual has an ASD. Rather, assessment relies on behavioral observations and comparison to criteria set forth by diagnostic systems such as the DSM-5 (APA, 2013). ASD assessment consists of two stages; the first is screening and the second is a comprehensive diagnostic evaluation (Strock, 2004). Screening is a brief assessment that is conducted to identify children with developmental difficulties who exhibit symptoms typical of ASD and are therefore in need of a more comprehensive evaluation. Screening, which requires less time and expertise than a full evaluation, often begins with the pediatrician or family physician during the child's routine visits; however, schools, child- welfare agencies, and early intervention programs also screen for ASD (Conrood & Stone, 2005). The American Academy of Pediatrics (AAP) recommends clinicians be cognizant of developmental delays and incorporate surveillance for any delays during regular well-child doctor visits at 9, 18, and 30 months. Identified concerns can then be followed-up with standardized developmental screening tests (Hyman et al., 2020).

Screening involves behavioral observations and may also include screening instruments such as checklists and parent and/or teacher questionnaires. Screening tools help provide information regarding developmental delays in cognitive development, language, and motor movements/skills; however, they should not be used in isolation to make a diagnosis. On the contrary, screening paves the way for referrals to more skilled professionals, which may then lead to a formal diagnosis from which intervention can be planned and financed.

There are several commonly used instruments that are employed for varying purposes in the screening process (CDC, 2024; Conrood & Stone, 2005). Level 1 screening measures are offered to all children, typically at pediatrician offices. Some of these are specifically designed to identify ASD; however, most are used to identify nonspecific developmental problems, such as cognitive, motor, or language problems. Level 2 autism-specific measures are designed to differentiate children who are more likely to have ASD than other developmental problems.

Although several individuals may be involved in the screening process, a formal diagnosis can only be made by a medical doctor, a licensed psychologist, or a multidisciplinary team which includes one or both of the aforementioned professionals. School counselors, teachers, speech therapists, occupational therapists, parents, and others who are not licensed psychologists or physicians cannot diagnose autism even though they may recognize the presence of ASD symptomatology (Waltz, 2002) and may play an important role in the assessment process. A formal diagnosis is typically rendered by way of a comprehensive diagnostic evaluation (Strock, 2004).

A comprehensive diagnostic evaluation is the second step in the process toward diagnosis. This thorough evaluation also includes the use of parent/caregiver questionnaires; however, it also involves clinical observations, including an FBA, and parent/caregiver interviews. The CDC (2024) has advised that no single source of information should serve alone for diagnostic purposes and one or more diagnostic scales may be used. The CDC identified the following as examples of screening tools for children aged 3 and older: *Ages and Stages Questionnaire* (*ASQ*), *Communication and Symbolic Behavior Scales* (*CSBS*), *Parents' Evaluation of Developmental Status* (*PEDS*), *Modified Checklist for Autism in Toddlers* (*M-CHAT*), and *Screening Tool for Autism in Toddlers and Young Children* (*STAT*). Examples of more comprehensive ASD diagnostic tools which may be part of the diagnostic process include: *Autism Diagnostic Interview-Revised* (*ADIR-R*), *Autism Diagnostic Observation Schedule* (*ADOS*), Childhood Autism Rating Scale (*CARS*), and the *Gilliam Autism Rating Scale, Second Edition (GARS-3).* All of these are discussed in more detail later in this chapter.

Autistic Regression

Most children who receive an ASD diagnosis demonstrate a gradually unfolding pattern of symptoms during their first 2 years of life (Stefanatos, 2008; Zwaigenbaum et al., 2015). Not all children with ASD demonstrate this pattern of symptoms, however. Research indicates that approximately 20% of children with ASD display a pattern characterized by regression in one or more domains of behavior or the worsening of previously reported ASD features (Bradley et al., 2016)). Stefanatos (2008) identifies three types of autistic regression. The most common type of autistic regression involves symptoms of ASD emerging during the first year of life but the saliency of these delays or deviations in behavior do not trigger parental concern until later in the developmental period (Dawson et al., 2007). In the second type, children demonstrate normal or near-normal early development but then exhibit an unexpected arrest or expansion in development, usually in their second year of life (Landa & Garrett-Mayer, 2006; Landa et al., 2007). The third type is illustrated by developmental regression or reversal of behavioral functioning in one or more domains (Lord et al., 2004). In this type, not only is there a cessation of skill acquisition but there is also a loss of previously acquired skills. This usually occurs between 15 and 30 months of age (Hoshino et al., 1987). Bradley et al. (2016) concluded that youth with a history of regression are more likely to have comorbid intellectual disability.

ASD Screening Instruments

Ages and Stages Questionnaire (ASQ). The *Ages and Stages Questionnaire, Third Edition* (*ASQ-3*, Squires et al., 2009) is a 30-item parent/caregiver-completed questionnaire designed to screen young children for developmental delays. With an age range from 1 to 5½ years, scores are provided on five dimensions: communication, gross motor, fine motor, problem solving, and personal-social. According to the test's authors it is intended to be a first step screening measure intended to assess the need for intervention services. While the measure is not designed specifically for autism screening, it has utility as an autism screener (Hanig, 2010), especially the communication and personal-social dimensions. Reviews of the psycho-metric qualities on the *ASQ-3* conclude that it is generally psychometrically sound with adequate support for its reliability and validity (Hanig, 2010, Valleley & Roane, 2010) although Velikonja et al. (2017) indicated caution when using translated versions. It should also be noted that its publication date of 2009 makes the standardization sample quite old and therefore should be considered a gross screen or possibly used for progress monitoring.

Parents' Evaluation of Developmental Status. The PEDS (Glascoe & Robertshaw, 2013) is a brief screening tool completed by parents/care-givers to identify concerns about children's language, motor, self-help, early academic skills, behavior, and social/emotional/mental health. The age range of the instrument is birth to 8 years. The PEDS can be used either as a screener or, in repeated administrations, to track progress. The PEDS was judged to be a useful screener with adequate reliability and validity (Campbell et al., 2016).

PDD Behavior Inventory-Screening Version. The *PDD Behavior Inventory-Screening Version* (*PDDBI-SV*; Cohen, 2011) is an 18-item abbreviated version of the *PDD Behavior Inventory* (*PDDBI*; Cohen & Sudhalter, 2005) designed as an ASD screen for children aged 18 months to 12 years, 5 months. The *PDDBI-SV* provides scores in two domains: social pragmatic problems and social approach behaviors as well as a composite score: social deficits. The author stresses that this measure is designed solely as a screen to help clinicians decide whether to pursue a more comprehensive assessment and should never be used for diagnostic purposes (Cohen, 2011). The *PDDBI-SV* was designed based on *DSM-IV-TR* criteria, not *DSM-5* criteria, and it assesses only the socialization component of ASD. The standardization and technical characteristics of the scale are limited which led to Barnard-Brak and Richman (2014) to recommend against its use. Shaw (2014a), however, concluded that it could be useful as an early identification screen, especially if used as a universal screen.

ASD Diagnostic Instruments

Autism Spectrum Rating Scales. The *Autism Spectrum Rating Scales* (*ASRS*; Goldstein & Naglieri, 2010) is a 70-item behavior rating scale designed to be easily administered to parents or teachers. In addition, there is a 15-item short form which may be used as a screen or tracking instrument and can be completed by informants in approximately 5 min. With an age range from 2 to 18, the *ASRS* yields a total score, two (social/communication and unusual behaviors for ages 2–5) or three (social/communication, unusual behaviors, and self-regulation for ages 6–18) subscales, and eight treatment subscales (peer socialization, adult socialization, social/emotional reciprocity, stereotypy, behavioral rigidity, sensory sensitivity, and attention/self-regulation for ages 2–5 or attention for ages 6–18) intended to aid in treatment planning and evaluation (Kluck, 2014). The ASRS was published in 2010 using DSM-IV-TR criteria, however, it has been updated to be consistent with DSM-5 criteria (Pearson Assessment, 2024). The intended purpose of the *ASRS* is to measure behaviors associated with autism spectrum disorders (Goldstein & Naglieri, 2010). One positive feature of *ASRS* development is that the standardization of the *ASRS* included both ASD and normally developing children. Overall, the test appears to be well developed with a good standardization sample, and strong reliability and validity (Shaw, 2014b). While the authors of the scales indicate that the *ASRS* can help guide diagnostic decisions as well as be used in treatment planning, ongoing monitoring of response to intervention, and program evaluation, Shaw concluded that the full *ASRS* is not a significant improvement in providing diagnostic information compared with other common ASD assessment instruments (e.g., ADI-R, ADOS, CARS). He also points out that norm-referenced measures such as the ASRS are insensitive to change over time reducing their utility in monitoring behavior change.

Autism Diagnostic Interview-Revised. The *ADI-R* (Rutter et al., 2003) is a semi-structured interview conducted with parents of individuals being evaluated for ASD. The interview can be used for diagnostic and treatment planning purposes for individuals aged 2 through adulthood (Rutter et al., 2003). It consists of 93 questions that are based on DSM-IV TR diagnostic criteria, but because the ADI-R is based on parental responses and the defining features of autism have not changed since the ADI-R was published in 2003, the publisher reports that it remains a valuable tool when administered by competent professionals. Scores are provided in three domains: language/communication, reciprocal social inter-actions, and repetitive behaviors/interests. The authors report excellent test-retest and inter-rater reliabilities (>0.9) and support for the validity of the scale, including the three factors identified above (Kim & Lord, 2012; Kim et al., 2013). Falkmer et al. (2013) concluded that the *ADI-R* is one of only three instruments with strong supporting evidence for its diagnostic accuracy. The *ADI-R* requires specific training for those administering the instrument but has been identified as a "gold standard" instrument in the assessment and diagnosis of ASD (Magaña & Smith, 2013) despite its lengthy administration time and high cost. The *ADI-R* has been translated into other languages (e.g., Spanish, Chinese, Japanese) and found to be generally equivalent to the English version in the assessment and diagnosis of ASD (e.g., Magaña & Smith, 2013; Sun et al., 2013; Tsuchiya et al., 2013). Kourtney and Lord (2022), Esler and Ruble (2015), and Kanne et al. (2008) all recommend it as one of the gold standard measurement tools for diagnosing ASD. The *ADI-R* is not recommended as a diagnostic tool for children below age 2 because of its poor ability to identify ASD at this age (Cox et al., 1999).

Autism Diagnostic Observation Schedule, Second Edition. The Autism Diagnostic Observation Schedule, Second Edition (ADOS-2) (Lord et al., 2012) is a play-based standardized instrument that assesses ASD symptomology (communication, social interaction, play, and restricted and repetitive behaviors) during a semi-structured interaction with an examiner. The *ADOS-2* includes five modules, each requiring 40–60 minutes to administer. The individual being evaluated is given only one module, selected on the level of their expressive language level and chronological age. Module 1 is for children 31 months and older who do not consistently use phrase-based speech. Module 2 is for children of any age who use phrase-based speech but lack verbal fluency. Module 3 is for verbally fluent children and young adolescents. Module 4 is for verbally fluent older adolescents and adults. In addition, there is a toddler module for children 12–30 months of age who do not consistently use phrase-based speech. Each module engages the examinee in a series of activities involving interactive stimulus materials. Scores are compared with cutoff scores to yield one of the three classifications: Autism, ASD, or non-ASD. The difference between the autism and ASD classifications is one of severity, with the former indicating more pronounced symptoms (i.e., DSM-5 Level 1). ADOS-2- specific training is recommended before administering this instrument. Translations are available in Czech, Danish, Dutch, Finnish, French, German, Italian, Norwegian, and Swedish. The *ADOS-2* is well studied, and the consensus is that it is a reliable and valid instrument to assess the presence of ASD (e.g., Bastiaansen et al., 2011; Falkmer et al., 2013; Gray et al., 2008). Falkmer and colleagues concluded that it was one of the only three instruments with strong supporting evidence for its diagnostic accuracy. Lebersfeld et al. (2021) conducted a systematic review and meta-analysis of the ADOS-2 and determined that the ADOS-2 exhibited high levels of sensitivity and specificity across settings, and it should be considered for any ASD evaluation. However, Maddox et al. (2017) cautioned that the ADOS-2 should be used with care as a diagnostic instrument with adults, particularly when the differential diagnosis includes the possibility of psychosis.

Childhood Autism Rating Scale, Second Edition. The *Childhood Autism Rating Scale, Second Edition* (*CARS-2*, Schopler et al., 2010) is a questionnaire used to identify behavioral symptoms of autism as part of the diagnostic process. Designed for ages 2 and higher, the *CARS-2* includes three forms: (a) Standard Version (CARS-2, ST, ages 2–5, or older if estimated IQ 79 or lower), (b) High-Functioning Version (CARS-2 HF, ages 6 and over with estimated IQ 80 or above), and (c) Questionnaire for Parents or Caregivers (unscored scale to assist in making ratings on the two other scales). For the ST and HF versions clinicians rate the individual on 15 items, using a 4-point scale. Ratings are based on frequency, intensity, peculiarity, and duration of the behavior in question. The ST and HF versions each address the following functional areas: (a) relating to people, (b) imitation (ST), (c) social-emotional understanding (HF), (d) emotional response (ST), (e) emotional expression and regulation of emotions (HF), (f) body use, (g) object use (ST), (h) object use in play (HF), (i) adaptation to change (ST), (j) adaptation to change/restricted interests (HF), (k) visual response, (l) listening response, (m) taste, smell, and touch response and use, (n) fear or nervousness (ST), (o) fear or anxiety (HF), (p) verbal communication, (q) nonverbal communication, (r) activity level (ST), (s) thinking/cognitive integration skills (HF), (t) level and consistency of intellectual response, and (u) general impressions.

The reliability and validity of the CARS and CARS-2 have been favorably evaluated by multiple researchers (e.g., Breidbord & Croudace, 2013; Malcolm, 2014; Magyar & Pandolfi, 2007; McLellan, 2014; Reszka et al., 2014) with Falkmer et al. (2013) concluding that it is one of the only three instruments with strong supporting evidence for its diagnostic accuracy. Dawkins et al. (2016) report that the diagnostic agreement of the CARS-2 is high for both DSM-IV and DSM-5 criteria for autism. Ji et al. (2023) concluded it has high concurrent validity with the ADOS-2 ($r = 0.864$, $p < 0.001$).

Gilliam Autism Rating Scale, Third Edition, GARS-3. The *Gilliam Autism Rating Scale, Third Edition* (*GARS-3*, Gilliam, 2013) is a behavioral checklist designed to identify persons with autism. The *GARS-3* is based on the DSM-5 diagnostic criteria for autism spectrum disorder (APA, 2013). It is designed to be completed by a parent, parents, or other caregivers/professionals familiar with the child's behavior and can be completed in a relatively short period of time and requires no professional training to administer.

The *GARS-3* consists of 56 items grouped into six subscales: Restrictive/Repetitive Behaviors, Social Interaction, Social Communication, Emotional Responses, Cognitive Style, and Maladaptive Speech. Psychometric information provided by the scale's publisher concludes that the *GARS-3* has high reliability and validity, as well as good sensitivity and specificity (Pro-Ed, 2024). Karren (2017) conducted a review of the *GARS-3* and concluded that the *GARS-3* is psychometrically sound overall.

PDD Behavior Inventory. The *PDDBI* (Cohen & Sudhalter, 2005) is designed to assess children aged 18 months to 12 years, 5 months. The *PDDBI* has parent and teacher forms and comes in standard (124 item) and extended (180 items) forms. The *PDDBI* standard rating form consists of six domains and the extended rating form consists of 10 domains (six maladaptive and four adaptive). Domain scores are divided into two sections: (a) approach/withdrawal problems and (b) receptive-expressive social communication abilities. Domain scores are grouped into five composite scores: (a) repetitive, ritualistic, and pragmatic problems; (b) approach/withdrawal problems (extended form only); (c) expressive social communication abilities; (d) receptive/expressive social communication abilities (extended form only); and (e) autism composite. While based on the *DSM-IV* criteria for pervasive developmental disorders, however, the majority of items also cover *DSM-5* criteria.

The standardization of the *PDDBI* is limited in size and diversity and there is some question as to the reliability and validity of the instrument (Hoff & Tobin, 2007) although Cohen et al. (2016) reported that the PDDBI sensitivity and specificity results were quite good, showing agreement with ADOS.A strength of the *PDDBI* is that it provides measures of both adaptive and maladaptive behaviors. While the authors indicate that the *PDDBI* can be useful in diagnosis and assessing response to intervention (Carey, 2007), its limitations suggest that other instruments (e.g., *CARS*) may be a better alternative. Please note that in doing library searches on the *PDDBI*, virtually all of the research identified is authored by the first author of the *PDDBI*.

Other Assessment

While ASD-specific measures are an essential element in the assessment and diagnosis of an ASD, they are by no means comprehensive if used as the sole measure. It is important that assessment leads not just to diagnosis but also to efficacious intervention and a variety of other measures may be needed on a case-by-case basis.

Functional Behavior Assessment. Functional behavior assessment (FBA) is essential to the link between assessment and intervention. An FBA attempts to identify the relationship between events in a person's environment and the occurrence of challenging behaviors in order to identify information about the purpose of behavior in order to develop an effective intervention (Cooper et al., 2020). The main outcomes of an FBA are a clear definition or description of the behavior(s); predictions as to the times and situations in which the behavior might or might not occur; and identification of what function the behavior(s) may serve (Rogers, 2001). The logic behind an FBA is that behavior occurs within a particular context and serves a specific purpose (i.e., positive reinforcement, negative reinforcement, automatic/sensory). Individuals engage in behaviors which maximize the likelihood that a desired outcome will result. Identifying the function of specific behaviors provides information that is essential to developing instructional strategies and supports to reduce or eliminate maladaptive behaviors and increasing the frequency of adaptive behaviors.

Functional assessment has been classified into three categories: indirect, descriptive, and experimental. Indirect FBA involves conducting an interview with parents/caregivers and/or the client to hypothesize the function of a behavior. The *Questions About Behavioral Function* (*QABF*) (Matson & Vollmer, 1995) is an indirect assessment tool with a significant amount of research supporting its use (Tarbox et al., 2009). Descriptive FBAs involve direct observation and measurement of the target behavior and environmental variables which are presumed to be functionally relevant (Cooper et al., 2020). The most common descriptive measure is an antecedent-behavior-consequence (ABC) observation. After data col- lection, antecedents, and consequences are analyzed and summarized to hypothesize the potential function of the behavior. Experimental functional assessments, also referred to as "functional analyses," involve direct manipulation of antecedents and consequences to the target behavior, in order to experimentally demonstrate a functional relationship between behavior and the environment. Tarbox et al. (2009) compared indirect, descriptive, and experimental functional assessments using seven children with autism. Results suggested that descriptive assessment did not produce conclusive results, whereas the indirect and experimental assessments generally did.

Practical Functional Assessment (PFA) has emerged as an alternative to traditional FBA methods. PFA, championed by Hanley et al. (2014), is lauded for its brevity, efficiency, and ability to establish client rapport. However, criticisms include its time-consuming nature and potential for irrelevant information (Fryling & Baires, 2016). Hanley (2012) provides a comprehensive overview of PFA, dispelling common myths about functional assessment and outlining strategies for overcoming implementation obstacles. He emphasizes the importance of synthesizing multiple sources of information to develop a nuanced understanding of behavioral functions. PFA has been found to be a, efficacious alternative to determining functions of behavior in multiple settings by a number of researchers including Jessel et al. (2016), Santiago et al. (2016), Slaton et al. (2017), Taylor et al. (2018), and Rajaraman et al. (2022).

Cognitive Functioning. A significant subset of children with ASD also has an intellectual disability (ID; Saunders et al., 2015). In addition, ASD and ID can present similarly, as children with either disorder may demonstrate difficulty with communication, social skills, and behavior (Johnson & Walker, 2006). Therefore, it is frequently important to get a measure of cognitive ability as part of a comprehensive ASD assessment. The *Wechsler Intelligence Scale for Children-Fifth Edition*

(*WISC-V*) and other Wechsler test (e.g., *Wechsler Preschool and Primary Scales of Intelligence-Fourth Edition, WPPSI-IV*) have been used in the ASD assessment process for many years, particularly for higher functioning individuals (Campbell et al., 2014). Other commonly used cognitive assessment measures include the *Woodcock-Johnson IV Tests of Cognitive Ability* (*WJ-III*) and the *Stanford-Binet Intelligence Scales, Fifth Edition* (*SB-5*). Due to communication deficits fundamental to an ASD diagnosis, language-related subtests on these scales may be depressed. Therefore, caution should be used in interpreting any global measure of cognitive ability generated by these instruments. Cognitive measures that are less reliant on language, such as *the Leiter International Performance Scale-Third Edition* (*Leiter-3*) or the *Universal Nonverbal Intelligence Test-2* (*UNIT-2*), should be considered when individuals with ASD present with significant language deficits (Al-Mazidi, 2023; Campbell et al., 2014).

Adaptive Behavior. In addition to deficits in intellectual functioning, an ID diagnosis also requires deficits in adaptive functioning (APA, 2013). The *DSM-5* defines adaptive functioning as "how well a person meets community standards of personal independence and social responsibility …" and "involves adaptive reasoning in three domains: conceptual, social, and practical" (p. 37). Measures such as the *Vineland Adaptive Behavior Scales, Third Edition* (*Vineland-III*) or the *Adaptive Behavior Assessment System, Third Edition* (*ABAS-3*) should also be considered. Tomanik et al. (2007) found that, even in the absence of ID and a cognitive measure, including a measure of adaptive behavior improved diagnostic accuracy from 75 to 84% from using the *ADI-R* and *ADOS* alone. A measure of adaptive behavior may also prove useful in program planning.

Communication. Assessment of communication skills is a funda- mental component of any ASD assessment. The scales discussed above under both screening and diagnostic assessment all contain a language/communication component as do measures of adaptive behavior (e.g., *Vineland*). As the goal of any assessment should be to not only diagnose but also direct subsequent interventions, a more detailed language assessment is recommended. In most cases this will be conducted by a speech-language pathologist (SLP) and include an assessment of receptive, expressive, and pragmatic language skills. An example of a standardized test that may be administered by an SLP is the *Clinical Evaluation of Language Fundamentals-Fifth Edition* (CELF-5; Wiig et al. 2013). This instrument provides a comprehensive evaluation of language, is helpful in determining eligibility for language services in schools and provides information which is useful in developing language-based interventions.

Social Skills. Another common area in which additional assessment may be needed for diagnostic and intervention planning purposes is social skills. As with communication deficits, social skill deficits are a core feature of autism and assessed on the screening and diagnostic measures discussed above. A more detailed assessment of social skills may be warranted in order to get a more in-depth understanding of the social functioning of the individual and as an aid to intervention development. Two common measures of social skills are the *Social Skills Rating Scale* (*SSRS*), now part of the *Social Skills Improvement System* (*SSIS*), and the *Preschool and*

Kindergarten Behavior Scale (*PKBS*). Wang et al. (2011) examined the usefulness of these scales with children with ASD. Results indicated that both measures were predictive of observations of behavior in the natural setting. However, their usefulness in detecting social skill progress over time or intervention outcomes was not satisfactory.

Summary and Conclusions

The assessment of autism spectrum disorders serves multiple purposes in preschool, early childhood, and adolescence (ages 3–18). First and foremost is diagnosis. While it is ideal for ASD to be diagnosed as early as possible, diagnosis prior to the age of 3 is not always possible. Factors such as autistic regression, cognitive development, and social emotional development may limit the manifestation of ASD symptomology until into the preschool and elementary school years. This is particularly evident with those children higher on the spectrum (ASD-Level 3). In addition to diagnosis, ASD assessment plays an important role in selecting intervention methodology and monitoring intervention effectiveness. The focus of diagnostic assessment is on identifying language delays, social skill deficits, and restricted, repetitive, and stereotyped patterns of behavior as these are the areas of functioning specified in the *DSM-5*.

Assessment relies on behavioral observations by psychologists or reports on behavior by parents, teachers, or other caregivers. ASD diagnosis involves a comparison of these behaviors to criteria set forth by diagnostic systems such as the *DSM-5* (APA, 2013) and consists of two stages: screening and comprehensive evaluation (Strock, 2004). Screening is a brief assessment that is conducted to identify children with developmental difficulties who exhibit symptoms typical of ASD and are therefore in need of a more comprehensive evaluation. Screening frequently involves behavioral observations and the use of screening instruments such as checklists and parent and/or teacher questionnaires. This chapter reviewed a number of screening instruments including the *ASQ-3* (Squires et al., 2009); the *PEDS* (Glascoe & Robertshaw, 2013); and the *PDDBI-SV* (Cohen, 2011). In addition to screening for diagnosis, each of these screening instruments can also be used to track an individual's response to intervention although these measures may not be sensitive enough to evaluate small increments of progress. Identifying and operationally defining specific target behaviors and conducting systematic behavioral observations would generally be considered a more sensitive response to intervention monitoring procedures.

This chapter also reviewed a number of diagnostic scales. These included the *Autism Spectrum Rating Scales* (*ASRS*; Goldstein & Naglieri, 2010), the *ADIR* (Rutter et al., 2003), the *ADOS- 2* (Lord et al., 2012), the *CARS-2* (Schopler et al., 2010), the *GARS- 3* (Gilliam, 2013), and the *PDDBI* (Cohen & Sudhalter, 2005). Of these, the *ADI-R*, the *ADOS-2*, and the CARS-2 have been identified as either "gold standard" instruments (Kanne et al., 2008; Magaña & Smith, 2013) or instruments with strong supporting evidence for their diagnostic accuracy (Falkmer et al., 2013). As with the screening instruments, these scales can be used for monitoring response to intervention/progress and assisting in program planning.

While ASD-specific measures such as the screening and diagnostic instruments mentioned above are an important element of ASD assessment, they should not be considered sufficient as the sole measure of ASD diagnosis. It is also important that assessment leads not just to diagnosis but also to efficacious intervention. Therefore, other instruments and procedures as well as input from other professionals are an important component of ASD assessment and diagnosis. It is also recommended that ASD diagnosis and program planning not be made by a sole professional but rather by a multidisciplinary team which may include professionals such as a pediatrician, psychologist, speech pathologist, and occupational therapist as needed based on the specific needs of the individual being assessed (Robertson et al., 2013). Information gathered from an FBA or PFA and assessment of cognitive, communicative, adaptive, and social/emotional functioning can all add to both diagnosis and program development.

References

Al-Mazidi, S. H. (2023). The physiology of cognition in autism spectrum disorder: Current and future challenges. *Cureus, 6*, e46581. https://doi.org/10.7759/cureus.46581

American Psychiatric Association. (2013). *Diagnostic and statistical manual of mental disorders* (5th ed.). Author.

Barnard-Brak, L., & Richman, D. M. (2014). Test review of the PDD behavior inventory-screening version. In J. F. Carlson, K. F. Geisinger, & J. L. Jonson (Eds.), *The nineteenth mental measurements yearbook* [electronic version]. Retrieved from the Burros Institute's Mental Measurements Yearbook online database.

Bastiaansen, J. A., Meffert, H., Hein, S., Huizinga, P., Ketelaars, C., Pijnenborg, B. A., Minderaa, R., Keysers, C., & de Bildt, A. (2011). Diagnosing autism spectrum disorders in adults: The use of *autism diagnostic observation schedule* (*ADOS*) module 4. *Journal of Autism and Developmental Disorders, 41*, 1256–1266. https://doi.org/10.1007/s10803-010-1157-x

Blumberg, S. J., Bramlett, M. D., Kogan, M. D., Schieve, L. A., Jones, J. R., & Lu, M. C. (2013). Changes in prevalence of parent-reported autism spectrum disorders in school-aged U.S. children: 2007 to 2011–12. *National Health Statistics Reports, 64*, 1–12.

Bradley, C. C., Boan, A. D., Cohen, A. P., Charles, J. M., & Carpenter, L. A. (2016). Reported history of developmental regression and restricted, repetitive behaviors in children with autism spectrum disorders. *Journal of Developmental Behavioral Pediatrics, 37*, 451–456. https://doi.org/10.1097/DBP.0000000000000316

Breidbord, J., & Croudace, T. J. (2013). Reliability generalization for childhood autism rating scale. *Journal of Autism and Developmental Disorders, 43*, 2855–2865. https://doi.org/10.1007/s10803-013-1832-9

Campbell, J. M., Ruble, L. A., & Hammond, R. K. (2014). Comprehensive developmental approach assessment model. In L. A. Wilkinson (Ed.), *Autism spectrum dis- order in children and adolescents: Evidence-based assessment and intervention* (pp. 51–73). American Psychological Association.

Campbell, J. M., Sheil, K. A., & Hammond, R. K. (2016). Screening methods. In J. L. Matson (Ed.), *Handbook of assessment and diagnosis of autism spectrum disorder. Autism and child psychopathology series* (pp. 65–86). Springer Nature. https://doi.org/10.1007/978-3-319-27171-2_5

Carey, K. (2007). Test review of the PDD behavior inventory. In K. F. Geisinger, R. A. Spies, J. F. Carlson, & B. S. Plake (Eds.), *The seventeenth mental measurements yearbook* [electronic version]. Retrieved from the Burros Institute's Mental Measurements Yearbook online database.

Centers for Disease Control and Prevention. (2014). Prevalence of autism spectrum disorder among children aged 8 years: Autism and developmental disabilities monitoring network, 11 sites, United States, 2010. *MMWR, 63*(2), 1–21.

Centers for Disease Control and Prevention. (2024). Autism spectrum disorder (ASD): *Clinical Screening for Autism Spectrum Disorder*. https://www.cdc.gov/autism/hcp/diagnosis/screening.html

Cohen, I. L. (2011). *PDD behavior inventory-screening version*. Psychological Assessment Resources, Inc.

Cohen, I. L., & Sudhalter, V. (2005). *PDD behavior inventory*. Psychological Assessment Resources, Inc.

Cohen, I. L., Liu, X., Hudson, M., Gillis, J., Cavalari, R. N., Romanczyk, R. G., Zarmel, B. Z., & Gardner, J. M. (2016). Using the PDD behavior inventory as a level 2 screener: A classification and regression trees analysis. *Journal of Autism and Developmental Disorders, 46*, 3006–3022. https://doi.org/10.1007/s10803-016-2843-0

Conrood, E. E., & Stone, W. L. (2005). Screening for autism in young children. In F. R. Volkmar, R. Paul, A. Klin, & D. Cohen (Eds.), *Handbook of autism and pervasive developmental disorders: Vol 2. Assessment, interventions, and policy* (3rd ed., pp. 707–720). Wiley.

Cooper, J. O., Heron, T. E., & Heward, W. L. (2020). *Applied behavior analysis* (3rd ed.). Upper Saddle River, NJ: Pearson Education.

Cox, A., Klein, K., Charman, T., Baird, G., Baron-Cohen, S., Swettenham, J., Drew, A., & Wheelwright, S. (1999). Autism spectrum disorders at 20 and 42 months of age: Stability of clinical and ADI-R diagnosis. *Journal of Child Psychology and Psychiatry, 40*, 719–732. https://doi.org/10.1111/1469-7610.00488

Dawkins, T., Meyer, A. T., & Van Bourgondien, M. E. (2016). The relationship between the childhood autism rating scale: Second edition and clinical diagnosis utilizing the DSM-IV-TR and the DSM-5. *Journal of Autism and Developmental Disorders, 46*, 3361–3368. https://doi.org/10.1007/s10803-016-2860-z

Dawson, G., Munson, J., Webb, S. J., Nalty, T., Abbott, R., & Toth, K. (2007). Rate of head growth decelerates and symptoms worsen in the second year of life in autism. *Biological Psychiatry, 61*, 458–464. https://doi.org/10.1016/j.biopsych.2006.07.016

Eikeseth, S., Smith, T., Jahr, K., & Eldevik, S. (2007). Outcome for children with autism who began intensive behavioral treatment between ages 4 and 7: A comparison controlled study. *Behavior Modification, 31*, 264–278. https://doi.org/10.1177/0145445506291396

Esler, A., & Ruble, L. (2015). DSM-5 diagnostic criteria for autism spectrum disorder with implications for school psychologists. *International Journal of School & Educational Psychology, 3*, 1–15. https://doi.org/10.1080/21683603.2014.890148

Falkmer, T., Anderson, K., Falkmer, M., & Horlin, C. (2013). Diagnostic procedures in autism spectrum dis- orders: A systematic literature review. *European Child & Adolescent Psychiatry, 22*, 329–340. https://doi.org/10.1007/s00787-013-0375-0

Fryling, M. J., & Baires, N. A. (2016). The practical importance of the distinction between open and closed-ended indirect assessments. *Behavior Analysis in Practice, 9*(2), 146–151. https://doi.org/10.1007/s40617-016-0115-2

Gilliam, J. E. (2013). *Gilliam autism rating scale* (3rd ed.) Pro-ed.

Glascoe, F. P., & Robertshaw, N. S. (2013). *Parents evaluation of developmental status*. PEDStest.com, LLC.

Goldstein, S., & Naglieri, J. (2010). *Autism spectrum rating scales*. Multi-Health Systems, Inc.

Gray, K. M., Tonge, B. J., & Sweeney, D. J. (2008). Using the autism diagnostic interview-revised and the autism diagnostic observation schedule with young children with developmental delay: Evaluating diagnostic validity. *Journal of Autism and Developmental Disorders, 38*, 657–667. https://doi.org/10.1007/s10803-007-0432-y

Hanig, K. M. (2010). Test review of the *Ages and Stages Questionnaire*: A parent completed child monitoring system, third edition. In R. A. Spies. J. F. Carlson.

Hanley, G. P. (2012). Functional assessment of problem behavior: Dispelling myths, overcoming implementation obstacles, and discovering new lore. *Behavior Analysis in Practice, 5*(1), 54–72. https://doi.org/10.1007/BF03391818

Hanley, G. P., Jin, C. S., Vanselow, N. R., & Hanratty, L. A. (2014). Producing meaningful improvements in problem behavior of children with autism via synthesized analyses and treatments. *Journal of Applied Behavior Analysis, 47*(1), 16–36. https://doi.org/10.1002/jaba.106

Hoff, K. E., & Tobin, R. M. (2007). Test review of the PDD behavior inventory. In K. F. Geisinger, R. A. Spies, J. F. Carlson, & B. S. Plake (Eds.), *The seventeenth mental measurements yearbook* [electronic version]. Retrieved from the Burros Institute's Mental Measurements Yearbook online database.

Hoshino, Y., Kaneko, M., Yashima, Y., Kumashiro, H., Volkmar, F., & Cohen, D. J. (1987). Clinical features of autistic children with setback course in their infancy. *Japanese Journal of Psychiatry and Neurology, 41*, 237–245. https://doi.org/10.1111/j.1440-1819.1987.tb00407.x

Hughes, M. M., Shaw, K. A., Patrick, M. E., DiRienzo, M., Bakian, A. V., Bilder, D. A., Durkin, M. S., Hudson, A., Spivey, M. H., DaWalt, L. S., Salinas, A., Schwenk, Y. D., Lopez, M., Baroud, T. M., & Maenner, M. J. (2023). Adolescents with autism spectrum disorder: Diagnostic patterns, co-occurring conditions, and transition planning. *Journal of Adolescent Health, 73*(2), 271–278. https://doi.org/10.1016/j.jadohealth.2022.12.010

Hyman, S. L., Levy, S. E., Myers, S. M., Council on children with disabilities, section on developmental and behavioral pediatrics, Kuo, D. Z., Apkon, S., Davidson, L. F., Ellerbeck, K. A., Foster, J. E. A., Noritz, G. N., O'Connor Leppert, M., Saunders, B. S., Stille, S., Yin, L., Weitzman, C. C., Jr, D. O., Levine, J. M., Peralta-Carcelen, A. M., Poon, J. K., Smith, P. J., Blum, N. J., Takayama, J. I., Baum, R., Voigt, R. G., & Bridgemohan, C. (2020). Identification, evaluation, and management of children with autism spectrum disorder. *Pediatrics, 145*, e20193447. https://doi.org/10.1542/peds.2019-3447

Jessel, J., Hanley, G. P., & Ghaemmaghami, M. (2016). Interview-informed synthesized contingency analyses: Thirty replications and reanalysis. *Journal of Applied Behavior Analysis, 49*(3), 576–595. https://doi.org/10.1002/jaba.316

Jeste, S., & Geschwind, D. (2014). Disentangling the heterogeneity of autism spectrum disorder through genetic findings. *Nature Reviews Neurology, 10*, 74–81. https://doi.org/10.1038/nrneurol.2013.278

Ji, S. I., Park, H., Yoon, S. A., & Hong, S. B. (2023). A validation study of the CARS-2 compared with the ADOS-2 in the diagnosis of autism spectrum disorder: A suggestion for cutoff scores. *Soa Chongsonyon Chongsin Uihak., 34*(1), 45–50. https://doi.org/10.5765/jkacap.220027

Johnson, C. P., & Walker, W. O., Jr. (2006). Mental retar- dation: Management and prognosis. *Journal of Developmental and Behavioral Pediatrics, 27*, 249–255. https://doi.org/10.1542/pir.27-7-249

Johnston, M. V., Ishida, A., Ishida, W. N., Matsushita, H. B., Nishimura, A., & Tsuji, M. (2009). Plasticity and injury in the developing brain. *Brain Development, 31*, 1–10. https://doi.org/10.1016/j.braindev.2008.03.014

Jorgenson, E. J. (2017). *Pretend play and children with autism spectrum disorder: Deficits and interventions.* Unpublished Honors Thesis. Appalachian State University, Boone, NC. https://api.semanticscholar.org/CorpusID:148773237

Kanne, S. M., Randolph, J. K., & Farmer, J. E. (2008). Diagnostic and assessment findings: A bridge to academic planning for children with autism spectrum dis- orders. *Neuropsychology Review, 18*, 367–384. https://doi.org/10.1007/s11065-008-9072-z

Karren, B. C. (2017). A test review: Gilliam, J. E. (2014). Gilliam Autism Rating Scale-Third Edition (GARS-3). *Journal of Psychoeducational Assessment, 35(3)*, 342–346. doi:https://doi.org/10.1177/0734282916635465

Kim, S. H., & Lord, C. (2012). New autism diagnostic interview-revised algorithms for toddlers and young preschoolers from 12 to 47 months of age. *Journal of Autism and Developmental Disorders, 42*, 82–93. https://doi.org/10.1007/s10803-011-1213-1

Kim, S. H., Thurm, A., Shumway, S., & Lord, C. (2013). Multisite study of new autism diagnostic interview- revised (ADI-R) algorithms for toddlers and young preschoolers. *Journal of Autism and Developmental Disorders, 43*, 1527–1538. https://doi.org/10.1007/s10803-012-1696-4

Kluck, A. S. (2014). Test review of the Autism Spectrum Rating Scales. In J. F. Carlson, K. F. Geisinger, & J. L. Jonson (Eds.), *The nineteenth mental measurements yearbook* [electronic version]. Retrieved from the Burros Institute's Mental Measurements Yearbook online database.

Kourtney, C., & Lord, C. (2022). Best practice assessments for autism spectrum disorders in schools. *Psychology in the Schools, 59*, 1454–1468. https://doi.org/10.1002/pits.22680

Landa, R., & Garrett-Mayer, E. (2006). Development in infants with autism spectrum disorders: A prospective study. *Journal of Child Psychology and Psychiatry, 47*, 629–638. https://doi.org/10.1111/j.1469-7610.2006.01531.x

Lebersfeld, J. B., Swanson, M., Clesi, C. D., & O'Kelley, S. E. (2021). Systematic review and meta-analysis of the clinical utility of the ADOS-2 and the ADI-R in diagnosing autism spectrum disorders in children. *Journal of Autism and Developmental Disorders, 51*, 4101–4114. https://doi.org/10.1007/s10803-020-04839-z

Little, S. G., & Akin-Little, A. (2016). Preschool, early childhood and adolescence. In J. Matson (Ed.), *Handbook of assessment and diagnosis of autism spectrum disorder* (pp. 175–190). Springer.

Lord, C., Rutter, M., DiLavore, P. C., Risi, S., Gotham, K., & Bishop, S. L. (2012). *Autism diagnostic observation schedule, second edition (ADOS-2)*. Western Psychological Services.

Lord, C., Shulman, C., & DiLavore, P. (2004). Regression and word loss in autistic spectrum disorders. *Journal of Child Psychology and Psychiatry and Allied Disciplines, 4*, 936–955. https://doi.org/10.1111/j.1469-7610.2004.t01-1-00287.x

Maddox, B. B., Brodkin, E. S., Calkins, M. E., Shea, K., Mullan, K., Hostager, J., Mandell, D. S., & Miller, J. S. (2017). The accuracy of the ADOS-2 in identifying autism among adults with complex psychiatric conditions. *Journal of Autism & Developmental Disorders, 47*(9), 2703–2709. https://doi.org/10.1007/s10803-017-3188-z

Maenner, M. J., Warren, Z., Williams, A. R. et al. (2023). Prevalence and Characteristics of Autism Spectrum Disorder Among Children Aged 8 Years–Autism and Developmental Disabilities Monitoring Network, 11 Sites, United States, *MMWR Surveillance Summary 2023*;72(No. SS-2):1–14. DOI: https://doi.org/10.15585/mmwr.ss7202a1

Magaña, S., & Smith, L. (2013). Are there differences in *ADI-R* lifetime scores between Latino and non-Latino adolescents and adults with autism spectrum disorders? *Journal of Autism and Developmental Disorders, 43*, 141–153.

Magyar, C. I., & Pandolfi, V. (2007). Factor structure evaluation of the childhood autism rating scale. *Journal of Autism and Developmental Disorders, 37*, 1787–1794. https://doi.org/10.1007/s10803-006-0313-9

Malcolm, K. K. (2014). *Test review of the Childhood autism rating scale, second edition.* In J. F. Carlson.

Manning, S. E., Davin, C. A., Barfield, W. D., Kotelchuck, M., Clements, K., Diop, H., Osbahr, T., & Smith, L. A. (2011). Early diagnoses of autism spectrum disorders in Massachusetts birth cohorts, 2001-2005. *Pediatrics, 127*, 1043–1051. https://doi.org/10.1542/peds.2010-2943

Matson, J. L., & Vollmer, T. (1995). *Questions about behavioral function (QABF).* Baton Rouge: http://www.disabilityconsultants.org

McLellan, M. J. (2014). Test review of the Childhood autism rating scale, second edition. In J. F. Carlson, K. F. Geisinger, & J. L. Jonson (Eds.), *The nineteenth mental measurements yearbook* [electronic version]. Retrieved from the Burros Institute's Mental Measurements Yearbook online database.

National Institute for Mental Health (2024). Autism spectrum disorder. https://www.nimh.nih.gov/health/topics/autism-spectrum-disorders-asd

Pearson Assessment (2024). *Autism Spectrum Rating Scales.* https://www.pearsonassessments.com/store/usassessments/en/Store/Professional-Assessments/Behavior/Autism-Spectrum-Rating-Scales/p/100000354.html?tab=product-details.

Pro-Ed (2024). *Gilliam Autism Rating Scale|Third Edition (GARS-3).* https://www.proedinc.com/Products/13780/gars3-gilliam-autism-rating-scalethird-edition.aspx

Rajaraman, A., Hanley, G. P., Gover, H. C., Ruppel, K. W., & Landa, R. K. (2022). On the reliability and treatment utility of the practical functional assessment process. *Behavior Analysis in Practice, 15*(3), 815–837. https://doi.org/10.1007/s40617-021-00665-6

Reszka, S. S., Boyd, B. A., McBee, M., Hume, K. A., & Odom, S. L. (2014). Brief report: Concurrent validity of autism symptom severity measures. *Journal of Autism and Developmental Disorders, 44*, 466–470. https://doi.org/10.1007/s10803-013-1879-7

Robertson, K., Stafford, T., Benedicto, J., & Hocking, N. (2013). Autism assessment: The Melton health model. *Journal of Paediatrics and Child Health, 49*, 1057–1062. https://doi.org/10.1111/jpc.12303

Rogers, E. L. (2001). Functional behavioral assessment and children with autism: Working as a team. *Focus on Autism and Other Developmental Disabilities, 16*, 228–231.

Rutter, M., Le Couteur, A., & Lord, C. (2003). Autism diagnostic interview-revised (ADI-R). *Western psychological services.*

Santiago, J. L., Hanley, G. P., Moore, K., & Jin, C. S. (2016). The generality of interview-informed functional analyses: Systematic replications in school and home. *Journal of Autism and Developmental Disorders, 46*(3), 797–811. https://doi.org/10.1007/s10803-015-2617-0

Saunders, B. S., Tilford, J. M., Fussell, J. J., Schulz, E. G., Casey, P. H., & Kuo, D. Z. (2015). Financial and employment impact of intellectual disability on families of children with autism. *Families, Systems & Health: The Journal of Collaborative Family Healthcare.* https://doi.org/10.1037/fsh0000102

Schopler, E., Van Bourgondien, M. E., Wellman, G. J., & Love, S. R. (2010). *Childhood autism rating scale* (2nd ed.). Western Psychological Services.

Shaw, S. R. (2014a). Test review of the PDD behavior inventory-screening version. In J. F. Carlson, K. F. Geisinger, & J. L. Jonson (Eds.), *The nineteenth mental measurements yearbook* [electronic version]. Retrieved from the Burros Institute's Mental Measurements Yearbook online database.

Shaw, S. R. (2014b). Test review of the autism spectrum rating scales. In J. F. Carlson, K. F. Geisinger, & J. L. Jonson (Eds.), *The nineteenth mental measurements yearbook* [electronic version]. Retrieved from the Burros Institute's Mental Measurements Yearbook online database.

Sheldrick, R. C., Carter, A. S., Eisenhower, A., Mackie, T. I., Cole, M. B., Hoch, N., Brunt, S., & Pedraza, F. M. (2022). Effectiveness of screening in early intervention settings to improve diagnosis of autism and reduce health disparities. *JAMA Pediatrics, 176*(3), 262–269. https://doi.org/10.1001/jamapediatrics.2021.5380

Slaton, J. D., Hanley, G. P., & Raftery, K. J. (2017). Interview-informed functional analyses: A comparison of synthesized and isolated components. *Journal of Applied Behavior Analysis, 50*, 252–277. https://doi.org/10.1002/jaba.384

Squires, J., Twombly, E., Bricker, D., & Potter, L. (2009). In H. Paul (Ed.), *Ages and stages questionnaire* (3rd ed.). Brookes Publishing Co.

Stefanatos, G. A. (2008). Regression in autistic spectrum disorders. *Neuropsychology Review, 18*, 305–319. https://doi.org/10.1007/s11065-008-9073-y

Strock, M. (2004). *Autism spectrum disorders (pervasive developmental disorders).* NIMH Publication No. NIH-04-5511. Bethesda, MD: National Institute of Mental Health, National Institutes of Health, U.S. Department of Health and Human Services.

Sun, X., Allison, C., Auyeung, B., Matthews, F. E., Baron-Cohen, S., & Brayne, C. (2013). What is available for case identification in autism research in mainland China? *Research in Autism Spectrum Disorders, 7*, 579–590. https://doi.org/10.1016/j.rasd.2012.11.003

Tarbox, J., Wilke, A. E., Najdowski, A. C., Findel-Pyles, R. S., Balasanyan, S., Caveney, A. C., Chilingaryan, V., King, D. M., Niehoff, s. M., Slease, K., & Tia, B. (2009). Comparing indirect, descriptive, and experimental functional assessments of challenging behavior in children with

autism. Journal of Developmental & Physical Disabilities, 21, 493–514. doi:https://doi.org/10.1007/s10882-009-9154-8.
Taylor, S. A., Phillips, K. J., & Gertzog, M. G. (2018). Use of synthesized analysis and informed treatment to promote school reintegration. *Behavioral Interventions, 33*, 364–379. https://doi.org/10.1002/bin.1640
Tomanik, S. S., Pearson, D. A., Loveland, K. A., Lane, D. M., & Shaw, J. B. (2007). Improving the reliability of autism diagnoses: Examining the utility of adaptive behavior. *Journal of Autism and Developmental Disorders, 37*, 921–928. https://doi.org/10.1007/s10803-006-0227-6
Tsuchiya, K. J., Matsumoto, K., Yagi, A., Inada, N., Kuroda, M., Inokuchi, E., Koyama, T., et al. (2013). Reliability and validity of autism diagnostic interview-revised, Japanese version. *Journal of Autism and Developmental Disorders, 43*, 643–662. https://doi.org/10.1007/s10803-012-1606-9
Valleley, R. J., & Roane, B. M. (2010). Test review of the ages and stages questionnaire: A parent completed child monitoring system, third edition. In R. A. Spies. J. F. Carlson, & K. F. Geisinger (Eds.), *The eighteenth mental measurements yearbook* [electronic version]. Retrieved from the Burros Institute's Mental Measurements Yearbook online database.
van't Hof, M., Tisseur, C., van Berckelear-Onnes, I., van Nieuwenhuyzen, A., Daniels, A. M., Deen, M., Hoek, H. W., & Ester, W. A. (2021). Age at autism spectrum disorder diagnosis: A systematic review and meta-analysis from 2012 to 2019. Autism, 25(4), 862–873. doi:https://doi.org/10.1177/1362361320971107.
Velikonja, T., Edbrooke-Childs, J., Calderon, A., Sleed, M., Brown, A., & Deighton, J. (2017). The psychometric properties of the ages & stages questionnaires for ages 2-2.5: A systematic review. *Child Care Health Development, 43*(1), 1–17. https://doi.org/10.1111/cch.12397
Volker, M. A., & Lopata, C. (2008). Autism: A review of biological bases, assessment, and intervention. *School Psychology Quarterly, 23*, 228–270. https://doi.org/10.1037/1045-3830.23.2.258
Waltz, M. (2002). *Autistic spectrum disorders: Finding a diagnosis and getting help*. O'Reilly & Associates.
Wang, H., Sandall, S. R., Davis, C. A., & Thomas, C. J. (2011). Social skills assessment in young children with autism: A comparison evaluation of the SSRS and PKBS. *Journal of Autism and Developmental Disorders, 41*, 1487–1495. https://doi.org/10.1007/s10803-010-1175-8
Wiig, E. H., Semel, E., & Secord, W. A. (2013). *Clinical evaluation of language fundamentals* (5th ed.). Pearson Assessment.
Zwaigenbaum, L., Bauman, M. L., Stone, W. L., Yirmiya, N., Estes, A., Hansen, R. L., McPartland, J C, Natowicz M R, Choueiri, R, Fein, D., Kasari, C., Pierce, K., Buie, T., Carter, A., Davis, P. A., Granpeesheh, D., Mailloux, Z., Newschaffer, C., Robins, D., Roley S. S., Wagner, S., & Wetherby A. (2015). Early identification of autism spectrum disorder: Recommendations for practice and research. Pediatrics, 136, S10–S40. doi:https://doi.org/10.1542/peds.2014-3667C.

Identification, Assessment, and Diagnosis of Autism in Adulthood

Aspasia Stacey Rabba, Lauren Taylor, Wenn Lawson, and Iliana Magiati

Abstract Substantial shifts have occurred in research and clinical practice in the last two decades towards improving identification, diagnosis, and understanding of autism in adults. One important aim of assessment of autistic people in adulthood is to identify, assess, and diagnose autism in adults who were not identified in childhood. Another important aim is to assess, understand, and support autistic adults' and older adults' strengths, needs, preferences, and to explore risk and enabling factors affecting their daily functioning, employment, education, social participation, health, and overall wellbeing and quality of life. Considering these two key aims of assessment in adulthood, in this chapter we critically summarize current guidance for the assessment and diagnosis of autism in adulthood; we then synthesize contemporary knowledge and approaches to assessment and assessment feedback adopting a strength-focused, person-centered, and neuro-affirming approach, in the following domains: social communication and interaction, behaviors and interests, intellectual, and executive functioning and cognitive styles, language and communication, adaptive functioning, behavior, mental health, and wellbeing. We also explore assessment during times of transition, for employment, and assessment relating to aging. In each of these domains, we discuss what to assess (i.e., what information is important to explore in the assessment) and how to assess (i.e., how to gather this information using a range of assessment approaches).

Keywords Autism · Adults/adulthood · Assessment · Diagnosis

A. S. Rabba (✉)
School of Educational Psychology and Counselling, Faculty of Education, Monash University, Clayton, VIC, Australia
e-mail: stacey.rabba@monash.edu

L. Taylor
Autism Association of Western Australia, Shenton Park, Perth, WA, Australia

W. Lawson
Curtin Autism Research Group, Curtin University, Perth, WA, Australia

I. Magiati
School of Psychological Science, The University of Western Australia, Perth, WA, Australia

J. L. Matson (ed.), *Assessment and Diagnosis in Autism*, Autism and Child Psychopathology Series, https://doi.org/10.1007/978-3-032-11802-8_6

Background and Aims of Assessment in Adulthood

In the last two decades, substantial shifts have occurred in research and clinical practice towards improving identification, diagnosis, and understanding of autism in adults (e.g., Gosling et al., 2022; Mason et al., 2021; Roestorf et al., 2022; Sáez-Suanes et al., 2022; Shattuck et al., 2020; Wright et al., 2019). However, there continue to be age-related inequalities in autism diagnosis (e.g., Brugha et al., 2011; Dietz et al., 2020; O'Nions et al., 2023). Many autistic adults are diagnosed later in life or remain unidentified, undiagnosed, and unsupported in adulthood for a range of reasons, including: subtle autistic presentations that become evident when demands exceed capacity; professionals' limited knowledge of the heterogeneity of autism; overrepresentation of males in autism research and services and limited—although emerging—understanding of autism in females and gender-diverse people. Access to diagnostic services is limited, stigma prevalent and diagnostic over-shadowing (diagnosing another condition, such as a mental health condition, but missing autism) is common (Green et al., 2019; Jones et al., 2014; Kentrou et al., 2024; Lai & Baron-Cohen, 2015). An autism diagnosis in adulthood can have many positive impacts (Davies et al., 2024a, 2024b), such as enabling individuals to make sense of their differences and lifelong difficulties, increasing self-understanding and acceptance, and facilitating access to accommodations, supports, and/or services (Gellini & Marczak, 2023; Lilley et al., 2022; Tan, 2018) that together improve quality of life, and enable autistic adults to live the life they want (Gellini & Marczak, 2024; Merrington et al., 2024; Pellicano & Heyworth, 2023; Tan, 2018). Therefore, *one important aim of assessment in adulthood is to identify, assess and diagnose autistic adults who were not identified or diagnosed in earlier life.*

In addition, while many autistic adults, including those who were diagnosed in childhood, are living fulfilling and productive lives, adult outcomes are highly variable, and many autistic adults have poor outcomes in adulthood, experiencing under- or unemployment, limited community participation/inclusion and high rates of co-occurring physical, mental health, and behavioral difficulties (see Mason et al., 2021). Thus, *a second important aim of assessment in adulthood is to assess, understand and support autistic individuals' strengths, needs, preferences, and to explore risk and enabling factors* affecting their daily functioning, independence, employment or education, social participation, and overall wellbeing. A strength-based, person-centered and needs-focused assessment approach is necessary, such that needs can be understood and supported, autistic autonomy and agency amplified, and wellbeing enhanced, to support people to flourish (Pellicano & Heyworth, 2023).

Considering these two key aims of assessment, in this chapter we first critically summarize current guidelines for the assessment and diagnosis of autism in adulthood. We then synthesize contemporary knowledge and approaches to the identification, assessment, and diagnosis of autism in adulthood by exploring *what to assess* (i.e., what information is important to explore during an assessment) and *how to assess* (i.e., how to gather this information using a range of assessment approaches).

Key Principles and Guidance for Autism Assessment and Diagnosis in Adulthood

Several international clinical guidelines have been published, which include key principles and good practice recommendations about autism assessment and diagnosis across the lifespan (e.g., Fuentes et al., 2021; Goodall et al., 2023; NICE, 2021; Whaikaha–Ministry of Disabled People, 2022). There is general agreement that regardless of the purpose of the assessment, the approach should be person- and family-centered, culturally responsive, strengths-based, and neuro-affirming (Goodall et al., 2023). As part of a good practice assessment, health professionals should gather detailed historical and current information relevant to the purpose of the assessment, and in the case of diagnostic assessments, use current versions of the Diagnostic and Statistical Manual of Mental Disorders, Fifth Edition, Text Revision (DSM-5-TR; APA, 2022) or the International Classification of Diseases—11th Revision (ICD-11; WHO, 2019).

An assessment for possible autism in adulthood should be considered when an adult presents with, or reports a history of:

(a) persistent difficulties in social interaction, social communication *or* highly focused or intense interests, repetitive behaviors, strong preference for routine and predictability and atypical sensory processing; and
(b) one or more of the following: (i) difficulties obtaining or sustaining education or employment or persistent difficulties with social relationships; (ii) a history of a neurodevelopmental or mental health condition/diagnosis; and/or (iii) past or present contact with mental health or learning disability services (NICE, 2021).

In adults with intellectual disabilities, autism may be considered when the adult presents with persistent difficulties in reciprocal social interaction and/or communication or with marked repetitive behaviors, strong preferences for routine and predictability, marked sensory sensitivities, or highly intense and focused interests, over and above those that may be expected based on their intellectual abilities (Fuentes et al., 2021).

To diagnose autism in adulthood and to facilitate differential diagnosis, clinicians require a high level of skill and experience, particularly around understanding autistic experiences across the lifespan and across age, gender, cognitive ability, and social contextual factors, as well as knowledge of neurotypical and neurodivergent development across the lifespan. For this reason, it is often recommended that comprehensive diagnostic assessments are conducted by a consensus multidisciplinary team comprised of professionals who have received training and are competent in autism assessment (Goodall et al., 2023; NICE, 2021).

The professionals involved in the assessment should gather detailed historical and current information that is relevant for the purpose of the assessment, and in the case of diagnostic assessments, to the diagnosis of autism using current versions of the DSM-5-TR (APA, 2022) or the ICD-11 (WHO, 2019).

A range of information gathering approaches and methods should be used in best-practice assessments (Goodall et al., 2023; NICE, 2021). These may include:

- reliable and valid screening and diagnostic procedures and tools, including self-report and informant-report checklists, and semi-standardized diagnostic instruments (see Whaikaha–Ministry of Disabled People, 2022; see also Bishop & Lord, 2023).
- focused and detailed interviews with the adult and significant others who know the person well.
- naturalistic and semi-structured observations of the adult in the clinic setting, and if indicated, in other environments (e.g., residential care, home, work).

As per the DSM-5-TR (APA, 2022) and other guidance (e.g., Fuentes et al., 2021), multiple assessment sessions, and/or sessions that are longer than standard, may be needed as part of assessment of autism in adulthood, especially when the assessment is complex, there are co-occurring conditions and/or autistic traits are subtle.

Assessment of Autistic Features and Characteristics

To make a clinical diagnosis of autism, the diagnostic criteria outlined in both the DSM-5-TR and the ICD-11 specify that the person must present with persistent difficulties in social communication and social interaction, and patterns of repetitive or highly focused interests, behaviors and activities. These must have been present in the early developmental period (childhood and adolescence) and across multiple contexts but may not manifest until social demands outweigh capacity. In addition, the autistic features must significantly limit or impair functioning or cause distress and cannot be better explained by another condition (APA, 2022; WHO, 2019). Therefore, both social communication and social interaction, and behavioral features of autism need to be comprehensively assessed, and alternative explanations for the person's differences be carefully considered as part of the assessment process.

What to Assess

Social Communication and Social Interaction

Clinicians should focus on gathering information about: (a) current and past social and emotional reciprocity, (b) non-verbal communication (including use and understanding of facial expressions, eye contact, gestures, and integration of verbal with non-verbal communication), and (c) the person's understanding of relationships and their ways of relating to others.

Importantly, when addressing each of these areas of social communication and social interaction, the clinician should gather *both* current and historical information about the person's strengths, differences and difficulties in a range of different social contexts. Specifically, information needs to be gathered about reciprocal social interactions currently and in childhood and adolescence; the frequency and quality of social initiations and responses; the adult's use, understanding, and integration of non-verbal communication; and past and current peer and romantic relationships across settings, in order to understand the patterns and persistence of social communication differences and difficulties across time and contexts.

In addition, it is important to assess social interaction, communication, and understanding of relationships relative to the person's intellectual and expressive language ability. Many adults with persistent language difficulties find aspects of social communication challenging, and their language differences may impact relationship development (e.g., Conti-Ramsden et al., 2006, 2013) and functional outcomes (e.g., Conti-Ramsden et al., 2018; Dubois et al., 2020). It is often hard to differentiate between profound developmental delays in social functioning and autistic social difficulties in individuals with intellectual disability (ID), especially those with severe and profound ID (Howlin, 2000; Thurm et al., 2019). Nevertheless, it is important to try to make this diagnostic determination, particularly for people with a mild to moderate ID, because the presence of a co-occurring autism diagnosis may have important implications for the person's support needs (Howlin, 2000). The assessment of social reciprocity and non-verbal social communication skills is critical to the differential diagnosis of autism from ID, as the social difficulties experienced by autistic people with ID are typically below expectations for their overall intellectual/developmental level.

Social-Emotional Reciprocity

Aspects of social emotional reciprocity that should be assessed include the way in which a person initiates and responds to social interactions, engages in conversation, and shares emotions and interests with others. Autistic adults differ from neurotypical adults in their social initiations and responses. For example, they may initiate few interactions, or social initiations may seem focused, pragmatic, direct, or scripted. Some may have a non-normative social approach, which can appear as a preference for focused social interactions that serve specific purposes (e.g., to find out information about a topic rather than making social enquiries). Some do not follow neurotypical social conventions or expectations, such as social greetings or reciprocal social chit-chat. Autistic adults may not share their interests with others or alternatively, they may share their interests and passions enthusiastically or in great detail without gauging the degree to which others' share their interest, which can be perceived by others as "dominating" in conversations. There may be qualitative differences and/or difficulties in the flexibility of social comments, so social initiations or responses may appear scripted. The degree to which autistic adults share and describe their emotional experiences may differ from neurotypical adults, as they may find it hard to articulate their emotions.

Non-verbal Social Communication

The extent to which the adult integrates non-verbal communication (i.e., gestures, speech, facial expressions, eye contact) during social interactions should be observed and explored. Both current and historical information should be gathered. When compared to neurotypical expectations, autistic people may have a smaller range of facial expressions, or their facial expressions may appear learnt or rehearsed. Some autistic adults may show facial expressions that appear mismatched to the social situation, such as smiling when discussing a subject typically considered serious. Eye contact may be limited, inconsistent, too intense, or well-rehearsed and learned through effortful control, and may be experienced as exhausting and uncomfortable by the autistic adult. Gestures may be reduced in range or exaggerated, or may appear learned or scripted, so they do not appear spontaneous to neurotypical people. Autistic adults may also have difficulties with integrating different modes of communication (e.g., using eye gaze, speaking, gesturing, and facial expressions flexibly, at the same time), which to the neurotypical observer can appear mis-timed and may contribute to social misunderstandings.

In addition, the person may find it hard to process or understand other people's facial expressions or body language. For example, the autistic person may consistently misinterpret others' facial expressions or have a highly analytical or structured approach to reading facial expressions, which may in turn contribute to relationship misunderstandings or communication breakdowns. An autistic adult may have explicitly taught themselves how to interpret other's non-verbal communication rather than developing this skill intuitively.

Understanding, Developing, and Maintaining Social Relationships

Autistic adults may engage in, maintain, and understand social relationships in ways that are different to neurotypical people. Some autistic adults have little social motivation so often prefer spending time by themselves. Many autistic adults are highly socially motivated when their relationships center around a common area of passion and interest, or when the social and sensory environments are not excessively taxing. Adjusting social behaviors in different contexts and with different people (for example an acquaintance, versus a close friend, a partner, or a colleague), may be difficult for some autistic individuals, many of whom make extensive conscious efforts to study and create detailed social rules and scripts, which may not be sufficiently flexible to manage different social interactions. Alternatively, an autistic person's behavior in social situations may be considered "socially inappropriate" by neurotypical individuals due to difficulties understanding or following typical social rules, conventions, intentions, or boundaries. Depending on age, cognitive and language level, understanding of relationships (such as friendships or romantic relationships) may be limited or different compared to neurotypical adults, and there may be differences and challenges navigating friendships or professional relationships for some autistic people. Consequently, sometimes autistic adults may come across as overly trusting socially or could be easily exploited, because they have difficulty understanding others' perspectives or malicious intent.

Patterns of Interests, Behaviors, and Activities, Including Sensory Features

Repetitive Speech, Behaviors, Interests, or Activities

The clinician should explore the nature, extent, intensity, and impact of repetitive or atypical speech in speaking adults (e.g., speech may be repetitive, appear overly formal, rehearsed, or learned, there may be idiosyncratic speech, or immediate or delayed echolalia). The clinician should also elicit specific past (in childhood and adolescence) and current examples of stereotyped or repetitive behaviors (also referred to as "stimming" behaviors, e.g., hand flapping, hand splays, hand/finger mannerisms, other atypical hand or whole-body posturing or movements, repetitive actions with objects, etc.). Autistic adults may have learned to suppress some of these behaviors, so it is important to ask about the presence of these in childhood and adolescence, as well as possible current engagement in these behaviors when alone.

Strong Preference for Routines and Predictability

Asking about the flexibility, impact and degree of distress associated with "change" provides insight into a person's strong preference for predictability and sameness and associated distress when there is unpredictability and change. These can include small changes in daily life, such as the way food is presented or objects organized on one's desk, as well as larger changes and life transitions, such as employment, living conditions, and family structure. Understanding the extent to which the person shows a strong preference for following rigid routines in daily life (e.g., highly routinized eating, clothing, daily routines), or routines that do not appear functional to a neurotypical person (e.g., following set sequences at work that cannot be altered even with the introduction of a more efficient approach etc.), as well as the extent to which they may find it hard to show flexible thinking patterns (for example, exploring if they have strong adherence to rules and experience distress when exceptions need to be made) are relevant for assessment and important to capture both currently and historically.

Highly Focused, Specialized, and/or Intense Interests

Highly focused or intense interests and passions in autism may range from highly specific or uncommon topics (e.g., sixteenth century calligraphy, airport departure, and landing schedules) to those that are more common in the general population (i.e., art, music, sport, animals, technology, nature, e.g., Grove et al., 2018). It is often the extent of the interest, deep knowledge, expertise, and intensity of engagement with, and discussion of, these interests that is different in autistic people compared to neurotypical people. It is also important that the quality and function of the interests be explored, as well as the degree to which an interest seems consistent with the person's age or developmental stage. Both the helpful and unhelpful impacts of the individual's interests need to be explored. Some autistic adults can be so immersed in their interest that everyday tasks (e.g., eating, undertaking domestic chores) may be forgotten. However, many autistic people have interests and passions that are often a great strength and that positively influence their motivation, learning and wellbeing, facilitate choice of studies and career, and/or enable social participation (Grove et al., 2018; Kapp et al., 2019; Lizon et al., 2024). These interests may remain consistent over time or change across the years, and most autistic adults have more than one intense interest, and thus information should be gathered about past and recent/current interests and passions.

Sensory Processing

Autistic adults often experience differences in the way in which they process information in one or more sensory systems (e.g., auditory, visual, tactile, taste, olfactory; e.g., MacLennan et al., 2022; Tavassoli et al., 2014a, 2014b). Under-responsiveness, such as showing limited reaction to pain (e.g., having a broken arm without noticing pain) and over-responsiveness (e.g., perceiving everyday sounds as painful) are common. Autistic people my also have an acute sense of hearing, where they notice everyday sounds that many other people would not. In addition, autistic adults may explore the sensory world in a way that differs from neurotypical adults (e.g., they might smell, stroke, or visually inspect objects in ways that are developmentally uncommon). Both early and current experiences of all sensory systems, and the everyday impact of sensory processing differences, must be explored during the assessment.

The person's perception of interoceptive cues, (i.e., their awareness of internal sensations and bodily states; Fiene & Brownlow, 2015), may also be relevant to an assessment in adulthood. Compared to neurotypical adults, some autistic adults are less aware of feelings of thirst, hunger, temperature, heartbeat, pain, vasomotor activity etc.; see Williams et al., 2023 for a review, and interoception may need to be assessed as part of a comprehensive assessment when there are difficulties with noticing and responding to internal cues.

How to Assess for Autistic Features in Adulthood

As autism is a neurodevelopmental condition, and autistic features are present across the person's life, clinicians need to obtain detailed information on both the *history* and *current* presentations of the core autistic characteristics. This information should be gathered from multiple informants, including lived experience from the adults themselves, and a developmental informant if available (e.g., a parent or other childhood caregiver, or a sibling or relative). Including other informants in the assessment process with the adult's consent is highly recommended wherever possible, as they can often provide insight into the developmental features of autism from childhood. However, their involvement may not always be feasible, and there may be circumstances in which it may be unhelpful to involve a family member. In these cases, the assessment should involve a review of other available relevant childhood information, such as school or health reports, to help establish the persistence and pervasiveness of the person's differences or difficulties over time. Information should also be obtained from multiple sources, such as standardized self- and other-report measures (e.g., checklists or clinical interviews) and direct naturalistic or semi-structured observations, ideally across settings, to understand the current presentation of the core autistic characteristics.

Screening for, and Identification of, Autistic Characteristics

Several self- and informant-report measures can facilitate the screening and initial identification of autistic social communication and behavioral patterns in adults without intellectual impairments and may be used as part of a comprehensive diagnostic assessment (see review by Wigham et al., 2019). These include the Social Responsiveness Scale for Adults (SRS-A; Constantino, 2012); the Social Communication Questionnaire Lifetime and Current forms (SCQ; Rutter et al., 2003a); the Ritvo Autism and Asperger Diagnostic Scale-14 Screen (RAADS; Eriksson et al., 2013); the Autism Spectrum Rating Scales (ASRS; Goldstein & Naglieri, 2009); the Autism Spectrum Quotient (AQ; Baron-Cohen et al., 2001) and the AQ-10 short version (Allison et al., 2012; Ashwood et al., 2016; Lundin et al., 2019); the Broad Autism Phenotype Questionnaire (BAPQ; Hurley et al., 2007), the Comprehensive Autistic Trait Inventory (CATI; English et al., 2021), and others (see Table 1 for a summary of all measures discussed in this chapter). A full description of the psychometric properties of each of these measures is beyond the scope of this chapter, but it is important to note that while abridged versions of the AQ and the RAADS-R have been developed (e.g., AQ-10; Allison et al., 2012; Eriksson et al., 2013), these measures have not been shown to adequately distinguish autism from other psychiatric conditions in adults (Jones et al., 2021; Kenny & Stansfield, 2016). Therefore, use of these tools can facilitate initial identification and referral for a more comprehensive assessment but may not have good predictive validity when used in psychiatric settings.

Two self-report scales developed to measure repetitive behaviors can provide information on patterns of behaviors, speech, interests, and activities. These include the Repetitive Behavior Questionnaire-Third Edition (RBQ-3; Jones et al., 2024) and the Repetitive Behavior Scale-Revised (RBS-R; Lam & Aman, 2007), both of which can be helpful in identifying the range and extent of repetitive or highly focused behaviors and interests.

Self-report measures, such as the Adolescent/Adult Sensory Profile (Brown & Dunn, 2002) or the Sensory Perception Quotient (SPQ; Tavassoli et al., 2014a), can be used to gather information about an individual's sensory interests and sensitivities. In addition, two measures of autistic sensory features have been identified as "appropriate for use with conditions" in a review by Gunderson et al., 2023: the Sensory Reactivity in Autism Spectrum (SR-AS; Elwin et al., 2016) and the Sensory Perception Quotient (Tavassoli et al., 2014a). While the overall scores may not always provide nuanced information about a person's sensory preferences, examining the item-level responses and exploring these further with the adult in a clinical interview can inform the diagnostic assessment.

Interoception could be explored with the Interoception Sensory Questionnaire (ISQ; Fiene et al., 2018; Suzman et al., 2021) or the Multidimensional Assessment of Interoceptive Awareness (MAIA-2; Mehling et al., 2018).

For adults with intellectual disabilities for whom autism may be considered, the SCQ has been found to be helpful in differentiating between individuals who are autistic from those who are not with cut-off score adjustments (Wigham et al., 2019). The Mini Psychiatric Assessment Schedule for Adults with Developmental Disabilities (Mini PAS-ADD; Moss, 2002a) includes a screening specifically for autism and could be used to aid the differential screening process, as can the Diagnostic Behavioral Assessment for Autism-Revised (di-BAS-R; Sappok et al., 2014).

Importantly, elevated scores on screening measures do not always indicate that a person is autistic, and similarly below cut-off scores do not always indicate no autism diagnosis. Furthermore, given the overlap in presentation across several different conditions (Lord & Bishop, 2021), not all traits endorsed in screening tools are specific to autism. Therefore, findings from screening measures *cannot, and should not, ever be used in isolation* to make clinical diagnostic decisions. The results of screening should never replace clinical judgment; they do, however, provide initial insight about an individual's profile of behaviors and can form a basis for further information gathering or referral for comprehensive diagnostic evaluation.

Clinical Interviewing

Clinical interviews should be conducted with the person being assessed as well as with other informants. The clinical interview provides clinicians with an opportunity to gather rich information and specific examples relating to past and current

Table 1 Summary table of assessment measures to consider in the diagnostic assessment of autism in adulthood

Domain of functioning assessed	Measures of autistic features and characteristics[a]
Screening of autistic features and characteristics	Autism Quotient (AQ; Baron-Cohen et al., 2001)[b] and AQ-10 short version (Allison et al., 2012) Autism Screen of the Mini Psychiatric Assessment Schedule for Adults with Developmental Disabilities (Mini PAS-ADD; Moss, 2002a)[c] Autism Spectrum Rating Scales (ASRS; Goldstein and Naglieri, 2009) Broad Autism Phenotype Questionnaire (BAPQ; Hurley et al., 2007)[b] Comprehensive Autistic Trait Inventory (CATI; English et al., 2021) Ritvo Autism and Asperger Diagnostic Scale-14 Screen (RAADS-14; Eriksson et al., 2013)[b] Empathy Quotient (EQ; Baron-Cohen et al., 2005)[b] Social Responsiveness Scale for Adults (SRS-A; Constantino, 2012)[b] Social Communication Questionnaire (SCQ; Rutter et al., 2003a)[b]
Diagnostic interview or observation aid tools for gathering information on autistic features and characteristics	Royal College of Psychiatrists (2001) structured diagnostic interview guide[c] (Berney et al., 2017) Ritvo Autism Asperger Diagnostic Scale-Revised (RITVO-R; Ritvo et al., 2011)[c] Adult Asperger Assessment (AAA; Baron-Cohen et al., 2005)[c] Asperger Syndrome Diagnostic Interview (AUTISM-I; Gillberg et al., 2001)[c] Diagnostic Behavioral Assessment for Autism-Revised (di-BAS-R; Sappok et al., 2014)[c] Diagnostic Autism Spectrum Interview (DASI; Young et al., 2020)

(continued)

Table 1 (continued)

Domain of functioning assessed	Measures of autistic features and characteristics[a]
	Autism Diagnostic Observation Schedule (ADOS-2; Lord et al., 2012)[c] Autism Diagnostic Interview-Revised (ADI-R; Rutter et al., 2003b)[c] Developmental, Dimensional, and Diagnostic Interview (3Di; Skuse et al., 2004)[c] Monteiro Interview Guidelines for Diagnosing the Autism Spectrum (MIGDAS-2; Monteiro & Stegall, 2018)[c] Diagnostic Interview for Social and Communication Disorders-11 (DISCO-11; Wing et al., 2002)[c] Autism Clinical Interview for Adults (ACIA; Wigham et al., 2020)[c]
Repetitive behaviors and sensory features	Adolescent/Adult Sensory Profile (Brown & Dunn, 2002)[b] Interoception Sensory Questionnaire (ISQ; Fiene et al., 2018)[b] Repetitive Behavior Scale-Revised (RBS-R; Lam & Aman, 2007)[b] Repetitive Behavior Questionnaire-Third Edition (RBQ-3; Jones et al., 2024) Sensory Perception Quotient (SPQ; Tavassoli et al., 2014a, 2014b)[b] Sensory Reactivity in Autism Spectrum (SR-AS; Elwin et al., 2016) Multidimensional Assessment of Interoceptive Awareness (MAIA-2; Mehling et al., 2018)
Social functioning and social coping strategies	Camouflaging Autistic Traits-Questionnaire (CAT-Q; Hull et al., 2019) Direct observations, information from adult, caregivers carers, and/or significant others

(continued)

Table 1 (continued)

Domain of functioning assessed	Measures of autistic features and characteristics[a]
Intellectual functioning	Kaufman Brief Intelligence Test—Second Edition Revised (Kaufman & Kaufman, 2022)[c] Leiter International Performance Scale, 3rd Edition (Roid et al., 2013)[c] Peabody Picture Vocabulary Test (PPVT-5; Dunn, 2018)[c] Stanford Binet Scales5th Edition (SB5; Roid, 2003)[c] Test of Non-verbal Intelligence (TONI-4; Brown et al., 2010)[c] Universal Non-verbal Intelligence Test (UNIT2; Bracken & McCallum, 2016)—Standardized to 21:11 years Wechsler Adult Intelligence Scale-Fifth Edition (WAIS-5; Wechsler, 2024)[c] Wechsler Abbreviated Scale of Intelligence-Second Edition (WASI-II; Wechsler, 2011)[c] Wechsler Non-verbal Scale of Ability (WNV; Wechsler & Naglieri, 2006)—Standardized up to 21:11 years
Executive functioning	Digits Forward and Backward subtests from the WAIS-5 Behavior Rating Inventory of Executive Function—Adult Version (BRIEF; Roth et al., 2005)[b] Delis-Kaplan Executive Functions System (D-KEFS; Delis et al., 2001)[c] Wisconsin Card Sorting Test (WCST; Grant & Berg, 1993)[c]
Adaptive functioning and Independence/life skills	Adaptive Behavior Assessment System-3rd Edition (ABAS-3; Harrison & Oakland, 2015)[b] International Classification of Functioning (ICF) Checklist (WHO, 2003) Scales of Independent Behavior-Revised (SIB-R; Bruininks et al., 1996)[b] Vineland Adaptive Behavior Scales-3rd Edition (VABS-3; Sparrow et al., 2016)[b,c] Waisman Activities of Daily Living Scale (Maenner et al., 2013)[b] World Health Organization Disability Assessment Schedule (WHODAS 2.0; Üstün, 2010)

(continued)

Table 1 (continued)

Domain of functioning assessed	Measures of autistic features and characteristics[a]
Cognitive styles and social cognition	Dispositional Adult Hyperfocus Questionnaire (Hupfeld et al., 2024) Edinburgh Social Cognitive Test (Baksh et al., 2020) Monotropism Questionnaire (Garau et al., 2023)
Language/verbal skills and communication	Clinical Evaluation of Language Fundamentals (CELF-5; Wiig et al., 2013)[c] Communication Checklist-Adult (CC-A; Whitehouse & Bishop, 2009) Informal or structured observations of communication/information from caregivers/carers Semi-structured or naturalistic observations of social communication in a range of social contexts (ADOS-2; Lord et al., 2012)[c]
Behavior	Achenbach System of Empirically Based Assessment (ASEBA; Achenback & Rescorla, 2003) for adults[b] Aberrant Behavior Checklist (ABC; Aman & Singh, 1986)[b] Developmental Behaviour Checklist-Adult version (DBC-A; Mohr et al., 2004)[b] Functional Analysis assessment approaches

(continued)

Table 1 (continued)

Domain of functioning assessed	Measures of autistic features and characteristics[a]
Mental health and wellbeing	Autism Spectrum Disorders-Comorbidity for Adults (ASD-CA; LoVullo & Matson, 2009)[b] Anxiety Scale for Autism-Adults (ASA-A; Rodgers et al., 2020) Beck Depression Inventory II (BDI-II; Williams et al., 2021)[b] Diagnostic Assessment for the Severely Handicapped-II (DASH-II; Matson, 1995)[c] Diagnostic Criteria for use with adults with Learning Disabilities (DC-LD; Royal College of Psychiatrists, 2001)[c] Diagnostic Manual Intellectual Disability (DM-ID; Fletcher et al., 2007)[c] Fear survey for Adults with Mental Retardation (Ramirez & Lukenbill, 2007)[b] Mood, Interest and Pleasure Questionnaire (MIPQ; Ross & Oliver, 2003)[b] Patient Health Questionnaire (PHQ-9; Arnold et al., 2020)[b] PERMA Profiler; Positive emotion, Engagement, Relationships, Meaning and Accomplishment wellbeing measure (Grosvenor et al., 2023) Psychiatric Assessment Schedule for Adults with Developmental Disabilities Checklist (PAS-ADD; Moss, 2002b)[c] and Mini-PAS-ADD (Moss, 2002a) Psychopathology in Autism Checklist (PAC; Helverschou et al., 2009) Self-report Depression Questionnaire (SRDQ; Reynolds & Baker, 1988)[b] Structured Clinical Interview of DSM Disorders Clinician Version (SCID-5-CV; First et al., 2016)[c] Suicidal Behaviours Questionnaire-Autism Spectrum Conditions (SBQ-ASC; Cassidy et al., 2021) Zung Self-Rating Anxiety Scale (Lindsay & Michie, 1988)[b]
Planning for transitions or employment/career planning	Adolescent and Adult Psychoeducational Profile (Mesibov et al., 1989) Community based Skills Assessment (CAS; Autism Speaks, 2014) TEACCH Transition assessment profile-second edition (TTAP; Mesibov et al., 1989) Transition Planning Inventory-Third Edition (TPI-3; Patton & Clark, 2021)

[a] Please note this list of measures is not exhaustive; [b] Self- or informant-report; [c] Clinician administered

Note Tests and measures should be selected considering the person's age, developmental age and verbal abilities, as well as the psychometric measurement properties

autistic social communication and interaction behaviors, interests, and activities. A detailed and comprehensive developmental history, exploring social and communication development and social interactions in childhood and adolescence, should be gathered to the extent that this is possible. The Autism Diagnostic Interview-Revised (ADI-R; Rutter, Le Couteur & Lord, 2003b) can be used to take a comprehensive developmental history of autistic characteristics. Despite generally strong psychometric properties, the agreement between the ADI-R and clinical diagnosis was poor in a study with autistic adults without intellectual disability (Fusar-Poli et al., 2017). The focus of the ADI-R is on the period between the ages of 4 and 5 years, which can make it difficult for informants to provide information due to the time elapsed between childhood and the adult assessment (Lai & Baron-Cohen, 2015).

Several other semi-structured diagnostic measures can be employed with cognitively able adults as part of a comprehensive diagnostic assessment. The Royal College of Psychiatrists in the UK (Berney et al., 2017) has produced a semi-structured diagnostic interview guide for the assessment of adults. The Diagnostic Interview for Social and Communication Disorders (DISCO-11; Wing et al., 2002) may be considered for more complex diagnostic assessments (NICE, 2021). Other structured or semi-structured diagnostic interviews include the Developmental, Dimensional, and Diagnostic Interview-Adult (3Di; Mandy et al., 2018; Skuse et al., 2004), the Adult Asperger Assessment (AAA; Baron-Cohen et al., 2005), and the Asperger Syndrome Diagnostic Interview (ASDI; Gillberg et al., 2001). More recently developed diagnostic tools may also be considered, such as the Autism Clinical Interview for Adults (ACIA; Wigham et al., 2020), the Monteiro Interview Guidelines for Diagnosing the Autism Spectrum (MIGDAS-2; Monteiro & Stegall, 2018) or the Diagnostic Autism Spectrum Interview (DASI; Young et al., 2020); however, there is currently only little or emerging research evidence supporting the predictive diagnostic validity of these tools (see Wigham et al., 2020).

Some autistic individuals may have developed compensating social strategies to mask (camouflage) their core social and behavioral autistic features, which may not be directly observable during a relatively brief assessment. Although such social strategies are not unique to autism, it may be useful to enquire, when clinically relevant, about the extent to which the adults may have learned to cope with social differences or difficulties through masking/camouflaging, and how they do so, to inform and corroborate the interviewing and observational information gathered. Questionnaires such as the Camouflaging Autistic Traits Questionnaire (CAT-Q; Hull et al., 2019; see Hannon et al., 2023 for a review) could be used to facilitate discussion about camouflaging. Completing the CAT-Q and probing with follow-up questions may provide useful psychosocial information on how, why, and when the autistic adults developed these strategies. However, because the CAT-Q is *not* an autism screening tool, and as not all autistic adults camouflage and many neurotypical adults also camouflage (see Ai et al., 2022, 2024a, 2024b; Hobson & Lee, 2023), the CAT-Q *should not* be used as a screening tool for autistic traits, but as a complementary tool to obtain insight into a person's efforts to hide autistic traits when clinically relevant.

Direct Observations

Observing the adult's social communication, interaction, and conversation skills during informal and semi-structured interactions with the clinician, family members, or others (e.g., in the waiting room, at reception) is a useful way to observe an adult's social and communication patterns, differences, and difficulties as part of a comprehensive assessment.

Some social communication and interaction patterns may be observed during the administration of the Autism Diagnostic Observation Schedule assessment (ADOS-2; Lord et al., 2012), a semi-structured observation specifically developed to assess social communication, social interaction, and behavior for people suspected of being autistic. The ADOS-2 is a reliable and valid tool but should never be used in isolation to inform diagnostic decision-making. Instead, the ADOS-2 should be used together with information obtained from the person and informants using the ADI-R or another clinical interview.

The diagnostic tools described in this section have been developed to *aid* the diagnostic process, not to replace clinical decision making (see Bishop & Lord, 2023). Clinicians should rely on their clinical judgement to determine which of the standardized measures of autistic traits should be included in the comprehensive diagnostic evaluation, based on the hypothesized differential diagnoses, age range, psychometric properties, and predictive diagnostic validity of the tools when considering their use.

Intellectual Functioning, Executive Functioning, and Cognitive Styles

In addition to assessing social, communication, and behavioral autistic characteristics, assessment of autistic or possibly autistic adults may also include comprehensive assessment of a range of domains of functioning and development, including intellectual functioning, cognitive styles and executive functioning when indicated.

What to Assess

Intellectual Functioning

When assessing for autism, a person's social communication and behavioral patterns should be considered with reference to their intellectual ability. In addition, an assessment of intellectual functioning can provide valuable information about adults' relative cognitive strengths and challenges, including in individuals who have successfully completed mainstream education, college, or university. As autistic individuals often have uneven cognitive profiles (Wilson, 2024), variability between different cognitive domains may help to explain strengths and challenges in everyday life. Understanding a person's cognitive profile can also inform the differential diagnosis of autism from ID, as many individuals with ID and autism have more uneven profiles of intellectual functioning than those with ID only, who often present with uniform intellectual profiles (see Wolf & Ventola, 2014).

Executive Functioning

While findings regarding the executive function (i.e., problem-solving, planning, organizing, response inhibition and initiation, cognitive flexibility, decision-making, and working memory) of autistic people compared to general population norms are mixed (Abbott et al., 2018; Davids et al., 2016; Lehnhardt et al., 2016; Nyden et al., 2010), the extant evidence indicates that many autistic adults experience executive functioning difficulties (Baldwin & Costley, 2016; Davids et al., 2016; see review by St. John et al. 2022), which can have a significant functional impact on everyday tasks at home, work, or in the community. Executive functioning strengths of autistic adults, such as excellent attention to detail or working memory, are currently less well understood (St John et al., 2022). Although autistic adults may perform well in primary memory tests, difficulties have been identified for some with other tasks that involve visual and auditory information and working memory (Nyden et al., 2010; St John et al., 2022). Assessing and describing the adult's profile of strengths and difficulties in executive functioning can help to identify daily functioning needs and the individualized supports required for those who present with executive function difficulties.

Cognitive Styles

Many of the core autistic features are related to underlying differences in the cognitive style of autistic people compared to neurotypical people. For example, difficulties with sharing emotions may be associated with alexithymia (difficulties in identifying and expressing emotions; see Kinnaird et al., 2019; Josyfon et al., 2023), and autistic social communication preferences may be related to differences in emotion and social perception (e.g., Sasson et al., 2020; Velikonja et al., 2019).

In addition, many autistic people have a monotropic disposition: autistic people tend to be monotropic in how their attention is utilized (single- or hyper-focused), whereas neurotypical people are often polytropic (dividing attention to several different things as a natural part of who they are, and moving through interests or shifting attention more easily; Dwyer et al., 2024; Lawson, 2011; Murray et al., 2005; Rapaport et al., 2024). A monotropic disposition can be both a strength and a challenge: it can positively impact flow states (Rapaport et al., 2024) and contribute to excellent hyper-focus, but it may also be associated with rumination, difficulties with or an inability to stop an action, thought, or activity, or with inertia (a prolonged mental state of being “stuck” resulting in physical inability to engage in activities a person may wish to do), which can be debilitating (Dwyer et al., 2024; Rapaport et al., 2024; Welch et al., 2020). Monotropism may explain some of the difficulties in social interactions between autistic and neurotypical people, due to autistic people’s difficulties noticing or shifting flexibly in response to others’ interests and focus. It could also explain how some executive functioning difficulties, such as forward thinking and shifting, may be difficult when attention is dominated by an existing area of focus. Therefore, recognizing and exploring differing cognitive styles can inform a comprehensive assessment for the purpose of diagnosis, as well as a person’s self-understanding and/or for the identification of cognitive strengths, needs, and accommodations.

How to Assess

Intellectual Functioning

A comprehensive assessment of intellectual abilities can be conducted using well-established measures that have been standardized for use with adults. These include the Wechsler Adult Intelligence Scale—Fifth Edition (WAIS-5; Wechsler, 2024), the briefer Wechsler Abbreviated Scale of Intelligence-Second Edition (WASI-II; Wechsler, 2011), the Stanford-Binet Scales-Fifth Edition (SB-5; Roid, 2003) or the Kaufman Brief Intelligence Test-Second Edition Revised (Kaufman & Kaufman, 2022).

While the Stanford-Binet and Wechsler scales can be used to assess cognitive skills in those with mild or moderate ID, they may not be suited to the assessment of individuals with severe or profound ID and/or very limited or no speech. In such cases, the Leiter International Performance Scale (Third Edition; Leiter-3; Roid et al., 2013), the Test of Non-verbal Intelligence (TONI-4; Brown et al., 2010) or the Wechsler Non-verbal Scale of Ability (WNV; Wechsler & Naglieri, 2006) could be considered. However, many of these measures have not been validated for use in autistic people, so clinicians need to use their clinical judgement in test selection and interpretation.

Executive Functioning

A range of measures can be used to assess a person’s executive functioning. These include the Delis-Kaplan Executive Functions System (D-KEFS; Delis et al., 2001), the Wisconsin Card Sorting Test (WCST; Grant & Berg, 1993), and the Behavior Rating Inventory of Executive Function-Adult questionnaire, which includes self-report and informant versions (BRIEF-A; Roth et al., 2005). Working memory can be assessed using the Digit Span subtests from the WAIS.

Other Cognitive Styles

Social cognition, emotional perception, and other social cognitive strengths, differences, and needs may be assessed, when indicated, through measures such as the Edinburgh Social Cognition Test (ESCoT; Baksh et al., 2020) or other social cognitive assessments (see Morrison et al., 2019 for a review). The recently developed Monotropism Questionnaire has shown preliminary good reliability and validity (Garau et al., 2023). The Dispositional Adult Hyperfocus Questionnaire (Hupfeld et al., 2024), which has recently been developed to measure hyper-focus, has promising psychometric properties in a general population sample, but has not been yet evaluated with autistic or ADHD adults.

Assessment of Independence and Life Skills

Autistic adults may often have adaptive skills (i.e., abilities to independently care for themselves, communicate or relate to others in everyday life) that are lower than expected for their intellectual functioning. This discrepancy may be more pronounced for autistic people without co-occurring intellectual disabilities than for those with intellectual disability and may be larger with increasing age (Alvares et al., 2020; Tillman & Prazak, 2019). Adaptive functioning difficulties can contribute to adjustment or emotional difficulties or to the breakdown of education, work, living arrangements, or relationships, and may affect parenting. Thus, it is helpful to assess the adaptive skills of autistic adults, especially those who present with or report difficulties living independently.

What to Assess

The International Classification of Functioning, Disability, and Health (ICF; WHO, 2001) is a universally accepted framework for describing an individual's functioning and disability (WHO, 2003) and includes four broad categories of functioning: (1) body functions and body structures (i.e., physiological and psychological functions and structures of body systems, such as pain, sleep, mental functions); (2) activities (e.g., learning, communication, mobility, eating, drinking) and participation (e.g., playing sports, working, interacting with peers, etc.); (3) environmental factors (e.g., physical, social, and attitudinal environmental factors influencing a person's life, including social supports and attitudes, adaptations, assisting technologies, etc.) and (4) personal factors (e.g., interests, motivations, priorities, and goals; see Schiariti et al., 2018), all of which can be explored as part of an assessment of functioning. The ICF Core Sets for Autism have been specifically developed to standardize the description of functional abilities, health, and disabilities of autistic people across multiple life dimensions (Bolte et al., 2014; Schiariti et al., 2018; de Schipper et al., 2015).

How to Assess Independence and Life Skills

Standardized assessments of adaptive behavior skills for people at all levels of intellectual ability, including those with ID, include the Vineland Adaptive Behavior Scales-Third Edition (VABS-3; Sparrow et al., 2016), the Adaptive Behavior Assessment System-3rd Edition (ABAS-3; Harrison & Oakland, 2015), the Scales of Independent Behavior-Revised (SIB-R; Bruininks et al., 1996), and the Waisman Activities of Daily Living Scale (Maenner et al., 2013).

The adult themselves and/or their caregivers can act as informants and the measures can be administered using either a structured interview or a checklist format. The World Health Organization Disability Assessment Schedule (WHODAS 2.0; Üstün, 2010) is a standardized measure that can be applied across sociocultural contexts and can be used along with the ICF Checklist (WHO, 2003), a practical tool that elicits information about an individual's functioning and disability.

Assessment of Language and Communication

What to Assess

It is important to assess communication strengths and difficulties, to identify whether the person's communication preferences can be explained by expressive (i.e., a person's ability to express themselves using words, symbols or signs) and/or receptive (i.e., a person's ability to understand words and sentences) language difficulties, and to address the DSM-5-TR specifier "with or without accompanying language impairment" (DSM-5-TR, 2022; see Rosen et al., 2021). A language assessment should be included as part of an autism diagnostic assessment when there is a clear history of early language delay or current indicators of possible language difficulties (e.g., word-finding difficulties or frequent grammatical errors; using short and simple sentences; having a smaller or less sophisticated vocabulary than expected for age, etc.). A language assessment also allows for the consideration of differential diagnoses such as developmental language disorder (DLD), an under-recognized neurodevelopmental condition often associated with learning and reading difficulties, and poor mental and physical health and vocational outcomes (Nudel et al., 2023).

A comprehensive language assessment often covers six language domains: syntax (grammar), semantics (vocabulary), phonology (speech sounds), morphology (word endings indicating grammatical relationships, e.g., the past tense marker -ed), discourse (narrative skills; conversation), and pragmatic language (the ways language is used in daily social interactions with others, including adapting language to context or social partner, or following "unspoken" conversation rules, inferencing, and figurative language), as difficulties in any one of these areas may indicate persistent language difficulties.

In autistic adults who speak, even when vocabulary and grammar are consistent with the adult's developmental level and intellectual functioning, there may be qualitative differences and/or difficulties in conversational skills (such as limited small talk or more matter-of-fact conversations, quality and flow of conversations, focus, and reciprocity of two-way interaction during conversation). Other differences may lie in semantic and pragmatic language (i.e., differences or difficulties initiating, organizing, selecting, and interpreting social communication through language), and in other language domains, such as in prosody (the quality and intonation of speech, which may be atypical, for example appearing somewhat monotonous or limited in variation).

How to Assess Language and Communication

Few standardized language assessments have norms that extend into the adult years. The informant-completed Communication Checklist-Adult (CC-A; Whitehouse & Bishop, 2009) can be used to screen for structural and pragmatic language difficulties in adults. The Peabody Picture Vocabulary Test (PPVT-5; Dunn, 2018) and the Expressive Vocabulary Test-3rd Edition (EVT-3; Williams, 2018), which assess single word receptive and expressive vocabulary respectively, have norms up to the age of 90 years. The fifth edition of the Clinical Evaluation of Language Fundamentals (CELF-5; Wiig et al., 2013) has an extended age range up to 22 years and may be useful with young adults. A person's social communication skills, and discrepancies between their vocabulary and pragmatic language ability, can be observed and assessed during naturalistic social contexts (Paul et al., 2014; American Speech-Language-Hearing Association, 2006). Information can also be gathered from the individual's communication partners and by "staging" communication contexts during the assessment, which may allow a person to demonstrate their communication strengths and needs (Wetherby et al., 2006).

Understanding and Assessing Behaviors that Challenge

Many autistic individuals may have difficulties regulating their own emotions (Cai et al., 2018; Conner et al., 2021). They may express emotional distress through behavioral responses that are challenging for others to understand and support, such as irritability, marked and persistent seemingly uncooperative behaviors, aggression, disruptive, or destructive behaviors towards the self, objects, or others (often referred to as meltdowns, outbursts or self-injurious behaviors); as well as freeze-like responses, characterized by withdrawal and retreat to inactivity or not speaking (described by autistic people as shutdowns; see National Autistic Society (NAS), 2020; Ambitious about Autism, 2022; Lewis & Stevens, 2023). Some of the co-occurring behavioral difficulties in autistic people have been described as Pathological Demand Avoidance (PDA), also referred to as Persistent Drive for Autonomy, which has been considered in recent years as a profile associated with autism (NAS, 2024; Kildahl et al., 2021; Lawson, 2020; O'Nions et al., 2013). PDA is characterized by persistent and marked resistance to or avoidance of everyday demands (see PDA society, n.d.), which can look like oppositional behavior. In PDA, demand avoidance is closely related to high levels of stress, anxiety and fear around uncertainty and the need for some control and autonomy, rather than to being defiant, oppositional, or spiteful, as seen in individuals with oppositional or conduct problem diagnoses (see Andrews & Istanffy, 2012).

Behaviors that challenge typically occur in the context of specific stimuli or contextual factors that result from interactions between individual, environmental and social factors, and reflect intense and distressed responses to overwhelming environmental, social, and/or sensory situations. Autistic people have identified various factors that contribute to these experiences and behaviors, such as high levels of distress, social demands, frustration, challenges with communication, small or major changes and transitions, overwhelming everyday life demands, aversive sensory overload and others (Lewis & Stevens, 2023; Welch et al., 2020). As these behaviors are often communicative and serve a purpose, it is important to investigate and understand the underlying function(s) of the behaviors and the factors contributing to their onset and maintenance before developing individualized and person-centered support plans that aim to change the contextual factors in which these occur.

How to Assess Behavior

Describing and understanding distressed behaviors is of paramount importance because of their significant impact on quality of life. A holistic, person-centered, functional assessment, and analysis can help identify and address the function(s) of specific behaviors. As part of a functional assessment, clinicians should explore all plausible explanations for the behavior, including anxiety, medical or psychiatric conditions, and individual and environmental factors; and conduct a functional analysis of individual and environmental triggering or maintaining factors to guide the development of positive behavior support plans (NICE, 2021; Goodall et al., 2023; see also Alim et al., 2014).

Information can be gathered from a range of environments and informants, including wherever possible the adult themselves, on: (i) factors that appear to be setting events or triggers (e.g., pain or illness, sensory issues, social or other demands, emotional difficulties, communication differences, anxiety, the care environment, etc.), and (ii) function, consequences and impact of the behavior (i.e., the functions served, helpful, and unhelpful ways of others' responding to the behavior, etc.), including risk assessment. The factors that may be evoking a specific behavior and the needs that person is trying to meet through the behavior can be identified by analyzing patterns and trends in behavior occurrence.

In many cases, a functional assessment is conducted through clinical interviews and direct observations. Although their content and standardization data are not always relevant for autistic individuals, the self- and informant-report versions of Achenbach System of Empirically Based Assessment checklists (ASEBA; Achenbach et al., 2003), which includes self-report and caregiver/informant-completed checklists for adults, could be used as part of an assessment of a person's behavior. For adults with ID, measures that mostly rely on information obtained from significant others and/or direct behavioral observations may be employed in the assessment. The Developmental Behavior Checklist-Adult version (DBC-A; Mohr et al., 2004) is a comprehensive and well-established screening measure of behaviors for individuals with ID and developmental disabilities. The Aberrant Behavior Checklist (ABC; Aman & Singh, 1986) is also a reliable and valid caregiver or clinician completed checklist measuring a range of behaviors in autistic people with ID (Halvorsen et al., 2024).

Understanding and Assessing Mental Health and Wellbeing

Compared to neurotypical individuals, autistic adults are over-represented in mental health settings and are diagnosed with significantly more mental health conditions (most commonly anxiety, depression, OCD, trauma-related presentations, eating or impulse control-related concerns; APA, 2022; Curnow et al., 2023; Hollocks et al., 2019; Lai et al., 2019; Lugnegard et al., 2011; Tromans et al., 2018; White et al., 2020). Similarities between observable autistic features and features of other neurodevelopmental and mental health conditions may contribute to diagnostic overshadowing and, consequently, to both missed and misdiagnoses (Au-Yeung et al., 2019; Bishop & Lord, 2023; Kentrou et al., 2024; Stavropoulos et al., 2022). Examples of common areas of diagnostic overshadowing between autistic and mental health presentations include: limited social initiations or social withdrawal, which could be presenting features in autism as well as social anxiety or depression; limited range of facial expressions and expression of affect, which could be an autistic characteristic and also a common presentation of low mood; strong preference for routines and rituals in autism which may resemble OCD compulsive behaviors, and others (Hofvander et al., 2009). Therefore, clinicians conducting comprehensive adult assessments should seek to identify and understand the person's emotional difficulties, including low mood and anxiety (Goodall et al., 2023; NICE, 2021) to ensure that autism is not missed; and that when present, co-occurring mental health conditions are also accurately identified in autistic people.

The outcome of a mental health assessment for an autistic adult should be an autism-informed biopsychosocial formulation, which is crucial to ensure that the person's mental health is understood in the context of neurocognitive, sensory, interpersonal, environmental, and psychosocial influences. The formulation should also capture the person's strengths, skills, preferences, resources, and supports (see Blainey et al., 2019; Cherewick & Matergia, 2024; Gaus, 2011).

What to Assess

When adults suspected of being autistic present to services with mental health concerns, the clinicians should obtain detailed information about the client's developmental, mental health, and psychosocial history to explore the extent to which persistent social, communication, and behavioral differences and difficulties associated with autism were present *before* the onset of the mental health concerns. The assessment should also include a careful exploration of individual biological, neurocognitive, and psychosocial adversity factors that may trigger or exacerbate mental health difficulties. These include obtaining information on family history of mental health difficulties and:

- neurocognitive factors that may increase one's likelihood of emotional distress (such as alexithymia, inflexible thinking styles, high need for predictability, high sensory sensitivities and overload etc.);
- psychological and sociocultural determinants of distress and wellbeing (including distressing family, interpersonal and/or care or support systems, recent changes or breakdown of family, employment or living arrangements, experiences of teasing, bullying, victimization, stigma, social isolation, abuse, coercion or neglect, all of which autistic people are disproportionately more likely to experience compared to neurotypical adults; e.g., Gibbs & Pellicano, 2022; Griffiths et al., 2019) and
- environmental and physical factors (e.g., illness, sleep, diet, medical condition, sensory or social overload, or under stimulation etc.).

The clinician then needs to carefully try to distinguish core autism-related features from psychiatric presentations for accurate differential diagnosis (see Stavropoulos & McPartland, 2022). Although some observable features are similar in autism and other mental health conditions, careful differential diagnosis requires the assessment of:

- the *onset* of mental health difficulties, i.e., social, communication, and behavioral patterns consistent with autism must be present during the person's childhood and adolescence, and prior to the onset of mental health concerns.
- the *form* and *focus* of observable behaviors: for example, common repetitive OCD behaviors often center around cleaning, checking, washing, hoarding, or ordering, whereas repetitive behaviors in autism often relate to intense interests and passions, body movements, or repetitive speech.
- the *function* of observed or reported features: for example, repetitive behaviors in OCD are typically driven by an underlying worry that something awful will happen

and cause distress (are ego-dystonic), whereas in autism repetitive behaviors are often driven by interests, need for repetition and a way to feel calmer and less distressed (are ego-syntonic; see Chew et al., 2021; McNeel et al., 2022; Ruzzano et al., 2015).

As part of the differential diagnostic process, clinicians should also gather information about features of autism that are specific to autism, and uncommon in other conditions. For example, intense and highly focused passions and interests are characteristic of autism and not a diagnostic feature of depression, ADHD, or other conditions. The assessment of mental health in autistic individuals with ID needs to be modified to consider intellectual disability, communication difficulties, and any additional impairments (Alim et al., 2014). As with any neurotypical individual, it is important to assess predisposing, precipitating, maintaining, and protective psychosocial and environmental factors in autistic adults to help develop a formulation and understanding of their situation (i.e., changes in residential setting or career; illness in the family, or in a supportive sibling, etc.), and how to move forward with supports beyond simply addressing individual or organic factors (see Deb et al., 2022; Magiati et al., 2014).

How to Assess Mental Health and Wellbeing

Identifying co-occurring mental health conditions in autistic people or differentiating between conditions cannot be achieved with quick or rigid use of screening tools. Currently, there is some, but limited, evidence of the reliability, validity, and clinical utility of some mental health screening tools with autistic adults. For example, the Patient Health Questionnaire (PHQ-9) (Arnold et al., 2020) and Beck Depression Inventory II (BDI-II; Williams et al., 2021) have been found to be useful when used with autistic adults. However, existing measures largely developed for the general population may have limitations when used with autistic or possibly autistic individuals (for example, use of language may be confusing, ambiguous or deficit-focused and autism-specific aspects of the construct being assessed are lacking; Nicolaidis et al., 2020).

The measures most commonly used for the assessment of mental health in autistic adults include the Psychopathology in Autism Checklist (PAC; Helverschou et al., 2009) and the Autism Spectrum Disorders-Comorbidity for Adults (ASD-CA; Matson & Boisjoli, 2008) (see Halvorsen et al., 2024, for a systematic review). Few measures of self-harm and suicidal ideation in autistic adults currently show potential for clinical use (Hedley et al., 2023; Newell et al., 2024).

Many autistic adults are insightful about, and can describe their mental health experiences, so self-reporting can be an important aspect of the information gathering process, with the caveat that some autistic adults may find it difficult to self-report due to verbal or cognitive impairments. Several self-report measures of mental health concerns, such as the Anxiety Scale for Autism-Adults (ASA-A; Rodgers et al.,

2020), the Suicidal Behaviors Questionnaire-Autism Spectrum Conditions (SBQ-ASC; Cassidy et al., 2021), and the PERMA Profiler (Positive emotion, Engagement, Relationships, Meaning, and Accomplishment) wellbeing measure (Grosvenor et al., 2023) have been developed with and for autistic adults (mostly with mild or no intellectual impairments). In addition to self-report, others who know the adult well and who can corroborate on the person's wellbeing and any recent changes can also contribute helpful information.

The Structured Clinical Interview for DSM Disorders Clinician Version (SCID-5-CV; First et al., 2016) can help gather detailed information about a range of psychiatric conditions from the adult or their caregiver/significant others, which may aid the differential diagnostic process. Clinicians may need to modify the interview by providing concrete definitions or explanations of items or by including visual aids and probing for both normative and autism-related mental health experiences (Kerns et al., 2014; Magiati et al., 2017; White et al. 2020; see Patel et al., 2023 for systematic review of measures in adults with intellectual disabilities).

The Psychiatric Assessment Schedule for Adults with Developmental Disabilities checklist (PAS-ADD; Moss, 2002b), the Autism Spectrum Disorders-Comorbidity for Adults (ASD-CA; LoVullo & Matson, 2009), and the informant rated Diagnostic Assessment for the Severely Handicapped-II for individuals with severe and profound ID (DASH-II; Matson, 1995) can aid the assessment of co-occurring mental health difficulties in autistic people with an ID. Assessment of psychiatric comorbidity in autistic individuals with ID may also be facilitated by standardized instruments such as the Diagnostic Criteria for use with adults with Learning Disabilities by the Royal College of Psychiatrists (DC-LD; Royal College of Psychiatrists, 2001) and the Diagnostic Manual-Intellectual Disability (DM-ID; Fletcher et al., 2007). A small number of self-report measures may be helpful with those who can respond to simplified items administered verbally, including the Self-Report Depression Questionnaire (SRDQ; Reynolds & Baker, 1988), the Mood, Interest, and Pleasure Questionnaire (MIPQ; Ross & Oliver, 2003), the Zung Self-Rating Anxiety Scale (Lindsay & Michie, 1988) and the Fear Survey for Adults with Mental Retardation (Ramirez & Lukenbill, 2007; see Kooijmans et al., 2022 for a review of adaptations of self-report measures).

Given the limitations of the available standardized assessments, one of the most clinically useful ways to identify the potential onset or worsening of a psychiatric or behavioral concern in autistic adults with and without ID is to determine whether there has been a sudden or gradual *change* in behavior or functioning compared to the person's usual baseline (Edwards et al., 2023). A *shift* in behavior (i.e., becoming more socially withdrawn or showing increased irritability) or the onset of *new* behaviors compared to their earlier functioning may suggest the onset of a co-occurring physical, behavioral, or mental health issues requiring further assessment.

For all clients with a presentation of depression, severely debilitating anxiety, self-harm or suicidal ideation, irrespective of their intellectual or verbal skills, a careful risk assessment and management plan needs to be developed and regularly reviewed (Goodall et al., 2023). This risk assessment should also consider any past, current, or likely future contact with the criminal justice system (Cheely et al., 2012; see Woodbury-Smith, 2014), as well as risks related to social vulnerability (e.g., deception or exploitation), breakdown of education, employment, or accommodation services.

Discussing Assessment Findings and Providing Feedback

What to Discuss

At least one feedback session should be planned as soon as possible after the assessment to discuss the assessment and its findings with the client (and their loved ones, if the adult wishes to involve others in the feedback meeting).

During the feedback appointment, the clinicians need to summarize the reasons for and aims of the assessment, and describe the assessments that were conducted and tools or approaches that were used. The diagnostic criteria used, and the diagnostic outcome(s) need to be clearly communicated to the client. Regardless of the diagnostic outcome, the clinician needs to explain the evidence that was gathered and how it was used to address the diagnostic criteria. Clinicians also need to share their clinical decision-making process with the client and the reasons for which they think the person meets or does not meet diagnostic criteria for autism. Any co-occurring or alternative diagnosis should also be discussed during the feedback appointment.

In some instances, the clinicians may not have arrived at any diagnostic decision. In this case, the outcome should also be discussed sensitively and clearly with the adult, and the clinician and person should create a collaborative plan for what needs to happen next (e.g., initiate a referral to specialist diagnostic service or other actions). In addition to discussions about the diagnostic decision, the clinician should discuss how the assessment findings can help the client and others better understand and make sense of their strengths and needs. Recommendations to be discussed with the adult may include accommodations and reasonable adjustments, supports and services, funding and financial supports possibly available, or any further assessments required to meet the adult's needs going forward.

For adults who are diagnosed as autistic following the assessment, it will be important to share information and resources about autism, specifically about autism in adulthood. Resources developed by or with autistic adults explaining autism and autistic adults' experiences are likely to be very helpful for newly diagnosed adults in navigating their new diagnosis and identity, as are links to autistic and/or autism organizations in the person's local area and/or country. Post-diagnostic supports for adults are currently limited, but emerging, and have been identified as very important by autistic adults (see Crane et al., 2021; Crowson et al., 2022; Wigham et al., 2023).

How to Feedback

The feedback session may elicit strong emotions from clients, both positive (e.g., hope, relief, compassion) and distressing (shock, anger, disappointment). For this reason, the style of oral and written communication needs to be clear, respectful, compassionate, and affirming. Regardless of the outcome, the feedback needs to be balanced, hopeful, and strength-focused and to include a discussion of the person's strengths, skills, talents, abilities and resources, alongside difficulties and identified needs.

Clinicians need to be honest while also avoiding overly technical, medical, or deficit-focused language (Pattison et al., 2022). If a diagnosis of autism is given, the clinicians should explore autism from a neuro-affirming perspective, as a neurological difference influencing the ways in which autistic people experience, process, and make sense of the world and other people, which comes with both strengths and challenges (Goodall et al., 2023). If a diagnosis of autism is not given, the clinicians should clearly and honestly explain the reasons they did not arrive at an autism diagnosis and check-in regarding the impact this may have on the adult, especially if the person self-identifies as autistic and may be feeling confused or frustrated as to why an autism diagnosis was not concluded.

Time and space should be set aside to discuss the recommendations clinicians believe should be made based on the assessment findings. The professionals involved in the feedback session need to provide opportunities for collaborative check-ins with the client and for summaries, and to create space for questions, reflections, and emotional processing. Some people may benefit from an additional follow-up session to consolidate the feedback findings and to discuss the client's questions (see Pattison et al., 2022).

Assessment for Life: Ongoing Assessment for Adults and Older Adults Who Are Autistic

Many, although not all, autistic adults will need varying levels of support, services, and resources at different points in their lives. This will largely depend on their skills, strengths, and needs and their social and environmental resources and stressors. As a result, assessment is often an ongoing process to aid understanding and ensure individualized supports are implemented and accessible.

Assessment as Part of Planning for Transitions

Many autistic adults share similar hopes and expectations for their lives as neurotypical individuals but may require others to understand that additional supports and accommodations, especially during stressful or transition periods, may be required to achieve their life goals. Particularly important time-points for an individualized assessment may be prior to major life transitions (e.g., from school to post-school education or vocational training; from living with family members to living with peers, alone or in residential settings; before and during the adult's first employment; when changing jobs; when anticipating a significant change in social support, such as ill health or aging of caregivers). Structured assessments, such as the TEACCH Transition assessment Profile-Second edition (TTAP; Mesibov et al., 1989) and the Transition Planning Inventory-Third Edition (TPI-3; Patton & Clark, 2021) may enable a systematic evaluation of skills at home, education, and/or work. A comprehensive Community based Skills Assessment (CSA; Autism Speaks, 2014) may also help facilitate a personalized plan and successful transition.

Assessment for Employment and Independent Living

Fewer autistic people of working age are in employment than other disabled people and people without disabilities (Buckland, 2024), and many of those who are working are underemployed (Davies et al., 2024a, 2024b). Therefore, assessment for employability and employment purposes may be particularly helpful for many autistic adults, and information should be gathered about the individual, family/social, work/organizational and broader systemic barriers, or facilitators to employment (Henninger & Lounds-Taylor, 2012). Facilitators can include a range of individual-related factors (for example, knowledge, skills, and talents relating to specific jobs, cognitive, and verbal communication skills, problem-solving, advocacy, and ability to seek help), environment- or context-specific factors (e.g., supportive families, coworkers, and friends, provisions of accommodations), and other organizational and systemic employment factors (e.g., training, coaching, supports, a good person-job match, workplace policies; see Black et al., 2020; Harmuth et al., 2018).

While traditional career planning assessments can be used to understand the autistic adult's strengths and needs in different employment settings, there is currently limited evidence of strong psychometric properties when these are used with autistic individuals (Murray et al., 2016). For autistic adults with ID, the Adolescent and Adult Psychoeducational Profile (Mesibov et al., 1989) assesses vocational, adaptive, leisure, communication, and interpersonal skills and can provide helpful recommendations for future planning for education, vocational training, or living arrangements.

Although many autistic people live on their own, with peers, partners or their own families, many also continue to live with their families well into their adult years. Assessment well before caregivers are no longer able or available to contribute, ideally in a proactive and planned way, can support decision-making regarding optimal living arrangements and independence centered on the adult's preferences and needs.

Assessment of Ageing Autistic Adults

While research relating to autism in older age has increased in recent years, little is currently known about the process of aging, cognitive decline and dementias, and even less about the care and support needs of autistic older adults (Roestorf et al., 2019, 2022). Physical and cognitive health, functioning and decline, daily living and independence, wellbeing, quality of life, social participation, and engagement (including continuing opportunities for productivity) are all important for healthy aging in autistic adults (Klein & Klinger, 2024). Future research and services need to prioritize developing assessments and understanding of the needs of older autistic adults and how to support them towards aging well.

Assessment in Adulthood: Summary and Conclusions

There are still gaps and limitations in our knowledge and provisions, despite major strides in research and clinical services for autistic adults in the last two decades. Although a growing number of professionals are developing the required expertise and skills to identify, assess, diagnose, and support autistic adults, diagnostic and support services continue to be scarce in many countries and settings. Given that research, training, resources (including validated assessment measures), and services remain limited, there remain considerable challenges in implementing best practices in assessment of autistic people in adulthood.

Nevertheless, the available evidence and best-practice guidelines for the assessment of autistic adults as outlined in this chapter highlight the importance of comprehensively assessing the individual's skills, strengths, needs, challenges, and preferences; of conducting assessments that are affirming, respectful to the autistic adult, and person-centered; and of carefully considering individual, family, social, employment and community environments, stressors, and facilitators, always aiming to support the autistic adult achieve their full potential, enhance their wellbeing, and thrive.

References

Abbott, P., Happé, F. G., & Charlton, R. A. (2018). Exploratory study of executive function abilities across the adult lifespan in individuals receiving an ASD diagnosis in adulthood. *Journal of Autism and Developmental Disorders, 48*(12), 4193–4206.

Achenbach, T. M., Rescorla, L. A., McConaughey, S., Pecora, P., Wetherbee, K., & Ruffle, T. (2003). Achenbach system of empirically based assessment. *Handbook of Psychological and Educational Assessment of Children: Personality, Behavior, and Context, 2*, 406–432.

Ai, W., Cunningham, W. A., & Lai, M. C. (2022). Reconsidering autistic 'camouflaging' as transactional impression management. *Trends in Cognitive Sciences, 26*(8), 631–645.

Ai, W., Cunningham, W. A., & Lai, M. C. (2024a). The dimensional structure of the Camouflaging Autistic Traits Questionnaire (CAT-Q) and predictors of camouflaging in a representative general population sample. *Comprehensive Psychiatry, 128*, Article 152434.

Ai, W., Cunningham, W. A., & Lai, M. C. (2024b). Camouflaging, internalized stigma, and mental health in the general population. *International Journal of Social Psychiatry, 70*(7), 1239–1253.

Alim, N., Paschos, D., & Hearn, M. (2014). Principles of clinical assessment. In E. Tsakanikos & J. McCarthy (Eds.), *Handbook of psychopathology in intellectual disability* (pp. 23–42). Springer Publications.

Allison, C., Auyeung, B., & Baron-Cohen, S. (2012). Toward brief "Red Flags" for autism screening: The short autism spectrum quotient and the short quantitative checklist for autism in toddlers in 1,000 cases and 3,000 controls. *Journal of American Academy of Child and Adolescent Psychiatry, 51*(2), 202–212.

Alvares, G. A., Bebbington, K., Cleary, D., Evans, K., Glasson, E. J., Maybery, M. T., Pillar, S., Uljarević, M., Varcin, K., Wray, J., & Whitehouse, A. J. (2020). The misnomer of 'high functioning autism': Intelligence is an imprecise predictor of functional abilities at diagnosis. *Autism, 24*(1), 221–232. https://doi.org/10.1177/1362361319852831

Aman, M. G., & Singh, N. N. (1986). *Aberrant Behavior Checklist*. Slosson Educational Publications.

Ambitious about Autism. (2022). *Meltdowns and shutdowns*. https://www.ambitiousaboutautism.org.uk/understanding-autism/behaviour/meltdowns-and-shutdowns

American Psychiatric Association. (2022). *Diagnostic and statistical manual of mental disorders* (5th ed., text rev.). https://doi.org/10.1176/appi.books.9780890425787

American Speech-Language-Hearing Association. (2006, March). *Guidelines for speech-language pathologists in diagnosis, assessment, and treatment of autism spectrum disorders across the life span*. http://www.asha.org/members/deskref-journal/deskref/default

Andrews, J. J. W., & Istvanffy, P. (Eds). (2012). *Conduct and oppositional defiant disorders, exceptional life journeys* (pp. 27–53). Elsevier. https://doi.org/10.1016/B978-0-12-385216-8.00002-3

Arnold, S. R., Uljarević, M., Hwang, Y. I., Richdale, A. L., Trollor, J. N., & Lawson, L. P. (2020). Brief report: Psychometric properties of the patient health questionaire-9 (PHQ-9) in autistic adults. *Journal of Autism and Developmental Disorders, 50*, 2217–2225.

Ashwood, K. L., Gillan, N., Horder, J., Hayward, H., Woodhouse, E., McEwen, F. S., Murphy, D. G., et al. (2016). Predicting the diagnosis of autism in adults using the Autism-Spectrum Quotient (AQ) questionnaire. *Psychological Medicine, 46*(12), 2595–2604.

Autism Speaks. (2014). *Community-based skills assessment (CSA): Developing a personalized transition plan*. https://autismspeaks.org/tool-kit/community-based-skills-assessment

Au-Yeung, S. K., Bradley, L., Robertson, A. E., Shaw, R., Baron-Cohen, S., & Cassidy, S. (2019). Experience of mental health diagnosis and perceived misdiagnosis in autistic, possibly autistic and non-autistic adults. *Autism, 23*(6), 1508–1518.

Baksh, R. A., Abrahams, S., Bertlich, M., Cameron, R., Jany, S., Dorrian, T., Auyeung, B., et al. (2020). Social cognition in adults with autism spectrum disorders: Validation of the Edinburgh Social Cognition Test (ESCoT). *The Clinical Neuropsychologist, 35*(7), 1275–1293. https://doi.org/10.1080/13854046.2020.1737236

Baldwin, S., & Costley, D. (2016). The experiences and needs of female adults with high-functioning autism spectrum disorder. *Autism, 20*(4), 483–495.

Baron-Cohen, S., Wheelwright, S., Robinson, J., & Woodbury-Smith, M. (2005). The Adult Asperger Assessment (AAA): A diagnostic method. *Journal of Autism and Developmental Disorders, 35*(6), 807–819.

Baron-Cohen, S., Wheelwright, S., Skinner, R., Martin, J., & Clubley, E. (2001). The Autism-Spectrum Quotient (AQ): Evidence from Asperger syndrome/high-functioning autism, males and females, scientists and mathematicians. *Journal of Autism and Developmental Disorders, 31*(1), 5–17.

Berney, T., Brugha, T., & Carpenter, P. (2017). *Royal College of Psychiatrists Interview Guide for the Diagnostic Assessment of Able Adults with Autism Spectrum Disorder (ASD).*
Bishop, S. L., & Lord, C. (2023). Commentary: Best practices and processes for assessment of autism spectrum disorder–the intended role of standardized diagnostic instruments. *Journal of Child Psychology and Psychiatry, 64*(5), 834–838.
Black, M. H., Mahdi, S., Milbourn, B., Scott, M., Gerber, A., Esposito, C., Girdler, S., et al. (2020). Multi-informant international perspectives on the facilitators and barriers to employment for autistic adults. *Autism Research, 13*(7), 1195–1214.
Blainey, S., et al. (2019). General Anxiety. In E. Chaplin (Ed.), *A clinician's guide to mental health conditions in adults with autism spectrum disorders: Assessment and interventions* (pp. 97–110). Jessica Kingsley Publishers.
Bölte, S., de Schipper, E., Robison, J. E., Wong, V. C., Selb, M., Singhal, N., dr Vries, P. J., & Zwaigenbaum, L. (2014). Classification of functioning and impairment: the development of ICF core sets for autism spectrum disorder. *Autism Research, 7*(1), 167–172.
Bracken, B. A., & McCallum, R. S. (2016). *Universal nonverbal intelligence test—Second Edition (UNIT2)* [Database record]. PsycTESTS. https://doi.org/10.1037/t79431-000
Brown, C., & Dunn, W. (2002). *Adolescent/Adult sensory profile manual*. Psychological Corporation.
Brown, L., Sherbenou, R. J., & Johnsen, S. K. (2010). *Test of nonverbal intelligence: TONI-4*. PRO-ED.
Brugha, T. S., McManus, S., Bankart, J., Scott, F., Purdon, S., et al. (2011). Epidemiology of autism spectrum disorders in adults in the community in England. *Archives of General Psychiatry, 68*(5), 459–465.
Bruininks, R. H., Woodcock, R., Weatherman, R., & Hill, B. (1996). *Scales of Independent Behavior-Revised: Comprehensive manual*. Riverside Publishing Company.
Buckland, R. (2024). The Buckland Review of Autism Employment Report and recommendations. Retrieved April 3, 2024. https://www.gov.uk/government/publications/the-buckland-review-of-autism-employment-report-and-recommendations/the-buckland-review-of-autism-employment-report-and-recommendations
Cai, R. Y., Richdale, A. L., Uljarević, M., Dissanayake, C., & Samson, A. C. (2018). Emotion regulation in autism spectrum disorder: Where we are and where we need to go. *Autism Research, 11*(7), 962–978. https://doi.org/10.1002/aur.1968
Cassidy, S. A., Bradley, L., Cogger-Ward, H., & Rodgers, J. (2021). Development and validation of the suicidal behaviours questionnaire-autism spectrum conditions in a community sample of autistic, possibly autistic and non-autistic adults. *Molecular Autism, 12*(1), 46.
Cheely, C. A., Carpenter, L. A., Letourneau, E. J., et al. (2012). The prevalence of youth with Autism Spectrum Disorders in the criminal justice system. *Journal of Autism and Developmental Disorders, 42*(9), 1856–1862.
Cherewick, M., & Matergia, M. (2024). Neurodiversity in practice: A conceptual model of autistic strengths and potential mechanisms of change to support positive mental health and wellbeing in autistic children and adolescents. *Advances in Neurodevelopmental Disorders, 8*(3), 408–422.
Chew, L., Sun, K. L., Sun, W., Wang, Z., Rajadas, J., Flores, R. E., Fung, L. K., et al. (2021). Association of serum allopregnanolone with restricted and repetitive behaviors in adult males with autism. *Psychoneuroendocrinology, 123*, Article 105039.
Conner, C. M., Golt, J., Shaffer, R., Righi, G., Siegel, M., & Mazefsky, C. A. (2021). Emotion dysregulation is substantially elevated in autism compared to the general population: Impact on psychiatric services. *Autism Research, 14*(1), 169–181.
Constantino, J. N. (2012). *Social responsiveness scale, Second edition.* (SRS-2). WPS.
Conti-Ramsden, G., Durkin, K., Toseeb, U., Botting, N., & Pickles, A. (2018). Education and employment outcomes of young adults with a history of developmental language disorder. *International Journal of Language & Communication Disorders, 53*(2), 237–255.

Conti-Ramsden, G., Mok, P. L., Pickles, A., & Durkin, K. (2013). Adolescents with a history of specific language impairment (SLI): Strengths and difficulties in social, emotional and behavioral functioning. *Research in Developmental Disabilities, 34*(11), 4161–4169.

Conti-Ramsden, G., Simkin, Z., & Botting, N. (2006). The prevalence of autistic spectrum disorders in adolescents with a history of specific language impairment (SLI). *Journal of Child Psychology and Psychiatry, 47*(6), 621–628.

Crane, L., Hearst, C., Ashworth, M., Davies, J., & Hill, E. L. (2021). Supporting newly identified or diagnosed autistic adults: An initial evaluation of an autistic-led programme. *Journal of Autism and Developmental Disorders, 51*, 892–905.

Crowson, S., Poole, D., Scargill, K., & Freeth, M. (2022). *Understanding the post-diagnostic support priorities of autistic adults in the UK: A co-produced modified Delphi study.*

Curnow, E., Rutherford, M., Maciver, D., Johnston, L., Prior, S., Boilson, M., Meff, T., et al. (2023). Mental health in autistic adults: A rapid review of prevalence of psychiatric disorders and umbrella review of the effectiveness of interventions within a neurodiversity informed perspective. *PLoS One, 18*(7), Article e0288275.

Davids, R. C., Groen, Y., Berg, I. J., Tucha, O. M., & van Balkom, I. D. (2016). Executive functions in older adults with autism spectrum disorder: Objective performance and subjective complaints. *Journal of Autism and Developmental Disorders, 46*, 2859–2873.

Davies, J., Cooper, K., Killick, E., Sam, E., Healy, M., Thompson, G., Mandy, W., Redmayne, B., & Crane, L. (2024a). Autistic identity: A systematic review of quantitative research. *Autism Research, 17*(5), 874–897. https://doi.org/10.1002/aur.3105

Davies, J., Romualdez, A. M., Malyan, D., Heasman, B., Livesey, A., Walker, A., Remington, A., et al. (2024b). Autistic adults' priorities for future autism employment research: Perspectives from the United Kingdom. *Autism in Adulthood, 6*(1), 72–85.

De Schipper, E., Lundequist, A., Coghill, D., de Vries, P. J., Granlund, M., Holtmann, M., Jonsson, U., Karande, S., Robison, J. E., Shulman, C., Singhal, N., Tonge, B., Wong, V. C., Zwaigenbaum, L., & Bölte, S. (2015). Ability and disability in autism spectrum disorder: A systematic literature review employing the international classification of functioning, disability and health-children and youth version. *Autism Research, 8*(6), 782–794. https://doi.org/10.1002/aur.1485

Deb, S., Perera, B., Krysta, K., Ozer, M., Bertelli, M., Novell, R., Wieland, J., & Sappok, T. (2022). The European guideline on the assessment and diagnosis of psychiatric disorders in adults with intellectual disabilities. *The European Journal of Psychiatry, 36*(1), 11–25.

Delis, D.C., Kaplan, E., & Kramer, J. H. (2001). *The Delis-Kaplan Executive Functions System (D-KEFS).* Pearson publications.

Dietz, P. M., Rose, C. E., McArthur, D., & Maenner, M. (2020). National and state estimates of adults with autism spectrum disorder. *Journal of Autism and Developmental Disorders, 50*(12), 4258–4266.

Dubois, P., St-Pierre, M. C., Desmarais, C., & Guay, F. (2020). Young adults with developmental language disorder: A systematic review of education, employment, and independent living outcomes. *Journal of Speech, Language, and Hearing Research, 63*(11), 3786–3800.

Dunn, D. M. (2018). Peabody picture vocabulary test fifth edition (PPVT-5). Minneapolis, MN.

Dwyer, P., Williams, Z. J., Lawson, W. B., & Rivera, S. M. (2024). A trans-diagnostic investigation of attention, hyper-focus, and monotropism in autism, attention dysregulation hyperactivity development, and the general population. *Neurodiversity, 2*. https://doi.org/10.1177/27546330241237883

Edwards, G., Tarver, J., Shelley, L., Bird, M., Hughes, J., Crawford, H., & Waite, J. (2023). Utilising interview methodology to inform the development of new clinical assessment tools for anxiety in autistic individuals who speak few or no words. *Journal of Autism and Developmental Disorders, 53*(6), 2328–2348.

Elwin, M., Schröder, A., Ek, L., & Kjellin, L. (2016). Development and pilot validation of a sensory reactivity scale for adults with high functioning autism spectrum conditions: Sensory Reactivity in Autism Spectrum (SR-AS). *Nordic Journal of Psychiatry, 70*(2), 103–110.

English, M. C., Gignac, G. E., Visser, T. A., Whitehouse, A. J., Enns, J. T., & Maybery, M. T. (2021). The comprehensive autistic trait inventory (CATI): Development and validation of a new measure of autistic traits in the general population. *Molecular Autism, 12*(1), 37.
Eriksson, J. M., Andersen, L. M. J., & Bejerot, S. (2013). RAADS-14 Screen: Validity of a screening tool for autism spectrum disorder in an adult psychiatric population. *Molecular Autism, 4*, 49.
Fiene, L., & Brownlow, C. (2015). Investigating interoception and body awareness in adults with and without autism spectrum disorder. *Autism Research, 8*(6), 709–716.
Fiene, L., Ireland, M. J., & Brownlow, C. (2018). The interoception sensory questionnaire (ISQ): A scale to measure interoceptive challenges in adults. *Journal of Autism and Developmental Disorders, 48*(10), 3354–3366.
First, M. B., Williams, J. B., Benjamin, L. S., & Spitzer, R. L. (2016). Structured clinical interview for DSM-5 personality disorders (SCID-5-PD). *Testkatalog, 30.*
Fletcher, R., Loschen, E., Stavrakaki, C., & First, M. (2007). DM-ID: diagnostic manual—intellectual disability: a textbook of diagnosis of mental disorders in persons with intellectual disability. *Journal of Mental Health Research in Intellectual Disabilities, 29.*
Fuentes, J., Hervás, A., Howlin, P., & (ESCAP ASD Working Party). (2021). ESCAP practice guidance for autism: a summary of evidence-based recommendations for diagnosis and treatment. *European Child & Adolescent Psychiatry, 30*(6), 961–984.
Fusar-Poli, L., Brondino, N., Rocchetti, M., Panisi, C., Provenzani, U., Damiani, S., & Politi, P. (2017). Diagnosing ASD in adults without ID: Accuracy of the ADOS-2 and the ADI-R. *Journal of Autism and Developmental Disorders, 47*, 3370–3379.
Garau, V., Murray, A. L., Woods, R., Chown, N., Hallett, S., Murray, F., Fletcher-Watson, S., et al. (2023). *Development and validation of a novel self-report measure of monotropism in autistic and non-autistic people: The monotropism questionnaire.*
Gaus, V. L. (2011). Adult Asperger syndrome and the utility of cognitive-behavioral therapy. *Journal of Contemporary Psychotherapy, 41*, 47–56.
Gellini, H., & Marczak, M. (2024). "I always knew I was different": Experiences of receiving a diagnosis of autistic spectrum disorder in adulthood—A meta-ethnographic systematic review. *Review Journal of Autism and Developmental Disorders, 11*(3), 620–639.
Gibbs, V., & Pellicano, E. (2023). 'Maybe we just seem like easy targets': A qualitative analysis of autistic adults' experiences of interpersonal violence. *Autism, 27*(7), 2021–2034.
Gillberg, C., Gillberng, C., Rastam, M., & Wentz, E. (2001). The Asperger syndrome (and high-functioning autism) Diagnostic Interview (AUTISMI): A preliminary study of a new structured clinical interview. *Autism, 5*(1), 57–66.
Goldstein, S., & Naglieri, J. A. (2009). *Autism spectrum rating scales (ASRS).* Multi-Health System.
Goodall, E., Dargue, N., Hinze, E., Sulek, R., Varcin, K., Waddington, H., Whitehouse, A. J. O., Wicks, R., Allen, G., Best, J., Eapen, V. Evans, K., Hiremath, M, Foster, W., Lawson, W., Toby, S., & Trembath, D. (2023). *National Guideline for the assessment and diagnosis of autism in Australia.* Autism CRC.
Gosling, C. J., Cartigny, A., Mellier, B. C., Solanes, A., Radua, J., & Delorme, R. (2022). Efficacy of psychosocial interventions for Autism spectrum disorder: An umbrella review. *Molecular Psychiatry, 27*(9), 3647–3656.
Grant, D. A., & Berg, E. A. (1993). *The Wisconsin Card Sorting Test (WCST).* WPS publishers.
Green, R. M., Travers, A. M., Howe, Y., & McDougle, C. J. (2019). Women and autism spectrum disorder: Diagnosis and implications for treatment of adolescents and adults. *Current Psychiatry Reports, 21*(4), 1–8.
Griffiths, S., Allison, C., Kenny, R., Holt, R., Smith, P., & Baron-Cohen, S. (2019). The vulnerability experiences quotient (VEQ): A study of vulnerability, mental health and life satisfaction in autistic adults. *Autism Research, 12*(10), 1516–1528.
Grosvenor, L. P., Errichetti, C. L., Holingue, C., Beasley, J. B., & Kalb, L. G. (2023). Self-report measurement of well-being in autistic adults: Psychometric properties of the PERMA profiler. *Autism in Adulthood, 5*(4), 401–410.

Grove, R., Hoekstra, R. A., Wierda, M., & Begeer, S. (2018). Special interests and subjective wellbeing in autistic adults. *Autism Research, 11*(5), 766–775.
Gunderson, J., Worthley, E., Byiers, B., Symons, F., & Wolff, J. (2023). Self and caregiver report measurement of sensory features in autism spectrum disorder: A systematic review of psychometric properties. *Journal of Neurodevelopmental Disorders, 15*(1), 5.
Halvorsen, M. B., Kildahl, A. N., Kaiser, S., Axelsdottir, B., Aman, M. G., & Helverschou, S. B. (2024). Applicability and Psychometric Properties of General Mental Health Assessment Tools in Autistic People: A Systematic Review. *Journal of Autism and Developmental Disorders*, 1–14.
Hannon, B., Mandy, W., & Hull, L. (2023). A comparison of methods for measuring camouflaging in autism. *Autism Research, 16*(1), 12–29.
Harmuth, E., Silletta, E., Bailey, A., Adams, T., Beck, C., & Barbic, S. P. (2018). Barriers and facilitators to employment for adults with autism: A scoping review. *Annals of International Occupational Therapy, 1*(1), 31–40.
Harrison, P., & Oakland, T. (2015). *Adaptive behavior assessment system—3rd edition (ABAS-3)*. Western Psychological Services.
Hedley, D., Batterham, P. J., Bury, S. M., Clapperton, A., Denney, K., Dissanayake, C., Stokes, M. A., et al. (2023). The Suicidal Ideation Attributes Scale-Modified (SIDAS-M): Development and preliminary validation of a new scale for the measurement of suicidal ideation in autistic adults. *Autism, 27*(4), 1115–1131.
Helverschou, S. B., Bakken, T. L., & Martinsen, H. (2009). The psychopathology in autism checklist (PAC): A pilot study. *Research in Autism Spectrum Disorders, 3*(1), 179–195.
Henninger, N. A., & Lounds-Taylor, J. (2012). Outcomes in adults with Autism Spectrum Disorders: A historical perspective. *Autism, 17*(1), 103–116.
Hobson, H. M., & Lee, A. (2023). Camouflaging in developmental language disorder: The views of speech and language pathologists and parents. *Communication Disorders Quarterly, 44*(4), 247–256. https://doi.org/10.1177/15257401221120937
Hofvander, B., Delorme, R., Chaste, P., Nyden, A., Wentz, E., et al. (2009). Psychiatric and psychosocial problems in adults with normal-intelligence autism spectrum disorders. *BMC Psychiatry, 9*, 35.
Hollocks, M. J., Lerh, J. W., Magiati, I., Meiser-Stedman, R., & Brugha, T. S. (2019). Anxiety and depression in adults with autism spectrum disorder: A systematic review and meta-analysis. *Psychological Medicine, 49*(4), 559–572.
Howlin, P. (2000). Autism and intellectual disability: Diagnostic and treatment issues. *Journal of the Royal Society of Medicine, 93*(7), 351–355.
Hull, L., Mandy, W., Lai, M. C., Baron-Cohen, S., Allison, C., Smith, P., & Petrides, K. V. (2019). Development and validation of the camouflaging autistic traits questionnaire (CAT-Q). *Journal of Autism and Developmental Disorders, 49*, 819–833.
Hupfeld, K., Osborne, J., Tran, Q., Hyatt, H., Abagis, T., & Shah, P. (2024). *Validation of the Dispositional Adult Hyperfocus Questionnaire (AHQ-D)*.
Hurley, R. S. E., Losh, M., Parlier, M., Reznick, J. S., & Piven, J. (2007). The broad autism phenotype questionnaire. *Journal of Autism and Developmental Disorders., 37*, 1679–1690.
Jones, L., Goddard, L., Hill, E. L., Henry, L. A., & Crane, L. (2014). Experiences of receiving a diagnosis of autism spectrum disorder: A survey of adults in the United Kingdom. *Journal of Autism and Developmental Disorders, 44*(12), 3033–3044.
Jones, C. R. G., Livingston, L. A., Fretwell, C., Uljarević, M., Carrington, S. J., Shah, P., & Leekam, S. R. (2024). Measuring self and informant perspectives of Restricted and Repetitive Behaviours (RRBs): Psychometric evaluation of the Repetitive Behaviours Questionnaire-3 (RBQ-3) in adult clinical practice and research settgs. *Molecular Autism, 15*(1), 24. https://doi.org/10.1186/s13229-024-00603-7
Jones, S. L., Johnson, M., Alty, B., & Adamou, M. (2021). The effectiveness of RAADS-R as a screening tool for adult ASD populations. *Autism Research and Treatment*. https://doi.org/10.1155/2021/9974791

Josyfon, E., Spain, D., Blackmore, C., Murphy, D., & Oakley, B. (2023, December). Alexithymia in adult autism clinic service-users: Relationships with sensory processing differences and mental health. *Healthcare, 11*(24), 3114. MDPI.
Kapp, S. K., Steward, R., Crane, L., Elliott, D., Elphick, C., Pellicano, E., & Russell, G. (2019). 'People should be allowed to do what they like': Autistic adults' views and experiences of stimming. *Autism, 23*(7), 1782–1792. https://doi.org/10.1177/1362361319829628
Kaufman, A. S., & Kaufman, N. L. (2022). *Kaufman brief intelligence test, Second edition revised*. Pearson.
Kenny, H., & Stansfield, A. J. (2016). How useful are the Adult Asperger Assessment and AQ-10 within an adult clinical population of all intellectual abilities? *Advances in Autism, 2*(3), 118–130.
Kentrou, V., Livingston, L. A., Grove, R., Hoekstra, R. A., & Begeer, S. (2024). Perceived misdiagnosis of psychiatric conditions in autistic adults. *EClinicalMedicine, 71*.
Kerns, C. M., Kendall, P. C., Berry, L., Souders, M. C., Franklin, M. E., Schultz, R. T., Herrington, J., et al. (2014). Traditional and atypical presentations of anxiety in youth with autism spectrum disorder. *Journal of Autism and Developmental Disorders, 44*, 2851–2861.
Kildahl, A. N., Helverschou, S. B., Rysstad, A. L., Wigaard, E., Hellerud, J. M., Ludvigsen, L. B., & Howlin, P. (2021). Pathological demand avoidance in children and adolescents: A systematic review. *Autism, 25*(8), 2162–2176. https://doi.org/10.1177/13623613211034382
Kinnaird, E., Stewart, C., & Tchanturia, K. (2019). Investigating alexithymia in autism: A systematic review and meta-analysis. *European Psychiatry, 55*, 80–89.
Klein, C. B., & Klinger, L. G. (2024, June). Aging well and autism: A narrative review and recommendations for future research. *Healthcare, 12*(12), 1207. MDPI.
Kooijmans, R., Mercera, G., Langdon, P. E., & Moonen, X. (2022). The adaptation of self-report measures to the needs of people with intellectual disabilities: A systematic review. *Clinical Psychology: Science and Practice, 29*(3), 250.
Lai, M. C., & Baron-Cohen, S. (2015). Identifying the lost generation of adults with autism spectrum conditions. *The Lancet Psychiatry, 2*(11), 1013–1027.
Lai, M. C., Kassee, C., Besney, R., Bonato, S., Hull, L., Mandy, W., Ameis, S. H., et al. (2019). Prevalence of co-occurring mental health diagnoses in the autism population: A systematic review and meta-analysis. *The Lancet Psychiatry, 6*(10), 819–829.
Lam, K. S. L., & Aman, M. G. (2007). The repetitive behavior scale-revised: Independent validation in individuals with autism spectrum disorders. *Journal of Autism and Developmental Disorders, 37*(5), 855–866.
Lawson, W. (2011). *The passionate mind: How people with autism learn*. Jessica Kingsley Publishers.
Lawson, W. B. (2020). Adaptive morphing and coping with social threat in autism: An autistic perspective. *Journal of Intellectual Disability-Diagnosis and Treatment, 8*(3), 519–526.
Lehnhardt, F. G., Falter, C. M., Gawronski, A., Pfeiffer, K., Tepest, R., Franklin, J., & Vogeley, K. (2016). Sex-related cognitive profile in autism spectrum disorders diagnosed late in life: Implications for the female autistic phenotype. *Journal of Autism and Developmental Disorders, 46*, 139–154.
Lewis, L. F., & Stevens, K. (2023). The lived experience of meltdowns for autistic adults. *Autism, 27*(6), 1817–1825. https://doi.org/10.1177/13623613221145783
Lilley, R., Lawson, W., Hall, G., Mahony, J., Clapham, H., Heyworth, M., Arnold, S. R., Trollor, J. N., Yudell, M., & Pellicano, E. (2022). 'A way to be me': Autobiographical reflections of autistic adults diagnosed in mid-to-late adulthood. *Autism, 26*(6), 1395–1408.
Lindsay, W. R., & Michie, A. M. (1988). Adaptatio of the Zung Self-rating scale for anxiety for people with a mental handicap. *Journal of Mental Deficiency Research, 32*, 485–490.
Lizon, M., Taels, L., & Vanheule, S. (2024). Specific interests as a social boundary and bridge: A qualitative interview study with autistic individuals. *Autism, 28*(5), 1150–1160. https://doi.org/10.1177/13623613231193532

Lord, C., & Bishop, S. L. (2021). Let's be clear that "autism spectrum disorder symptoms" are not always related to autism spectrum disorder. *American Journal of Psychiatry, 178*(8), 680–682.
Lord, C., Rutter, M., & DiLavore, P.C. (2012). *Autism Diagnostic Observation Schedule, Second edition* (ADOS-2). Western Psychological Services.
LoVullo, S. V., & Matson, J. J. (2009). Comorbid psychopathology in adults with autism spectrum disorders and intellectual disabilities. *Research in Developmental Disabilities, 30*, 1288–1296.
Lugnegard, T., Hallerback, M., & Gillberg, C. (2011). Psychiatric comorbidity in young adults with a clinical diagnosis of Asperger syndrome. *Research in Developmental Disabilities, 32*(5), 1910–1917.
Lundin, A., Kosidou, K., & Dalman, C. (2019). Measuring autism traits in the adult general population with the brief autism-spectrum quotient, AQ-10: Findings from the Stockholm public health cohort. *Journal of Autism and Developmental Disorders, 49*, 773–780.
MacLennan, K., O'Brien, S., & Tavassoli, T. (2022). In our own words: The complex sensory experiences of autistic adults. *Journal of Autism and Developmental Disorders, 52*(7), 3061–3075.
Maenner, M. J., Smith, L. E., Hong, J., Makuch, R., Greenberg, J., & Mailick, M. R. (2013). An evaluation of an activities of daily living scale for adolescents and adults with developmental disabilities. *Disability and Health Journal, 6*(1), 8–17.
Magiati, I., Ozsivadjian, A., & Kerns, C. M. (2017). Phenomenology and presentation of anxiety in autism spectrum disorder. In *Anxiety in children and adolescents with autism spectrum disorder* (pp. 33–54). Academic Press.
Magiati, I., Tsakanikos, E., & Howlin, P. (2014). Psychological and social factors. In E. Tsakanikos & J. McCarthy (Eds.), *Handbook of psychopathology in intellectual disability: Research, practice, and policy* (pp. 123–143). Springer Publications.
Mandy, W., Clarke, K., McKenner, M., Strydom, A., Crabtree, J., Lai, M. C., Allison, C., Baron-Cohen, S., & Skuse, D. (2018). Assessing autism in adults: An evaluation of the developmental, dimensional and diagnostic interview—Adult version (3Di adult). *Journal of Autism and Developmental Disorders, 48*, 549–560.
Mason, D., Capp, S. J., Stewart, G. R., Kempton, M. J., Glaser, K., Howlin, P., & Happé, F. (2021). A meta-analysis of outcome studies of autistic adults: Quantifying effect size, quality, and meta-regression. *Journal of Autism and Developmental Disorders, 51*, 3165–3179.
Matson, J. L. (1995). *The diagnostic assessment for the severely handicapped revised (DASH-II).* Disability Consultants, LLC.
Matson, J. L., & Boisjoli, J. A. (2008). Autism spectrum disorders in adults with intellectual disability and comorbid psychopathology: Scale development and reliability of the ASD-CA. *Research in Autism Spectrum Disorders, 2*(2), 276–287.
McNeel, M. M., Grebe, S. C., Clayton, R. J., Schneider, S. C., Viana, A. G., Mire, S. S., Omar, Y., Goodman, W. K., & Storch, E. A. (2022). Autism spectrum disorder versus obsessive-compulsive disorder and Tourette's disorder. In K. K. M. Stavropoulos & J. C. McPartland (Eds.), *Differential diagnosis of autism spectrum disorder* (p. 18). Oxford University Press. https://doi.org/10.1093/med-psych/9780197516881.003.0008
Mehling, W. E., Acree, M., Stewart, A., Silas, J., & Jones, A. (2018). The multidimensional assessment of interoceptive awareness, version 2 (MAIA-2). *PLoS One, 13*(12), Article e0208034.
Merrington, H., Gibbs, V., Haas, K., Clark, T., Robinson, A., Al Ansari, M., & Pellicano, E. (2024). What matters most? An exploration of quality of life through the everyday experiences of autistic young people and adults. *Autism in Adulthood.*
Mesibov, G., Schopler, E., & Caison, W. (1989). The adolescent and adult psychoeducational profile: Assessment of adolescents and adults with severe developmental handicaps. *Journal of Autism and Developmental Disorders, 19*(1), 33–40.

Mohr, C., Tonge, B., Einfeld, S., & Gray, K. (2004). The developmental behaviour checklist for adults: A new contribution to the assessment of psychopathology in people with intellectual disability (ID). *Journal of Intellectual Disability Research, 48*(4–5), 319.

Monteiro, M. J., & Stegall, S. (2018). *MIGDAS-2: Monteiro interview guidelines for diagnosing the Autism Spectrum.* WPS Publishing.

Morrison, K. E., Pinkham, A. E., Kelsven, S., Ludwig, K., Penn, D. L., & Sasson, N. J. (2019). Psychometric evaluation of social cognitive measures for adults with autism. *Autism Research: Official Journal of the International Society for Autism Research, 12*(5), 766–778. https://doi.org/10.1002/aur.2084

Moss, S. C. (2002a). *The mini PAS-ADD intervention assessment pack.* Pavilion Press.

Moss, S. C. (2002b). *The PAS-ADD checklist* (revised). Pavilion.

Murray, N., Hatfield, M., Falkmer, M., & Falkmer, T. (2016). Evaluation of career planning tools for use with individuals with autism spectrum disorder: A systematic review. *Research in Autism Spectrum Disorders, 23*, 188–202.

Murray, D., Lesser, M., & Lawson, W. (2005). Attention, monotropism and the diagnostic criteria for autism. *Autism, 9*(2), 139–156.

National Autistic Society (NAS). (2020). *Meltdowns—A guide for all audiences.* https://www.autism.org.uk/advice-and-guidance/topics/behaviour/meltdowns/all-audiences

National Autistic Society (NAS). (2024, April 15). *Demand avoidance.* https://www.autism.org.uk/advice-and-guidance/topics/behaviour/demand-avoidance

National Institute of Clinical Excellence (NICE). (2021). *Autism: recognition, referral, diagnosis and management of adults on the autism spectrum.* NHS Evidence. http://www.nice.org.uk/guidance/cg142.

Newell, V., Townsend, E., Richards, C., & Cassidy, S. (2024). Measurement properties of tools used to assess self-harm in autistic and general population adults. *Clinical Psychology Review*, 102412.

Nicolaidis, C., Raymaker, D. M., McDonald, K. E., Lund, E. M., Leotti, S., Kapp, S. K., Zhen, K. Y., et al. (2020). Creating accessible survey instruments for use with autistic adults and people with intellectual disability: Lessons learned and recommendations. *Autism in Adulthood, 2*(1), 61–76.

Nudel, R., Christensen, R. V., Kalnak, N., Schwinn, M., Banasik, K., Dinh, K. M., DBDS Genomic Consortium, et al. (2023). Developmental language disorder–a comprehensive study of more than 46,000 individuals. *Psychiatry Research, 323*, 115171.

Nydén, A., Niklasson, L., Stahlberg, O., Anckarsater, H., Wentz, E., Rastam, M., & Gillberg, C. (2010). Adults with autism spectrum disorders and ADHD neuropsychological aspects. *Research in Developmental Disabilities, 31*(6), 1659–1668.

O'Nions, E., et al. (2013). Pathological demand avoidance: Exploring the behavioural profile. *Autism, 18*(5), 538–544.

O'Nions, E., Petersen, I., Buckman, J. E., Charlton, R., Cooper, C., Corbett, A., ... & Stott, J. (2023). Autism in England: Assessing underdiagnosis in a population-based cohort study of prospectively collected primary care data. *The Lancet Regional Health–Europe*, 29.

Patel, M., Lee, J. Y., & Scior, K. (2023). Psychometric properties of measures designed to assess common mental health problems and wellbeing in adults with intellectual disabilities: A systematic review. *Journal of Intellectual Disability Research, 67*(5), 397–414.

Pathological Demand Avoidance (PDA) Society. (n.d). *What is PDA? A guide to the Pathological Demand Avoidance profile of autism.* https://www.pdasociety.org.uk/wp-content/uploads/2021/04/What-is-PDA-booklet-website-v2.1.pdf

Pattison, E., Ure, A., Mittiga, S. R., Williams, K., & Freeman, N. C. (2022). The feedback session of an autism assessment: A scoping review of clinical practice guideline recommendations. *Journal of Autism and Developmental Disorders, 52*(4), 1821–1840.

Patton J. R. & Clark G. M. (2021). *Transition planning inventory–Third Edition, complete kit*. PRO-ED.

Paul, R., Landa, R., & Simmons, E. (2014). Assessing and treating communication. In J. McPartland, A. Klin, & F. Volkmar (Eds.), *Asperger syndrome: Assessing and treating high functioning autism spectrum disorder* (2nd ed., pp. 103–142). Guilford Press.

Pellicano, E., & Heyworth, M. (2023). The foundations of autistic flourishing. *Current Psychiatry Reports, 25*(9), 419–427.

Ramirez, S. Z., & Lukenbill, J. F. (2007). Development of the fear survey for adults with mental retardation. *Research in Developmental Disabilities, 28*, 225–237.

Rapaport, H., Clapham, H., Adams, J., Lawson, W., Porayska-Pomsta, K., & Pellicano, E. (2024). "In a state of flow": A qualitative examination of autistic adults' phenomenological experiences of task immersion. *Autism in Adulthood, 6*(3), 362–373.

Reynolds, W. M., & Baker, J. A. (1988). Assessment of depression in persons with mental retardation. *American Journal of Mental Retardation: AJMR, 93*(1), 93–103.

Ritvo, R. A., Ritvo, E. R., Guthrie, D., Ritvo, M. J., Hufnagel, D. H., et al. (2011). The Ritvo Autism Asperger Diagnostic Scale-Revised (RAADS-R): A scale to assist the diagnosis of autism spectrum disorder in adults: An international validation study. *Journal of Autism and Developmental Disorders, 41*, 1076–1089.

Rodgers, J., Farquhar, K., Mason, D., Brice, S., Wigham, S., Ingham, B., Parr, J. R., et al. (2020). Development and initial evaluation of the anxiety scale for autism-adults. *Autism in Adulthood, 2*(1), 24–33.

Roestorf, A., Bowler, D. M., Deserno, M. K., Howlin, P., Klinger, L., McConachie, H., Geurts, H. M., et al. (2019). "Older adults with ASD: The consequences of aging". Insights from a series of special interest group meetings held at the International Society for Autism Research 2016–2017. *Research in Autism Spectrum Disorders, 63*, 3–12.

Roestorf, A., Howlin, P., & Bowler, D. M. (2022). Ageing and autism: A longitudinal follow-up study of mental health and quality of life in autistic adults. *Frontiers in Psychology, 13*, Article 741213. https://doi.org/10.3389/fpsyg.2022.741213

Roid, G. H. (2003). *Stanford-Binet intelligence scales-Fifth Edition*. Riverside Publishing.

Roid, G. H., Miller, L. J., Pomplun, M., & Koch, C. (2013). *Leiter international performance scale-third edition*. Stoelting Company.

Rosen, N. E., Lord, C., & Volkmar, F. R. (2021). The diagnosis of autism: From Kanner to DSM-III to DSM-5 and beyond. *Journal of Autism and Developmental Disorders, 51*, 4253–4270.

Ross, E., & Oliver, C. (2003). Preliminary analysis of the psychometric properties of the Mood, Interest & Pleasure Questionnaire (MIPQ) for adults with severe and profound learning disabilities. *British Journal of Clinical Psychology, 42*(1), 81–93.

Roth, R. M., Isquith, P. K., & Gioia, G. A. (2005). Behavior rating inventory of executive function®—Adult version. *Archives of Clinical Neuropsychology*.

Royal College of Psychiatrists. (2001). *DC-LD: Diagnostic criteria for learning disability: Diagnostic criteria for psychiatric disorders for use with adults with learning disabilities/mental retardation*. RCPsych Publications.

Rutter, M., Bailey, A., & Lord, C. (2003a). *SCQ: The social communication questionnaire*. Western Psychological Services.

Rutter, M., Le Couteur, A., & Lord, C. (2003b). ADI-R. *Autism diagnostic interview revised. Manual*. Western Psychological Services.

Ruzzano, L., Borsboom, D., & Geurts, H. M. (2015). Repetitive behaviors in autism and obsessive—Compulsive disorder: New perspectives from a network analysis. *Journal of Autism and Developmental Disorders, 45*, 192–202.

Sáez-Suanes, G. P., & Álvarez-Couto, M. (2022). Factors associated with quality of life in adults with autism spectrum disorder: A systematic review. *Review Journal of Autism and Developmental Disorders, 9*(3), 307–319.

Sappok, T., Gaul, I., Bergmann, T., Dziobek, I., Bolte, S., et al. (2014). The diagnostic behavioral assessment for autism spectrum disorder-revised: A screening instrument for adults with intellectual disability suspected of autism spectrum disorders. *Research in Autism Spectrum Disorders, 8*, 362–375.

Sasson, N. J., Morrison, K. E., Kelsven, S., & Pinkham, A. E. (2020). Social cognition as a predictor of functional and social skills in autistic adults without intellectual disability. *Autism Research, 13*(2), 259–270.

Schiariti, V., Mahdi, S., & Bölte, S. (2018). International classification of functioning, disability and health core sets for cerebral palsy, autism spectrum disorder, and attention-deficit–hyperactivity disorder. *Developmental Medicine & Child Neurology, 60*(9), 933–941.

Shattuck, P. T., Garfield, T., Roux, A. M. et al. (2020). Services for adults with autism spectrum disorder: A systems perspective. *Current Psychiatry Reports, 22*, 13. https://doi.org/10.1007/s11920-020-1136-7

Skuse, D., Warrington, R., Bishop, D., Chowdhury, U., Lau, J., Mandy, W., & Place, M. (2004). The developmental, dimensional and diagnostic interview (3di): A novel computerized assessment for autism spectrum disorders. *Journal of the American Academy of Child & Adolescent Psychiatry, 43*(5), 548–558.

Sparrow, S., Cicchetti, D., & Saulnier, C. (2016). *Vineland adaptive behavior scales–Third Edition (Vineland-3)*. Pearson.

Stavropoulos, K. K., & McPartland, J. C. (Eds.). (2022). *Differential diagnosis of autism spectrum disorder*. Oxford University Press.

St. John, T., Woods, S., Bode, T., Ritter, C., & Estes, A. (2022). A review of executive functioning challenges and strengths in autistic adults. *The Clinical Neuropsychologist, 36*(5), 1116–1147.

Suzman, E., Williams, Z. J., Feldman, J. I., Failla, M., Cascio, C. J., Wallace, M. T., Woynaroski, T. G., et al. (2021). Psychometric validation and refinement of the Interoception Sensory Questionnaire (ISQ) in adolescents and adults on the autism spectrum. *Molecular Autism, 12*(1), 42.

Tan, C. D. (2018). "I'm a normal autistic person, not an abnormal neurotypical": Autism spectrum disorder diagnosis as biographical illumination. *Social Science & Medicine, 197*, 161–167.

Tavassoli, T., Hoekstra, R. A., & Baron-Cohen, S. (2014a). The Sensory Perception Quotient (SPQ): Development and validation of a new sensory questionnaire for adults with and without autism. *Molecular Autism, 5*, 29.

Tavassoli, T., Miller, L. J., Schoen, S. A., Nielsen, D. M., & Baron-Cohen, S. (2014b). Sensory over-responsivity in adults with autism spectrum conditions. *Autism, 18*(4), 428–432. https://doi.org/10.1177/1362361313477246

Thurm, A., Farmer, C., Salzman, E., Lord, C., & Bishop, S. (2019). State of the field: Differentiating intellectual disability from autism spectrum disorder. *Frontiers in Psychiatry, 10*, 526.

Tillman, K. S., & Prazak, M. (2019). Friendship club: Development and implementation of a 12-week social skills group curriculum. *Counselling and Psychotherapy Research, 19*(2), 158–166.

Tromans, S., Chester, V., Kiani, R., Alexander, R., & Brugha, T. (2018). The prevalence of autism spectrum disorders in adult psychiatric inpatients: A systematic review. *Clinical Practice and Epidemiology in Mental Health: CP & EMH, 14*, 177.

Üstün, T. B. (Ed.). (2010). *Measuring health and disability: Manual for WHO disability assessment schedule WHODAS 2.0*. World Health Organization.

Velikonja, T., Fett, A. K., & Velthorst, E. (2019). Patterns of nonsocial and social cognitive functioning in adults with autism spectrum disorder: A systematic review and meta-analysis. *JAMA Psychiatry, 76*(2), 135–151.

Whaikaha–Ministry of Disabled People. (2022). *Aotearoa New Zealand autism guideline: He waka huia takiwātanga rau, Third edition*. https://www.whaikaha.govt.nz/about-us/programmes-strategies-and-studies/guidelines/nz-autism-guideline#scroll-to-2

Wechsler, D. (2011). *Wechsler abbreviated scale of intelligence-Second Edition (WASI-II)* [Database record]. *APA PsycTests.* https://doi.org/10.1037/t15171-000

Wechsler, D. (2024). *Wechsler adult intelligence scale—Fifth Edition (WAIS-5).* https://www.pearsonassessments.com/store/usassessments/en/Store/Professional-Assessments/Cognition-%26-Neuro/Wechsler-Adult-Intelligence-Scale-%7C-Fifth-Edition/p/P100071002.html?tab=overview

Wechsler, D., & Naglieri, J. A. (2006). Wechsler nonverbal scale of ability (WNV) [Database record]. *APA PsycTests.* https://doi.org/10.1037/t15176-000

Welch, C., Cameron, D., Fitch, M., and Polatajko, H. (2020). Living in autistic bodies: bloggers discuss movement control and arousal regulation. *Disability Rehabilitation,* 1–9. https://doi.org/10.1080/09638288.2020.1729872

Wetherby, A., Diehl, S., et al. (2006). *Guidelines for Speech-language pathologists in diagnosis, assessment, and treatment of autism spectrum disorders across the life span.* American Speech Language Hearing Association (ASHA).

White, S. W., Maddox, B. B., & Mazefsky, C. A. (Eds.). (2020). *The Oxford handbook of autism and co-occurring psychiatric conditions.* Oxford University Press.

Whitehouse, A. J. O., & Bishop, D. V. M. (2009). *Communication checklist—Adult.* Pearson.

Wigham, S., Ingham, B., Le Couteur, A., Berney, T., Ensum, I., & Parr, J. R. (2020). Development and initial utility of the autism clinical interview for adults: A new adult autism diagnostic measure. *Autism in Adulthood, 2*(1), 42–47.

Wigham, S., Ingham, B., Le Couteur, A., Wilson, C., Ensum, I., & Parr, J. R. (2023). Consensus statements on optimal adult post-autism diagnosis support and services: Delphi process following a UK survey of autistic adults, relatives and clinicians. *Autism, 27*(2), 344–355.

Wigham, S., Rodgers, J., Berney, T., Le Couteur, A., Ingham, B., & Parr, J. R. (2019). Psychometric properties of questionnaires and diagnostic measures for autism spectrum disorders in adults: A systematic review. *Autism: The International Journal of Research and Practice, 23*(2), 287–305. https://doi.org/10.1177/1362361317748245

Wiig, E. H., Semel, E., & Secord, W. A. (2013). *The clinical evaluation of language fundamentals, 5th edition (CELF-5).* Pearson publications.

Williams, K. T. (2018). *Expressive vocabulary test, third edition (EVT-3).* https://www.pearsonclinical.com.au/store/auassessments/en/Store/Professional-Assessments/Academic-Learning/Expressive-Vocabulary-Test%2C-3rd-Edition/p/P100010103.html?tab=training

Williams, Z. J., Everaert, J., & Gotham, K. O. (2021). Measuring depression in autistic adults: Psychometric validation of the Beck Depression Inventory–II. *Assessment, 28*(3), 858–876.

Williams, Z. J., Suzman, E., Bordman, S. L., Markfeld, J. E., Kaiser, S. M., Dunham, K. A., Zoltowski, A. R., Failla, M. D., Cascio, C. J., & Woynaroski, T. G. (2023). Characterizing interoceptive differences in autism: A systematic review and meta-analysis of case–control studies. *Journal of Autism and Developmental Disorders, 53*(3), 947–962. https://doi.org/10.1007/s10803-022-05656-2

Wilson, A. C. (2024). Cognitive profile in autism and ADHD: A meta-analysis of performance on the WAIS-IV and WISC-V. *Archives of Clinical Neuropsychology, 39*(4), 498–515.

Wing, L., Leekam, S. R., Libby, S. J., Gould, J., & Larcombe, M. (2002). The diagnostic interview for social and communication disorders: Background, inter-rater reliability and clinical use. *Journal of Child Psychology and Psychiatry, 43*(3), 307–325.

Wolf, J. M., & Ventola, P. (2014). Assessment and treatment planning in adults with autism spectrum disorders. In *Adolescents and adults with autism spectrum disorders* (pp. 283–298). Springer New York.

Woodbury-Smith, M. (2014). Editorial: Autism and illegal behaviors. *Journal of Autism and Developmental Disorders, 44*(11), 2679–2681.

World Health Organization. (2001). *The world health report 2001: Mental health: New understanding, new hope.*

World Health Organization. (2003). *The world health report 2003: Shaping the future.* World Health Organization.

World Health Organization. (2019). *International statistical classification of diseases and related health problems* (11th ed.). https://icd.who.int/

Wright, S. D., Wright, C. A., D'Astous, V., & Wadsworth, A. M. (2019). Autism aging. *Gerontology & Geriatrics Education, 40*(3), 322–338.

Young, S., Hollingdale, J., Absoud, M., Bolton, P., Branney, P., Colley, W., Craze, E., Dave, M., Deeley, W., Farrag, E., Gudjonsson, G., Hill, P., Liang, H. I., Murphy, C., Mackintosh, P., Murin, M., O'Regan, F., Ougrin, D., Rios, P., … Woodhouse, E. (2020). Guidance for identification and treatment of individuals with attention deficit/hyperactivity disorder and autism spectrum disorder based upon expert consensus. *BMC Medicine, 18*, 1–29.

Comprehensive Feeding Assessment for Individuals on the Autism Spectrum: Exploring Multidisciplinary Approaches with Emphasis on Individual and Cultural Considerations

Hannah Young, Meg Stone-Heaberlin, Jill C. Fodstad, Ashley McGinn, and Maura L. Rouse Altman

Abstract Adequate nutrition is key for healthy growth and development. Unfortunately, for individuals on the autism spectrum, feeding difficulties are a common concern and, therefore, their growth and development may be compromised by inadequate nutrition. Given the chronic and pervasive nature of feeding and other associated eating difficulties in the autistic community, interventions to improve nutrition are needed. Before proper treatment can occur, a comprehensive behavioral, medical, and developmental feeding assessment should occur. The purpose of this chapter is to discuss the value of working within a multidisciplinary team for assessing feeding difficulties in autistic individuals. We review the various provider roles during a multidisciplinary feeding assessment when formulating targeted interventions. Further, we discuss the importance of considering the role of the individual and their family, as

H. Young (✉)
Division of Behavioral Medicine and Clinical Psychology, Cincinnati Children's Hospital Medical Center, Cincinnati, OH, USA
e-mail: hannah.young@cchmc.org

M. Stone-Heaberlin
University of Cincinnati College of Medicine, Cincinnati, OH, USA

Department of Pediatrics, Cincinnati Children's Hospital Medical Center, Cincinnati, USA

M. Stone-Heaberlin
e-mail: megan.stone@cchmc.org

J. C. Fodstad
Department of Psychiatry, Indiana University School of Medicine, Indianapolis, IN, USA
e-mail: jfodstad@iu.edu

Indiana University Health, Indianapolis, IN, USA

A. McGinn · M. L. R. Altman
Department of Pediatrics, Indiana University School of Medicine, Indianapolis, USA
e-mail: amcginn@iu.edu

M. L. R. Altman
e-mail: rousem@iu.edu

J. L. Matson (ed.), *Assessment and Diagnosis in Autism*, Autism and Child Psychopathology Series, https://doi.org/10.1007/978-3-032-11802-8_7

well as their preferences, values, and family culture when formulating an assessment plan.

Keywords Autism · Feeding disorders · Feeding assessment · Multidisciplinary team

Common Feeding Disorders in Autism

While not a core diagnostic symptom of Autism Spectrum Disorder (autism), feeding and mealtime difficulties are a common concern of caregivers. Estimates of feeding/eating difficulties in children with autism range from 50% to 90% (Baraskewich et al., 2021). Feeding difficulties in individuals on the autism spectrum are often chronic (Rodrigues et al., 2023; Suarez et al., 2014), and their presence impacts the quality of life not just for the person but also their family or caregivers. Food selectivity is the most common eating problem for individuals on the autism spectrum and includes refusal of entire food groups (e.g., fruits, vegetables, and proteins), restricted food variety (e.g., starches, snack, or processed foods), and excessive or selective intake (Bandini et al., 2010; Sharp et al., 2013).

Additional feeding difficulties are reported to occur across the autistic community. Food avoidance, also noted to occur in autistic children and adults, is the refusal to eat all or most developmentally appropriate foods presented. Avoidant/Restrictive Food Intake Disorder (ARFID), a severe form of food avoidance introduced in the Diagnostic and Statistical Manual of Mental Disorders, Fifth Edition (DSM-5; American Psychiatric Association, 2013), occurs when food avoidance or refusal reaches a chronic and pervasive level resulting in energy and nutritional deficits that has the potential to impact overall psychosocial functioning. Further, autistic individuals may have strong preferences in their eating or feeding habits including specific methods of food preparation or presentation, or mealtime rituals (e.g., insisting on same color plate, presenting food in a specific order, specific brands of food) (Twachtman-Reilly et al., 2008; Williams et al., 2000). Rumination, or the non-purposeful regurgitation of recently ingested food from the stomach to the mouth, is a serious feeding problem with associated health risks (e.g., malnutrition, weight loss, dehydration, tooth decay, choking and gastrointestinal bleeding, aspiration risk, decreased caloric intake; Lang et al., 2011; Seiverling et al., 2020). Additionally, Pica, the ingestion of non-food items without nutritional value (Fields et al., 2021), is more commonly seen in autistic individuals with co-occurring intellectual disability and, when present, can have potentially serious health impacts (Matson et al., 2011). Lastly, behavior problems, including aggression and tantrums, may also be associated with feeding especially when non-preferred foods are presented (Provost et al., 2010). Due to behavioral and cognitive rigidity, autistics are more likely to refuse to try new foods, eat smaller amounts and less variety, state they do not like a food without trying it, and/or be less interested in eating food and instead drink primarily liquids (Kozak et al., 2023). Depending on the severity or restrictedness of the feeding problems, it may limit the individual and family from participating in community activities or meals and can increase family stress (Thullen & Bonsall, 2017).

There is disagreement about the strength of correlation between having a diagnosis of autism and the severity of co-occurring feeding problems. There is some support to suggest that individuals with lower nonverbal intelligence, those with more internalizing and externalizing behavior problems, and individuals with more sensory differences may also experience more feeding problems (Page et al., 2022). Several possible causes of feeding problems have been suggested. For example, autistic individuals commonly experience sensory differences including under-responsivity and/or over-responsivity (Kozak et al., 2023) or struggle with feeding, in part, due to behavioral and cognitive rigidity (Johnson et al., 2014). Social communication differences, a hallmark of autism, may account for feeding difficulties. Individuals with autism may be less motivated by the social aspects of a meal and less able to imitate positive feeding habits modeled by others at the table (van Dijk et al., 2021). Further, Kral et al. (2015) wrote that feeding problems can be closely related to the behaviors of parents who may avoid mealtimes (due to stress) or attempt to force their children to eat. Additionally, food selection provided by parents may also play a role. As an example, Wallace and colleagues (2018) argue that feeding problems are cyclical. When children restrict the food they eat, a parent buys a narrower variety of foods, which children then eat. This then creates a cascading effect to multiple body systems, including the potential for oral motor deficits because they are not using as many chewing muscles and/or an increase in gastrointestinal problems due to a narrowed diet. Individuals with feeding problems and autism generally have more gastrointestinal problems such as abdominal pain and constipation (Leader et al., 2020).

There are a variety of other consequences of poor feeding. Individuals with autism and feeding problems are at higher risk for nutritional deficiency and stunted growth (Bandini et al., 2010; Sharp et al., 2013), as they typically eat fewer fruits and vegetables and ingest lower amounts of calcium and protein (Sharp et al., 2013). Many prefer carbohydrates and high fat foods (Wallace et al., 2018), leading to concerns for obesity (Kral et al., 2015).

Regardless of how or why, or what type, of feeding problems occur in those on the autism spectrum, these difficulties occur at a high rate causing concern by parents and caregivers. This chapter focuses on assessing feeding problems in the autistic population. A first step is examining the value of a multidisciplinary team assessment and considering the role different disciplines have in the assessment process. Finally, the chapter also examines individual considerations that need to be made in feeding assessment and highlights the importance of culturally responsive care.

The Importance of a Multidisciplinary Approach

Feeding disorders are multifaceted in etiology and presentation; therefore, having several disciplines involved in assessment and treatment is best practice (Goday et al., 2019). Disciplines typically included in the team include physicians, registered dieticians, psychologists, behavior analysts, occupational therapists, speech-language pathologists, social workers, the individual themselves, and the caregivers of that individual with feeding difficulties (Goday et al., 2019). Each discipline has an important role to play, and including their expertise can be vital in ensuring that the team has a complete understanding to the medical, physical, developmental, diagnosis-specific, and psychosocial factors that contribute to the individual's feeding difficulties and should be addressed in any comprehensive treatment plan. Furthermore, the individual themselves and their family also have an important role and should be involved collaboratively with assessment, goal setting, and intervention.

Medical Support and Assessment

Primary Care

When caregivers express concern regarding their child's nutrition, weight, or ability to eat or self-feed, they typically seek guidance from their pediatric or primary care physician (PCP). As a result, the PCP often serves as the initial point of contact for assessing and managing feeding and eating concerns. Whether functioning as part of a multidisciplinary feeding team or independently, the PCP conducts an initial comprehensive physical examination to identify any active medical conditions, motor concerns, anatomical abnormalities, or other physiological or biopsychosocial factors contributing to the feeding difficulties (Beaudry-Bellefeuille et al., 2021; Dharmaraj et al., 2023).

During the physical examination, a full developmental (including prenatal, birth, and postnatal), medical, and feeding/dietary history is collected (Kleinert, 2017). This process involves clarifying the presence of a motor disability or delay (e.g., cerebral palsy, spina bifida, and fine motor delay), constipation, and/or sleep patterns that may affect eating or feeding habits. Screening for food allergies or syndromes contributing to the presenting difficulties can indicate the need for further testing to assess if there is an inability to digest or metabolize certain proteins. Additionally, it is important to note any prescribed medications with known side effects impacting appetite, ability to swallow, or quality of taste sensations, and then identify strategies to manage these factors in treatment. Anthropometric parameters such as height, weight, head circumference (for young children), and body mass index (BMI) are calculated to evaluate the nutritional status, growth pattern relative to age-and height-based normative data, and overall health and development. Identifying if the person is underweight (BMI for age <5th percentile), overweight (BMI for age, 85th–94th percentile), or obese (BMI for age >95th percentile) is important as all are associated with negative health and developmental outcomes (Bass & Eneli, 2015; Rudolf & Logan, 2005). Reviewing individual and family eating preferences, mealtime habits, and normal diet aids can also assist in identifying if nutritional deficiencies exist. Cataloging foods consistently eaten across food groups may be particularly important as individuals on the autism spectrum are more likely to be of minimally adequate anthropometric status but may not consume a nutritiously diverse diet due to extreme food selectivity or ARFID (Esteban-Figuerola et al., 2019; Zimmer et al., 2012).

Given the diagnostic complexity of autism, the PCP must adopt a higher level of scrutiny during the medical work-up and a lower threshold for making referrals to subspecialists for added consultation and testing. A thorough anatomical assessment should occur, beginning with the mouth and moving through the esophagus, stomach, intestines, and associated systems. The PCP performs an oral-facial examination to assess symmetry; shape and height of the hard and soft palate; movement of the tongue, lips, jaw, and velum; cranial nerves; and the ability to manage secretions to identify any sign of pain, neurologic, or anatomical abnormality. Those with a history of prematurity, intubation, and/or chronic respiratory problems should be referred to an otolaryngologist for evaluation of the airway structure and vocal cord function. Current presence or history of spitting up, gagging, multiple swallows, wet voice, vomiting, discomfort while eating, or choking should trigger concerns for aspiration or other esophageal pathology including gastroesophageal reflux disease (GERD; Buie et al., 2010). The PCP also completes an abdominal, cardiorespiratory, and neurologic exam to assess for abnormalities that could affect the ability to self-feed or eat successfully.

Following the physical examination, the PCP may order blood work, an endoscopy and x-ray of the upper digestive tract, a fiberoptic endoscopic evaluation of swallow, or consultation requests from collaborating specialists. Medical referrals that may be considered include gastroenterology, dentistry, hematology, cardiology, nephrology, endocrinology, pulmonology, neurology, and/or genetics. These additional tests aim to identify nutritional deficiencies, inflammatory and allergic processes, anatomic abnormalities, and functional deficits, among others, contributing to feeding difficulties, informing treatment planning, and ongoing monitoring. While some interventions can be managed fully with primary care, the ideal solution for many cases involves a referral to multidisciplinary feeding clinics where multiple providers work collaboratively to assess the presenting problem. At this stage, the PCP continues to assess outcomes, monitor physical health and growth, provide family support, and coordinate referrals as needed.

Gastroenterology

Gastrointestinal (GI) difficulties are prevalent within the autistic community, with reported rates ranging from 46% to 84% in children (Leader et al., 2022). Common co-occurring GI problems include food intolerance or sensitivities, gut motility issues, insufficient digestive enzyme activity, nausea or vomiting, chronic constipation, diarrhea, GERD, abdominal discomfort or inflammation, and/or failure to thrive. The etiology of these difficulties is multifaceted, stemming from inherent features of autism (e.g., rigidity, food selectivity, sensory processing difficulties) and the elevated prevalence of certain co-occurring conditions (e.g., genetic mutations or variations, gut microbiota imbalance, immune system dysfunction, impaired gut-brain axis; Al-Beltagi et al., 2023). Further, due to expressive language difficulties and sensory processing difference in the autism population, GI conditions may present atypically (e.g., gritting teeth, facial grimacing, pica, applying pressure to the abdomen, disordered sleep, unusual posturing, or sudden and unexplained, irritability, self-injury, or aggression; Buie et al., 2010). Given the increased prevalence of and unique presentation of GI difficulties in those on the autism spectrum, research underscores the importance of assessing or addressing digestive concerns before developing treatments targeting feeding difficulties (Al-Beltagi et al., 2023).

A gastroenterologist plays a vital role when feeding and eating are impacted by issues related to the GI tract. The assessment process for potential GI abnormalities varies based on the presenting symptoms. When maldigestion or malabsorption is suspected, a gastroenterologist typically conducts relevant laboratory tests and performs an upper endoscopy (i.e., esophagogastroduodenoscopy or EGD) to measure disaccharidases, which are digestive enzymes in the gut. Individuals with swallowing difficulties or showing signs of esophageal pathology (e.g., spitting up, gagging, or vomiting during or after meals; eating discomfort; texture limited to liquids or purees) should be evaluated for esophageal inflammation. In cases of odynophagia (i.e., pain or burning sensation during swallowing), an upper GI contrast study is performed to assess the anatomy and motility of the upper GI tract. An EGD may also be necessary to biopsy the enteric mucosa and examine for signs of eosinophilic esophagitis, including esophageal rings, linear furrows, white plaques, or exudates. A pH probe may be recommended to quantify reflux for diagnosing GERD, and some may require esophageal manometry to evaluate upper GI tract motility. Based upon results from these various assessments, the gastroenterologist may prescribe and monitor the outcomes of "acid blockade" medications, such as proton pump inhibitors or histamine-2 antagonists, to support esophageal healing (Dipasquale et al., 2022). In instances where acid blocker medications are ineffective at reducing esophageal and upper GI abnormalities, a gastroenterologist can assist the team in making decisions regarding further treatment options like off-label use of Baclofen, topical steroid or monoclonal antibodies (for eosinophilic esophagitis), anti-reflux surgery, or enteral feeding (Berg & Khlevner, 2021; Hungin et al., 2019; Rossetti et al., 2020).

For individuals whose feeding difficulties may be related to bowel abnormalities such as constipation, diarrhea, abdominal bloating or pain, chronic flatulence, or inflammatory bowel pathology, a gastroenterologist can aid in assessing, diagnosing, and addressing contributing factors. Functional constipation, stool withholding, and poor bowel control often seen in autistic individuals can improve through laxatives, family support, and behavioral toileting strategies (Seidler et al., 2022). However, in cases where constipation and bowel issues persist despite negative allergy test results, dietary modifications, behavioral toilet training, laxatives, and fiber supplementation trials, further diagnostic testing and medical interventions may be necessary (Al-Beltagi et al., 2023). Depending upon concerns, a gastroenterologist may order anorectal testing with manometry, a balloon expulsion test, barium or magnetic resonance defecography, intestinal endoscopy, abdominal x-rays or CT scan, enteroscopy, colonoscopy, or a digital rectal exam (Tran & Sintusek, 2023). These assessments can help find anatomical abnormalities or significant pathology, including structural disorders, fecal impaction, colon transit and motility dysfunction, or irritable bowel syndrome. Based upon results from these assessments, the gastroenterologist may prescribe targeted medications to address bowel inflammation and pain, accelerate GI motility, promote more water and sodium secretions in the gut, and reduce constipation (e.g., guanylate cyclase C-receptor agonists, serotonin agonists, sodium/hydrogen exchanger isoform 3-inhibitors), and also determine if anal irrigation/fecal disimpaction or surgery (e.g., percutaneous cecostomy and Malone appendicostomy) are necessary (Włodarczyk et al., 2021).

Dietary Support

A registered dietician is often part of the multidisciplinary team that evaluates an individual's feeding behaviors and their impact on health and development. In partnership with the PCP, a dietician may assess feeding concerns by reviewing data collected from food records, blood screening, and anthropometric measures, such as height, weight, and body mass index (BMI) (Ptomey & Wittenbrook, 2015). These assessment methods help clinicians understand the dietary diversity of what a person is consuming, if they have nutritional deficiencies, and if their growth is impacted by their feeding behaviors (Ptomey & Wittenbrook, 2015).

As mentioned, food selectivity is one of the most common feeding problems associated with autism (Cermak et al., 2010). Approximately two-thirds of children with autism and food selectivity do not consume vegetables and just under one-third of children do not consume fruit (Sharp et al., 2018). Dieticians partner with physicians to order blood screening, which can be used to evaluate for nutritional inadequacies in individuals with identified low dietary diversity or clinical symptoms of nutritional deficiency (Van Hoorn et al., 2023). Autistic individuals have been found to consume less calcium, fewer servings of dairy, and less vitamins E and B6 compared to peers (Herndon et al., 2009). These limited food preferences can result in decreased dietary diversity, measured by using food records over the course of one to three days and adding up the number foods or food groups consumed (Ruel, 2003). Additional dietary diversity measures have been developed to more specifically evaluate the number of servings from different food groups compared to the recommended dietary guidelines (Ruel, 2003). If concerns are noted for limited dietary diversity, clinicians may recommend multi-nutrient oral supplementation to support the person's nutritional needs. Individuals who are not able to consume enough calories by mouth may require nasogastric tube or gastrostomy tube (g-tube) feedings (Dharmaraj et al.,

2023), and a dietician would collaborate with other medical professionals (e.g., pediatrician, gastroenterology) for a full medical work-up to place, monitor, and make adjustments to enteral feedings to ensure the individual's nutritional needs are met.

Speech-Language Pathologist (SLP)

A speech-language pathologist (SLP)'s role in feeding disorder assessment may include the evaluation of swallowing concerns and possible aspiration. SLPs also investigate if the individual has oral motor concerns that are influencing the way a person uses their lips, teeth, and jaw while eating (Dharmaraj et al., 2023).

Oral-Motor Dysfunction/Dysphagia

A clinical interview, physical exam, or feeding observation may indicate concern for oral-motor dysfunction. Indicators include drooling excessively, abnormal muscle tone, excessive gagging or choking, and difficulty meeting expected feeding milestones (Dharmaraj et al., 2023). Evaluating oral-motor function starts with assessing a person's facial features and symmetry, in addition to the position and movement of the lips, jaw, and tongue. Laryngeal functions, such as vocal pitch, quality, and intensity are also considered (Dharmaraj et al., 2023). Additionally, oral reflexes and nonnutritive sucking are evaluated in young infants (Arvedson, 2008; Dharmaraj et al., 2023).

Dysphagia is characterized by challenges swallowing, or transitioning food and/or liquids from the mouth to the esophagus when eating (Dharmaraj et al., 2023). These difficulties can occur at four different stages of the swallowing process including, the oral stage (when food or liquid enters the mouth until it moves over the tongue), initiation of the swallow, pharyngeal phase (from the beginning of the swallow until the chewed food enters the esophagus), and finally the esophageal phase (which starts and ends at the upper and lower esophageal sphincters; Arvedson, 2008). There are also multiple levels of dysphasia, from complete dysphasia that includes difficulty swallowing all food textures, to dysphasia with only liquids with low viscosity (Dharmaraj et al., 2023). These swallowing difficulties can result in aspiration, which is when food, liquid, or saliva get below the trachea and into the lungs (Arvedson, 2008; Calvo et al., 2016). Aspiration can increase risk for pneumonia (Kelly et al., 2007; Weir et al., 2007) and other health complications, such as chronic airway disease and lung damage (Miller, 2011).

Video Fluoroscopy Swallow Study

A video fluoroscopic swallow study (VFSS) is often completed by a SLP in partnership with a radiologist or specialist to identify dysphagia. This involves x-ray video recording of an individual chewing and swallowing food and liquids (bolus) containing barium and observing it move from the person's mouth through the pharynx and into the esophagus. This measure can help assess the function of the esophagus, identify reflux, and structural abnormalities (Dharmaraj et al., 2023). The SLP can identify if there are instances of aspiration and determine if this occurs before, during, or after the person swallows. SLPs also identify the consistency of the liquids or foods that are consumed leading to aspiration (Arvedson, 2008). Limitations of the VFSS include radiation exposure; however, the dose is considered very low (Matsuo & Palmer, 2016). It is also not recommended for infants and very young children with limited oral feeding skills (Miller, 2011).

Fiberoptic Endoscopic Evaluation of Swallow

A fiberoptic endoscopic evaluation of swallow (FEES) is another measure that can be used to investigate concerns for dysphagia. This assessment involves placing a small endoscope through the nose and down into the pharynx and larynx to evaluate their functioning. This allows for the evaluation of the person's ability to manage oral secretions and spontaneous swallowing (Miller, 2011). There are limitations in the FEES related to the assessment of the oral and esophageal phases; however, it has advantages in identifying structural differences in the pharynx of children compared to the VFSS (Miller & Wilging, 2019).

Occupational Therapy (OT)

Individuals with autism are more likely to have challenges with oral-sensory processing (Chistol et al., 2018), which can be evaluated by an occupational therapist (OT). Oral-sensory difficulties include orally sorting out foods of different textures, holding food in the cheek or under the tongue to avoid swallowing, vomiting related to specific textures, and gagging when foods approach or touch the lips (Arvedson, 2008). Occupational therapists often use a combination of parent interview, medical record review, questionnaires, and direct observation to evaluate feeding skills and inform treatment (Rabaey et al., 2023). *The Sensory Processing Measure* (SPM; Parham et al., 2021) is a standardized measure that includes caregiver and teacher questionnaires to gain information about six different sensory systems including tactile, olfactory, and gustatory systems. The *Sensory Profile-2* (SP-2; Dunn, 2014) also includes caregiver and teacher questionnaires that can be used by occupational therapists to gain additional information regarding a child's sensory differences related to feeding (i.e., touch, oral sensory, and their experience in different environments).

While not all sensory differences can be noted during informant-based measures, the OT should also make note of any other sensory differences during clinical observation or parent interview that may be impacting the feeding or eating success of the individual on the autism spectrum. Oral over-responsiveness, under-responsiveness, and oral-seeking behaviors are additional sensory differences often noted in autistics that may relate to nutritional intake difficulties. Oral over-responsiveness includes aversions to food textures that results in increased food selectivity. Under-responsiveness is associated with decreased sensation resulting in over-stuffing behavior. Oral-seeking behavior includes putting a variety of items in the mouth for oral stimulation (Cermak et al., 2010). Additional sensory sensitivities to smell and noise can also be part of the mealtime environment influencing behaviors (Cermak et al., 2010).

In addition to sensory differences, children with feeding difficulties may also have motor skill delays that are impacting their feeding success. Occupational therapists can specifically evaluate a child's motor skills related to feeding, such as picking up small pieces of food, grasping utensils, and holding a cup. These observations may be made during direct observation or difficulties may be noted during a caregiver interview. Further evaluation of a child's fine motor and gross motor skills are commonly evaluated with standardized measures such as the Bruininks-Oseretsky Test of Motor Proficiency, 2nd edition (BOT-2; Bruininks & Bruininks, 2005) which is used with children ages 4 through twenty-one. The fine motor portion includes assessment of fine motor precision and integration, manual dexterity, and upper-limb coordination. In younger children, ages birth to five, the Peabody Developmental Motor Scales-Third Edition (PDMS-3; Folio & Fewell, 2023) includes five core subtests to evaluate a child's eye-hand coordination, hand manipulation, object control skills, body transport, and body control. Evaluation of a child's motor skills that may impact feeding success should be completed before developing a feeding intervention.

Psychological and Behavioral Assessment

Autistic individuals may display distinctive feeding difficulties and atypical feeding behaviors including food selectivity, food avoidance, problems associated with rigidity or rituals, challenging behaviors during mealtime, and pica. Assuming that medical and/or physiological concerns are ruled out as a primary contributing factor, feeding problems should be assessed from the psychological and behavioral perspective. In these instances, psychologists and Board Certified Behavior Analysts (BCBA) are often included on the feeding assessment team due to the expertise in behavioral science and understanding of cognitive-behavioral strategies that can promote change in behavior over time.

A psychologist and/or BCBA can perform a variety of assessments to gather data about the feeding problem and determine the function, or reason, it occurs. Factors such as the individual's behavior, caregiver's behavior, type of behavior (e.g., aggression, self-injury, tantrums, inappropriate mealtime behavior, negative vocalizations/ language), and severity of that behavior are all considered (Kleinert, 2017). Once the function (e.g., tangible, escape, attention, automatic) is identified, specific techniques and strategies are put into place to modify the mealtime environment (e.g., structure, setting, caregivers, or family members involved) to decrease the problematic behavior. Additional feeding goals often focus on increasing the variety and/or amount of food eaten by the individual.

Variables related to the maintenance of problematic feeding behavior are often identified through a combination of behavioral assessment strategies including indirect questionnaires or logs, direct observation, and functional analysis. These assessments primarily focus on the autistic individual's feeding behavior, but often look at the interaction between the individual and caregiver during mealtime.

Indirect Questionnaires, Logs, and Caregiver Interview

Several indirect assessment procedures can help in identifying variables related to the individual's feeding problem. Indirect measures, most often completed by the primary caregiver, are an ideal and collaborative component in the assessment of feeding difficulties, as they provide the caregiver's impression of the feeding problem and common factors affecting success in the home mealtime environment. A variety of indirect measures exist and have been utilized by clinicians for decades.

The *Aut-Eat Questionnaire* (AEQ; Gal et al., 2022) is a relatively new caregiver-report questionnaire used to assess the breadth of eating problems and feeding profile of children with autism between the ages of 3 and 8. The questionnaire includes six categories of eating problems: chewing and swallowing problems, eating avoidance, eating selectivity, eating sameness and rituals, over-eating, and problem behavior during mealtime, as well as a food list eaten by the child, that is subdivided into specific food categories (Gal et al., 2022). The *Brief Autism Mealtime Behavior Inventory* (BAMBI; Lukens & Linscheid, 2008) and the revised *Brief Assessment of Mealtime Behavior in Children* (BAMBIC; Hendy et al., 2013) were designed for the clinical assessment of feeding behavior in individuals with autism aged 18 months old to 17 years old. These tools provide an overall feeding problem severity score, as well as scores on three subscales: limited food variety, food refusal, and disruptive behavior. Each subscale matches to common feeding problems and aids in determining treatment outcomes. Additionally, the SWedish Eating Assessment (SWEAA) (Karlsson et al., 2013) is self-reported structured questionnaire with 81 items, which was normed on autistic individuals ages 15 and 25 years old. Finally, the inclusion of an indirect, caregiver-report functional assessment measure or interview may also provide critical information to assist with developing hypotheses on factors that influence or maintain feeding behavior in the home environment. The *Questions about Behavioral Function* (QABF; Matson & Vollmer, 1995) is a caregiver report measure used to hypothesize functions of problem behaviors in individuals with autism and co-occurring intellectual disability. It is unique in its usefulness in assessing the functions of feeding and mealtime-related problem behavior using caregiver input (Matson et al., 2005).

Several other caregiver-report measures have been commonly used when assessing feeding difficulties in the autism population, although these were not normed on individuals on the autism spectrum specifically. The *Screening Tool of Feeding Problems* (STEP; Matson & Kuhn, 2001) is a widely used 23-item scale for individuals ages 2–18 that targets specific feeding problems, such as food selectivity (by type or texture), eating too quickly, vomiting, and pushing food away. The STEP includes five subscales corresponding to aspiration risk, food selectivity, feeding and eating skills, problem behaviors during mealtimes, and nutrition. While not specific to autistic individuals, the STEP is suitable for this population given the wide range of feeding problems often observed in autism, especially in those with co-occurring intellectual disability. Additionally, the *Children's Eating Behavior Inventory* (CEBI; Archer et al., 1991), *Behavioral Pediatrics Feeding Assessment Scale* (BPFAS; Crist & Napier-Phillips, 2001), *Parent Mealtime Action Scale* (PMAS; Hendy et al., 2009), and *Mealtime Behavior Questionnaire* (MBQ; Berlin et al., 2010) are caregiver-report measures that assist with identifying child, caregiver, and family factors that contribute to feeding and mealtime problems. Again, while not specific to autism, their recognition of the many variables that influence a person's feeding and mealtime habits may be beneficial for including in the initial assessment process.

In addition to indirect questionnaires that identify and categorize specific feeding or mealtime behaviors, identifying the individual's food preferences and current consumption level can be beneficial. This can be done through a clinical interview with the family, as well as the individual, if appropriate. Further, clinicians can use one of a variety of structured inventories (e.g., Aponte & Romanczyk, 2016; Bandini et al., 2010; Pizzo et al., 2009) to determine which foods to target during intervention by asking caregivers about the foods their family regularly consumes, relevant cultural practices, and the individual's current food preferences. Foods targeted for intervention include those relevant to the family or culture and/or those important to the autistic individual's preferences or nutrition. Oftentimes, including a registered dietician during this step is helpful with ensuring adequate representation of food groups and consideration for calories consumed. The *Food Preference Inventory* (FPI; Willet, 1998) is used to identify target foods for intervention, and it can be used as a treatment outcome measure. The FPI includes 154 items across seven food categories (i.e., fruits, vegetables, proteins, starches, dairy, miscellaneous/snacks, and combination foods). Autistic individuals and/or their caregivers rate their consumption level of various foods using a Likert-type scale (never, with prodding, willing, favorite, or not applicable). The FPI then provides a food selectivity score for each food category, as well as an overall total selectivity score.

Though less formal, a food log or journal is another indirect measure used to assess feeding difficulties. The individual an/or caregivers document information regarding the individual's feeding habits, including time of meals, duration of meals, foods accepted or rejected, and quantity of food ingested. It is also important to document external factors that occur during family mealtime (e.g. distractions in the home, siblings, media, or television, etc.) which must be incorporated into and accounted for, yet are rarely witnessed in a clinical setting. Best practice suggests a data collection period of consecutive days lasting 1–2 weeks prior to treatment (Harvey et al., 2015).

Direct Observation

Another way to assess feeding difficulties involves clinical observation of a meal involving the autistic individual and the primary caregiver. This naturalistic observation provides valuable information regarding mealtime behaviors and interactions. It assists in determining both antecedents and consequences that maintain the problematic feeding behaviors. During the observation, the caregiver presents preferred and non-preferred foods while the psychologist or BCBA records specific mealtimes behaviors, including foods accepted or refused, the individual's behavior, and caregiver responses to appropriate and inappropriate behaviors (Aponte & Romanczyk, 2016; Gale et al., 2011; Piazza et al., 2003; Silverman, 2015). This observation can occur in the clinic or at home. Telemedicine is a relatively new but effective modality for clinicians to observe naturalistic mealtime behaviors in the home (Peterson et al., 2021). Some researchers have discussed using direct observations of the individual eating either as a self-feeder (if able to do so) or with a clinician-feeder. Often in this assessment, a selection of foods from different food groups and/or of different texture levels are presented to the individual and data is taken on the number of bites accepted (Ahearn et al., 2001). Regardless, outcomes from direct mealtime observations are beneficial for treatment planning, as well as monitoring progress over time.

Functional Analysis

A functional analysis (FA) is a formalized, evidence-based process of observing and collecting data on an individual's behaviors and interactions with others. This direct assessment involves the systematic manipulation of antecedents and consequences to determine their influence on targeted behaviors (Iwata et al., 1994; Oliver et al., 2015; Roscoe et al., 2015). Investigators have explored the utility of FA as it relates to feeding disorders and other mealtime difficulties in individuals with autism with or without co-occurring intellectual disability (Hodges et al., 2020; Oliver et al., 2015; Roscoe et al., 2015). FAs identify variables that maintain problematic feeding behaviors, which aides in determining function-based interventions. While time-consuming, a FA is a more ideal assessment strategy compared to indirect, non-experimental methods, or even direct observation of a mealtime, as it is an objective method to measure outcomes when directly manipulating the environment and feeder behavior (caregiver or clinician) in response to the individual's behaviors (Thompson & Iwata, 2007). In general, FA is optimized when used in combination with other behavioral assessment strategies and is best for unclear or complicated cases.

A FA for feeding and mealtime behaviors is led by a psychologist or BCBA and includes a series of control and test conditions. Test conditions (i.e., attention, escape, tangible) are designed to mimic the consequences (or responses) caregivers most often use during meals. In the attention condition, the clinician provides verbal or physical attention each time the person engages in the target feeding behavior (e.g., expulsions, batting at the spoon, head turning). During the escape condition, the clinician allows the individual to take a brief break from eating following the target behavior. Finally, during the tangible condition, the clinician provides a toy, activity, or another food item when the individual engages in the target feeding behavior. Across most research using FA methods, escape from the mealtime, or the demand of consuming non-preferred or new foods, is the most common function of feeding problems for individuals with autism (Kirkwood et al., 2021; Piazza et al., 2003). Conversely, many have noted that escape from sensory aspects of the food (e.g., texture, temperature, smell, etc.; Nadon et al., 2011; Sharp et al., 2013) or other psychologically/physiologically related concerns (e.g., perceived pain, fear of choking; (Twachtman-Reilly et al., 2008) may be under-detected in those with autism, and should also be considered.

Supporting Family Involvement

During the multidisciplinary assessment process, it is important for team members to consider how parenting an individual with autism can impact the family (Chan & Leung, 2020). In many cultures, mealtimes are weaved into family tradition and associated with wellbeing and positive health outcomes (Le Moal et al., 2021). However, families of individuals on the spectrum may experience additional challenges and stress that impact the family unit (Thullen & Bonsall, 2017). Further, autism-related assessments and interventions are costly (Tinelli et al., 2023). Thus, social workers can play an important role on the assessment team because of their specialized expertise in family-centered care and their focus on supporting caregivers. In order to ensure the family's ability to participate in the feeding assessment and the treatment plan to the fullest, it is important to recognize and attempt to alleviate caregiver stress, financial constraints, and other limitations (e.g., transportation, food scarcity). Thus, social work can play a crucial role in coordinating care among the team and other specialists, providing knowledge, and accessing valuable resources that can ultimately improve outcomes. Social workers should be embedded in each step of feeding assessment to ensure that the autistic individual and the family are heard and supported, serve as an advocate, and ensure that the assessment process does not cause undue or unexpected emotional or financial burden.

Culturally Responsive Practices and Honoring the Individual

Research supports that people want to have a trust-based relationship with their providers (Taylor et al., 2015). Thus, providers should seek to understand the experiences of the autistic individual and their family to build trust and ultimately engage in a collaborative feeding assessment process.

Cultural Considerations

When providing services, it is important for the team to acknowledge and respect the diversity and identities of the individual and their family. As part of their typical assessment procedures, providers should seek to understand the perspective, family and cultural background, and other identities of the individual and incorporate the person's strengths when developing a plan for assessment. This individual and family-centered approach can also help the team prepare for and discuss openly any potential barriers to assessment or treatment (e.g., readiness to change, language differences, cultural dietary preferences, or family communication style). A collaborative and trusting relationship among the feeding team has been shown to drive better outcomes (McCafferty & McCutcheon, 2021).

Feeding practices are unique between different racial and ethnic cultures, but also within cultures. Variability in feeding practices includes types of food, rituals and routines around eating, and beliefs about health and nutrition (Davis-McFarland, 2008). Therefore, providers should first taking the time to understand the person's culture and beliefs, as this will provide insight about the best path forward for assessing feeding difficulties. Providers should also strive to provide culturally responsive care by examining and working through their own biases or beliefs.

Understanding Neurodiversity and Respecting Autonomy

Neurodiversity refers to the reality that diverse minds and brains exist (Walker, 2014). The neurodiversity approach highlights the importance of honoring differences instead of focusing on deficits; respecting neurodiverse culture and value; and incorporating neurodivergent minds in the development and execution of research, assessment, and treatment (Rutherford & Johnston, 2023). Historically, goals have been initiated and designed by individuals who identify as *neurotypical*, which may not respect nor align with autistic culture or preferences. The medical model, an approach used traditionally and for decades, assumes that there is something "wrong" or "broken" in the person with the disability, which ultimately leads to *ableism* (i.e., discrimination in favor of able-bodied people; Mathur et al., 2024).

The social model on disabilities re-conceptualizes the approach to care into social, cultural, and political constructs but continues to recognize the presence of impaired functioning (Mathur et al., 2024). The social model acknowledges that the differences in understanding disability result from different cultural contexts leading to a shift in how assessment or treatment are implemented (Mathur et al., 2024). Instead, a strengths-based and collaborative approach to care should be used. By recognizing autistic culture broadly, as well as the individual's preferences and abilities, realistic goals, and objectives can be developed (Mathur et al., 2024). When it comes to assessing food consumption or food variety to improve nutritional needs, the person's health is the utmost goal. However, the family and the individual should be stakeholders in the decision-making process regarding the assessments completed, which foods to be targeted, and the eventual treatment priorities.

Conclusion

Using a multidisciplinary approach to feeding allows for relevant disciplines to assess feeding difficulties through collaboration (Goday et al., 2019) and is individual and family-centered. Given the complexity of feeding difficulties for individuals on the spectrum, the team approach can minimize resources required from the family to receive treatment (e.g., limiting number of clinic visits; Arvedson, 2008). Additionally, collaborating and providing education to the individual and their family about the assessment process brings in the individual and their caregivers as stakeholders on the team and offers a rational for treatment. This ultimately can increase the family's fidelity to implementation and generalization outside of the clinic. Most importantly, team members should honor preferences unique to the individual and family as they relate to feeding assessment, and maintain open communication throughout the assessment process to ensure that the individual and the family are a part of the decision-making team.

References

Ahearn, W. H., Castine, T., Nault, K., & Green, G. (2001). An assessment of food acceptance in children with autism or pervasive developmental disorder-not otherwise specified. *Journal of Autism and Developmental Disorders, 31*(5), 505–511. https://doi.org/10.1023/a:1012221026124

Al-Beltagi, M., Saeed, N. K., Bediwy, A. S., Elbeltagi, R., & Alhawamdeh, R. (2023). Role of gastrointestinal health in managing children with autism spectrum disorder. *World Journal of Clinical Pediatrics, 12*(4), 171–196. https://doi.org/10.5409/wjcp.v12.i4.171

American Psychiatric Association. (2013). *Diagnostic and statistical manual of mental disorders* (5th ed.). https://doi.org/10.1176/appi.books.9780890425596

Aponte, C. A., & Romanczyk, R. G. (2016). Assessment of feeding problems in children with autism spectrum disorder. *Research in Autism Spectrum Disorders, 21*, 61–72. https://doi.org/10.1016/j.rasd.2015.09.007

Archer, L. A., Rosenbaum, P. L., & Streiner, D. L. (1991). The children's eating behavior inventory: Reliability and validity results. *Journal of Pediatric Psychology, 16*(5), 629–642. https://doi.org/10.1093/jpepsy/16.5.629

Arvedson, J. C. (2008). Assessment of pediatric dysphagia and feeding disorders: Clinical and instrumental approaches. *Developmental Disabilities Research Reviews, 14*(2), 118–127. https://doi.org/10.1002/ddrr.17

Bandini, L. G., Anderson, S. E., Curtin, C., Cermak, S., Evans, E. W., Scampini, R., Maslin, M., & Must, A. (2010). Food selectivity in children with autism spectrum disorders and typically developing children. *The Journal of Pediatrics, 157*(2), 259–264. https://doi.org/10.1016/j.jpeds.2010.02.013

Baraskewich, J., von Ranson, K. M., McCrimmon, A., & McMorris, C. A. (2021). Feeding and eating problems in children and adolescents with autism: A scoping review. *Autism: The International Journal of Research and Practice, 25*(6), 1505–1519. https://doi.org/10.1177/1362361321995631

Bass, R., & Eneli, I. (2015). Severe childhood obesity: An under-recognised and growing health problem. *Postgraduate Medical Journal, 91*(1081), 639–645. https://doi.org/10.1136/postgradmedj-2014-133033

Beaudry-Bellefeuille, I., Pomoni, M., Welch, A., Moriyón-Iglesias, T., Suárez-González, M., & Ramos-Polo, E. (2021). Multidisciplinary approach to assessment and intervention of feeding problems in children with autism spectrum disorders: A clinical perspective. *Irish Journal of Occupational Therapy, 49*(2), 77–83. https://doi.org/10.1108/IJOT-12-2020-0019

Berg, E. A., & Khlevner, J. (2021). Treatment of gastroesophageal reflux disease in children. *Pediatrics in Review, 42*(1), 51–53. https://doi.org/10.1542/pir.2020-001602

Berlin, K. S., Davies, W. H., Silverman, A. H., Woods, D. W., Fischer, E. A., & Rudolph, C. D. (2010). Assessing children's mealtime problems with the Mealtime Behavior Questionnaire. *Children's Health Care, 39*(2), 142–156. https://doi.org/10.1080/02739611003679956

Bruininks, R. H., & Bruininks B. D. (2005). *Bruininks-Oseretsky Test of motor proficiency* (2nd ed.; BOT-2). Pearson.

Buie, T., Campbell, D. B., Fuchs, G. J., Furuta, G. T., Levy, J., Vandewater, J., Whitaker, A. H., Atkins, D., Bauman, M. L., Beaudet, A. L., Carr, E. G., Gershon, M. D., Hyman, S. L., Jirapinyo, P., Jyonouchi, H., Kooros, K., Kushak, R., Levitt, P., Levy, S. E., … Winter, H. (2010). Evaluation, diagnosis, and treatment of gastrointestinal disorders in individuals with ASDs: A consensus report. *Pediatrics, 125*(Suppl. 1), S1–18. https://doi.org/10.1542/peds.2009-1878C

Calvo, I., Conway, A., Henriques, F., & Walshe, M. (2016). Diagnostic accuracy of the clinical feeding evaluation in detecting aspiration in children: A systematic review. *Developmental Medicine & Child Neurology, 58*(6), 541–553. https://doi.org/10.1111/dmcn.13058

Cermak, S. A., Curtin, C., & Bandini, L. G. (2010). Food selectivity and sensory sensitivity in children with autism spectrum disorders. *Journal of the American Dietetic Association, 110*(2), 238–246. https://doi.org/10.1016/j.jada.2009.10.032

Chan, K. K. S., & Leung, D. C. K. (2020). The impact of child autistic symptoms on parental marital relationship: Parenting and coparenting processes as mediating mechanisms. *Autism Research: Official Journal of the International Society for Autism Research, 13*(9), 1516–1526. https://doi.org/10.1002/aur.2297

Chistol, L. T., Bandini, L. G., Must, A., Phillips, S., Cermak, S. A., & Curtin, C. (2018). Sensory sensitivity and food selectivity in children with autism spectrum disorder. *Journal of Autism and Developmental Disorders, 48*(2), 583–591. https://doi.org/10.1007/s10803-017-3340-9

Crist, W., & Napier-Phillips, A. (2001). Mealtime behaviors of young children: A comparison of normative and clinical data. *Journal of Developmental and Behavioral Pediatrics: JDBP, 22*(5), 279–286. https://doi.org/10.1097/00004703-200110000-00001

Davis-McFarland, E. (2008). Family and cultural issues in a school swallowing and feeding program. *Language, Speech & Hearing Services in Schools, 39*(2), 199–213. https://doi.org/10.1044/0161-1461(2008/020)

Dharmaraj, R., Elmaoued, R., Alkhouri, R., Vohra, P., & Castillo, R. O. (2023). Evaluation and management of pediatric feeding disorder. *Gastrointestinal Disorders, 5*(1), Article 1. https://doi.org/10.3390/gidisord5010008

Dipasquale, V., Cicala, G., Spina, E., & Romano, C. (2022). A narrative review on efficacy and safety of proton pump inhibitors in children. *Frontiers in Pharmacology, 13*, 839972. https://doi.org/10.3389/fphar.2022.839972

Dunn, W. (2014) *Sensory profile 2*. Pearson.

Esteban-Figuerola, P., Canals, J., Fernández-Cao, J. C., & Arija Val, V. (2019). Differences in food consumption and nutritional intake between children with autism spectrum disorders and typically developing children: A meta-analysis. *Autism: The International Journal of Research and Practice, 23*(5), 1079–1095. https://doi.org/10.1177/1362361318794179

Fields, V. L., Soke, G. N., Reynolds, A., Tian, L. H., Wiggins, L., Maenner, M., DiGuiseppi, C., Kral, T. V. E., Hightshoe, K., & Schieve, L. A. (2021). Pica, autism, and other disabilities. *Pediatrics, 147*(2), e20200462. https://doi.org/10.1542/peds.2020-0462

Folio, M. R., & Fewell, R. (2023). *Peabody Developmental Motor Scales* (3rd ed.; PDMS-3). Pearson.

Gal, E., Gal-Mishael, R., Vissoker, R. E., Hedley, D., Bury, S. M., & Stolar, O. (2022). Eating challenges in children with autism spectrum disorder: Development and validation of the "Aut-Eat" Questionnaire (AEQ). *Journal of Autism and Developmental Disorders, 52*(2), 811–822. https://doi.org/10.1007/s10803-021-04978-x

Gale, C. M., Eikeseth, S., & Rudrud, E. (2011). Functional assessment and behavioural intervention for eating difficulties in children with autism: A study conducted in the natural environment using parents and ABA tutors as therapists. *Journal of Autism and Developmental Disorders, 41*(10), 1383–1396. https://doi.org/10.1007/s10803-010-1167-8

Goday, P. S., Huh, S. Y., Silverman, A., Lukens, C. T., Dodrill, P., Cohen, S. S., Delaney, A. L., Feuling, M. B., Noel, R. J., Gisel, E., Kenzer, A., Kessler, D. B., Kraus de Camargo, O., Browne, J., & Phalen, J. A. (2019). Pediatric feeding disorder: Consensus definition and conceptual framework. *Journal of Pediatric Gastroenterology and Nutrition, 68*(1), 124–129. https://doi.org/10.1097/MPG.0000000000002188

Harvey, L., Bryant-Waugh, R., Watkins, B., & Meyer, C. (2015). Parental perceptions of childhood feeding problems. *Journal of Child Health Care: For Professionals Working with Children in the Hospital and Community, 19*(3), 392–401. https://doi.org/10.1177/1367493513509422

Hendy, H. M., Seiverling, L., Lukens, C. T., & Williams, K. E. (2013). Brief assessment of meal-time behavior in children: Psychometrics and association with child characteristics and parent responses. *Children's Health Care, 42*(1), 1–14. https://doi.org/10.1080/02739615.2013.753799

Hendy, H. M., Williams, K. E., Camise, T. S., Eckman, N., & Hedemann, A. (2009). The Parent Mealtime Action Scale (PMAS). Development and association with children's diet and weight. *Appetite, 52*(2), 328–339. https://doi.org/10.1016/j.appet.2008.11.003

Herndon, A. C., DiGuiseppi, C., Johnson, S. L., Leiferman, J., & Reynolds, A. (2009). Does nutritional intake differ between children with autism spectrum disorders and children with typical development? *Journal of Autism and Developmental Disorders, 39*(2), 212–222. https://doi.org/10.1007/s10803-008-0606-2

Hodges, A., Davis, T. N., & Kirkpatrick, M. (2020). A review of the literature on the functional analysis of inappropriate mealtime behavior. *Behavior Modification, 44*(1), 137–154. https://doi.org/10.1177/0145445518794368

Hungin, A. P. S., Molloy-Bland, M., & Scarpignato, C. (2019). Revisiting Montreal: New insights into symptoms and their causes, and implications for the future of GERD. *The American Journal of Gastroenterology, 114*(3), 414–421. https://doi.org/10.1038/s41395-018-0287-1

Iwata, B. A., Dorsey, M. F., Slifer, K. J., Bauman, K. E., & Richman, G. S. (1994). Toward a functional analysis of self-injury. *Journal of Applied Behavior Analysis, 27*(2), 197–209. https://doi.org/10.1901/jaba.1994.27-197

Johnson, C. R., Turner, K., Stewart, P. A., Schmidt, B., Shui, A., Macklin, E., Reynolds, A., James, J., Johnson, S. L., Manning Courtney, P., & Hyman, S. L. (2014). Relationships between feeding

problems, behavioral characteristics and nutritional quality in children with ASD. *Journal of Autism and Developmental Disorders, 44*(9), 2175–2184. https://doi.org/10.1007/s10803-014-2095-9
Karlsson, L., Råstam, M., & Wentz, E. (2013). The SWedish Eating Assessment for Autism spectrum disorders (SWEAA)-Validation of a self-report questionnaire targeting eating disturbances within the autism spectrum. *Research in Developmental Disabilities, 34*(7), 2224–2233. https://doi.org/10.1016/j.ridd.2013.03.035
Kelly, A. M., Drinnan, M. J., & Leslie, P. (2007). Assessing penetration and aspiration: How do videofluoroscopy and fiberoptic endoscopic evaluation of swallowing compare? *The Laryngoscope, 117*(10), 1723–1727. https://doi.org/10.1097/MLG.0b013e318123ee6a
Kirkwood, C. A., Piazza, C. C., & Peterson, K. M. (2021). A comparison of function- and nonfunction-based extinction treatments for inappropriate mealtime behavior. *Journal of Applied Behavior Analysis, 54*(3), 928–945. https://doi.org/10.1002/jaba.825
Kleinert, J. Or. (2017). Pediatric feeding disorders and severe developmental disabilities. *Seminars in Speech and Language, 38*(2), 116–125. https://doi.org/10.1055/s-0037-1599109
Kozak, A., Czepczor-Bernat, K., Modrzejewska, J., Modrzejewska, A., Matusik, E., & Matusik, P. (2023). Avoidant/Restrictive Food Disorder (ARFID), food neophobia, other eating-related behaviours and feeding practices among children with autism spectrum disorder and in non-clinical sample: A preliminary study. *International Journal of Environmental Research and Public Health, 20*(10), 5822. https://doi.org/10.3390/ijerph20105822
Kral, T. V. E., Souders, M. C., Tompkins, V. H., Remiker, A. M., Eriksen, W. T., & Pinto-Martin, J. A. (2015). Child eating behaviors and caregiver feeding practices in children with autism spectrum disorders. *Public Health Nursing (Boston, MA), 32*(5), 488–497. https://doi.org/10.1111/phn.12146
Lang, R., Mulloy, A., Giesbers, S., Pfeiffer, B., Delaune, E., Didden, R., Sigafoos, J., Lancioni, G., & O'Reilly, M. (2011). Behavioral interventions for rumination and operant vomiting in individuals with intellectual disabilities: A systematic review. *Research in Developmental Disabilities, 32*(6), 2193–2205. https://doi.org/10.1016/j.ridd.2011.06.011
Le Moal, F., Michaud, M., Hartwick-Pflaum, C. A., Middleton, G., Mallon, I., & Coveney, J. (2021). Beyond the normative family meal promotion: A narrative review of qualitative results about ordinary domestic commensality. *International Journal of Environmental Research and Public Health, 18*(6), 3186. https://doi.org/10.3390/ijerph18063186
Leader, G., Abberton, C., Cunningham, S., Gilmartin, K., Grudzien, M., Higgins, E., Joshi, L., Whelan, S., & Mannion, A. (2022). Gastrointestinal symptoms in autism spectrum disorder: A systematic review. *Nutrients, 14*(7), 1471. https://doi.org/10.3390/nu14071471
Leader, G., Tuohy, E., Chen, J. L., Mannion, A., & Gilroy, S. P. (2020). Feeding problems, gastrointestinal symptoms, challenging behavior and sensory issues in children and adolescents with autism spectrum disorder. *Journal of Autism and Developmental Disorders, 50*(4), 1401–1410. https://doi.org/10.1007/s10803-019-04357-7
Lukens, C. T., & Linscheid, T. R. (2008). Development and validation of an inventory to assess mealtime behavior problems in children with autism. *Journal of Autism and Developmental Disorders, 38*(2), 342–352. https://doi.org/10.1007/s10803-007-0401-5
Mathur, S., Renz, E., & Tarbox, J. (2024). Affirming neurodiversity within applied behavior analysis. *Behavior Analysis in Practice*. https://doi.org/10.1007/s40617-024-00907-3
Matson, J. L., Belva, B., Hattier, M. A., & Matson, M. L. (2011). Pica in persons with developmental disabilities: Characteristics, diagnosis, and assessment. *Research in Autism Spectrum Disorders, 5*(4), 1459–1464. https://doi.org/10.1016/j.rasd.2011.02.006
Matson, J. L., & Kuhn, D. E. (2001). Identifying feeding problems in mentally retarded persons: Development and reliability of the screening tool of feeding problems (STEP). *Research in Developmental Disabilities, 22*(2), 165–172. https://doi.org/10.1016/s0891-4222(01)00065-8
Matson, J. L., Mayville, S. B., Kuhn, D. E., Sturmey, P., Laud, R., & Cooper, C. (2005). The behavioral function of feeding problems as assessed by the questions about behavioral function

(QABF). *Research in Developmental Disabilities, 26*(4), 399–408. https://doi.org/10.1016/j.ridd.2004.11.008

Matson, J. L., & Vollmer, T. (1995). *The Questions About Behavioral Function (QABF).* Scientific Publishers.

Matsuo, K., & Palmer, J. B. (2016). Video fluoroscopic techniques for the study of Oral Food Processing. *Current Opinion in Food Science, 9*, 1–10. https://doi.org/10.1016/j.cofs.2016.03.004

McCafferty, P., & McCutcheon, J. (2021). Parenting a child with autism: Considering the stresses, supports and implications for social work practice. *Child Care in Practice, 27*(4), 389–405. https://doi.org/10.1080/13575279.2020.1765145

Miller, C. K. (2011). Aspiration and swallowing dysfunction in pediatric patients. *ICAN: Infant, Child, & Adolescent Nutrition, 3*(6), 336–343. https://doi.org/10.1177/1941406411423967

Miller, C. K., & Wilging, J. P. (2019). Fiberoptic endoscopic evaluation of swallowing in infants and children: Protocol, safety, and clinical efficacy: 25 years of experience. *Annals of Otology, Rhinology & Laryngology*, 1–13. https://doi.org/10.1177/0003489419893720

Nadon, G., Feldman, D. E., Dunn, W., & Gisel, E. (2011). Association of sensory processing and eating problems in children with autism spectrum disorders. *Autism Research and Treatment, 2011*, 541926. https://doi.org/10.1155/2011/541926

Oliver, A. C., Pratt, L. A., & Normand, M. P. (2015). A survey of functional behavior assessment methods used by behavior analysts in practice. *Journal of Applied Behavior Analysis, 48*(4), 817–829. https://doi.org/10.1002/jaba.256

Page, S. D., Souders, M. C., Kral, T. V. E., Chao, A. M., & Pinto-Martin, J. (2022). Correlates of feeding difficulties among children with autism spectrum disorder: A systematic review. *Journal of Autism and Developmental Disorders, 52*(1), 255–274. https://doi.org/10.1007/s10803-021-04947-4

Parham, L. D., Ecker, C. L., Kuhaneck, H., Henry, D. A., & Glennon, T. J. (2021). Sensory Processing Measure (2nd ed.; SPM-2). WPS.

Peterson, K. M., Ibañez, V. F., Volkert, V. M., Zeleny, J. R., Engler, C. W., & Piazza, C. C. (2021). Using telehealth to provide outpatient follow-up to children with avoidant/restrictive food intake disorder. *Journal of Applied Behavior Analysis, 54*(1), 6–24. https://doi.org/10.1002/jaba.794

Piazza, C. C., Patel, M. R., Gulotta, C. S., Sevin, B. M., & Layer, S. A. (2003). On the relative contributions of positive reinforcement and escape extinction in the treatment of food refusal. *Journal of Applied Behavior Analysis, 36*(3), 309–324. https://doi.org/10.1901/jaba.2003.36-309

Pizzo, B., Williams, K. E., Paul, C., & Riegel, K. (2009). Jump start exit criterion: Exploring a new model of service delivery for the treatment of childhood feeding problems. *Behavioral Interventions, 24*(3), 195–203. https://doi.org/10.1002/bin.285

Provost, B., Crowe, T. K., Osbourn, P. L., McClain, C., & Skipper, B. J. (2010). Mealtime behaviors of preschool children: Comparison of children with autism spectrum disorder and children with typical development. *Physical & Occupational Therapy in Pediatrics, 30*(3), 220–233. https://doi.org/10.3109/01942631003757669

Ptomey, L. T., & Wittenbrook, W. (2015). Position of the academy of nutrition and dietetics: Nutrition services for individuals with intellectual and developmental disabilities and special health care needs. *Journal of the Academy of Nutrition and Dietetics, 115*(4), 593–608. https://doi.org/10.1016/j.jand.2015.02.002

Rabaey, P. A., Barlow, K., Jama, H., & Lehr, V. (2023). Investigation of assessment tools in the area of pediatric feeding evaluation: A mixed-methods study. *American Journal of Occupational Therapy, 77*(4), 7704205110. https://doi.org/10.5014/ajot.2023.050040. PMID: 37498961.

Rodrigues, J. V. S., Poli, M. C. F., Petrilli, P. H., Dornelles, R. C. M., Turcio, K. H., & Theodoro, L. H. (2023). Food selectivity and neophobia in children with autism spectrum disorder and neurotypical development: A systematic review. *Nutrition Reviews, 81*(8), 1034–1050. https://doi.org/10.1093/nutrit/nuac112

Roscoe, E. M., Phillips, K. M., Kelly, M. A., Farber, R., & Dube, W. V. (2015). A statewide survey assessing practitioners' use and perceived utility of functional assessment. *Journal of Applied Behavior Analysis, 48*(4), 830–844. https://doi.org/10.1002/jaba.259

Rossetti, D., Isoldi, S., & Oliva, S. (2020). Eosinophilic esophagitis: Update on diagnosis and treatment in pediatric patients. *Paediatric Drugs, 22*(4), 343–356. https://doi.org/10.1007/s40272-020-00398-z

Rudolf, M. C. J., & Logan, S. (2005). What is the long term outcome for children who fail to thrive? A systematic review. *Archives of Disease in Childhood, 90*(9), 925–931. https://doi.org/10.1136/adc.2004.050179

Ruel, M. T. (2003). Operationalizing dietary diversity: A review of measurement issues and research priorities. *The Journal of Nutrition, 133*(11), 3911S-3926S. https://doi.org/10.1093/jn/133.11.3911S

Rutherford, M., & Johnston, L. (2023). Perspective chapter: Rethinking autism assessment, diagnosis, and intervention within a neurodevelopmental pathway framework. *IntechOpen.* https://doi.org/10.5772/intechopen.108784

Seidler, G. R., Knaus, M. E., Beyene, T. J., Ahmad, H., Lu, P. L., Gasior, A. C., Halaweish, I., & Wood, R. J. (2022). Impact of neurodevelopmental disorders on bowel management outcomes in children with functional constipation. *Journal of Pediatric Gastroenterology and Nutrition, 75*(3), 286–292. https://doi.org/10.1097/MPG.0000000000003517

Seiverling, L., Hendy, H. M., Yusupova, S., Kaczor, A., Panora, J., & Rodriguez, J. (2020). Improvements in children's feeding behavior after intensive interdisciplinary behavioral treatment: Comparisons by developmental and medical status. *Behavior Modification, 44*(6), 891–908. https://doi.org/10.1177/0145445519865170

Sharp, W. G., Berry, R. C., McCracken, C., Nuhu, N. N., Marvel, E., Saulnier, C. A., Klin, A., Jones, W., & Jaquess, D. L. (2013). Feeding problems and nutrient intake in children with autism spectrum disorders: A meta-analysis and comprehensive review of the literature. *Journal of Autism and Developmental Disorders, 43*(9), 2159–2173. https://doi.org/10.1007/s10803-013-1771-5

Sharp, W. G., Postorino, V., McCracken, C. E., Berry, R. C., Criado, K. K., Burrell, T. L., & Scahill, L. (2018). Dietary intake, nutrient status, and growth parameters in children with autism spectrum disorder and severe food selectivity: An electronic medical record review. *Journal of the Academy of Nutrition and Dietetics, 118*(10), 1943–1950. https://doi.org/10.1016/j.jand.2018.05.005

Silverman, A. H. (2015). Behavioral management of feeding disorders of childhood. *Annals of Nutrition & Metabolism, 66*(Suppl. 5), 33–42. https://doi.org/10.1159/000381375

Suarez, M. A., Nelson, N. W., & Curtis, A. B. (2014). Longitudinal follow-up of factors associated with food selectivity in children with autism spectrum disorders. *Autism: The International Journal of Research and Practice, 18*(8), 924–932. https://doi.org/10.1177/1362361313499457

Taylor, C. M., Wernimont, S. M., Northstone, K., & Emmett, P. M. (2015). Picky/fussy eating in children: Review of definitions, assessment, prevalence and dietary intakes. *Appetite, 95*, 349–359. https://doi.org/10.1016/j.appet.2015.07.026

Thompson, R. H., & Iwata, B. A. (2007). A comparison of outcomes from descriptive and functional analyses of problem behavior. *Journal of Applied Behavior Analysis, 40*(2), 333–338. https://doi.org/10.1901/jaba.2007.56-06

Thullen, M., & Bonsall, A. (2017). Co-parenting quality, parenting stress, and feeding challenges in families with a child diagnosed with autism spectrum disorder. *Journal of Autism and Developmental Disorders, 47*(3), 878–886. https://doi.org/10.1007/s10803-016-2988-x

Tinelli, M., Roddy, A., Knapp, M., Arango, C., Mendez, M. A., Cusack, J., Murphy, D., Canitano, R., Oakley, B., & Quoidbach, V. (2023). Economic analysis of early intervention for autistic children: Findings from four case studies in England, Ireland, Italy, and Spain. *European Psychiatry: THe Journal of the Association of European Psychiatrists, 66*(1), e76. https://doi.org/10.1192/j.eurpsy.2023.2449

Tran, D. L., & Sintusek, P. (2023). Functional constipation in children: What physicians should know. *World Journal of Gastroenterology, 29*(8), 1261–1288. https://doi.org/10.3748/wjg.v29.i8.1261

Twachtman-Reilly, J., Amaral, S. C., & Zebrowski, P. P. (2008). Addressing feeding disorders in children on the autism spectrum in school-based settings: Physiological and behavioral issues. *Language, Speech, and Hearing Services in Schools, 39*(2), 261–272. https://doi.org/10.1044/0161-1461(2008/025)

van Dijk, M. W. G., Buruma, M. E., & Blijd-Hoogewys, E. M. A. (2021). Detecting feeding problems in young children with autism spectrum disorder. *Journal of Autism and Developmental Disorders, 51*(11), 4115–4127. https://doi.org/10.1007/s10803-021-04869-1

Van Hoorn, M., Feuling, M. B., Allen, K., Berry, R., Brown, S., Sullivan, C. M., & Goday, P. S. (2023). Evaluation and management of reduced dietary diversity in children with pediatric feeding disorder. *Journal of Autism and Developmental Disorders, 53*(3), 1290–1297. https://doi.org/10.1007/s10803-022-05715-8

Walker, N. (2014). *Neurodiversity: Some basic terms & definitions.*

Wallace, G. L., Llewellyn, C., Fildes, A., & Ronald, A. (2018). Autism spectrum disorder and food neophobia: Clinical and subclinical links. *The American Journal of Clinical Nutrition, 108*(4), 701–707. https://doi.org/10.1093/ajcn/nqy163

Weir, K., McMahon, S., Barry, L., Ware, R., Masters, I. B., & Chang, A. B. (2007). Oropharyngeal aspiration and pneumonia in children. *Pediatric Pulmonology, 42*(11), 1024–1031. https://doi.org/10.1002/ppul.20687

Willett, W. (1998). Food frequency methods. In *Nutritional Epidemiology* (2nd ed., pp. 69–91). Oxford University Press.

Williams, P. G., Dalrymple, N., & Neal, J. (2000). Eating habits of children with autism. *Pediatric Nursing, 26*(3), 259–264.

Włodarczyk, J., Waśniewska, A., Fichna, J., Dziki, A., Dziki, Ł., & Włodarczyk, M. (2021). Current overview on clinical management of chronic constipation. *Journal of Clinical Medicine, 10*(8), 1738. https://doi.org/10.3390/jcm10081738

Zimmer, M. H., Hart, L. C., Manning-Courtney, P., Murray, D. S., Bing, N. M., & Summer, S. (2012). Food variety as a predictor of nutritional status among children with autism. *Journal of Autism and Developmental Disorders, 42*(4), 549–556. https://doi.org/10.1007/s10803-011-1268-z

Assessing Sleep Problems in Children with Autism Spectrum Disorder

Terry Katz, Beth A. Malow, and Ann M. Reynolds

Abstract This chapter examines sleep in children with autism spectrum disorder (ASD). Up to 80% of children with ASD have co-occurring sleep problems, and poor sleep has been associated with difficulties in autistic characteristics, cognition, mood, attention, behavior, and adaptive functioning. Sleep disorders in children with ASD include insomnia, sleep-related breathing disorders, parasomnias, rapid eye movement associated abnormalities, rhythmic movement disorders, and restless legs syndrome. Sleep surveys, sleep diaries, actigraphy, and polysomnography may be used to evaluate sleep problems. Assessment of sleep problems must also include a review of potential contributing medical factors. Helping children prepare for a successful sleep study often involves advance preparation and desensitization. Effective intervention strategies include behavioral sleep education and the use of exogenous melatonin.

Keywords Insomnia · Sleep-related breathing disorders · Parasomnias · Restless legs syndrome · Sleep surveys · Sleep diaries · Actigraphy · Polysomnography · Behavioral sleep education · Melatonin

T. Katz (✉) · A. M. Reynolds
Department of Pediatrics, Children's Hospital Colorado, University of Colorado School of Medicine, Aurora, CO, USA
e-mail: terry.katz@cuanschutz.edu

B. A. Malow
Department of Neurology, Vanderbilt University Medical Center, Nashville, TN, USA

J. L. Matson (ed.), *Assessment and Diagnosis in Autism*, Autism and Child Psychopathology Series, https://doi.org/10.1007/978-3-032-11802-8_8

Prevalence of Sleep Problems in Individuals with ASD

Sleep problems in children with autism spectrum disorder[1] (ASD) occurs much more frequently than in the general population. While up to 80% of children with ASD have co-occurring sleep problems (Souders et al., 2017), the prevalence rate for children with typical development is 9% to 50%. (Couturier et al., 2005; Krakowiak et al., 2008; Richdale & Schreck, 2009; Souders et al., 2009). While the frequency of sleep problems in all children with developmental disabilities is high, children with ASD are more likely to have sleep problems than children with other developmental disabilities (Schreck & Mulick, 2000; Wiggs & Stores, 1996), and insomnia is a common difficulty (Cortese et al., 2020; Johnson & Zarrinnegar, 2021).

The association between age and level of cognition and the presence of sleep problems is also different for children with ASD than for individuals with other developmental disabilities. In a sample of 2–5-year-olds, Reynolds et al. (2019) found that while sleep problems were common in all children, there was a higher prevalence of sleep problems in children with ASD compared to children with developmental delays without ASD or children in the general population. While younger age and lower cognitive level are associated with higher rates of sleep problems in children with other developmental disabilities, these associations are not necessarily present in children with ASD (Krakowiak et al., 2008; Malow et al., 2006; Richdale, 1999). This difference may be related, in part, to the significant heterogeneity that is seen in autism. While some research finds no age-related differences in sleep problems of children with ASD, other research has documented that parents of children who are younger than 8 years of age report more severe sleep concerns than parents of children who are older (Richdale & Prior, 1995).

Sleep problems are also present in autistic adolescents and adults (Gail Williams et al., 2004; Limoges et al., 2005). While there is strong evidence that autistic individuals across all age groups have significant difficulties with sleep, the types of sleep problems that are evident may vary. Older children and adolescents have more problems falling asleep and staying asleep during the night, while younger children demonstrate greater bedtime resistance, sleep anxiety, parasomnias, and night waking (Oyane & Bjorvatn, 2005).

[1] We recognize that identity-first language is preferred by many people in the autism community (Bottema-Beutel et al., 2021) while others (including many parents of children with autism) prefer person-first language. We are following the recommendations of the National Institutes of Health (NIH) and will use person-first language when writing about children and a mix of person-first and identity-first language when writing about adults or autistic individuals generally (National Institutes of Health, 2023).

Effects of Sleep Problems

Sleep problems may have profound and far-reaching implications for the individual who is experiencing difficulties as well as for family members (American Academy of Sleep Medicine, 2014). Poor sleep in typically developing children has been associated with difficulties in cognition, mood, attention, and behavior (Armstrong et al., 1994; Kataria et al., 1987; Pollock, 1994; Zuckerman et al., 1987). Studies have also associated negative mood, irritability, self-injury, and aggression to poor sleep in children with developmental disabilities (Clements et al., 1986; Quine, 1991).

The relationship between sleep and daytime functioning has also been documented in children with ASD (Schreck, 2021). Difficulties with anxiety (May et al., 2015; Uren et al., 2019), mood (DeVincent et al., 2007), attention (Roussis et al., 2021), activity level (Goldman et al., 2009; Mazurek & Sohl, 2016), and aggressive behavior have been correlated with sleep problems (Mayes & Calhoun, 2009; Mazurek & Sohl, 2016; Shui et al., 2018). Daytime behavioral challenges and delays in adaptive behavior and functional skills are more common in children with ASD and co-occurring sleep problems than in children with ASD who do not have sleep problems (Lamônica et al., 2021; Sikora et al., 2012; Taylor et al., 2012; Veatch et al., 2017).

Poor sleep in children with ASD has been related to autistic behaviors including difficulties with social interaction, repetitive behavior, self-injury, the need for sameness, and sensory difficulties (Gabriels et al., 2005; Goldman et al., 2009, 2011; Malow et al., 2006; Mazurek & Petroski, 2015; Schreck et al., 2004a; Tzischinsky et al., 2018). These associations may highlight the bidirectional nature of sleep in ASD. Children with more autistic traits may have more sleep problems; conversely, sleep problems may lead to increased autistic behavior.

Sleep problems in children with developmental disabilities have also been associated with disruptions in parental sleep as well as higher levels of maternal stress (Quine, 1991). The importance of good sleep has also been related to the overall quality of life for children with developmental disabilities and their families (Didden & Sigafoos, 2001; Didden et al., 2002; Robinson & Richdale, 2004). Researchers have found that sleep problems in children with ASD are associated with increased parental stress (Bernardi et al., 2023; Doo & Wing, 2006; Hodge et al., 2013; Mannion & Leader, 2023); anxiety, (Foody et al., 2015; Mannion & Leader, 2023) and depression (Leader et al., 2022; Mannion & Leader, 2023; Meltzer, 2011).

Types of Sleep Disorders

Identification of sleep disorders in children with ASD is a critical step in providing appropriate treatment.

Insomnia

Insomnia is characterized by difficulty initiating and/or maintaining sleep, and symptoms of insomnia are the main sleep concern reported by parents of children with ASD. According to data compiled through parent-completed questionnaires and sleep diaries, common symptoms of insomnia in children with ASD include prolonged sleep latency (the amount of time it takes to fall asleep), increased bedtime resistance, decreased sleep efficiency (time actually asleep in relation to time in bed), decreased sleep duration, poor continuity, and increased nighttime awakenings (Couturier et al., 2005; Gail Williams et al., 2004; Krakowiak et al., 2008; Richdale, 1999). Children with ASD often experience both sleep onset insomnia (difficulty falling asleep) and sleep maintenance insomnia (difficulty staying asleep), although sleep onset insomnia is more common (Gail Williams et al., 2004; Krakowiak et al., 2008).

It is important to consider the variety of factors that may contribute to insomnia in ASD.

Biological Considerations. While sleep habits and behavior may be a primary factor, there may also be a host of other causes that may be simultaneously contributing to this difficulty. Neurobiological factors including aberrations in neurotransmitter systems that promote sleep and establish a regular sleep-wake cycle may play a role in sleep problems in children with ASD. Several neurotransmitters that play a role in sleep regulation have also been associated with ASD. Melatonin is a sleep-promoting substance that is regulated by exposure to light and is released by the pineal gland (Gooley & Saper, 2011). It is synthesized from serotonin (Lin-Dyken & Dyken, 2002), and there are reports of abnormal platelet serotonin levels in children with ASD (Rapin & Katzman, 1998). The relation between hyperserotonemia and sleep warrants additional investigation (Portas et al., 2000). Melatonin secretion has been noted to be low in individuals with ASD (Kulman et al., 2000; Melke et al., 2008; Nir et al., 1995; Tordjman et al., 2005), although one study performing overnight sampling documented normal blood levels in children responding to supplemental melatonin for sleep-onset delay (Goldman et al., 2014). Goldman et al. (2017) also found that dim light melatonin onsets (DLMOs) were not different for adolescents and young adults with and without ASD. In another study, the level of the major metabolite of melatonin was directly related to the level of deep sleep in children with ASD (Leu et al., 2011). A decrease in melatonin may be related to low activity of the last enzyme in the melatonin syntheses pathway: acetylserotonin-*O*-methyltransferase (ASMT). While the research is far from conclusive, some findings suggest that ASMT variability may contribute to abnormalities in the syntheses of serotonin to melatonin. In a study involving children with ASD, Jonsson and colleagues studied all the genes involved in the melatonin pathway and found mutations in regulatory regions in 3 genes: ASMT, melatonin receptor 1A, and melatonin receptor 1B (Jonsson et al., 2010). Other researchers have also found a higher rate of abnormalities in ASMT in children with ASD compared with controls as well as ASMT polymorphisms and lower levels of ASMT activity in children with ASD (Cai et al., 2008). There is also evidence, however, to suggest that there is no difference in ASMT variants (Toma et al., 2007). Melatonin is primarily metabolized by the liver enzyme, cytochrome P450 1A2 (*CYP1A2*) (Arendt, 1998; Arendt et al., 1985). Slow-metabolizing alleles in *CYP1A2* has been postulated to contribute to sleep problems in ASD (Braam et al., 2010, 2013; Veatch et al., 2015). One mechanism that reconciles the presence of normal melatonin levels with low ASMT transcript production is that these same children have reduced CYP1A2 metabolic activity. Veatch and colleagues observed an association between lower levels of ASMT transcript production and reduced CYP1A2 metabolic activity in children with ASD and co-occurring sleep-onset delay responding to supplemental melatonin. (Veatch et al., 2015) Of note, treatment of insomnia with melatonin in children with ASD has been found to be beneficial in a number of well-controlled studies (Cortesi et al., 2012; Garstang & Wallis, 2006; Giannotti et al., 2006; Johnson & Zarrinnegar, 2021; Malow et al., 2012a; Souders et al., 2017; Wright et al., 2011).

Anxiety and overarousal are common difficulties in children with ASD, and these factors may affect their sleep (Mazurek & Petroski, 2015; Richdale & Baglin, 2015). Children and adolescents have been characterized as having high levels of arousal before sleep (Baker et al., 2019; Richdale et al., 2014). Cortisol is a stress hormone that is associated with sleep problems. Researchers indicate that children without ASD who have sleep problems have elevated cortisol levels when they first fall asleep and in the early stages of sleep (Rodenbeck et al., 2002). Adults and children with ASD have been found to have reduced evening cortisol (Baker et al., 2019) and reduction in the normal diurnal slope of cortisol has been associated with stress and sensory difficulties (Corbett et al., 2009). Taken together, this suggests that a dysregulated hypothalamic–pituitary-adrenal axis (Baker et al., 2019; Taylor & Corbett, 2014) may, in turn, may affect sleep.

Medical Factors. There are several medical factors that may also contribute to difficulties with sleep initiation and maintenance. Medical conditions that may cause discomfort or pain may contribute to disrupted sleep. It may be especially important to consider medical conditions that may interfere with sleep when working with individuals with ASD who are minimally verbal and who may not be able to describe physical symptoms that may be causing interruptions to their sleep. Gastrointestinal problems are common in children with ASD (Holingue et al., 2018), and these include diarrhea, constipation, abdominal pain, and gastroesophageal reflux disease related symptoms (Buie et al., 2010). Restrepo and colleagues (2020) found that GI symptoms are more common in children ages 2 to 3.5 years than in those in children without ASD. They also found that children with ASD were more likely to experience multiple GI symptoms and that GI symptoms were associated with sleep problems as well as other co-occurring difficulties. Other researchers have also demonstrated a strong link between GI dysfunction and sleep in children with ASD (Aldinger et al., 2015; McCue et al., 2017). Neumeyer et al. (2019) found a significant correlation between constipation and sleep problems in children with ASD ages 5 years and under. Eosinophilic esophagitis (EoE) is one of the most common esophageal diseases and has been related to sleep problems including insomnia (Siriwat et al., 2020). Sohn et al. (2021) found that a high prevalence of ASD and developmental disabilities in children with EoE.

Pain may also make sleep difficult. Tudor and colleagues (2015) found an association between specific sleep problems (sleep duration, parasomnias, and sleep-disordered breathing) and pain in children with ASD. Pain may be multifactorial. One important consideration is dental pain. Jaber (2011) found that children ages 6 to 16 years with autism had a higher prevalence of caries, poorer oral hygiene, and greater unmet need for dental treatment than children without autism. Ferrazzano et al. (2020) found that children with ASD are also more prone to dental injury and gingivitis.

Asthma (Cukic et al., 2011) and allergic rhinitis (D'Elia et al., 2022) may affect sleep. Other medical factors that may affect sleep include allergies, reactive airway disease, and eczema. While researchers have not found a higher incidence of overall allergies or asthma in children with ASD, they have found that increased stereotypies are associated with allergies in children with ASD, and food allergies are more highly associated with ASD in children (Lyall et al., 2015). Additionally, Fishbein et al. (2021) found that 66.9% of children ages 5–17 years with atopic dermatitis also had sleep problems, and a meta-analysis found a significant correlation between autism and atopic dermatitis (Tsai et al., 2020).

Primary sleep conditions such as sleep-disordered breathing and restless leg syndrome may also result in poor sleep (these will be discussed in more detail later in this chapter). Thus, a thorough assessment of medical conditions is an essential component of a sleep evaluation. Reynolds and Malow worked with the Autism Treatment Network to develop a comprehensive screening checklist for medical conditions associated with sleep problems (Reynolds & Malow, 2011). The checklist is intended to be used by clinicians when interviewing families and includes questions related to reflux, constipation, abdominal pain, seizures, sleep-disordered breathing, asthma, sinusitis, dental issues, eczema, nutrition, sensitivity to sensory input, restless sleep, and current medications. A physical examination is also part of this screening and includes consideration of tonsil size, hypotonia, nasal congestion or signs of allergic rhinitis, dental issues, wheezing, and eczema or dry, itchy skin. We provide more information about this checklist later in this chapter.

Co-occurring Psychiatric Conditions. Autistic individuals may have co-occurring psychiatric conditions that may impact sleep. Symptoms of anxiety, depression, attention-deficit/hyperactivity disorder (ADHD), and obsessive-compulsive disorder may contribute to insomnia (Veatch et al., 2017). The impact of sleep and psychiatric conditions may be bidirectional as poor sleep may also intensify psychiatric symptomatology. Approximately a third of children with ASD have a co-occurring diagnosis of ADHD (Simonoff et al., 2008), and children with ADHD often have sleep problems (Singh & Zimmerman, 2015). Researchers have also found a connection between symptoms of inattention and hyperactivity and poor sleep in children with ASD (Devincent et al., 2007; Goldman et al., 2011).

Anxiety is a common difficulty in children with ASD; van Steensel and colleagues (2011) completed a meta-analysis and concluded that 39.6% of children with ASD had symptoms or an anxiety diagnosis. Anxiety may be associated with hyperarousal (Monk et al., 2001), and research has shown that sensory over-responsivity is associated with sleep problems. A child who is anxious may have difficulty falling asleep because of generalized anxiety, specific fears or concerns, or separation issues that make it difficult to fall asleep at night. Mazurek and Petroski (2015) found that anxiety and sensory over-responsivity was associated with bedtime resistance, sleep-onset delay, sleep duration, sleep anxiety, and night wakings.

Mood disorders including depression and bipolar disorders co-occur with autism spectrum disorders (Simonoff et al., 2008, 2012), and research has demonstrated that difficulties with anxiety and mood in autistic individuals is associated with sleep problems (Mayes & Calhoun, 2009; Wiggs & Stores, 2004). Individuals with obsessive-compulsive disorder may need to engage in long and complex rituals that prolong bedtime and result in shortened sleep. Depression may result in an individual waking up very early in the morning and not being able to return to sleep. An individual with bipolar disorder may experience an overall decrease in the need for sleep (Gold & Sylvia, 2016).

Medications. When considering the ways in which a psychiatric condition may impact sleep, it may also be necessary to address the role of psychotropic medications in sleep. A child with ADHD may have difficulty settling for the night but may also have difficulty falling asleep because of the impact of taking a stimulant medication to address symptoms of ADHD during the day (Sangal et al., 2006). In addition to the ADHD medication interfering with sleep, it can also suppress appetite. A child taking a stimulant may wake up at night due to being hungry. In addition, medications used to treat other conditions such as seizures may disrupt sleep (Liguori et al., 2021).

Characteristics of Autism. There are defining characteristics of ASD which may also contribute to insomnia. Difficulties with understanding social cues may make it difficult to understand parental and societal expectations for getting ready for bed and falling asleep. Struggles with both verbal and nonverbal communication may also make it hard to help children learn a bedtime routine. An insistence on sameness and struggles with transition and change may also make it hard to prepare for bedtime. Moving from wakefulness and engagement in daytime (and potentially stimulating) activities to relaxing and sleep-promoting activities requires flexibility and the ability to handle transitions and change. This may be particularly difficult for individuals with ASD who often have difficulty with transitions and flexibility. Individuals who have a strong need to engage in specific activities or focus on certain topics may also have difficulty ending these activities at bedtime and may thus have trouble winding down for the night and relaxing for bed. They may also obsess about their restricted interests or worries about the school day. Hyper-reactivity to sensory input may also contribute to difficulties falling asleep. Sensitivity to noises, textures, or other sensations in the environment, for example, may interfere with falling asleep at night. Careful consideration of a child's sleep environment including bedding and pajamas may be beneficial. Additionally, children with ASD may have difficulty with self-regulation and may easily become hyperaroused. High states of arousal will then lead to struggles with settling and establishing a relaxed state that is needed to initiate and maintain sleep.

Sleep-Disordered Breathing

Sleep-related breathing disorders (SDB) include several chronic conditions in which difficulties in breathing occur many times during the night. Symptoms may include snoring, gasping and pauses in breathing. Research using laboratory or portable home testing indicates that approximately 2% of children ages 8 to 11 years, 4% of adult men, and 2% of adult women have sleep-disordered breathing (Rosen et al., 2003; Young et al., 1993). Zaffanello et al. (2023) recently completed a literature review that examined studies on SDB and children with ASD and concluded that there was a high incidence of SDB in this population. Tomkies et al. (2019) completed a retrospective case review of children with ASD ages 2 to 18 years who completed a sleep study over a six-year period. Out of a total of 45 children, 26 (58%) had obstructive sleep apnea (OSA) and 9 children had severe obstructive sleep apnea. Of note, 33% of the children were obese, and obesity is a risk factor, especially for severe OSA in children with ASD (Tomkies et al., 2019). Children with ASD are at greater risk for obesity due to difficulties with feeding (Eow et al., 2022) and decreased physical activity (McCoy & Morgan, 2020). Low muscle tone has been associated with ASD (Ming et al., 2007) and this may also be a risk factor for OSA (Zaffanello et al., 2023).

Children at risk for OSA will likely need to complete a sleep study (polysomnography or PSG). Many aspects of a PSG may be difficult for children with ASD as this involves staying overnight at a sleep center or hospital and tolerating the placement of multiple electrodes and sensors. This can be very difficult for children with sensory sensitivities as well as for children who have difficulty tolerating changes in routine. There are, however, many strategies that can be employed to help an individual successfully complete the procedure (Zaffanello et al., 2023). More information about sleep studies and preparation for successful completion of the procedure may be found later in this chapter. Adenotonsillectomy is considered the preferred treatment for OSA (Marcus et al., 2012), and studies have documented improvement in daytime behavior in children with ASD following adenotonsillectomy (Murata et al., 2017). Some individuals may also benefit from positive airway pressure (PAP). This involves providing air pressure through an individual's airway and requires wearing a full-face mask, a nasal mask, or a nasal pillow. Compliance with wearing a PAP mask and tolerating the air pressure can be challenging for many individuals (King et al., 2014). Behavioral strategies including desensitization can help improve adherence (Slifer et al., 2019). More information about this is provided later in this chapter.

Parasomnias

Parasomnias are common in childhood with over 80% of preschool-age children experiencing parasomnia events (Kotagal, 2008) and include non-rapid eye movement (NREM) arousal disorders, sleep terrors, sleepwalking, and confusional arousals. Parasomnias may be related to sleep deprivation and may be a sign that medical conditions are impacting the quality of sleep. They tend to occur during the first half of the night during N3 sleep (deep, slow-wave sleep). It is important to distinguish between sleep terrors and nightmares (Leung et al., 2020). Key points to consider include timing of the event (early in the night vs. late) and how responsive a child is during an episode (children are not responsive during a parasomnia but alert very quickly if they are awakened from a bad dream.) It is also important to distinguish parasomnias from nocturnal seizures (Leung et al., 2020). There is some evidence to indicate that parasomnias are more common in children with ASD than in other groups, but the findings are not consistent (Honomichl et al., 2002; Patzold et al., 1998; Richdale & Prior, 1995; Schreck & Mulick, 2000).

Rapid Eye Movement Associated Sleep Abnormalities

Rapid eye movement (REM) sleep primarily occurs during the second half of the night and is the sleep phase in which most dreams occur. Normal physiologic generalized muscle paralysis occurs during REM sleep. REM sleep behavior disorder (RBD) is characterized by individuals acting out their dreams. This is a rare disorder, and it has been documented in one case series of children who were studied using polysomnography (Thirumalai et al., 2002). A larger polysomnography study that excluded children who were taking psychotropic medications did not document REM sleep without atonia or RBD (Malow et al., 2006). Selective Serotonin Reuptake Inhibitors (SSRIs) are often prescribed for individuals with ASD, and these psychotropic medications can affect REM sleep and can occur in association with REM sleep behavior disorder (Mahowald, 2011).

Rhythmic Movement Disorders

Rhythmic movement disorders typically involve repetitive whole-body movements, limb rocking, rolling, or head banging. These behaviors usually occur during the transition from wakefulness to sleep (Hoban, 2003), but may often be seen at the start of bedtime or during sustained sleep. They are most common in infants and toddlers but may persist in older children and adolescents with ASD and other developmental disorders (Lam & Veeravigrom, 2023).

Restless Legs Syndrome

Restless legs syndrome (RLS) is a neurological sensory motor disorder that involves the urge to move the legs during times of rest or inactivity. The diagnostic criteria for pediatric-onset RLS describe a condition in which children have an urge to move their legs; this urge may be accompanied by uncomfortable leg sensations, but this may not always occur. The urge to move their legs starts or becomes worse during periods of inactivity or rest, and movement, including walking or stretching, may help reduce the urge. The urge for individuals to move their legs during rest or inactivity primarily occurs in the evening or night (Picchietti et al., 2013). This may result in difficulties settling and falling asleep at bedtime and may present as insomnia or bedtime refusal (DelRosso et al., 2024). DelRosso and colleagues (2024) note that most children with RLS also describe having leg discomfort during the day and explain that this may be associated with the number of hours children sit during a school day.

An RLS diagnosis is based on clinical features, and thus a sleep study is not needed to make the diagnosis (DelRosso et al., 2024). It may be missed by medical care providers as symptoms may be intermittent and mild (DelRosso et al., 2024). Diagnostic criteria state that symptoms need to be described by children in their own words. This may be difficult for young children as well as individuals with language delays. It may thus be particularly difficult to make this diagnosis in children with ASD who have problems with communication. RLS is associated with excessive daytime sleepiness (Yalcinkaya et al., 2021), school problems, irritability, aggression, inattentiveness, and mood changes (DelRosso et al., 2023).

DelRosso and colleagues (2024) describe the steps in an evaluation of RLS which includes a comprehensive history, physical examination, and information about a child's bedtime routine and habits. They note the importance of asking about family history. Research indicates that 40–92% of children with RLS have family members with this condition (Jiménez-Jiménez et al., 2018; Walters et al., 2013). Knowing about family history may be particularly important when assessing for restless sleep in children who have difficulty describing their symptoms.

Periodic limb movements of sleep (PLMS) include repetitive limb movements in sleep that may be disruptive to sleep. Symptoms of both RLS and PLMS may contribute to a number of sleep problems including difficulty falling asleep and staying asleep as well as restless sleep throughout the night (American Academy of Sleep Medicine, 2014; Armstrong et al., 1994). A diagnosis of PLMS is dependent on data obtained during a polysomnography (PSG) and does not require any self-report. Studies indicate that 63% to 74% of children with RLS have an elevated frequency of periodic limb movements (Picchietti et al., 2009; Simakajornboon et al., 2009). Thus, while a sleep study is not indicated for RLS, information about PLMs that are obtained during this procedure may provide helpful diagnostic information (DelRosso et al., 2024; Walters et al., 1994).

The prevalence of RLS varies in the general adult population from 5 to 15% (Phillips et al., 2000). A pediatric population-based study found a prevalence of restless legs syndrome in 2% of 8-to-17-year-olds (Picchietti et al., 2007). There is a significant association of pediatric RLS with ADHD seen in approximately 13% to 25% of pediatric RLS cases (Kotagal & Silber, 2004; Muhle et al., 2008; Picchietti et al., 2007; Yilmaz et al., 2011) and 25% of ADHD cases (Oner et al., 2007; Pullen et al., 2011; Silvestri et al., 2007; Wiggs et al., 2005). Difficulties with mood and anxiety have also been linked to a diagnosis of RLS in children (Pullen et al., 2011).

Latif et al. (2002) found a very high prevalence of iron deficiency in children with ASD. In a study that looked at the effect of iron treatment in children with ASD, Dosman et al. (2007) found that 77% of their sample of 33 children had restless sleep at baseline. Gail Williams et al. (2004) found that 40% of their sample had restless sleep. Studies indicate that decreased iron stores are associated with RLS symptoms (Aul et al., 1998; Sun et al., 1998), and iron deficiency is common in children with ASD (Dosman et al., 2007; Hergüner et al., 2012). This may be due, in part, to the limited and restricted diets of children with ASD (Esposito et al., 2023); as many as 70% to 90% of children with ASD have atypical feeding behaviors (Ahearn et al., 2001; Nieminen-von Wendt et al., 2005; Schreck & Williams, 2006; Schreck et al., 2004b). To date, there has not been research on rates of RLS in ASD. Based on chart review, Youssef et al. (2013), found that 47% of children with ASD had PLMS when compared to 8% in the general population. As noted above, there are many challenges associated with having individuals with ASD complete a PSG study, and this may lead to difficulties detecting PLMS in this population.

Restless Sleep Disorder (RSD) is associated with low-normal ferritin levels. Large, frequent movements during sleep are present as well as difficulties with daytime functioning. Daytime difficulties may include sleepiness, changes in mood, and high activity level. RSD is diagnosed through polysomnography and is treated with iron supplementation (DelRosso et al., 2021, 2023). Children and adolescents with this disorder may have increased nighttime awakenings (DelRosso et al., 2018).

Currently, there are no FDA-approved medications for the management of RLS in children. Serum ferritin is the best indicator for iron deficiency and current evidence indicates that a clinical goal of serum ferritin levels above 50 ng/ml can help alleviate symptoms of RLS and PLMS (DelRosso et al., 2024). DelRosso and colleagues (2024) provide an algorithm for the evaluation of RLS in children and recommend treatment with oral ferrous sulfate for children whose serum ferritin levels are below 50 ng/ml. The International Restless Legs Syndrome Study Group has published guidelines on the treatment of RLS using iron supplementation in children and states that evidence supporting this intervention remains insufficient (Allen et al., 2018; DelRosso et al., 2024). Despite inconclusive evidence, iron supplementation remains a recommended therapy for children with RLS and low iron stores (DelRosso & Bruni, 2019; DelRosso et al., 2024; Earley, 2003). Treatment for RLS may also involve sleep education to improve sleep habits (DelRosso et al., 2024), avoiding caffeine (Amos et al., 2014), getting exercise or taking walks in the afternoon or a few hours before bedtime (DelRosso et al., 2024) and leg massages before bed (Bega & Malkani, 2016). The use of weighted blankets or cooling or heating pads may also be helpful (DelRosso et al., 2024).

Assessment of Sleep Problems

An obvious, but often overlooked, first step in determining whether an individual with an ASD has any sleep problems is to ask if this is a concern. Many individuals with ASD and their families are overwhelmed by many difficulties. These may include difficult daytime behaviors as well as struggles in negotiating complex medical, funding, and educational systems. Families are often dealing with so many difficulties, that it is easy to push sleep concerns to the side. Additionally, many individuals with ASD have long-standing difficulties with sleep; their families may have grown accustomed to their sleep patterns and may not realize that improvements are possible. Thus, it is important to directly ask autistic adolescents or adults (or parents of children with ASD), specific questions about sleep as they may not volunteer these concerns.

Sleep Surveys

There are several surveys and questionnaires that are designed to evaluate a child's sleep habits, sleep problems, and medical concerns that may be related to sleep. Most of these questionnaires were not originally designed for use with children with ASD. However, many have been used extensively with children with autism, have been validated with this population, and may serve as useful screening devices that can guide treatment and intervention.

Sleep Habits and Sleep Quality. While designed for use with typically developing children, the Children's Sleep Habits Questionnaire (CSHQ) (Owens et al., 2000b) has been used extensively with children with ASD. The CSHQ was originally validated on a sample of children ages 4–10 years. It has been used in studies assessing sleep problems in children with ASD including toddlers and preschoolers (Goodlin-Jones et al., 2008) as well as adolescents (Goldman et al., 2011; Goldman et al., 2012b). The CSHQ consists of 45 items that ask parents to report on their children's sleep behaviors over the past month. Most of the questions are answered on a 3-point scale (1 = rarely, 2 = sometimes, 3 = usually). A total score is calculated as well as the following subscale scores: sleep anxiety, sleep duration, sleep-onset delay, night wakings, bedtime resistance, sleep-disordered breathing, parasomnias, and daytime sleepiness. Parents are also asked to rate whether each behavior being queried is a problem or whether it is not a problem. The CSHQ was originally validated on a community sample of 469 children, and results from this sample are often used as normative data in research studies. A total score of 41 is the clinical cut-off for sleep problems (Owens et al., 2000b).

Katz et al. (2018) examined the factor structure of the CSHQ in children with ASD. They looked at CSHQ data from 2872 children enrolled in the Autism Speaks Autism Treatment Network. Results indicated that an abbreviated 23-item version of the CSHQ may be used to assess sleep in children with ASD. The CSHQ-Autism has four factors: Sleep Initiation and Duration, Sleep Anxiety, Night Wakings/Parasomnias, and Daytime Alertness. Internal consistencies ranged from 0.67 to 0.81. Cut-off values for the CSHQ-Autism total score were 34, 35, 33, and 35 for the 2–3, 4–10, 11–17, and 2–17-years age groups, respectively. All cut-off scores performed with moderate to high sensitivity (76.6–82.4%) and moderate specificity (69.1–75.5%), while the original CSHQ cut-off of 41 had high sensitivity (89.9–93.0%) but low specificity (42.6–57.7%). The CSHQ-autism had significantly higher specificity but lower sensitivity than the original CSHQ cut-off of 41 in all age groups (Shui et al., 2021).

Other researchers have also explored the factor structure of the CSHQ in children with ASD. Johnson et al. (2016) looked at CSHQ data from 310 children ages (mean age 4.7 years) and derived five factors (Sleep Routine Problems, Insufficient Sleep, Sleep-onset Association Problems, Parasomnia/Sleep-disordered breathing, and Sleep Anxiety). Internal consistency ranged from 0.87 to 0.50. Zaidman-Zait et al. (2020) looked at the factor structure of the CSHQ in 281 children with ASD ages 4–5. Their 5-factor solution included Bedtime Routine, Sleep Onset and Duration, Night Wakening, Sleep-Disordered Breathing, and Morning Waking.

Hatch and colleagues (2021) looked at the CHSQ in children with and without ASD ages 2–4 years and found that a factor of 7 items that included sleep initiation and nighttime awakening items allowed for comparison between children with and without ASD. They concluded that comparisons for other CSHQ items between the two groups were not appropriate.

The Sleep Committee of the Autism Speaks Autism Treatment Network used expert consensus to develop a practice pathway that captures best practices for the identification, evaluation, and management of insomnia in children and adolescents with autism (Malow et al., 2012b). The guidelines are geared toward general pediatricians, primary care providers, and autism medical specialists. Practitioners are advised to screen all children with ASD for insomnia. Screening may be accomplished by asking a series of questions that target insomnia from the CSHQ and determining if the parent considers these to be a problem. The questions are as follows: (1) child falls asleep within 20 min after going to bed; (2) child falls asleep in parent's or sibling's bed. (3) child sleeps too little; and (4) child awakens once during the night. The practice pathway also stresses the importance of addressing any medical issues that may be impacting sleep, and a questionnaire that helps identify underlying medical conditions is provided. The pathway was updated (Galion et al., 2023) with a focus on night wakings. More about the updated pathway is presented later in this chapter.

There are over 300 pediatric sleep questionnaires (Meltzer et al., 2020). The CSHQ and other commonly used questionnaires that examine behavioral and medical aspects of sleep are summarized in Table 1.

Some sleep questionnaires focus specifically on sleep initiation, maintenance, and quality. The Children's Sleep Wake Scale (LeBourgeois & Harsch, 2001) is a 40 item, 1-month retrospective parent-report measure that has five subscales: going to bed, falling asleep, awakening, reinitiating sleep, and wakefulness. It is designed for

Table 1 Sleep questionnaires

Name	Description	Respondent
BEARS (Owens & Dalzell, 2005)	Assesses 5 sleep domains: B = Bedtime problems (difficulty going to bed and falling asleep); E = Excessive daytime sleepiness; A = Awakenings during the night; R = Regularity and duration of sleep; S = Snoring. For ages 5 to 18 years	Parent and adolescent self-report
Children's sleep habits questionnaire (Owens et al., 2000b)	45 items; 8 subscales including bedtime resistance, sleep-onset delay, sleep duration, sleep anxiety, night wakings, parasomnias, sleep-disordered breathing, and daytime sleepiness. The measure been used with children with ASD ages 2 to 17 years	Parent report
Pediatric sleep questionnaire (Chervin et al., 2000)	69 items; 8 subscales including sleep-related breathing disorders, daytime sleepiness, snoring, and inattention. Ages 2–18 years	Parent report
Pittsburgh sleep quality index (Buysse et al., 1989)	19 items; 7 "component scores": subjective sleep quality, sleep latency, sleep duration, habitual sleep efficiency, sleep disturbances, use of sleeping medication, and daytime dysfunction (there are five additional questions rated by the respondent's roommate or bed partner that are not scored); the measure was originally normed on individuals ages 24–83 years; it has been validated on adolescents and young adults and has been used with autistic individuals	Self-report
Patient Reported Outcome Measurement Information System (PROMIS) Sleep Disturbance Instruments (Bevans et al., 2019; Forrest et al., 2018)	There are several forms for adults and children, including parent proxy forms and a computerized adaptive test. The pediatric self-report is for children ages 8 to 17; the parent proxy report is for parents of children ages 5 to 17. Researchers have validated the self-report measure for children (ages 8 to 17) with chronic illnesses and neurodevelopmental disabilities including ASD and without intellectual or developmental delay (Meltzer et al., 2020)	Self-report and parent report
Simonds & Parraga sleep questionnaire (Simonds & Parraga, 1982)	51 items; the measure is structured in two parts. Part 1 queries sleep quantity and quality. Part 2 assesses specific sleep disorders. 36 items assess bedtime resistance/struggles, sleep-onset delay, parasomnias, sleep-disordered breathing, sleep anxiety, and daytime sleepiness. For children ages 5–18; modified versions have been used with ASD and other developmental delays (Wiggs & Stores, 2004)	Parent report
Sleep disturbance scale for children (Bruni et al., 1996)	26 items; 6 subscales including sleep initiation and maintenance, daytime sleepiness, sleep-disordered breathing, sleep arousal. Ages 5–15 years. The measure has been used with individuals with ASD	Parent report

(continued)

Table 1 (continued)

Name	Description	Respondent
Sleep habits survey (Wolfson et al., 2003)	63 items; 3 subscales including school performance, daytime sleepiness, sleep/wake behavior problems. Ages 10–19 years. The measure has been used by individuals with ASD	Adolescent self-report
Sleep self report (Owens et al., 2000a)	18 items assessing sleep habits, problems falling asleep, sleep duration, night waking, daytime sleepiness. Ages 7–12 years	Child self-report

children ages 2–8 years of age. LeBourgeois has also developed an adolescent self-report measure of sleep initiation and maintenance (LeBourgeois et al., 2005). The Adolescent Sleep Wake Scale is a 28-item questionnaire designed for adolescents ages 12–18; it is a one-month retrospective report that includes 28 items. There are five subscales: going to bed, falling asleep, awakening, reinitiating sleep, and wakefulness.

The Family Inventory of Sleep Habits (FISH) (Malow et al., 2009) is specifically designed for parents of children with autism spectrum disorders ages 4 to 10 years. The items on the FISH assess daytime behaviors that may influence sleep and are amenable to change. Thus, the measure may yield provide information that can guide behavioral intervention. The items address daytime habits (such as exercise, or caffeine intake later in the day), pre-bedtime habits (including engagement in stimulating activities), sleep setting (amount of light and noise in the bedroom), presence (or lack) of a bedtime routine, and parental behaviors (such as remaining with a child until he or she is asleep.) Some of the items focus on sleep behaviors that are particularly relevant for children with ASD such as needing to wear pajamas made from certain fabrics. For each item the parent is asked to indicate how often the behavior was true during the last month on a five-point scale (1 = never, 2 = occasionally, 3 = sometimes, 4 = usually, 5 = always.) The FISH has been validated as a 12-item scale, although a full version contains 22 items.

The Pediatric Sleep Clinical Global Impressions Scale (Malow et al., 2016a) is a clinician-based measure that is designed to measure insomnia in children with ASD. Questions include the child's ability to fall asleep and remain sleeping independently, bedtime resistance, sleep-onset delay, night awakening, parental satisfaction with their child's current sleep patterns, family functioning as affected by their child's current sleep patterns, and the clinician's overall concern with the child's sleep.

Other sleep habits questionnaires are not specifically geared toward children with ASD but can still provide important information. The Children's Sleep Hygiene Scale (LeBourgeois & Harsch, 2001; Harsh et al., 2002) and the Bedtime Routines Questionnaire (Henderson & Jordan, 2010) are brief surveys that provide information about bedtime routines and activities and the sleep environment. Both questionnaires are parent-report measures for parents of children ages 2–8. The Adolescent Sleep Hygiene Scale (Storfer-Isser et al., 2013) is an adolescent-report measure for individuals ages 12–18; it was modified from the Children's Sleep Hygiene Scale and examines behaviors that may interfere with good sleep. These include consumption of caffeine close to bedtime and level of activity before bed.

Daytime Sleepiness. At times it may be important to specifically assess daytime sleepiness. This may be especially important when examining behaviors that may be indicative of sleep-disordered breathing. Behaviors that may indicate sleepiness (versus just being tired) during the day may include falling sleep during daytime activities and overall level of alertness. The Pediatric Daytime Sleepiness Scale (Drake et al., 2003; Nixon et al., 2006) has been validated in children ages 5 to 15 years. It is an 8 item self-report measure that includes questions related to drowsiness, alertness, feeling the need for more sleep, and daytime hyperactivity. The Epworth Sleepiness Scale (Johns, 1991) was first designed as a measure for adults. A modified version for adolescents, The Epworth Sleepiness Scale-Revised for Children, (Melendres et al., 2004; Moore et al., 2009) assesses behaviors that are more applicable to teens than to adults. For example, there are items that look at sleepiness while taking a test. This questionnaire may be completed by parents or by adolescents and is designed for children and adolescents from age 2 to 18 years. The Cleveland Adolescent Sleep Questionnaire (Spilsbury et al., 2007) is a self-report measure for teens ages 11–17 years. Owens and her colleagues have also developed a teacher-survey (The Teacher's Daytime Sleepiness Questionnaire) (Owens et al., 2000c) to assess classroom behaviors of children ages 4–10 years that may be indicative of poor sleep.

Lewandowksi et al. (2011) and Spruyt and Gozal (2011) provide excellent reviews of parent and child-report sleep measures. Sen and Spruyt (2020) have updated the 2011 review and include newly developed measures. These authors describe several limitations of these measures and note that most of these measures need additional information about their reliability and validity. As noted above, most of these measures have not been validated for use with autistic individuals. Additionally, they have not been validated across diverse cultures or ethnic groups. When used clinically, it is important to review responses to survey questions in person to better understand and confirm any sleep problems that may be present.

General Assessment of Child Behaviors. In addition to using surveys that focus exclusively on sleep and sleep-related behavior, clinicians and researchers may use questionnaires that look at a variety of daytime behaviors and provide some information about sleep. Clinicians may find these questionnaires helpful as an initial screening tool although they will not cover all aspects of sleep that should be examined.

The Child Behavior Checklist (Achenbach & Rescoria, 2000) is a parent-report measure of childhood behavioral difficulties including symptoms that are consistent with an ASD diagnosis. It is the most common screening measure for psychopathology that is used by pediatric psychologists (Holmbeck et al., 2008). Children are rated in terms of internalizing and externalizing behavior; similar questions are grouped into subscales or syndrome scales. There is a version for preschoolers (ages 18 months to 5 years) and a version for children ages 6 to 18 years of age. The preschool version includes a scale for sleep problems that includes 7 items (doesn't want to sleep alone, has trouble getting to sleep, nightmares, resists going to sleep, sleeps less than most children during day and/or night, talks or cries out in sleep, wakes often at night.) The CBCL for ages 6–18 years includes multiple items that assess various aspects of sleep, but these items do not form a validated sleep scale on the CBCL. The 7 items include nightmares, overtired without good reason, sleeps less than most kids, sleeps more than most kids during the day/or night, talks or walks in sleep, trouble sleeping, and wets the bed. Parents rate their children for how true each item is currently or within the past 6 months using a 3-point scale (0 = not true, 1 = somewhat or sometimes true, 2 = very true or often true.) Research has supported the use of the CBCL as a tool in epidemiological or archival studies that do not include a more comprehensive sleep measure. It may also be useful for clinicians who do not use other validated sleep measures in their practice (Becker et al., 2015). Becker et al. found that individual CBCL items were generally associated with sleep scales on validated sleep measures and with sleep disorder diagnoses. The CBCL sleep composite was associated with total scores on other sleep-specific measures. Some (but not all) CBCL items are also associated with other measures of sleep. For example, the item "trouble sleeping" has been found to be correlated with sleep information obtained from diaries as well as actigraphy data (Gregory et al., 2011). While the CBCL does not cover important aspects of sleep problems (including those secondary to co-occurring medical conditions) and will not provide a thorough evaluation of sleep problems, it does provide the opportunity to have standardized sleep scores for younger children and to directly compare sleep problems to daytime behavior.

Other measures of daytime behavior also include some sleep items. Some of these measures are: the Behavior Assessment System for Children, Second Edition, (Reynolds & Kamphaus, 2004) which includes 2–4 items depending on the age of the child being assessed; the Child Depression Inventory (Kovacs et al., 2003) which includes 2 items; the Pediatric Quality of Life (Varni et al., 2003) which includes 1 item; and the Parental Concerns Questionnaire (McGrew et al., 2007) which includes 1 item. These questionnaires should not, of course, be relied upon for a screening of sleep problems, but they may provide a means to begin to identify whether there are concerns about a child's sleep and to compare sleep problems to other aspects of a child's functioning. Screening for daytime behavioral difficulties may also help determine whether a more comprehensive psychiatric evaluation is indicated. Psychiatric conditions such as anxiety, bipolar disorder, and depression can affect sleep and may be exacerbated by sleep problems. Thus, consideration of these psychiatric co-occurring conditions should also be part of a comprehensive sleep evaluation.

Sleep Diaries

Information about sleep may also be obtained using logs, sleep diaries, and homework sheets (Spruyt & Gozal, 2011). These parent or self-report measures are ideally completed just before bed and first thing in the morning. Parents, children, and adolescents with age-appropriate reading and writing skills may complete this information.

Diaries or sleep logs include a variety of information. Respondents may be asked to record when a child goes to bed, total time asleep, and when a child wakes up in the morning. The number of nighttime wakings, the time at which they occur, and the length of time a child is awake is often recorded. Sleep logs may also include times that a child gets out of his or her bed. Children may complete sleep logs that require them to record when they went to bed and how many minutes it took them to fall asleep. Information about daytime functioning including fatigue during the day and naps may also be gathered. This information can be used for an initial assessment as well as an evaluation of the effectiveness of an intervention. Observing and recording information about daytime and nighttime routines and behaviors may often help parents become aware of effective strategies and invested in implementing beneficial techniques. At times, information from sleep diaries or logs is paired with information that is acquired through actigraphy (discussed below.) Table 2 lists the type of information that can be gathered through sleep diaries, homework, or logs.

There are a variety of sleep diaries and logs available, but none have been evaluated for their psychometric properties. The National Sleep Foundation has a sleep diary that includes information about daytime behavior: https://www.thensf.org/nsf-sleep-diary/ (National Sleep Foundation, n.d.). As Spruyt and Gozal (2011) note, there is no standardized format for sleep diaries. The wording, order of questions, format, number of questions, information requested, and time frame for completing diaries varies from study to study. Spruyt and Gozal (2011) make key points about using diaries or logs. They correctly note that daily recording and/or rating of nighttime behavior will be more time intensive yet more valid than recording weekly or monthly information. They also note that specific questions may raise an awareness of nighttime behavior or patterns. It is important to confirm that families understand how to complete a sleep log and to consider whether a family can reasonably gather

Table 2 Sleep diaries, sleep logs, and homework

Daytime Habits: Timing of caffeine intake, exposure to morning light, exercise, naps
Evening Habits: Timing of dinner, television, computers, electronics, video games, homework, exercise, other stimulating activities, relaxing activities, lowering of lights
Sleep Setting: Description and evaluation of location, sensory components (e.g., noise level, temperature, light), potential distractions (e.g., electronic devices, toys, materials related to focused interests)
Bedtime Routine: Time to start and finish, evaluation of consistency and inclusion of calm and relaxing activities
Use of visual supports: Are visual schedules or other visual aids used to help a child fall asleep?
Bedtime: What time is bedtime and is it consistent each night including weekends?
Sleep Resistance: How long does it take to fall asleep? What happens once a child is in bed? What are parental responses?
Night Wakings: How many? How long do they last? Does child leave the bed? What are parental responses?
Wake Time: What time is wake time and is it consistent each night including weekends?

and complete the required information. Spruyt and Gozal (2011) also state that it is advisable to have respondents demonstrate their understanding of what is expected, the importance of the information gathered, and the need for precision. They note that it is easy to create logs or diaries that may make it appealing and simple to complete and raise the possibility of creating programs that will allow the use of electronic (computer or mobile) logs with reminders for completion. Children and adolescents may respond well to the use of computers with interactive touch screens. Spruyt and Gozal were not addressing the needs of children with ASD, but using such tools might be highly appealing to technology-minded individuals on the autism spectrum.

Actigraphy

Sleep diaries may be used in combination with actigraphy. This involves recording movement using a miniaturized watch-like device containing an accelerometer that is worn on the wrist during sleep. The actigraph records body movement and this data is interpreted by computer algorithms as periods of sleep and wake. Information about sleep onset, sleep offset, sleep latency, total sleep duration, and wake after sleep onset may also be gathered. The actigraph can collect data continuously over an extended period (often 3 days to 2 weeks and in some cases even longer). Data that is collected are then downloaded to a computer for analysis. New actigraphy devices, algorithms for interpreting data, and operating procedures are frequently being developed, and there is no consensus about which of these are best (Alder et al., 2020). There are also differences in the sensitivity settings that are used during data analysis. Sadeh and Acebo (2002) detail the ways in which actigraphy has become an essential tool in sleep research and sleep medicine. They advise new users to carefully review the scientific literature on each instrument that is being considered to determine which device, mode of operation and scoring algorithm will be most suitable for a researcher or clinician's needs. There are now many devices that are designed to measure physical activity that may also be used to obtain information about sleep, and there are also computer apps on tablets and cell phones that may do the same.

There have been multiple studies that have documented the adequacy of using actigraphy to differentiate clinical groups and to identify some sleep-wake disorders; Morgenthaler et al., (2007) detail practice parameters for the use of actigraphy in clinical practice. Meltzer et al. (2012) provide a thorough review on the validity of actigraphy in children. Actigraphy is a useful measure of change in sleep patterns and can thus help document the effectiveness of sleep interventions, and it can be used for research and clinical purposes. Since it allows for data collection at home, it may provide sleep data that is obtained in a more naturalistic setting than a laboratory (Beebe et al., 2008; Blackwell et al., 2011; Goldman et al., 2009; Goldman et al., 2012a; Peterson et al., 2012). The most common alternative to actigraphy is polysomnography (see below for more information about this.) Polysomnography is expensive and thus usually only includes data from a single night's stay in a sleep laboratory. Actigraphy can provide many days or weeks of data and may provide a more representative sample of sleep than what may be obtained during a night of sleep in an unfamiliar setting while wearing multiple monitors and recording devices.

As with any sleep measure, there are some limitations associated with actigraphy. Most validation studies have been conducted in sleep laboratories while research and clinical studies are conducted in the home where there is less control over factors that are not directly related to sleep (Sadeh & Acebo, 2002). For example, someone who is watching television very quietly may be scored as being asleep. Detailed information from daily logs is thus very important when interpreting actigraph data. Information about bedtime, wake time, when the actigraph is worn and not worn, and external motion (such as riding in a car), or unusual events will be critical when interpreting results (Sadeh & Acebo, 2002). Increased wakefulness during the night also decreases the accuracy of information obtained from actigraphy, and decreased accuracy has been well-documented in individuals with insomnia (Chambers, 1994; Hauri & Wisbey, 1992). Quiet wakefulness while in bed can be miscoded as sleep, and actigraphy has also been documented as less accurate in people with movement disorders (Hauri & Wisbey, 1992). Overall, actigraphy results will vary as a function of age, sex, physical health, and mental health (Sadeh & Acebo, 2002). Thus, the usefulness of actigraphy to compare sleep between different groups may be limited. By contrast, actigraphy data may be very useful for within-subjects designs that assess various factors including treatment efficacy (Sadeh & Acebo, 2002.)

Actigraphy with children poses specific challenges. Children may be curious about how a device works, and this curiosity may result in damaged devices or inaccurate data. Children with ASD may have difficulty wearing an actigraph device on their wrist due to sensory sensitivity or because wearing a watch may be a new and thus stressful experience. Malow and her colleagues have developed effective techniques to help children with ASD and their families successfully use actigraphy (Adkins et al., 2012). They have piloted the use of an actigraph device that is placed in a tight pocket on a child's shoulder. This alternative placement may be used with children who cannot tolerate wearing an actigraph device on their wrist. This pocket placement was initially developed by Souders and colleagues (2009). Pilot results indicate that shoulder placement is promising and worthy of further study. Malow and her colleagues have also developed several strategies to increase caregiver knowledge and skills in obtaining actigraphy data (Fawkes et al., 2014). They found that a one-hour structured parent training session resulted in an increase in scorable actigraphy data. Training included information on how to accurately complete sleep and actigraphy diary forms and the importance of having a child wear the actigraph watch each night. They were careful to review with parents when to mark bedtime and specifically discussed the difference between activities that are part of a bedtime routine (before a parent says goodnight to a child) and activities that occur after a child should be trying to fall asleep (after saying goodnight and turning off lights). The training included examples that emphasized when to press the event marker, the importance of placing the device on their children for at least an hour before bedtime, and the need to leave the device on after waking. Training also included a short quiz to verify caregiver understanding of the material that was presented. Quiz scores that were lower than 80% resulted in a review of any necessary information.

While it may be challenging for children with ASD to wear an actigraph device, there are several strategies that may help. As noted above, some children respond well to the opportunity to wear an actigraph watch in a shoulder pocket. At times, a slow and gradual approach may be beneficial. Children can be desensitized to wearing something on their wrist. A hierarchy of materials to be placed on the wrist can be devised (e.g., start with a thin piece of string followed by a piece of cloth, then gradually move to items that more closely approximate a watch) and a child can practice and be rewarded for wearing objects on their wrist. Some children may prefer a particular watchband that has a particular color, sensation, or design. Some children respond well to learning about actigraphy and become interested and motivated to learn about their sleep patterns. Using a visual schedule at bedtime and including activities related to the actigraph watch can also help children comply with the procedure. Validity of actigraph data may differ depending on the scoring algorithm and actigraph that is being used. There are some potential artifacts of measurement that can lead to inaccurate results, and actigraphy is not adequate for diagnosis in individuals with motor disorders or high motility during sleep.

Polysomnography

A critical component of an adequate sleep assessment must include a review of any potential medical contributions to poor sleep. Use of Reynolds and Malow's (2011) medical conditions questionnaire is an important first step in determining whether there are any medical factors that are impacting sleep. These questions can be incorporated into a review of systems that can lead to medical treatment and determination if a sleep study is needed. Please see Table 3 for a checklist of medical co-occurring conditions that should be assessed.

Sleep Study Overview. A sleep study or polysomnography (PSG) is indicated if a child is noted to have snoring more than 2 nights per week, in addition to one of the following: physical signs on exam; daytime symptoms such as difficulty with attention and learning; or gasping, labored breathing, pauses in breathing, or abnormal posture during sleep. Epilepsy may also disrupt sleep and if there is a concern about possible sleep-related seizures, a sleep study with electroencephalogram (EEG) may be warranted. Sleep studies may also be used to determine if an individual has leg movements or if the child has excessive daytime somnolence (Kotagal et al., 2012).

PSG has been called the "gold standard" for assessing sleep. Individuals spend the night in a sleep laboratory where physiological measures are gathered. These include measures of brain activity (electroencephalography), eye movements (electrooculography), muscle activity (electromyography), and heart rhythm (electrocardiography.) Oxygen levels, airflow, and carbon dioxide levels are monitored throughout the night.

To gather these data, sensors are placed on an individual's head, chin, legs, chest, and area near the eyes. The sensors are usually held in place with gels secured with

Table 3 Screening checklist for medical conditions associated with sleep problems[a]

Gastrointestinal: Current or past symptoms of reflux, constipation, abdominal pain during the day or at night
Seizures and Other Nighttime events: Frequency of nighttime seizures, unusual events (behaviors or movements during the night)
Sleep-Disordered Breathing: Snoring, loud breathing, gasping for breath, stops breathing, allergies, nasal congestion
Asthma/Sinusitis: Coughing at night
Pain/Itching/Discomfort: Regular dental visits, tooth or gum pain, eczema/dry itchy skin, hunger at night, sensory sensitivity (light, sounds, textures, smells)
Nutrition: eat at least 1–2 oz of meat per day, take vitamins with iron
Restless sleep: signs of restless sleep, leg pains or "growing pains," frequent leg movements during sleep, or unusual feelings involving the legs when in bed
Medication: Note all medications currently being used and potential side effects
Physical exam: Large tonsils, hypotonia, nasal congestion or signs of allergic rhinitis, dental issues, wheezing, eczema, and dry or itchy skin

[a] Modified from Reynolds and Malow (2011)

tape or mesh netting. A person's head also needs to be wrapped with gauze to hold the sensors in place. Belts are wrapped around a child's chest and stomach. Pulse oximeter sensors are placed on fingers or toes to monitor oxygen, and a flow sensor and nasal cannula are used. It can take between 30 to 90 min to fully prepare an individual for a sleep study. While the procedure is not painful, it can be stressful and difficult for individuals with ASD who also have sensory sensitivities and who need to adjust to sleeping in a new environment. It is important to note, however, that with careful preparation, most children with ASD can successfully complete a sleep study.

Preparation and Desensitization. One of the first steps to take in preparing a child with ASD for a sleep study is to become familiar with the process. Reviewing a social story that includes photographs or other visual images of the sleep study may be helpful. The Vanderbilt Kennedy Center has developed a very helpful toolkit that includes a social story, visual supports, and concrete suggestions to help prepare a child for a sleep study (Vanderbilt Kennedy Center et al., 2014). Some children enjoy learning about the technical aspects of the study. If possible, use pictures and/or videos from the sleep laboratory where the study will take place. Many sleep centers have produced videos that explain each step of a sleep study. A visit to the sleep lab sometime before the sleep study occurs can also be helpful. Some children may require several visits to get used to the idea of being in the lab. If possible, a child might be able to practice some of the procedures during a brief visit. Ending on a positive note is important, and providing rewards is often a useful strategy. Some individuals will also require systematic desensitization to specific aspects of the sleep study. They may need help to tolerate some of the sensory sensations involved in a sleep study such as having electrodes placed on their head.

During the actual preparation for the sleep study, it may help to provide distractions and comfort objects. Saving a special toy or materials related to a focused interest may also help a child sit through the preparation process. Sensory toys including squeeze balls or oil and water timers may be calming. Allowing a child to watch a special video or play a cherished electronic game may be useful strategies. A visual schedule that depicts each step may help a child track and tolerate the procedure. Rewards may be paired with successfully completing each step. Whenever possible, try to offer a child some choices during the preparation. This may involve choosing which small prize or sticker he or she can earn. If possible, it might involve choosing which electrode will go on next. It helps tremendously if all the adults involved (parents and providers) remain calm and matter of fact throughout the preparation. Zaremba and colleagues (Zaremba et al., 2005) have detailed several strategies geared toward helping children successfully complete a sleep study. They advocate a flexible approach, the use of child-friendly terms instead of medical terminology, the use of distractors, implementation of coping strategies, appropriate modeling of parental behavior, and ongoing praise and reassurance. Baughn et al. (2020) used a Six Sigma framework (define, measure, analyze, improve and control) to improve the pediatric polysomnography experience for patients. They also consulted with their Patient and Family Advisory Council and implemented strategies that included child-life specialists, distraction kits that were available during hook-up, consideration of age-appropriate check-in times, patient education, use of motivational rewards, and modifications to their consultation room and waiting rooms.

Split-Night Sleep Studies. Some sleep labs will complete what is called a "**split-night PSG with CPAP titration**." They will evaluate a child for sleep apnea during the first part of the night. If it is determined that a child has moderate to severe sleep apnea and requires continuous positive airway pressure (CPAP), technicians in the lab may use the second half of the night to obtain information about the level of CPAP pressure that will be required to treat the apnea. Beck and Marcus (2009) advise against this practice with pediatric patients. There has, however, been some research supporting this approach for children (Gerdung et al., 2022). We are not aware of any research about the implementation of this practice in children with ASD. While this may be an efficient use of sleep lab resources, it is not a good strategy for most children with ASD. As noted above, children with ASD often need a great deal of preparation to successfully complete a sleep study. As Beck and Marcus (2009) note, having a CPAP mask placed during the middle of the night may be very upsetting for a child and may make future CPAP compliance much more difficult. A slow, gradual introduction to CPAP that includes desensitization will likely be much more successful. Many children need time to learn to use a CPAP device. These devices are masks that are worn on the face and use air pressure to open airways to allow for uninterrupted breathing. Many individuals (including adults without developmental disorders) find it difficult to adjust to wearing CPAP masks. The same techniques that help children complete a sleep study are also used to teach children to comply with CPAP treatment. Thus, a slow and gradual strategy that includes social stories, systematic desensitization, distraction, and rewards should be used. Once a child can use a CPAP device without difficulty, a second sleep study can be scheduled to determine the proper titration levels.

Home Testing

Given the many difficulties associated with overnight sleep studies in a sleep lab, alternative methods of determining whether someone has sleep apnea is understandably appealing. This may be especially true for children with ASD who have difficulties with transitions and changes in routine. Home sleep apnea studies (HSAT) have become more common for adults. The American Academy of Sleep Medicine released a position paper in 2017 (Kirk et al., 2017) that states that HSAT is not recommended for the diagnosis of OSA in children. They also indicated that clinicians should make the final decision about this and should consider diagnostic tools that are available as well as treatment options. They noted some of the difficulties with home testing of children including difficulties with identification of specific apnea criteria and parents' ability to properly place sensors during the night. Ingram et al. (2023) provide a summary of research studies about HSAT in children and report mixed results including difficulties ruling-out sleep-disordered breathing (Westenberg et al., 2021) and challenges with correct sensor placement during the home-study (Lildal et al., 2021). Researchers have also shown that telehealth support and the availability of an online video attending technician may be helpful strategies (Green et al., 2022; Griffiths et al., 2022).

Wearables

The Sleep Research Society requested a review of wearable sleep-tracking devices (de Zambotti et al., 2023). The extensive review concludes that while wearable sleep-tracking devices may potentially provide beneficial data and contribute to an understanding of an individual's sleep, there continue to be significant limitations that need to be addressed.

As Ingram et al., (2023) note, the use of consumer sleep devices is changing rapidly. There has been frequent introduction of new devices as well as improvements to existing devices. Families frequently purchase sleep-monitoring devices and apps. The American Academy of Sleep Medicine's Consumer and Clinical Technology committee published a position statement about consumer sleep technology (CST; Khosla et al., 2018). The authors note that the use of consumer sleep technology may improve patient engagement, increase the awareness of the importance of sleep and the need for evaluation and treatment, and add to the quality of interactions with families. They note that "understanding the capabilities and limitations of CST is crucial." Schutte-Rodin et al. (2021) has developed a checklist for clinicians to help them evaluate a sleep product; some of the items on the checklist include awareness of FDA terms, familiarity with sleep term definitions across devices and apps, and their use with specific populations. The AASM has also developed and support the following online resource (#SleepTechnology) that is available on for members on the AASM website: https://aasm.org/consumer-clinical-sleep-technology/

Treatment

Behavioral Sleep Education. Research has established that behavioral sleep education is an effective approach to help improve the sleep of children with ASD (Cortesi et al., 2012; Loring et al., 2018; Papadopoulos et al., 2019). Hunter et al. (2020) completed a systematic review that shows that behavioral sleep interventions for children and adolescents with ASD may also lead to positive changes in daytime functioning and well-being. While it is important to address medical and psychiatric disorders, families will also benefit from information that can help improve sleep habits. The practice pathway developed by Malow and her colleagues notes that medical contributors to poor sleep may be assessed and treated concomitantly with a sleep education program (Galion et al., 2023; Malow et al., 2012b). Similarly, Williams Buckley et al. (2020) advise that in addition to determining if coexisting conditions or medications may be affecting sleep, clinicians should consider behavioral strategies as a primary treatment approach. Clinical judgment along with consultation with a family will help determine whether it is best to sequentially assess medical and behavioral contributors to poor sleep or whether a simultaneous approach is best.

Johnson and her colleagues (Johnson et al., 2013) used a manualized parent training program to address sleep problems in young children with ASD and found that it resulted in better sleep based on parental report. Malow et al. (2014) demonstrated that providing parents with sleep education results in improvements as measured by actigraphy in sleep-onset delay in children with ASD. Parents were taught about the importance of daytime habits, evening habits, sleep environment, and bedtime routines. Some of the basic concepts covered in each of these areas are described in Table 4. Many children with ASD respond very well to the use of visual information to help them with routines, manage transitions, and understand parental expectations. The sleep education provided in the Malow et al. (2014) study emphasized the use of visual schedules and other visual supports. The importance of helping children learn to fall asleep independently was also stressed. An important aspect to consider when working with families of children with ASD is that techniques often must be modified and individualized for the child and the family. Malow and colleagues have also established that educational materials for families (including pamphlets, videos, and books) may be effective (Malow et al., 2021b; Malow et al., 2016b). It is important to partner with the family to come up with strategies that will work best.

Resources are available to help families of children with ASD who are experiencing sleep problems. Autism Speaks has online toolkits related to sleep and

Table 4 Fundamentals of healthy sleep practices for children with ASD

Daytime Behaviors: Consideration of exercise, caffeine consumption, presence and timing of naps, bedroom use
Evening Habits: Reduce stimulation, light, stress, exposure to electronics
Bedtime Routine: Implementation of a calm and consistent set of bedtime activities
Sleep Environment: Appraisal of light, temperature, noise, and other sensory input

the use of visual supports (Autism Speaks, n.d.). Materials that may be used to construct pictures schedules for bedtime routines and other visual supports are also provided and may be found at https://www.autismspeaks.org/tool-kit. The books *Sleep Better! A Guide to Improving Sleep in Children with Special Needs* by V. Mark Durand (2013), *Solving Sleep Problems in Children With Autism Spectrum Disorders: A Guide for Frazzled Families* by Katz and Malow (2014) and *Sleep Well on the Autism Spectrum* by Kenneth Aitken (2014) all provide useful information for families.

When providing sleep education to parents, clinicians may use a variety of behavioral strategies. Some examples include extinction and gradual extinction (systematically ignoring undesirable bedtime behaviors). These strategies are often helpful when addressing bedtime resistance and waking during the night (Vriend et al., 2011; Weiskop et al., 2001). Fading parental presence involves having a parent gradually move farther and farther away from their child while they are falling asleep, and this helps children learn to fall asleep independently (Schreck, 2001). Fading other sleep onset associations (such as watching shows on television or a device) is often needed, and parent education about the basics of sleep can be very helpful. Children who are anxious and have difficulty with separation may benefit from using a "bedtime pass" (Friman et al., 1999). This is a card that may be exchanged for contact with a parent during the night. If a child does not use their pass, they can exchange it for a prize in the morning. It can provide comfort to a child who has difficulty with separation and establish a way to reward children for staying in bed. Other forms of positive reinforcement may also be used to encourage desired sleep habits in children with ASD and other developmental disabilities (Allen et al., 2013). Educating families about the ways in which electronic media may affect their children's sleep is also an important component of effective sleep education (Mazurek et al., 2016). MacDonald and colleagues (2021) demonstrated that community therapists can be trained to successfully deliver effective sleep education to families of children with ASD. Their promising results provide evidence that access to effective sleep education may be available to families in rural and underserved communities who may not have access to care in academic medical centers.

Most research on behavioral sleep interventions for children with autism has focused on providing education and support to parents. While there is research demonstrating the effectiveness of working directly with typically developing children to help them sleep better, there is little research examining the benefits of this approach with autistic youth. McCrae et al. (2020) provided cognitive-behavioral sleep interventions directly to children with autism and showed that this is a promising approach. Van Deurs and colleagues (2021) also showed that children and youth with autism ages 9 to 15 can benefit from direct intervention to address their sleep problems. The authors noted that parental involvement was also necessary for successful implementation.

Melatonin. Research indicates that the use of melatonin may be helpful in treating sleep problems in children with ASD (Braam et al., 2009; Malow et al., 2012a; Paavonen et al., 2003). As noted earlier, endogenous melatonin helps regulate our sleep-wake cycles. Synthetic melatonin is available as a dietary supplement. Melatonin may be particularly helpful in addressing difficulties with sleep-onset latency, especially when it is paired with behavioral intervention. Williams Buckley and colleagues (2020) recommend using melatonin if behavioral intervention has not improved sleep. They caution that co-occurring conditions and current medications also need to be reviewed. They advise that parents and children and youth need to be aware of potential side effects and the lack of long-term safety data. They suggest starting with a low dose of melatonin and recommend using pharmaceutical-grade melatonin if it is available.

The Food and Drug Administration (FDA) does not regulate supplements and it is thus not officially approved for any indication (Savage et al., 2024). Erland and Saxena (2017) analyzed 31 melatonin supplements and found that the amount of melatonin in supplements ranged from −83% to +478% of what was described on the bottle. They also found that lot-to-lot variation within a specific product varied as much as 465%. The authors found that more than 71% of the supplements did not meet label claims and note that an additional 26% of the products contained serotonin (which is a controlled substance that is used in the treatment of several neurological disorders). Savage and colleagues (2024) note that supplements with approval from the United States Pharmacopeia ("USP verified") may help assure correct dosing and quality (What the Letters "USP" Mean on the Label of Your Medicine, 2015).

Members of the Autism Treatment Network/Autism Intervention Research Network on Physical Health (ATN/AIR-P) have updated their practice pathway to specifically address difficulties with night waking (Galion et al., 2023). The authors note that night wakings may be related to medical concerns. They suggest that after addressing medical concerns and implementing behavioral strategies, use of extended-release melatonin may be indicated. The authors note that children who have difficulty swallowing pills may need intervention to learn this skill before they can try using this supplement. Malow, Findling and et al., (2021a, 2021b) found that long-term use (up to two years) of extended-release melatonin in children and adolescents with ASD was effective and safe.

Prescription Medications. Other pharmacologic treatments may be warranted when behavioral therapy and melatonin do not result in improved sleep. There are medications that have been used clinically, but there is a paucity of research that can be used to inform the use of these medications in children with ASD. Owens (2023) states behavioral intervention should be considered first-line therapy for children with sleep problems. She outlines a general approach for deciding about pharmacological intervention and recommends considering efficacy, side effects, safety, and ethical considerations. She notes that the child's age, the type of sleep problem, whether the sleep problem is acute or chronic, existence of co-occurring conditions, and information about concurrent use of prescription and nonprescription medications are all important considerations. Owens (2023) describes that most prescription medications for insomnia (such as benzodiazepines and nonbenzodiazepine receptor agonists) have been trialed in adults and notes that there is a paucity of information about their efficacy and safety in children. Additionally, there are prescription medications that are commonly used off-label for insomnia in children. These include alpha-adrenergic agonists (used to treat behaviors associated with ADHD), antidepressants, atypical antidepressants, and selective serotonin reuptake inhibitors.

Novel Treatments. Esposito and colleagues provide a narrative review of non-pharmacological interventions and over-the counter treatments for sleep problems in children with ASD (Esposito et al., 2020). Their review includes sleep education, behavioral interventions, complementary and alternative medicine (special mattresses and blankets, massage, aromatherapy, yoga, and physical therapy). They also review over-the counter medications and supplements (which will not be summarized in the current chapter). They provide an excellent overview of sleep behavioral interventions. They note that behavioral intervention is effective and conclude that since there is no evidence about the superiority of one technique over another, it is important to work together with parents to develop a behavioral plan. They conclude that there is no strong evidence to recommend the use of weighted blankets and vests, mattress-based technologies, massage, aromatherapy, yoga, sports, and physical activity to help with sleep. Williams Buckley and colleagues (2020) also agree about the lack of research evidence supporting the use of weighted blankets or specialized mattress technology. Williams Buckley et al. (2020) note that there are no serious adverse events associated with blanket use and that some families may find it worthwhile to try this approach. Esposito et al. (2020) note that some of these techniques (namely mattress-based technologies, yoga therapy, massage, and physical therapy) have been examined in small clinical trials and there were no adverse effects of these strategies; thus, while families should be informed about the lack of research evidence regarding these strategies, they may be worth trying in some situations.

Telehealth. The use of telehealth services to provide sleep intervention to children with ASD is a growing and promising field (Ellison et al., 2021). Use of telehealth services increased significantly during the Covid-19 pandemic (Taylor et al., 2021). Johnson and colleagues (2023) provided a manualized behavioral parent sleep education program to families of children ages 2 to 7. The authors found that this approach was effective in addressing sleep problems. They note that this approach may help increase access to services for many families. Other researchers have also shown that addressing sleep problems in children with ASD via telehealth is effective (Davenport et al., 2021; McCrae et al., 2021). Lewis et al., (2023) describe the need for telehealth delivery and note that during the COVID-19 pandemic children with autism had increased difficulties with sleep. They note that behavioral sleep interventions are well suited to telehealth delivery and state that providing intervention remotely is an important option for many families.

Summary

Evaluation of sleep problems in children with ASD is a critical and often overlooked component of ensuring an effective treatment plan. Poor sleep can have a profound effect on daytime functioning and may have medical implications as well. It also can have a significant impact on the quality of life of the family. The first step in assessing a child's sleep involves determining if a parent has any concerns about their child's sleep. Getting detailed information or a sleep history can be accomplished by interviewing parents, reviewing their responses to a standardized questionnaire, or both. When talking with parents of children with autism about their sleep problems, it is important to ask specific questions and give clear indication that this is a critical aspect of their child's development. Key information includes knowing how long it takes a child to fall asleep, whether a child can fall asleep independently, the amount of sleep a child gets in a 24-h period, and how often a child awakens during the night. Knowing about daytime functioning and sleepiness during the day is also important, and interview data and information obtained from questionnaires such as the Child Behavior Checklist may be useful. The Family Inventory of Sleep Habits may provide data that will be needed to help families develop behavioral strategies that will promote good sleep. Sleep questionnaires such as the Child Sleep Habits Questionnaire may also provide critical information about sleep behaviors and medical issues. It may often be necessary to address both behavioral and medical concerns. Strategies to address behavioral difficulties may be implemented while medical co-occurring conditions are being considered. In addition to a medical screening, the use of actigraphy or polysomnography may be indicated to assess some primary sleep disorders.

References

Achenbach, T., & Rescoria, L. (2000). *Child behavior checklist*. ASEBA.

Adkins, K. W., Goldman, S. E., Fawkes, D., Surdyka, K., Wang, L., Song, Y., & Malow, B. A. (2012). A pilot study of shoulder placement for actigraphy in children. *Behavioral Sleep Medicine, 10*(2), 138–147. https://doi.org/10.1080/15402002.2011.596598

Ahearn, W. H., Castine, T., Nault, K., & Green, G. (2001). An assessment of food acceptance in children with autism or pervasive developmental disorder-not otherwise specified. *Journal of Autism and Developmental Disorders, 31*(5), 505–511. https://doi.org/10.1023/a:1012221026124

Aitken, K. J. (2014). *Sleep well on the autism spectrum: How to recognise common sleep problems, choose the right treatment, and get you or your child sleeping soundly*. Jessica Kingsley Publishers.

Alder, M. L., Ye, F., Run, F., Bagai, K., Fawkes, D. B., Peterson, B. T., & Malow, B. A. (2020). Application of a novel actigraphy algorithm to detect movement and sleep/wake patterns in children with autism spectrum disorder. *Sleep Medicine, 71*, 28–34. https://doi.org/10.1016/j.sleep.2020.02.020

Aldinger, K. A., Lane, C. J., Veenstra-VanderWeele, J., & Levitt, P. (2015). Patterns of risk for multiple co-occurring medical conditions replicate across distinct cohorts of children with autism spectrum disorder. *Autism Research, 8*(6), 771–781. https://doi.org/10.1002/aur.1492

Allen, K. D., Kuhn, B. R., DeHaai, K. A., & Wallace, D. P. (2013). Evaluation of a behavioral treatment package to reduce sleep problems in children with Angelman Syndrome. *Research in Developmental Disabilities, 34*(1), 676–686. https://doi.org/10.1016/j.ridd.2012.10.001

Allen, R. P., Picchietti, D. L., Auerbach, M., Cho, Y. W., Connor, J. R., Earley, C. J., Garcia-Borreguero, D., Kotagal, S., Manconi, M., Ondo, W., Ulfberg, J., Winkelman, J. W., & International Restless Legs Syndrome Study Group (IRLSSG), 2018 Allen, R. P., Picchietti, D. L., Auerbach, M., Cho, Y. W., Connor, J. R., Earley, C. J., Garcia-Borreguero, D., Kotagal, S., Manconi, M., Ondo, W., Ulfberg, J., Winkelman, J. W., & International Restless Legs Syndrome Study Group (IRLSSG). (2018). Evidence-based and consensus clinical practice guidelines for the iron treatment of restless legs syndrome/Willis-Ekbom disease in adults and children: an IRLSSG task force report. *Sleep Medicine, 41*, 27–44. https://doi.org/10.1016/j.sleep.2017.11.1126

American Academy of Sleep Medicine. (2014). *The international classification of sleep disorders: Diagnostic and coding manual* (3rd ed.). Author.

Amos, L. B., Grekowicz, M. L., Kuhn, E. M., Olstad, J. D., Collins, M. M., Norins, N. A., & D'Andrea, L. A. (2014). Treatment of pediatric restless legs syndrome. *Clinical Pediatrics, 53*(4), 331–336. https://doi.org/10.1177/0009922813507997

Arendt, J. (1998). Melatonin and the pineal gland: Influence on mammalian seasonal and circadian physiology. *Reviews of Reproduction, 3*(1), 13–22. https://doi.org/10.1530/ror.0.0030013

Arendt, J., Bojkowski, C., Franey, C., Wright, J., & Marks, V. (1985). Immunoassay of 6-hydroxymelatonin sulfate in human plasma and urine: Abolition of the urinary 24-hour rhythm with atenolol. *Journal of Clinical Endocrinology & Metabolism, 60*(6), 1166–1173. https://doi.org/10.1210/jcem-60-6-1166

Armstrong, K. L., Quinn, R. A., & Dadds, M. R. (1994). The sleep patterns of normal children. *Medical Journal of Australia, 161*(3), 202–206. https://doi.org/10.5694/j.1326-5377.1994.tb127383.x

Aul, E. A., Davis, B. J., & Rodnitzky, R. L. (1998). The importance of formal serum iron studies in the assessment of restless legs syndrome. *Neurology, 51*(3), 912. https://doi.org/10.1212/wnl.51.3.912

Autism Speaks. (n.d.). *Tool Kits | Autism Speaks*. Retrieved November 27, 2025 from https://www.autismspeaks.org/tool-kit

Baker, E. K., Richdale, A. L., Hazi, A., & Prendergast, L. A. (2019). Assessing a hyperarousal hypothesis of insomnia in adults with autism spectrum disorder. *Autism Research, 12*(6), 897–910. https://doi.org/10.1002/aur.2094

Baughn, J. M., Lechner, H. G., Herold, D. L., Brown, V. A., Moore, W. R., Harris, C. D., Stehr, H. I., Sorensen, C. M., Cleveland, E. J., Akason, J. D., Morgenthaler, T. I., & Lloyd, R. M. (2020). Enhancing the patient and family experience during pediatric sleep studies. *Journal of Clinical Sleep Medicine, 16*(7), 1037–1043. https://doi.org/10.5664/jcsm.8386

Beck, S. E., & Marcus, C. L. (2009). Pediatric polysomnography. *Sleep Medicine Clinics, 4*(3), 393–406. https://doi.org/10.1016/j.jsmc.2009.04.007

Becker, S. P., Ramsey, R. R., & Byars, K. C. (2015). Convergent validity of the child behavior checklist sleep items with validated sleep measures and sleep disorder diagnoses in children and adolescents referred to a sleep disorders center. *Sleep Medicine, 16*(1), 79–86. https://doi.org/10.1016/j.sleep.2014.09.008

Beebe, D. W., Fallone, G., Godiwala, N., Flanigan, M., Martin, D., Schaffner, L., & Amin, R. (2008). Feasibility and behavioral effects of an at-home multi-night sleep restriction protocol for adolescents. *Journal of Child Psychology and Psychiatry, 49*(9), 915–923. https://doi.org/10.1111/j.1469-7610.2008.01885.x

Bega, D., & Malkani, R. (2016). Alternative treatment of restless legs syndrome: An overview of the evidence for mind-body interventions, lifestyle interventions, and neutraceuticals. *Sleep Medicine, 17*, 99–105. https://doi.org/10.1016/j.sleep.2015.09.009
Bernardi, K., Prono, F., Bruni, G., Panerai, S., Ferri, R., & Bruni, O. (2023). Sleep disturbances in subjects with autism spectrum disorder: A parental perspective. *Sleep Medicine, 110*, 220–224. https://doi.org/10.1016/j.sleep.2023.08.020
Bevans, K. B., Meltzer, L. J., De La Motte, A., Kratchman, A., Viél, D., & Forrest, C. B. (2019). Qualitative development and content validation of the PROMIS pediatric sleep health items. *Behavioral Sleep Medicine, 17*(5), 657–671. https://doi.org/10.1080/15402002.2018.1461102
Blackwell, T., Ancoli-Israel, S., Redline, S., & Stone, K. (2011). Factors that may influence the classification of sleep-wake by wrist actigraphy: The MrOS sleep study. *Journal of Clinical Sleep Medicine, 7*(4), 357–367. https://doi.org/10.5664/JCSM.1190
Bottema-Beutel, K., Kapp, S. K., Lester, J. N., Sasson, N. J., & Hand, B. N. (2021). Avoiding ableist language: Suggestions for autism researchers. *Autism in Adulthood, 3*(1), 18–29. https://doi.org/10.1089/aut.2020.0014
Braam, W., Geijlswijk, I. V., Keijzer, H., Smits, M. G., Didden, R., & Curfs, L. M. (2010). Loss of response to melatonin treatment is associated with slow melatonin metabolism: Loss of response to melatonin treatment. *Journal of Intellectual Disability Research, 54*(6), 547–555. https://doi.org/10.1111/j.1365-2788.2010.01283.x
Braam, W., Keijzer, H., Struijker Boudier, H., Didden, R., Smits, M., & Curfs, L. (2013). CYP1A2 polymorphisms in slow melatonin metabolisers: A possible relationship with autism spectrum disorder? *Journal of Intellectual Disability Research, 57*(11), 993–1000. https://doi.org/10.1111/j.1365-2788.2012.01595.x
Braam, W., Smits, M. G., Didden, R., Korzilius, H., Geijlswijk, I. M., & Curfs, L. M. (2009). Exogenous melatonin for sleep problems in individuals with intellectual disability: A meta-analysis. *Developmental Medicine and Child Neurology, 51*(5), 340–349. https://doi.org/10.1111/j.1469-8749.2008.03244.x
Bruni, O., Ottaviano, S., Guidetti, V., Romoli, M., Innocenzi, M., Cortesi, F., & Giannotti, F. (1996). The Sleep Disturbance Scale for Children (SDSC) construction and validation of an instrument to evaluate sleep disturbances in childhood and adolescence. *Journal of Sleep Research, 5*(4), 251–261. https://doi.org/10.1111/j.1365-2869.1996.00251.x
Buie, T., Fuchs III, G. J., Furuta, G. T., Kooros, K., Levy, J., Lewis, J. D., Wershil, B. K., & Winter, H. (2010). Recommendations for evaluation and treatment of common gastrointestinal problems in children with ASDs. *Pediatrics, 125*(Supplement 1), S19–S29. https://doi.org/10.1542/peds.2009-1878D
Buysse, D. J., Reynolds, C. F., 3rd., Monk, T. H., Berman, S. R., & Kupfer, D. J. (1989). The Pittsburgh sleep quality index: A new instrument for psychiatric practice and research. *Psychiatry Research, 28*(2), 193–213. https://doi.org/10.1016/0165-1781(89)90047-4
Cai, G., Edelmann, L., Goldsmith, J. E., Cohen, N., Nakamine, A., Reichert, J. G., Hoffman, E. J., Zurawiecki, D. M., Silverman, J. M., Hollander, E., Soorya, L., & Buxbaum, J. D. (2008). Multiplex ligation-dependent probe amplification for genetic screening in autism spectrum disorders: Efficient identification of known microduplications and identification of a novel microduplication in ASMT. *BMC Medical Genomics, 1*(50). https://doi.org/10.1186/1755-8794-1-50
Chambers, M. J. (1994). Actigraphy and insomnia–a closer look. *Sleep, 17*(5), 405–408.
Chervin, R. D., Hedger, K., Dillon, J. E., & Pituch, K. J. (2000). Pediatric Sleep Questionnaire (PSQ): Validity and reliability of scales for sleep-disordered breathing, snoring, sleepiness, and behavioral problems. *Sleep Medicine, 1*(1), 21–32. https://doi.org/10.1016/s1389-9457(99)00009-x
Clements, J., Wing, L., & Dunn, G. (1986). Sleep problems in handicapped children: A preliminary study. *Journal of Child Psychology and Psychiatry, 27*(3), 399–407. https://doi.org/10.1111/j.1469-7610.1986.tb01841.x

Corbett, B. A., Schupp, C. W., Levine, S., & Mendoza, S. (2009). Comparing cortisol, stress, and sensory sensitivity in children with autism. *Autism Research, 2*(1), 39–49. https://doi.org/10.1002/aur.64

Cortese, S., Wang, F., Angriman, M., Masi, G., & Bruni, O. (2020). Sleep disorders in children and adolescents with autism spectrum disorder: Diagnosis, epidemiology, and management. *CNS Drugs, 34*(4), 415–423. https://doi.org/10.1007/s40263-020-00710-y

Cortesi, F., Giannotti, F., Sebastiani, T., Panunzi, S., & Valente, D. (2012). Controlled-release melatonin, singly and combined with cognitive behavioural therapy, for persistent insomnia in children with autism spectrum disorders: A randomized placebo-controlled trial. *Journal of Sleep Research, 21*(6), 700–709. https://doi.org/10.1111/j.1365-2869.2012.01021.x

Couturier, J. L., Speechley, K. N., Steele, M., Norman, R., Stringer, B., & Nicolson, R. (2005). Parental perception of sleep problems in children of normal intelligence with pervasive developmental disorders: Prevalence, severity, and pattern. *Journal of the American Academy of Child and Adolescent Psychiatry, 44*(8), 815–822. https://doi.org/10.1097/01.chi.0000166377.22651.87

Cukic, V., Lovre, V., & Dragisic, D. (2011). Sleep disorders in patients with bronchial asthma. *Materia Socio-Medica, 23*(4), 235–237. https://doi.org/10.5455/msm.2011.23.235-237

Davenport, M. A., Berry, J. R., Mazurek, M. O., & McCrae, C. S. (2021). Using telehealth to deliver family-based cognitive behavioral treatment of insomnia in a school-aged child with autism spectrum disorder. *Journal of Cognitive Psychotherapy, 35*(4), 235–254. https://doi.org/10.1891/JCPSY-D-20-00062

D'Elia, C., Gozal, D., Bruni, O., Goudouris, E., Meira, E., & Cruz, M. (2022). Allergic rhinitis and sleep disorders in children - coexistence and reciprocal interactions. *Jornal De Pediatria, 98*(5), 444–454. https://doi.org/10.1016/j.jped.2021.11.010

DelRosso, L., & Bruni, O. (2019). Treatment of pediatric restless legs syndrome. *Advances in Pharmacology (San Diego, Calif.), 84*, 237–253. https://doi.org/10.1016/bs.apha.2018.11.001

DelRosso, L. M., Bruni, O., & Ferri, R. (2018). Restless sleep disorder in children: A pilot study on a tentative new diagnostic category. *Sleep, 41*(8), zsy102.

DelRosso, L. M., Mogavero, M. P., Baroni, A., Bruni, O., & Ferri, R. (2024). Restless legs syndrome in children and adolescents. *The Psychiatric Clinics of North America, 47*(1), 147–161. https://doi.org/10.1016/j.psc.2023.06.010

DelRosso, L. M., Mogavero, M. P., Bruni, O., & Ferri, R. (2023). Restless legs syndrome and restless sleep disorder in children. *Sleep Medicine Clinics, 18*(2), 201–212. https://doi.org/10.1016/j.jsmc.2023.01.008

DelRosso, L. M., Silvestri, R., & Ferri, R. (2021). Restless sleep disorder. *Sleep Medicine Clinics, 16*(2), 381–387. https://doi.org/10.1016/j.jsmc.2021.03.003

DeVincent, C. J., Gadow, K. D., Delosh, D., & Geller, L. (2007). Sleep disturbance and its relation to DSM-IV psychiatric symptoms in preschool-age children with pervasive developmental disorder and community controls. *Journal of Child Neurology, 22*(2), 161–169. https://doi.org/10.1177/0883073807300310

de Zambotti, M., Goldstein, C., Cook, J., Menghini, L., Altini, M., Cheng, P., & Robillard, R. (2023). State of the science and recommendations for using wearable technology in sleep and circadian research. *Sleep*, zsad325. https://doi.org/10.1093/sleep/zsad325

Didden, R., Korzilius, H., van Aperlo, B., van Overloop, C., & de Vries, M. (2002). Sleep problems and daytime problem behaviours in children with intellectual disability. *Journal of Intellectual Disability Research, 46*(Pt 7), 537–547. https://doi.org/10.1046/j.1365-2788.2002.00404.x

Didden, R., & Sigafoos, J. (2001). A review of the nature and treatment of sleep disorders in individuals with developmental disabilities. *Research in Developmental Disabilities, 22*(4), 255–272. https://doi.org/10.1016/s0891-4222(01)00071-3

Doo, S., & Wing, Y. K. (2006). Sleep problems of children with pervasive developmental disorders: Correlation with parental stress. *Developmental Medicine and Child Neurology, 48*(8), 650–655. https://doi.org/10.1017/S001216220600137X

Dosman, C. F., Brian, J. A., Drmic, I. E., Senthilselvan, A., Harford, M. M., Smith, R. W., Sharieff, W., Zlotkin, S. H., Moldofsky, H., & Roberts, S. W. (2007). Children with autism: Effect of iron supplementation on sleep and ferritin. *Pediatric Neurology, 36*(3), 152–158. https://doi.org/10.1016/j.pediatrneurol.2006.11.004

Drake, C., Nickel, C., Burduvali, E., Roth, T., Jefferson, C., & Pietro, B. (2003). The Pediatric Daytime Sleepiness Scale (PDSS): Sleep habits and school outcomes in middle-school children. *Sleep, 26*(4), 455–458.

Durand, V. M. (2013). *Sleep better!: A guide to improving sleep for children with special needs* (2nd ed.). Paul H. Brookes Pub. Co.

Earley C. J. (2003). Clinical practice. Restless legs syndrome. *The New England Journal of Medicine, 348*(21), 2103–2109. https://doi.org/10.1056/NEJMcp021288

Ellison, K. S., Guidry, J., Picou, P., Adenuga, P., & Davis, T. E., 3rd. (2021). Telehealth and autism prior to and in the age of COVID-19: A systematic and critical review of the last decade. *Clinical Child and Family Psychology Review, 24*(3), 599–630. https://doi.org/10.1007/s10567-021-00358-0

Eow, S. Y., Gan, W. Y., Lim, P. Y., Awang, H., & Mohd Shariff, Z. (2022). Parental feeding practices and child-related factors are associated with overweight and obesity in children and adolescents with autism spectrum disorder. *Journal of Autism and Developmental Disorders, 52*(8), 3655–3667. https://doi.org/10.1007/s10803-021-05247-7

Erland, L. A., & Saxena, P. K. (2017). Melatonin natural health products and supplements: Presence of serotonin and significant variability of melatonin content. *Journal of Clinical Sleep Medicine, 13*(2), 275–281. https://doi.org/10.5664/jcsm.6462

Esposito, D., Belli, A., Ferri, R., & Bruni, O. (2020). Sleeping without prescription: Management of sleep disorders in children with autism with non-pharmacological interventions and over-the-counter treatments. *Brain Sciences, 10*(7), 441. https://doi.org/10.3390/brainsci10070441

Esposito, M., Mirizzi, P., Fadda, R., Pirollo, C., Ricciardi, O., Mazza, M., & Valenti, M. (2023). Food selectivity in children with autism: Guidelines for assessment and clinical interventions. *International Journal of Environmental Research and Public Health, 20*(6), 5092. https://doi.org/10.3390/ijerph20065092

Fawkes, D. B., Malow, B. A., Weiss, S. K., Reynolds, A., Loh, A., Adkins, K., Wofford, D., Wyatt, A. D., & Goldman, S. E. (2014). Conducting actigraphy research in children with neurodevelopmental disorders–a practical approach. *Behavioral Sleep Medicine*. https://doi.org/10.1080/15402002.2013.854245

Ferrazzano, G. F., Salerno, C., Bravaccio, C., Ingenito, A., Sangianantoni, G., & Cantile, T. (2020). Autism spectrum disorders and oral health status: Review of the literature. *European Journal of Paediatric Dentistry, 21*(1), 9–12. https://doi.org/10.23804/ejpd.2020.21.01.02

Fishbein, A. B., Cheng, B. T., Tilley, C. C., Begolka, W. S., Carle, A. C., Forrest, C. B., Zee, P. C., Paller, A. S., & Griffith, J. W. (2021). Sleep disturbance in school-aged children with atopic dermatitis: Prevalence and severity in a cross-sectional sample. *The Journal of Allergy and Clinical Immunology. In Practice, 9*(8), 3120–3129.e3. https://doi.org/10.1016/j.jaip.2021.04.064

Foody, C., James, J. E., & Leader, G. (2015). Parenting stress, salivary biomarkers, and ambulatory blood pressure: A comparison between mothers and fathers of children with autism spectrum disorders. *Journal of Autism and Developmental Disorders, 45*, 1084–1095. https://doi.org/10.1007/s10803-014-2263-y

Forrest, C. B., Meltzer, L. J., Marcus, C. L., de la Motte, A., Kratchman, A., Buysse, D. J., Pilkonis, P. A., Becker, B. D., & Bevans, K. B. (2018). Development and validation of the PROMIS pediatric sleep disturbance and sleep-related impairment item banks. *Sleep, 41*(6). https://doi.org/10.1093/sleep/zsy054

Friman, P. C., Hoff, K. E., Schnoes, C., Freeman, K. A., Woods, D. W., & Blum, N. (1999). The bedtime pass: An approach to bedtime crying and leaving the room. *Archives of Pediatrics & Adolescent Medicine, 153*(10), 1027–1029. https://doi.org/10.1001/archpedi.153.10.1027

Gabriels, R. L., Cuccaro, M. L., Hill, D. E., Ivers, B. J., & Goldson, E. (2005). Repetitive behaviors in autism: Relationships with associated clinical features. *Research in Developmental Disabilities, 26*(2), 169–181. https://doi.org/10.1016/j.ridd.2004.05.003

Gail Williams, P., Sears, L. L., & Allard, A. (2004). Sleep problems in children with autism. *Journal of Sleep Research, 13*(3), 265–268. https://doi.org/10.1111/j.1365-2869.2004.00405.x

Galion, A. W., Farmer, J. G., Connolly, H. V., Allhusen, V. D., Bennett, A., Coury, D. L., … & Autism Treatment Network/Autism Intervention Research Network on Physical Health (ATN/AIR-P) Sleep Committee, 2023 Galion, A. W., Farmer, J. G., Connolly, H. V., Allhusen, V. D., Bennett, A., Coury, D. L., Lam, J., Neumeyer, A. M., Sohl, K., Witmans, M., Malow, B. A., & Autism Treatment Network/Autism Intervention Research Network on Physical Health (ATN/AIR-P) Sleep Committee. (2023). A practice pathway for the treatment of night wakings in children with autism spectrum disorder. *Journal of Autism and Developmental Disorders*, 1–20. https://doi.org/10.1007/s10803-023-06026-2

Garstang, J., & Wallis, M. (2006). Randomized controlled trial of melatonin for children with autism spectrum disorders and sleep problems. *Child: Care, Health, and Development, 32*(5), 585–589. https://doi.org/10.1111/j.1365-2214.2006.00616.x

Gerdung, C. A., Castro-Codesal, M. L., Nettel-Aguirre, A., Kam, K., Hanly, P. J., MacLean, J. E., & Bendiak, G. N. (2022). Feasibility of split night polysomnography in children to diagnose and treat sleep related breathing disorders. *Sleep Medicine, 96*, 107–112. https://doi.org/10.1016/j.sleep.2022.05.011

Giannotti, F., Cortesi, F., Cerquiglini, A., & Bernabei, P. (2006). An open-label study of controlled-release melatonin in treatment of sleep disorders in children with autism. *Journal of Autism and Developmental Disorders, 36*(6), 741–752. https://doi.org/10.1007/s10803-006-0116-z

Gold, A. K., & Sylvia, L. G. (2016). The role of sleep in bipolar disorder. *Nature and Science of Sleep, 8*, 207–214. https://doi.org/10.2147/NSS.S85754

Goldman, S. E., Adkins, K. W., Calcutt, M., Carter, M. D., Goodpaster, R. L., Wang, L., Burgess, H. J., Hachey, D. L., Malow, B. A., & Shi, Y. (2014). Melatonin in children with autism spectrum disorders: Endogenous and pharmacokinetic profiles in relation to sleep. *Journal of Autism and Developmental Disorders, 44*(10), 2525–2535. https://doi.org/10.1007/s10803-014-2123-9

Goldman, S. E., Alder, M. L., Burgess, H. J., Corbett, B. A., Hundley, R., Wofford, D., Fawkes, D. B., Wang, L., Laudenslager, M. L., & Malow, B. A. (2017). Characterizing sleep in adolescents and adults with autism spectrum disorders. *Journal of Autism and Developmental Disorders, 47*(6), 1682–1695. https://doi.org/10.1007/s10803-017-3089-1

Goldman, S. E., Bichell, T., Surdyka, K., & Malow, B. A. (2012a). Sleep in children and adolescents with Angelman syndrome: Association with parent sleep and stress. *Journal of Intellectual Disability Research, 56*(6), 600–608. https://doi.org/10.1111/j.1365-2788.2011.01499.x

Goldman, S. E., McGrew, S., Johnson, K. P., Richdale, A. L., Clemons, T., & Malow, B. A. (2011). Sleep is associated with problem behaviors in children and adolescents with autism spectrum disorders. *Research in Autism Spectrum Disorders, 5*(3), 1223–1229. https://doi.org/10.1016/j.rasd.2011.01.010

Goldman, S. E., Richdale, A. L., Clemons, T., & Malow, B. A. (2012b). Parental sleep concerns in autism spectrum disorders: Variations from childhood to adolescence. *Journal of Autism and Developmental Disorders, 42*(4), 531–538. https://doi.org/10.1007/s10803-011-1270-5

Goldman, S. E., Surdyka, K., Cuevas, R., Adkins, K., Wang, L., & Malow, B. A. (2009). Defining the sleep phenotype in children with autism. *Developmental Neuropsychology, 34*(5), 580–573. https://doi.org/10.1080/87565640903133509

Goodlin-Jones, B. L., Sitnick, S. L., Tang, K., Liu, J., & Anders, T. F. (2008). The children's sleep habits questionnaire in toddlers and preschool children. *Journal of Developmental and Behavioral Pediatrics, 29*(2), 82–88. https://doi.org/10.1097/dbp.0b013e318163c39a

Gooley, J. J., & Saper, C. B. (2011). Anatomy of the mammalian circadian system. In M. H. Kryger, T. Roth, & W. C. Dement (Eds.), *Principles and practice of sleep medicine*. Saunders/Elsevier. https://doi.org/10.1016/B978-0-323-24288-2.00033-7

Green, A., Nagel, N., Kemer, L., & Dagan, Y. (2022). Comparing in-lab full polysomnography for diagnosing sleep apnea in children to Home Sleep Apnea Tests (HSAT) with an online video attending technician. *Sleep and Biological Rhythms, 20*(3), 397–401. https://doi.org/10.1007/s41105-022-00384-7

Gregory, A. M., Cousins, J. C., Forbes, E. E., Trubnick, L., Ryan, N. D., Axelson, D. A., Birmaher, B., Sadeh, A., & Dahl, R. E. (2011). Sleep items in the child behavior checklist: A comparison with sleep diaries, actigraphy, and polysomnography. *Journal of the American Academy of Child and Adolescent Psychiatry, 50*(5), 499–507. https://doi.org/10.1016/j.jaac.2011.02.003

Griffiths, A., Mukushi, A., & Adams, A. M. (2022). Telehealth-supported level 2 pediatric home polysomnography. *Journal of Clinical Sleep Medicine, 18*(7), 1815–1821. https://doi.org/10.5664/jcsm.9982

Harsh, J. R., Easley, A., & LeBourgeois, M. K. (2002). A measure of children's sleep hygiene. *Sleep, 25*, A316.

Hatch, B., Nordahl, C. W., Schwichtenberg, A. J., Ozonoff, S., & Miller, M. (2021). Factor structure of the children's sleep habits questionnaire in young children with and without autism. *Journal of Autism and Developmental Disorders, 51*(9), 3126–3137. https://doi.org/10.1007/s10803-020-04752-5

Hauri, P. J., & Wisbey, J. (1992). Wrist actigraphy in insomnia. *Sleep, 15*(4), 293–301. https://doi.org/10.1093/sleep/15.4.293

Henderson, J. A., & Jordan, S. S. (2010). Development and preliminary evaluation of the Bedtime Routines Questionnaire. *Journal of Psychopathology and Behavioral Assessment, 32*(2), 271–280. https://doi.org/10.1007/s10862-009-9143-3

Hergüner, S., Keleşoğlu, F. M., Tanıdır, C., & Çöpür, M. (2012). Ferritin and iron levels in children with autistic disorder. *European Journal of Pediatrics, 171*(1), 143–146. https://doi.org/10.1007/s00431-011-1506-6

Hoban, T. F. (2003). Rhythmic movement disorder in childhood. *CNS Spectrums, 8*(2), 135–138. https://doi.org/10.1017/s1092852900018368

Hodge, D., Hoffman, C. D., Sweeney, D. P., & Riggs, M. L. (2013). Relationship between children's sleep and mental health in mothers of children with and without autism. *Journal of Autism and Developmental Disorders, 43*(4), 956–963. https://doi.org/10.1007/s10803-012-1639-0

Holingue, C., Newill, C., Lee, L. C., Pasricha, P. J., & Daniele Fallin, M. (2018). Gastrointestinal symptoms in autism spectrum disorder: A review of the literature on ascertainment and prevalence. *Autism Research, 11*(1), 24–36. https://doi.org/10.1002/aur.1854

Holmbeck, G. N., Thill, A. W., Bachanas, P., Garber, J., Miller, K. B., Abad, M., Bruno, E. F., Carter, J. S., David-Ferdon, C., Jandasek, B., Mennuti-Washburn, J. E., & Zukerman, J. (2008). Evidence-based assessment in pediatric psychology: Measures of psychosocial adjustment and psychopathology. *Journal of Pediatric Psychology, 33*, 958–980. https://doi.org/10.1093/jpepsy/jsm059

Honomichl, R. D., Goodlin-Jones, B. L., Burnham, M. M., Hansen, R. L., & Anders, T. F. (2002). Secretin and sleep in children with autism. *Child Psychiatry & Human Development, 33*(2), 107–123. https://doi.org/10.1023/a:1020778108068

Hunter, J. E., McLay, L. K., France, K. G., & Blampied, N. M. (2020). Systematic review of the collateral effects of behavioral sleep interventions in children and adolescents with autism spectrum disorder. *Research in Autism Spectrum Disorders, 79*, Article 101677. https://doi.org/10.1016/j.rasd.2020.101677

Ingram, D. G., Cranford, T. A., & Al-Shawwa, B. (2023). Sleep technology. *Sleep Medicine Clinics.*

Jaber, M. A. (2011). Dental caries experience, oral health status and treatment needs of dental patients with autism. *Journal of Applied Oral Science, 19*, 212–217. https://doi.org/10.1590/s1678-77572011000300006

Jiménez-Jiménez, F. J., Alonso-Navarro, H., García-Martín, E., & Agúndez, J. A. (2018). Genetics of restless legs syndrome: An update. *Sleep Medicine Reviews, 39*, 108–121. https://doi.org/10.1016/j.smrv.2017.08.002

Johns, M. W. (1991). A new method for measuring daytime sleepiness: The epworth sleepiness scale. *Sleep, 14*(6), 540–545. https://doi.org/10.1093/sleep/14.6.540

Johnson, C. R., Barto, L., Worley, S., Rothstein, R., & Alder, M. L. (2023). Telehealth parent training for sleep disturbances in young children with autism spectrum disorder: A randomized controlled trial. *Sleep Medicine, 111*, 208–219. https://doi.org/10.1016/j.sleep.2023.08.033

Johnson, C. R., DeMand, A., Lecavalier, L., Smith, T., Aman, M., Foldes, E., & Scahill, L. (2016). Psychometric properties of the children's sleep habits questionnaire in children with autism spectrum disorder. *Sleep Medicine, 20*, 5–11. https://doi.org/10.1016/j.sleep.2015.12.005

Johnson, C. R., Turner, K. S., Foldes, E., Brooks, M. M., Kronk, R., & Wiggs, L. (2013). Behavioral parent training to address sleep disturbances in young children with autism spectrum disorder: A pilot trial. *Sleep Medicine, 14*(10), 995–1004. https://doi.org/10.1016/j.sleep.2013.05.013

Johnson, K. P., & Zarrinnegar, P. (2021). Autism spectrum disorder and sleep. *Child and Adolescent Psychiatric Clinics of North America, 30*(1), 195–208. https://doi.org/10.1016/j.chc.2020.08.012

Jonsson, L., Ljunggren, E., Bremer, A., Pedersen, C., Landén, M., Thuresson, K., Giacobini, M., & Melke, J. (2010). Mutation screening of melatonin-related genes in patients with autism spectrum disorders. *BMC Medical Genomics, 3*, 10. https://doi.org/10.1186/1755-8794-3-10.doi:10.1186/1755-8794-3-10

Kataria, S., Swanson, M., & Trevathan, G. (1987). Persistence of sleep disturbances in preschool children. *Journal of Pediatrics*. https://doi.org/10.1016/S0022-3476(87)80571-1

Katz, T., & Malow, B. A. (2014). *Solving sleep problems in children with autism spectrum disorders: A guide for frazzled families*. Woodbine House Inc.

Katz, T., Shui, A. M., Johnson, C. R., Richdale, A. L., Reynolds, A. M., Scahill, L., & Malow, B. A. (2018). Modification of the children's sleep habits questionnaire for children with autism spectrum disorder. *Journal of Autism and Developmental Disorders, 48*(8), 2629–2641. https://doi.org/10.1007/s10803-018-3520-2

Khosla, S., Deak, M. C., Gault, D., Goldstein, C. A., Hwang, D., Kwon, Y., O'Hearn, D., Schutte-Rodin, S., Yurcheshen, M., Rosen, I. M., Kirsch, D. B., & Rowley, J. A. (2018). Consumer sleep technology: an American academy of sleep medicine position statement. *Journal of Clinical Sleep Medicine, 14*(5), 877–880. https://doi.org/10.5664/jcsm.7128

King, M. S., Xanthopoulos, M. S., & Marcus, C. L. (2014). Improving positive airway pressure adherence in children. *Sleep Medicine Clinics, 9*(2), 219–234. https://doi.org/10.1016/j.jsmc.2014.02.003

Kirk, V., Baughn, J., D'Andrea, L., Friedman, N., Galion, A., Garetz, S., Hassan, F., Wrede, J., Harrod, C. G., & Malhotra, R. K. (2017). American academy of sleep medicine position paper for the use of a home sleep apnea test for the diagnosis of OSA in children. *Journal of Clinical Sleep Medicine, 13*(10), 1199–1203. https://doi.org/10.5664/jcsm.6772

Kotagal, S. (2008). Parasomnias of childhood. *Current Opinion in Pediatrics, 20*(6), 659–665. https://doi.org/10.1097/MOP.0b013e328316bd9d

Kotagal, S., Nichols, C. D., Grigg-Damberger, M. M., Marcus, C. L., Witmans, M. B., Kirk, V. G., Hoban, T. F., & D'Andrea, L. A. (2012). Non-respiratory indications for polysomnography and related procedures in children: An evidence-based review. *Sleep, 35*(11), 1451–1466. https://doi.org/10.5665/sleep.2188

Kotagal, S., & Silber, M. H. (2004). Childhood-onset restless legs syndrome. *Annals of Neurology, 56*(6), 803–807. https://doi.org/10.1002/ana.20292

Kovacs, M., MHS, S., & Multi-Health Systems. (2003). *Children's depression inventory 2(CDI2)*. Multi-Health Systems, Inc.

Krakowiak, P., Goodlin-Jones, B., Hertz-Picciotto, I., Croen, L. A., & Hansen, R. L. (2008). Sleep problems in children with autism spectrum disorders, developmental delays, and typical development: A population-based study. *Journal of Sleep Research, 17*(2), 197–206. https://doi.org/10.1111/j.1365-2869.2008.00650.x

Kulman, G., Lissoni, P., Rovelli, F., Roselli, M. G., Brivio, F., & Sequeri, P. (2000). Evidence of pineal endocrine hypofunction in autistic children. *Neuroendocrinology Letters, 21*(1), 31–34.

Lam, N., & Veeravigrom, M. (2023). Sleep-related rhythmic movement disorder in children: A mini-review. *Frontiers in Neurology, 14*, 1165130. https://doi.org/10.3389/fneur.2023.1165130
Lamônica, D. A. C., Giacheti, C. M., Dias Hayssi Haduo, M., Dias Dos Santos, M. J., da Silva, N. C., & Pinato, L. (2021). Sleep quality, functional skills, and communication in preschool-aged children with autism spectrum disorder. *Research in Developmental Disabilities, 116*, 104024. https://doi.org/10.1016/j.ridd.2021.104024
Latif, A., Heinz, P., & Cook, R. (2002). Iron deficiency in autism and Asperger syndrome. *Autism, 6*(1), 103–114. https://doi.org/10.1177/1362361302006001008
Leader, G., Glynn, C., Kirkpatrick, B., Chen, J. L., O'Súilleabháin, P. S., & Mannion, A. (2022). Familial sleep and autism spectrum disorder: A pilot actigraphy study of sleep quality, quality of life and psychological distress. *Irish Journal of Psychological Medicine, 39*(3), 261–271. https://doi.org/10.1017/ipm.2021.24
LeBourgeois, M. K., Giannotti, F., Cortesi, F., Wolfson, A. R., & Harsh, J. (2005). The relationship between reported sleep quality and sleep hygiene in Italian and American adolescents. *Pediatrics, 115*(1), 257–259. https://doi.org/10.1542/peds.2004-0815H
LeBourgeois, M. K., & Harsch, J. R. (2001). A new research measure for children's sleep. *Sleep, 24*, A213–A214.
Leu, R. M., Beyderman, L., Botzolakis, E. J., Surdyka, K., Wang, L., & Malow, B. A. (2011). Relation of melatonin to sleep architecture in children with autism. *Journal of Autism and Developmental Disorders, 41*(4), 427–433. https://doi.org/10.1007/s10803-010-1072-1
Leung, A. K. C., Leung, A. A. M., Wong, A. H. C., & Hon, K. L. (2020). Sleep terrors: An updated review. *Current Pediatric Reviews, 16*(3), 176–182. https://doi.org/10.2174/157339631566619 1014152136
Lewandowski, A. S., Toliver-Sokol, M., & Palermo, T. M. (2011). Evidence-based review of subjective pediatric sleep measures. *Journal of Pediatric Psychology, 36*(7), 780–793. https://doi.org/10.1093/jpepsy/jsq119
Lewis, S., Papadopoulos, N., Mantilla, A., Hiscock, H., Whelan, M., McGillivray, J., & Rinehart, N. (2023). The impact of COVID-19 on sleep for autistic children: A systematic review. *Research in Autism Spectrum Disorders, 102*, Article 102110. https://doi.org/10.1016/j.rasd.2023.102110
Liguori, C., Toledo, M., & Kothare, S. (2021). Effects of anti-seizure medications on sleep architecture and daytime sleepiness in patients with epilepsy: A literature review. *Sleep Medicine Reviews, 60*, Article 101559. https://doi.org/10.1016/j.smrv.2021.101559
Lildal, T. K., Bertelsen, J. B., & Ovesen, T. (2021). Feasibility of conducting type III home sleep apnoea test in children. *Acta Oto-Laryngologica, 141*(7), 707–713. https://doi.org/10.1080/000 16489.2021.1930152
Limoges, E., Mottron, L., Bolduc, C., Berthiaume, C., & Godbout, R. (2005). Atypical sleep architecture and the autism phenotype. *Brain, 128*(Pt 5).
Lin-Dyken, D. C., & Dyken, M. E. (2002). Use of melatonin in young children for sleep disorders. *Infants and Young Children, 15*(2), 20–37.
Loring, W. A. L., Johnston, R., Shui, A. M., & Malow, B. A. (2018). Impact of a brief behavioral intervention for insomnia on daytime behaviors in adolescents with autism spectrum disorders. *Journal of Contemporary Psychotherapy, 48*, 165–177 https://doi.org/10.1007/s10879-018-9381-3
Lyall, K., Van de Water, J., Ashwood, P., & Hertz-Picciotto, I. (2015). Asthma and allergies in children with autism spectrum disorders: Results from the CHARGE study. *Autism Research, 8*(5), 567–574. https://doi.org/10.1002/aur.1471
MacDonald, L. L., Gray, L., Loring, W., Wyatt, A., Bonnet, K., Schlund, D., Gaston, M. L., & Malow, B. A. (2021). A community-based sleep educational intervention for children with autism spectrum disorder. *Research in Autism Spectrum Disorders, 81*, Article 101719. https://doi.org/10.1016/j.rasd.2020.101719
Mahowald, M. W. (2011). REM sleep parasomnias. In M. H. Kryger, T. Roth, & W. C. Dement (Eds.), *Principles and Practice of Sleep Medicine* (pp. 1083–1097). Saunders/Elsevier.

Malow, B. A., Adkins, K. W., McGrew, S. G., Wang, L., Goldman, S. E., Fawkes, D., & Burnette, C. (2012a). Melatonin for sleep in children with autism: A controlled trial examining dose, tolerability, and outcomes. *Journal of Autism and Developmental Disorders, 42*(8), 1729–1737. https://doi.org/10.1007/s10803-011-1418-3

Malow, B. A., Byars, K., Johnson, K., Weiss, S., Bernal, P., Goldman, S. E., Panzer, R., Coury, D. L., Glaze, D. G., & Sleep Committee of the Autism Treatment Network. (2012b). A practice pathway for the identification, evaluation, and management of insomnia in children and adolescents with autism spectrum disorders. *Pediatrics, 130*, S106–124.

Malow, B. A., Adkins, K. W., Reynolds, A., Weiss, S. K., Loh, A., Fawkes, D., Katz, T., Goldman, S. E., Madduri, N., Hundley, R., & Clemons, T. (2014). Parent-based sleep education for children with autism spectrum disorders. *Journal of Autism and Developmental Disorders, 44*(1), 216–228. https://doi.org/10.1007/s10803-013-1866-z

Malow, B. A., Connolly, H. V., Weiss, S. K., Halbower, A., Goldman, S., Hyman, S. L., & Reynolds, A. M. (2016a). The pediatric sleep clinical global impressions scale—A new tool to measure pediatric insomnia in autism spectrum disorders. *Journal of Developmental & Behavioral Pediatrics, 37*(5), 370–376. https://doi.org/10.1542/peds.2012-0900I

Malow, B. A., Crowe, C., Henderson, L., McGrew, S. G., Wang, L., Song, Y., & Stone, W. L. (2009). A sleep habits questionnaire for children with autism spectrum disorders. *Journal of Child Neurology, 24*(1), 19–24. https://doi.org/10.1177/0883073808321044

Malow, B. A., Findling, R. L., Schroder, C. M., Maras, A., Breddy, J., Nir, T., Zisapel, N., & Gringras, P. (2021a). Sleep, growth, and puberty after 2 years of prolonged-release Melatonin in children with autism spectrum disorder. *Journal of the American Academy of Child and Adolescent Psychiatry, 60*(2), 252–261.e3. https://doi.org/10.1016/j.jaac.2019.12.007

Malow, B. A., Galion, A., Lu, F., Kennedy, N., Lawrence, C. E., Tassone, A., O'Neal, L., Wilson, T. M., Parker, R. A., Harris, P. A., & Neumeyer, A. M. (2021b). A REDCap-based model for online interventional research: Parent sleep education in autism. *Journal of Clinical and Translational Science, 5*(1), e138. https://doi.org/10.1017/cts.2021.798

Malow, B. A., MacDonald, L. L., Fawkes, D. B., Alder, M. L., & Katz, T. (2016b). Teaching children with autism spectrum disorder how to sleep better: A pilot educational program for parents. *Clinical Practice in Pediatric Psychology, 4*(2), 125. https://doi.org/10.1037/cpp0000138

Malow, B. A., Marzec, M. L., McGrew, S. G., Wang, L., Henderson, L. M., & Stone, W. L. (2006). Characterizing sleep in children with autism spectrum disorders: A multidimensional approach. *Sleep, 29*(12), 1563–1571. https://doi.org/10.1093/sleep/29.12.1563

Mannion, A., & Leader, G. (2023). Relationship between child sleep problems in autism spectrum disorder and parent mental health and well-being. *Sleep Medicine, 109*, 4–10. https://doi.org/10.1016/j.sleep.2023.05.009

Marcus, C. L., Brooks, L. J., Draper, K. A., Gozal, D., Halbower, A. C., Jones, J., Schechter, M. S., Ward, S. D., Sheldon, S. H., Shiffman, R. N., Lehmann, C., Spruyt, K., & American Academy of Pediatrics. (2012). Diagnosis and management of childhood obstructive sleep apnea syndrome. *Pediatrics, 130*(3), e714–e755. https://doi.org/10.1542/peds.2012-1672

Mayes, S. D., & Calhoun, S. L. (2009). Variables related to sleep problems in children with autism. *Research in Autism Spectrum Disorders, 3*(4), 931–941. https://doi.org/10.1016/j.rasd.2009.04.002

May, T., Cornish, K., Conduit, R., Rajaratnam, S. M., & Rinehart, N. J. (2015). Sleep in high-functioning children with autism: Longitudinal developmental change and associations with behavior problems. *Behavioral Sleep Medicine, 13*(1), 2–18. https://doi.org/10.1080/15402002.2013.829064

Mazurek, M. O., Engelhardt, C. R., Hilgard, J., & Sohl, K. (2016). Bedtime electronic media use and sleep in children with autism spectrum disorder. *Journal of Developmental & Behavioral Pediatrics, 37*(7), 525–531. https://doi.org/10.1097/DBP.0000000000000314

Mazurek, M. O., & Petroski, G. F. (2015). Sleep problems in children with autism spectrum disorder: Examining the contributions of sensory over-responsivity and anxiety. *Sleep Medicine, 16*(2), 270–279. https://doi.org/10.1016/j.sleep.2014.11.006

Mazurek, M. O., & Sohl, K. (2016). Sleep and behavioral problems in children with autism spectrum disorder. *Journal of Autism and Developmental Disorders, 46*, 1906–1915. https://doi.org/10.1007/s10803-016-2723-7

McCoy, S. M., & Morgan, K. (2020). Obesity, physical activity, and sedentary behaviors in adolescents with autism spectrum disorder compared with typically developing peers. *Autism, 24*(2), 387–399. https://doi.org/10.1177/1362361319861579

McCrae, C. S., Chan, W. S., Curtis, A. F., Deroche, C. B., Munoz, M., Takamatsu, S., Muckerman, J. E., Takahashi, N., McCann, D., McGovney, K., Sahota, P., & Mazurek, M. O. (2020). Cognitive behavioral treatment of insomnia in school-aged children with autism spectrum disorder: A pilot feasibility study. *Autism Research, 13*(1), 167–176. https://doi.org/10.1002/aur.2204

McCrae, C. S., Chan, W. S., Curtis, A. F., Nair, N., Deroche, C. B., Munoz, M., Takamatsu, S., McLean, D., Davenport, M., Muckerman, J. E., Takahashi, N., McCann, D., McGovney, K., Sahota, P., & Mazurek, M. O. (2021). Telehealth cognitive behavioral therapy for insomnia in children with autism spectrum disorder: A pilot examining feasibility, satisfaction, and preliminary findings. *Autism, 25*(3), 667–680. https://doi.org/10.1177/1362361320949078

McCue, L. M., Flick, L. H., Twyman, K. A., & Xian, H. (2017). Gastrointestinal dysfunctions as a risk factor for sleep disorders in children with idiopathic autism spectrum disorder: A retrospective cohort study. *Autism, 21*(8), 1010–1020. https://doi.org/10.1177/1362361316667061

McGrew, S., Malow, B. A., Henderson, L., Wang, L., Song, Y., & Stone, W. L. (2007). Developmental and behavioral questionnaire for autism spectrum disorders. *Pediatric Neurology, 37*(2), 108–116. https://doi.org/10.1016/j.pediatrneurol.2007.04.013

Melendres, M. C., Lutz, J. M., Rubin, R. E., & Marcus, C. L. (2004). Daytime sleepiness and hyperactivity in children with suspected sleep-disordered breathing. *Pediatrics, 114*(3), 768–775. https://doi.org/10.1542/peds.2004-0730

Melke, J., Botros, H. G., Chaste, P., Betancur, C., Nygren, G., Anckarsäter, H., Rastam, M., Ståhlberg, O., Gillberg, I. C., Delorme, R., Chabane, N., & Bourgeron, T. (2008). Abnormal melatonin synthesis in autism spectrum disorders. *Molecular Psychiatry, 13*(1), 90–98. https://doi.org/10.1038/sj.mp.4002016

Meltzer, L. J. (2011). Factors associated with depressive symptoms in parents of children with autism spectrum disorders. *Research in Autism Spectrum Disorders, 5*(1), 361–367. https://doi.org/10.1016/j.rasd.2010.05.001

Meltzer, L. J., Forrest, C. B., de la Motte, A., & Bevans, K. B. (2020). Clinical validity of the PROMIS pediatric sleep measures across populations of children with chronic illnesses and neurodevelopment disorders. *Journal of Pediatric Psychology, 45*(3), 319–327. https://doi.org/10.1093/jpepsy/jsz088

Meltzer, L. J., Montgomery-Downs, H. E., Insana, S. P., & Walsh, C. M. (2012). Use of actigraphy for assessment in pediatric sleep research. *Sleep Medicine Reviews, 16*(5), 793–796. https://doi.org/10.1016/j.smrv.2011.10.002

Ming, X., Brimacombe, M., & Wagner, G. C. (2007). Prevalence of motor impairment in autism spectrum disorders. *Brain and Development, 29*(9), 565–570. https://doi.org/10.1016/j.braindev.2007.03.002

Monk, C., Kovelenko, P., Ellman, L. M., Sloan, R. P., Bagiella, E., Gorman, J. M., & Pine, D. S. (2001). Enhanced stress reactivity in paediatric anxiety disorders: Implications for future cardiovascular health. *The International Journal of Neuropsychopharmacology, 4*(2), 199–206. https://doi.org/10.1017/S146114570100236X

Moore, M., Kirchner, H. L., Drotar, D., Johnson, N., Rosen, C., Ancoli-Israel, S., & Redline, S. (2009). Relationships among sleepiness, sleep time, and psychological functioning in adolescents. *Journal of Pediatric Psychology, 34*(10), 1175–1183. https://doi.org/10.1093/jpepsy/jsp039

Morgenthaler, T., Alessi, C., Friedman, L., Owens, J., Kapur, V., Boehlecke, B., Brown, T., Chesson Jr, A., Coleman, J., Lee-Chiong, T., Pancer, J., & Swick, T. J. (2007). Practice parameters for the use of actigraphy in the assessment of sleep and sleep disorders: An update for 2007. *Sleep, 30*(4), 519–529. https://doi.org/10.1093/sleep/30.4.519

Muhle, H., Neumann, A., Lohmann-Hedrich, K., Lohnau, T., Lu, Y., Winkler, S., Waltz, S., Fischenbeck, A., Kramer, P. L., Klein, C., & Stephani, U. (2008). Childhood-onset restless legs syndrome: Clinical and genetic features of 22 families. *Movement Disorders, 23*(8), 1113–1121. https://doi.org/10.1002/mds.22016

Murata, E., Mohri, I., Kato-Nishimura, K., Iimura, J., Ogawa, M., Tachibana, M., Ohno, Y., & Taniike, M. (2017). Evaluation of behavioral change after adenotonsillectomy for obstructive sleep apnea in children with autism spectrum disorder. *Research in Developmental Disabilities, 65*, 127–139. https://doi.org/10.1016/j.ridd.2017.04.012

National Institutes of Health. (2023). Writing respectfully: Person first and identity-first language by Shannon Wooldridge, public affairs specialist, IH office of communications and public liaison. Retrieved January 20, 2024 from https://www.nih.gov/about-nih/what-we-do/science-health-public-trust/perspectives/writing-respectfully-person-first-identity-first-language

National Sleep Foundation. (n.d.). *Sleep diary*. Retrieved November 27, 2025 from https://www.thensf.org/nsf-sleep-diary/

Neumeyer, A. M., Anixt, J., Chan, J., Perrin, J. M., Murray, D., Coury, D. L., Bennett, A., Farmer, J., & Parker, R. A. (2019). Identifying associations among co-occurring medical conditions in children with autism spectrum disorders. *Academic Pediatrics, 19*(3), 300–306. https://doi.org/10.1016/j.acap.2018.06.014

Nieminen-von Wendt, T. N., Paavonen, J. E., Ylisaukko-Oja, T., Sarenius, S., Källman, T., Järvelä, I., & Wendt, L. V. (2005). Subjective face recognition difficulties, aberrant sensibility, sleeping disturbances and aberrant eating habits in families with Asperger syndrome. *BMC Psychiatry, 5*(1), 20. https://doi.org/10.1186/1471-244X-5-20

Nir, I., Meir, D., Zilber, N., Knobler, H., Hadjez, J., & Lerner, Y. (1995). Brief report: Circadian melatonin, thyroid-stimulating hormone, prolactin, and cortisol levels in serum of young adults with autism. *Journal of Autism and Developmental Disorders, 25*(6), 641–654. https://doi.org/10.1007/BF02178193

Nixon, G. M., Wawruszak, M., Verginis, N., & Davey, M. J. (2006). The pediatric daytime sleepiness scale in elementary school children. *Sleep Medicine, 7*, S71–S72.

Oner, P., Dirik, E. B., Taner, Y., Caykoylu, A., & Anlar, O. (2007). Association between low serum ferritin and restless legs syndrome in patients with attention deficit hyperactivity disorder. *Tohoku Journal of Experimental Medicine, 213*(3), 269–276. https://doi.org/10.1620/tjem.213.269

Owens, J. A. (2023). Pharmacotherapy for insomnia in children and adolescents: A rational approach. *UpToDate*. Retrieved November 27, 2025 from https://www.uptodate.com/contents/pharmacotherapy-for-insomnia-in-children-and-adolescents-a-rational-approach

Owens, J. A., & Dalzell, V. (2005). Use of the 'BEARS' sleep screening tool in a pediatric residents' continuity clinic: A pilot study. *Sleep Medicine, 6*(1), 63–69. https://doi.org/10.1016/j.sleep.2004.07.015

Owens, J. A., Maxim, R., Nobile, C., McGuinn, M., & Msall, M. (2000a). Parental and self-report of sleep in children with attention-deficit/hyperactivity disorder. *Archives of Pediatric Adolescent Medicine, 154*(6), 549–555. https://doi.org/10.1001/archpedi.154.6.549

Owens, J. A., Spirito, A., & McGuinn, M. (2000b). The Children's Sleep Habits Questionnaire (CSHQ): Psychometric properties of a survey instrument for school-aged children. *Sleep, 23*(8), 1043–1051.

Owens, J. A., Spirito, A., McGuinn, M., & Nobile, C. (2000c). Sleep habits and sleep disturbance in elementary school-aged children. *Journal of Developmental and Behavioral Pediatrics, 21*(1), 27–36. https://doi.org/10.1097/00004703-200002000-00005

Oyane, N. M. F., & Bjorvatn, B. (2005). Sleep disturbances in adolescents and young adults with autism and Asperger syndrome. *Autism, 9*(1), 83–94. https://doi.org/10.1177/1362361305049031

Paavonen, E. J., Wendt, T. N., Vanhala, R., Aronen, E. T., & Wendt, L. V. (2003). Effectiveness of melatonin in the treatment of sleep disturbances in children with Asperger disorder. *Journal of Child and Adolescent Psychopharmacology, 13*(1), 83–95. https://doi.org/10.1089/104454603321666225

Papadopoulos, N., Sciberras, E., Hiscock, H., Mulraney, M., McGillivray, J., & Rinehart, N. (2019). The efficacy of a brief behavioral sleep intervention in school-aged children with ADHD and comorbid autism spectrum disorder. *Journal of Attention Disorders, 23*(4), 341–350. https://doi.org/10.1177/1087054714568565

Patzold, L. M., Richdale, A. L., & Tonge, B. J. (1998). An investigation into sleep characteristics of children with autism and Asperger's disorder. *Journal of Paediatrics and Child Health, 34*(6), 528–533. https://doi.org/10.1046/j.1440-1754.1998.00291.x

Peterson, B., Chiao, P., Pickering, E., Freeman, J., Zammit, G., Ding, Y., & Badura, L. L. (2012). Comparison of actigraphy and polysomnography to assess effects of zolpidem in a clinical research unit. *Sleep Medicine, 13*(4), 419–424. https://doi.org/10.1016/j.sleep.2011.12.003

Phillips, B., Young, T., Finn, L., Asher, K., Hening, W. A., & Purvis, C. (2000). Epidemiology of restless legs symptoms in adults. *Archives of Internal Medicine, 160*(14), 2137–2141. https://doi.org/10.1001/archinte.160.14.2137

Picchietti, D., Allen, R. P., Walters, A. S., Davidson, J. E., Myers, A., & Ferini-Strambi, L. (2007). Restless legs syndrome: Prevalence and impact in children and adolescents The Peds REST Study. *Pediatrics, 120*(2), 253–266. https://doi.org/10.1542/peds.2006-2767

Picchietti, D. L., Bruni, O., de Weerd, A., Durmer, J. S., Kotagal, S., Owens, J. A., Simakajornboon, N., & International Restless Legs Syndrome Study Group (IRLSSG), 2013 Picchietti, D. L., Bruni, O., de Weerd, A., Durmer, J. S., Kotagal, S., Owens, J. A., Simakajornboon, N., & International Restless Legs Syndrome Study Group (IRLSSG). (2013). Pediatric restless legs syndrome diagnostic criteria: an update by the International Restless Legs Syndrome Study Group. *Sleep Medicine, 14*(12), 1253–1259. https://doi.org/10.1016/j.sleep.2013.08.778

Picchietti, D. L., Rajendran, R. R., Wilson, M. P., & Picchietti, M. A. (2009). Pediatric restless legs syndrome and periodic limb movement disorder: Parent-child pairs. *Sleep Medicine, 10*(8), 925–931. https://doi.org/10.1016/j.sleep.2008.10.006

Pollock, J. I. (1994). Night-waking at five years of age: Predictors and prognosis. *Journal of Child Psychology and Psychiatry, 35*(4), 699–708. https://doi.org/10.1111/j.1469-7610.1994.tb01215.x

Portas, C. M., Bjorvatn, B., & Ursin, R. (2000). Serotonin and the sleep/wake cycle: Special emphasis on microdialysis studies. *Progress in Neurobiology, 60*(1), 13–25. https://doi.org/10.1016/s0301-0082(98)00097-5

Pullen, S. J., Wall, C. A., Angstman, E. R., Munitz, G. E., & Kotagal, S. (2011). Psychiatric comorbidity in children and adolescents with restless legs syndrome: A retrospective study. *Journal of Clinical Sleep Medicine, 7*(6), 587–596. https://doi.org/10.5664/jcsm.1456

Quine, L. (1991). Sleep problems in children with mental handicap. *Journal of Mental Deficiency Research, 35*(Pt 4), 269–290. https://doi.org/10.1111/j.1365-2788.1991.tb00402.x

Rapin, I., & Katzman, R. (1998). Neurobiology of autism. *Annals of Neurology, 43*(1), 7–14. https://doi.org/10.1002/ana.410430106

Restrepo, B., Angkustsiri, K., Taylor, S. L., Rogers, S. J., Cabral, J., Heath, B., Hechtman, A., Solomon, M., Ashwood, P., Amaral, D. G., & Nordahl, C. W. (2020). Developmental–behavioral profiles in children with autism spectrum disorder and co-occurring gastrointestinal symptoms. *Autism Research, 13*(10), 1778–1789. https://doi.org/10.1002/aur.2354

Reynolds, A. M., & Malow, B. A. (2011). Sleep and autism spectrum disorders. *Pediatric Clinics of North America, 58*(3), 685–698. https://doi.org/10.1016/j.pcl.2011.03.009

Reynolds, A. M., Soke, G. N., Sabourin, K. R., Hepburn, S., Katz, T., Wiggins, L. D., Schieve, L. A., & Levy, S. E. (2019). Sleep problems in 2- to 5-year-olds with autism spectrum disorder and other developmental delays. *Pediatrics, 143*(3), Article e20180492. https://doi.org/10.1542/peds.2018-0492

Reynolds, C. R., & Kamphaus, R. W. (2004). *BASC 2, Behavior assessment system for children*. American Guidance Service.
Richdale, A. L. (1999). Sleep problems in autism: Prevalence, cause, and intervention. *Developmental Medicine and Child Neurology, 41*(1), 60–66. https://doi.org/10.1017/s0012162299000122
Richdale, A. L., & Baglin, C. L. (2015). Self-report and caregiver-report of sleep and psychopathology in children with high-functioning autism spectrum disorder: A pilot study. *Developmental Neurorehabilitation, 18*(4), 272–279. https://doi.org/10.3109/17518423.2013.829534
Richdale, A. L., Baker, E., Short, M., & Gradisar, M. (2014). The role of insomnia, pre-sleep arousal and psychopathology symptoms in daytime impairment in adolescents with high-functioning autism spectrum disorder. *Sleep Medicine, 15*(9), 1082–1088. https://doi.org/10.1016/j.sleep.2014.05.005
Richdale, A. L., & Prior, M. R. (1995). The sleep/wake rhythm in children with autism. *European Child & Adolescent Psychiatry, 4*(3), 175–186. https://doi.org/10.1007/BF01980456
Richdale, A. L., & Schreck, K. A. (2009). Sleep problems in autism spectrum disorders: Prevalence, nature, possible biopsychosocial aetiologies. *Sleep Medicine Reviews, 13*(6), 403–411. https://doi.org/10.1016/j.smrv.2009.02.003
Robinson, A. M., & Richdale, A. L. (2004). Sleep problems in children with an intellectual disability: Parental perceptions of sleep problems, and views of treatment effectiveness. *Child: Care, Health and Development*, *30*(2), 139–150. https://doi.org/10.1111/j.1365-2214.2004.00395.x
Rodenbeck, A., Huether, G., Rüther, E., & Hajak, G. (2002). Interactions between evening and nocturnal cortisol secretion and sleep parameters in patients with severe chronic primary insomnia. *Neuroscience Letters, 324*(2), 159–163. https://doi.org/10.1016/s0304-3940(02)00192-1
Rosen, C. L., Larkin, E. K., Kirchner, H. L., Emancipator, J. L., Bivins, S. F., Surovec, S. A., Martin, R. J., & Redline, S. (2003). Prevalence and risk factors for sleep-disordered breathing in 8- to 11-year-old children: Association with race and prematurity. *Journal of Pediatrics, 142*(4), 383–389. https://doi.org/10.1067/mpd.2003.28
Roussis, S., Richdale, A. L., Katz, T., Malow, B. A., Barbaro, J., & Sadka, N. (2021). Behaviour, cognition, and autism symptoms and their relationship with sleep problem severity in young children with autism spectrum disorder. *Research in Autism Spectrum Disorders, 83*, Article 101743. https://doi.org/10.1016/j.rasd.2021.101743
Sadeh, A., & Acebo, C. (2002). The role of actigraphy in sleep medicine. *Sleep Medicine Reviews, 6*(2), 113–124. https://doi.org/10.1053/smrv.2001.0182
Sangal, R. B., Owens, J., Allen, A. J., Sutton, V., Schuh, K., & Kelsey, D. (2006). Effects of atomoxetine and methylphenidate on sleep in children with ADHD. *Sleep, 29*(12), 1573–1585. https://doi.org/10.1093/sleep/29.12.1573
Savage, R. A., Zafar, N., Yohannan, S., & Miller, J. M. M. (2024). Melatonin. In *StatPearls*. StatPearls Publishing. Available from: https://www.ncbi.nlm.nih.gov/books/NBK534823/
Schreck, K. A. (2001). Behavioral treatments for sleep problems in autism: Empirically supported or just universally accepted? *Behavioral Interventions: Theory & Practice in Residential & Community-Based Clinical Programs, 16*(4), 265–278. https://doi.org/10.1002/bin.98
Schreck, K. A. (2021). Sleep quantity and quality as predictors of behavior and mental health issues for children and adolescents with autism. *Research in Autism Spectrum Disorders, 84*, Article 101767. https://doi.org/10.1016/j.rasd.2021.101767
Schreck, K. A., & Mulick, J. A. (2000). Parental report of sleep problems in children with autism. *Journal of Autism and Developmental Disorders, 30*(2), 127–135. https://doi.org/10.1023/a:1005407622050
Schreck, K. A., Mulick, J. A., & Smith, A. F. (2004a). Sleep problems as possible predictors of intensified symptoms of autism. *Research in Developmental Disabilities*, *25*(1), 57–66. https://doi.org/10.1016/j.ridd.2003.04.007

Schreck, K. A., & Williams, K. (2006). Food preferences and factors influencing food selectivity for children with autism spectrum disorders. *Research in Developmental Disabilities, 27*(4), 353–363. https://doi.org/10.1016/j.ridd.2005.03.005

Schreck, K. A., Williams, K., & Smith, A. F. (2004b). A comparison of eating behaviors between children with and without autism. *Journal of Autism and Developmental Disorders, 34*(4), 433–438. https://doi.org/10.1023/b:jadd.0000037419.78531.86

Schutte-Rodin, S., Deak, M. C., Khosla, S., Goldstein, C. A., Yurcheshen, M., Chiang, A., Gault, D., Kern, J., O'Hearn, D., Ryals, S., Verma, N., & Ramar, K. (2021). Evaluating consumer and clinical sleep technologies: An American Academy of Sleep Medicine update. *Journal of Clinical Sleep Medicine, 17*(11), 2275–2282. https://doi.org/10.5664/jcsm.9580

Sen, T., & Spruyt, K. (2020). Pediatric sleep tools: An updated literature review. *Frontiers in Psychiatry, 11*, 317. https://doi.org/10.3389/fpsyt.2020.00317

Shui, A. M., Katz, T., Malow, B. A., & Mazurek, M. O. (2018). Predicting sleep problems in children with autism spectrum disorders. *Research in Developmental Disabilities, 83*, 270–279. https://doi.org/10.1016/j.ridd.2018.10.002

Shui, A. M., Richdale, A. L., & Katz, T. (2021). Evaluating sleep quality using the CSHQ-Autism. *Sleep Medicine, 87*, 69–76. https://doi.org/10.1016/j.sleep.2021.08.022

Sikora, D. M., Johnson, K., Clemons, T., & Katz, T. (2012). The relationship between sleep problems and daytime behavior in children of different ages with autism spectrum disorders. *Pediatrics, 130*(Suppl 2), S83-90. https://doi.org/10.1542/peds.2012-0900F

Silvestri, R., Gagliano, A., Calarese, T., Aricò, I., Cedro, C., Condurso, R., & Tortorella, G. (2007). Ictal and interictal EEG abnormalities in ADHD children recorded over night by video-polysomnography. *Epilepsy Research, 75*(2–3), 130–137. https://doi.org/10.1016/j.eplepsyres.2007.05.007

Simakajornboon, N., Kheirandish-Gozal, L., & Gozal, D. (2009). Diagnosis and management of restless legs syndrome in children. *Sleep Medicine Reviews, 13*(2), 149–156. https://doi.org/10.1016/j.smrv.2008.12.002

Simonds, J. F., & Parraga, H. (1982). Prevalence of sleep disorders and sleep behaviors in children and adolescents. *Journal of the American Academy of Child & Adolescent Psychiatry*. https://doi.org/10.1016/s0002-7138(09)60942-0

Simonoff, E., Jones, C. R., Pickles, A., Happé, F., Baird, G., & Charman, T. (2012). Severe mood problems in adolescents with autism spectrum disorder. *Journal of Child Psychology and Psychiatr, 53*(11), 1157–1166. https://doi.org/10.1111/j.1469-7610.2012.02600.x

Simonoff, E., Pickles, A., Charman, T., Chandler, S., Loucas, T., & Baird, G. (2008). Psychiatric disorders in children with autism spectrum disorders: Prevalence, comorbidity, and associated factors in a population-derived sample. *Journal of the American Academy of Child and Adolescent Psychiatry, 47*(8), 921–929. https://doi.org/10.1097/CHI.0b013e318179964f

Singh, K., & Zimmerman, A. W. (2015). Sleep in autism spectrum disorder and attention deficit hyperactivity disorder. *Seminars in Pediatric Neurology, 22*(2), 113–125. https://doi.org/10.1016/j.spen.2015.03.006

Siriwat, R., Gurbani, N., Xu, Y., Hossain, M. M., & Simakajornboon, N. (2020). Sleep manifestations, sleep architecture in children with Eosinophilic esophagitis presenting to a sleep clinic. *Sleep Medicine, 68*, 160–166. https://doi.org/10.1016/j.sleep.2019.08.018

Slifer, K. J., Tunney, M. A., & Paasch, V. (2019). Behavioral intervention for positive airway pressure (CPAP/BPAP) desensitization. *Sleep in Children with Neurodevelopmental Disabilities: An Evidence-Based Guide*, 373–382.

Sohn, J. K., Barnes, B. H., Al-Hazaymeh, A., Sauer, B. G., & McGowan, E. C. (2021). High prevalence of developmental disorders in pediatric eosinophilic esophagitis (EoE): A single-center observational study. *The Journal of Allergy and Clinical Immunology: In Practice, 9*(2), 1032–1034.e1. https://doi.org/10.1016/j.jaip.2020.09.032

Souders, M. C., Mason, T. B., Valladares, O., Bucan, M., Levy, S. E., Mandell, D. S., Weaver, T. E., & Pinto-Martin, J. (2009). Sleep behaviors and sleep quality in children with autism spectrum disorders. *Sleep, 32*(12), 1566–1578. https://doi.org/10.1093/sleep/32.12.1566

Souders, M. C., Zavodny, S., Eriksen, W., Sinko, R., Connell, J., Kerns, C., Schaaf, R., & Pinto-Martin, J. (2017). Sleep in children with autism spectrum disorder. *Current Psychiatry Reports, 19*(6), 34. https://doi.org/10.1007/s11920-017-0782-x

Spilsbury, J. C., Drotar, D., Rose, C. L., & Redline, S. (2007). The Cleveland adolescent sleepiness questionnaire: A new measure to assess excessive daytime sleepiness in adolescents. *Journal of Clinical Sleep Medicine, 3*(6), 603–612.

Spruyt, K., & Gozal, D. (2011). Pediatric sleep questionnaires as diagnostic or epidemiological tools: A review of currently available instruments. *Sleep Medicine Reviews, 15*(1), 19–32. https://doi.org/10.1016/j.smrv.2010.07.005

Storfer-Isser, A., LeBourgeois, M. K., Harsh, J., Tompsett, C. J., & Redline, S. (2013). Psychometric properties of the adolescent sleep hygiene scale. *Journal of Sleep Research, 22*(6), 707–716. https://doi.org/10.1111/jsr.12059

Sun, E. R., Chen, C. A., Ho, G., Earley, C. J., & Allen, R. P. (1998). Iron and the restless legs syndrome. *Sleep, 21*(4), 371–377.

Taylor, A., Caffery, L. J., Gesesew, H. A., King, A., Bassal, A. R., Ford, K., Kealey, J., Maeder, A., McGuirk, M., Parkes, D., & Ward, P. R. (2021). How Australian health care services adapted to telehealth during the COVID-19 pandemic: A survey of telehealth professionals. *Frontiers in Public Health, 9*, Article 648009. https://doi.org/10.3389/fpubh.2021.648009

Taylor, J. L., & Corbett, B. A. (2014). A review of rhythm and responsiveness of cortisol in individuals with autism spectrum disorders. *Psychoneuroendocrinology, 49*, 207–228. https://doi.org/10.1016/j.psyneuen.2014.07.015

Taylor, M. A., Schreck, K. A., & Mulick, J. A. (2012). Sleep disruption as a correlate to cognitive and adaptive behavior problems in autism spectrum disorders. *Research in Developmental Disabilities, 33*(5), 1408–1417. https://doi.org/10.1016/j.ridd.2012.03.013

Thirumalai, S. S., Shubin, R. A., & Robinson, R. (2002). Rapid eye movement sleep behavior disorder in children with autism. *Journal of Child Neurology, 17*(3), 173–178. https://doi.org/10.1177/088307380201700304

Toma, C., Rossi, M., Sousa, I., Blasi, F., Bacchelli, E., Alen, R., Vanhala, R., Monaco, A. P., Järvelä, I., & Maestrini, E. (2007). Is ASMT a susceptibility gene for autism spectrum disorders? A replication study in European populations. *Molecular Psychiatry, 12*(11), 977–979. https://doi.org/10.1038/sj.mp.4002069

Tomkies, A., Johnson, R. F., Shah, G., Caraballo, M., Evans, P., & Mitchell, R. B. (2019). Obstructive sleep Apnea in children with autism. *Journal of Clinical Sleep Medicine, 15*(10), 1469–1476. https://doi.org/10.5664/jcsm.7978

Tordjman, S., Anderson, G. M., Pichard, N., Charbuy, H., & Touitou, Y. (2005). Nocturnal excretion of 6-sulphatoxymelatonin in children and adolescents with autistic disorder. *Biological Psychiatry, 57*(2), 134–138. https://doi.org/10.1016/j.biopsych.2004.11.003

Tsai, T. Y., Chao, Y. C., Hsieh, C. Y., & Huang, Y. C. (2020). Association between atopic dermatitis and autism spectrum disorder: A systematic review and meta-analysis. *Acta Dermato-Venereologica, 100*(10), adv00146. https://doi.org/10.2340/00015555-3501

Tudor, M. E., Walsh, C. E., Mulder, E. C., & Lerner, M. D. (2015). Pain as a predictor of sleep problems in youth with autism spectrum disorders. *Autism, 19*(3), 292–300. https://doi.org/10.1177/1362361313518994

Tzischinsky, O., Meiri, G., Manelis, L., Bar-Sinai, A., Flusser, H., Michaelovski, A., Zivan, O., Ilan, M., Faroy, M., Menashe, I., & Dinstein, I. (2018). Sleep disturbances are associated with specific sensory sensitivities in children with autism. *Molecular Autism, 9*, 22. https://doi.org/10.1186/s13229-018-0206-8

Uren, J., Richdale, A. L., Cotton, S. M., & Whitehouse, A. J. O. (2019). Sleep problems and anxiety from 2 to 8 years and the influence of autistic traits: A longitudinal study. *European Child & Adolescent Psychiatry, 28*(8), 1117–1127. https://doi.org/10.1007/s00787-019-01275-y

Vanderbilt Kennedy Center, Makowiec, K., Thompson, A., & Stevens, J. (2014, June). *Helping your child with intellectual/developmental disability prepare for a sleep study*. Retrieved November 27, 2025 from https://vkc.vumc.org/assets/files/resources/sleepstudy.pdf

van Deurs, J. R., France, K. G., McLay, L. K., & Blampied, N. M. (2021). Cognitive-behavioral treatment of sleep disturbance in children and adolescents with autism: Eight case studies using functional behavior assessment. *Research in Autism Spectrum Disorders, 86*, Article 101823. https://doi.org/10.1016/j.rasd.2021.101823

van Steensel, F. J., Bögels, S. M., & Perrin, S. (2011). Anxiety disorders in children and adolescents with autistic spectrum disorders: A meta-analysis. *Clinical Child and Family Psychology Review, 14*(3), 302–317. https://doi.org/10.1007/s10567-011-0097-0

Varni, J. W., Burwinkle, T. M., Seid, M., & Skarr, D. (2003). The PedsQL™* 4.0 as a pediatric population health measure: Feasibility, reliability, and validity. *Ambulatory Pediatrics, 3*(6), 329–341. https://doi.org/10.1367/1539-4409(2003)003<0329:tpaapp>2.0.co;2

Veatch, O. J., Pendergast, J. S., Allen, M. J., Leu, R. M., Johnson, C. H., Elsea, S. H., & Malow, B. A. (2015). Genetic variation in melatonin pathway enzymes in children with autism spectrum disorder and comorbid sleep onset delay. *Journal of Autism and Developmental Disorders, 45*(1), 100–110. https://doi.org/10.1007/s10803-014-2197-4

Veatch, O. J., Sutcliffe, J. S., Warren, Z. E., Keenan, B. T., Potter, M. H., & Malow, B. A. (2017). Shorter sleep duration is associated with social impairment and comorbidities in ASD. *Autism Research, 10*(7), 1221–1238. https://doi.org/10.1002/aur.1765

Vriend, J. L., Corkum, P. V., Moon, E. C., & Smith, I. M. (2011). Behavioral interventions for sleep problems in children with autism spectrum disorders: Current findings and future directions. *Journal of Pediatric Psychology, 36*(9), 1017–1029. https://doi.org/10.1093/jpepsy/jsr044

Walters, A. S., Gabelia, D., & Frauscher, B. (2013). Restless legs syndrome (Willis-Ekbom disease) and growing pains: Are they the same thing? A side-by-side comparison of the diagnostic criteria for both and recommendations for future research. *Sleep Medicine, 14*(12), 1247–1252. https://doi.org/10.1016/j.sleep.2013.07.013

Walters, A. S., Picchietti, D. L., Ehrenberg, B. L., & Wagner, M. L. (1994). Restless legs syndrome in childhood and adolescence. *Pediatric Neurology, 11*(3), 241–245. https://doi.org/10.1016/0887-8994(94)90110-4

What the Letters "USP" Mean on the Label of Your Medicine | Quality Matters | U.S. Pharmacopeia Blog. (2015). Retrieved February 11, 2024 from https://qualitymatters.usp.org/what-letters-usp-mean-label-your-medicine#:~:text=The%20law%20elevated%20the%20public,differing%20from%20%E2%80%9Cthe%20standard%20of

Weiskop, S., Matthews, J., & Richdale, A. (2001). Treatment of sleep problems in a 5-year-old boy with autism using behavioural principles. *Autism, 5*(2), 209–221. https://doi.org/10.1177/1362361301005002009

Westenberg, J. N., Petrof, B. J., Noel, F., Zielinski, D., Constantin, E., Oskoui, M., & Kaminska, M. (2021). Validation of home portable monitoring for the diagnosis of sleep-disordered breathing in adolescents and adults with neuromuscular disorders. *Journal of Clinical Sleep Medicine, 17*(8), 1579–1590. https://doi.org/10.5664/jcsm.9254

Wiggs, L., Montgomery, P., & Stores, G. (2005). Actigraphic and parent reports of sleep patterns and sleep disorders in children with subtypes of attention-deficit hyperactivity disorder. *Sleep, 28*(11), 1437–1445. https://doi.org/10.1093/sleep/28.11.1437

Wiggs, L., & Stores, G. (1996). Severe sleep disturbance and daytime challenging behavior in children with severe learning disabilities. *Journal of Intellectual Disability Research, 40*(Pt 6), 518–528. https://doi.org/10.1046/j.1365-2788.1996.799799.x

Wiggs, L., & Stores, G. (2004). Sleep patterns and sleep disorders in children with autistic spectrum disorders: Insights using parent report and actigraphy. *Developmental Medicine and Child Neurology, 46*(6), 372–380. https://doi.org/10.1017/s0012162204000611

Williams Buckley, A., Hirtz, D., Oskoui, M., Armstrong, M. J., Batra, A., Bridgemohan, C., Coury, D., Dawson, G., Donley, D., Findling, R. L., Gaughan, T., Gloss, D., Gronseth, G., Kessler, R., Merillat, S., Michelson, D., Owens, J., Pringsheim, T., Sikich, L., Stahmer, A., & Ashwal, S. (2020). Practice guideline: Treatment for insomnia and disrupted sleep behavior in children and adolescents with autism spectrum disorder: Report of the Guideline Development, Dissemination, and Implementation Subcommittee of the American Academy of Neurology. *Neurology, 94*(9), 392–404. https://doi.org/10.1212/WNL.0000000000009033

Wolfson, A. R., Carskadon, M. A., Acebo, C., Seifer, R., Fallone, G., Labyak, S. E., & Martin, J. L. (2003). Evidence for the validity of a sleep habits survey for adolescents. *Sleep, 26*(2), 213–216. https://doi.org/10.1093/sleep/26.2.213

Wright, B., Sims, D., Smart, S., Alwazeer, A., Alderson-Day, B., Allgar, V., & Miles, J. (2011). Melatonin versus placebo in children with autism spectrum conditions and severe sleep problems not amenable to behaviour management strategies: A Randomised controlled crossover trial. *Journal of Autism and Developmental Disorders, 41*(2), 145–184. https://doi.org/10.1007/s10803-010-1036-5

Yalcinkaya, B. C., Amirov, C. B., Saltik, S., & Senel, G. B. (2021). Restless legs syndrome in pediatric onset multiple sclerosis. *Multiple Sclerosis and Related Disorders, 56*, Article 103295. https://doi.org/10.1016/j.msard.2021.103295

Yilmaz, K., Kilincaslan, A., Aydin, N., & Kor, D. (2011). Prevalence and correlates of restless legs syndrome in adolescents. *Developmental Medicine and Child Neurology, 53*(1), 40–47. https://doi.org/10.1111/j.1469-8749.2010.03796.x

Young, T., Palta, M., Dempsey, J., Skatrud, J., Weber, S., & Badr, S. (1993). The occurrence of sleep-disordered breathing among middle-aged adults. *New England Journal of Medicine, 328*(17), 1230–1235. https://doi.org/10.1056/NEJM199304293281704

Youssef, J., Singh, K., Huntington, N., Becker, R., & Kothare, S. V. (2013). Relationship of serum ferritin levels to sleep fragmentation and periodic limb movements of sleep on polysomnography in autism spectrum disorders. *Pediatric Neurology, 49*(4), 274–278. https://doi.org/10.1016/j.pediatrneurol.2013.06.012

Zaffanello, M., Piacentini, G., Nosetti, L., & Zoccante, L. (2023). Sleep disordered breathing in children with autism spectrum disorder: An in-depth review of correlations and complexities. *Children, 10*(10), 1609. https://doi.org/10.3390/children10101609

Zaidman-Zait, A., Zwaigenbaum, L., Duku, E., Bennett, T., Szatmari, P., Mirenda, P., Smith, I., Vaillancourt, T., Volden, J., Waddell, C., Kerns, C., Elsabbagh, M., Georgiades, S., Ungar, W. J., Fombonne, E., & Roberts, W. (2020). Factor analysis of the children's sleep habits questionnaire among preschool children with autism spectrum disorder. *Research in Developmental Disabilities, 97*, Article 103548. https://doi.org/10.1016/j.ridd.2019.103548

Zaremba, E. K., Barkey, M. E., Mesa, C., Sanniti, K., & Rosen, C. L. (2005). Making polysomnography more "child friendly": A family-centered care approach. *Journal of Clinical Sleep Medicine, 1*(2), 189–198.

Zuckerman, B., Stevenson, J., & Bailey, V. (1987). Sleep problems in early childhood: Continuities, predictive factors, and behavioral correlates. *Pediatrics, 80*(5), 664–671.

Intelligence

Chieko Kanai, Gabor Toth, and Hirokazu Doi

Abstract The Intelligence chapter initially explores the relationship between Intelligence Quotient (IQ) and Autism Spectrum Disorders (ASD). It introduces recent developmental and intelligence tests used in Japan, organized by developmental stages, and emphasizes the importance of ASD assessments. Additionally, the chapter investigates differences in traits between children and adults through studies on Intelligence Quotient in individuals with ASD.

Next parts of the Intelligence chapter explore the complex interrelationships between ASD, Intellectual Disability (ID), and cognitive functions. It provides an in-depth analysis of recent research methods, neurological science advances, genetic and environmental factors, and the impact of early social experiences on cognitive development. The text discusses the co-occurrence of ASD and ID, highlighting their shared and distinct etiological factors, the influence of sensory processing disorders, and the significance of early detection and intervention. It also examines genetic and epigenetic research contributions to understanding ASD and ID, emphasizing the need for comprehensive therapeutic approaches and educational placements for affected individuals.

Last parts of the Intelligence chapter explore the association between neural function/morphology and intellectual ability in people with ASD. Exiting EEG/MEG studies indicated a potential link between ID and dysregulation of cortical excitability

---

Three authors are Equal Authorship.

C. Kanai (✉)
Child Development and Education, Faculty of Humanities, Wayo Women's University, Chiba, Japan
e-mail: c-kanai@wayo.ac.jp

G. Toth
Department of Education and Child Studies, Faculty of Arts and Sciences, Sagami Women's University, Kanagawa, Japan
e-mail: toth_gabor@isc.sagami-wu.ac.jp

H. Doi
Department of Information and Management Systems Engineering, Nagaoka University of Technology, Niigata, Japan
e-mail: doidoih@vos.nagaokaut.ac.jp

J. L. Matson (ed.), *Assessment and Diagnosis in Autism*, Autism and Child Psychopathology Series, https://doi.org/10.1007/978-3-032-11802-8_9

in children with ASD. Functional connectivity studies raised the possibility that differential neural networks contribute to intellectual function between individuals with and without ASD. However, the number of relevant studies is relatively small, and as such considerable effort is required to elucidate the neurophysiological basis of intellectual function in people with ASD.

Keywords Autism Spectrum Disorders · Assessment · Intelligence Quotient · Intellectual development · Cognitive functioning · Sensory processing · Intelligence · EEG · Spectral power · Functional connectivity

Assessment for Intelligence Quotient

Assessment for Intelligence Quotient for ASD

The assessment of intelligence, encompassing both verbal and nonverbal abilities, is a crucial aspect in the field of ASD. Intellectual tests are employed to quantify intelligence, allowing for the identification of individuals' cognitive strengths and weaknesses. Moreover, these tests facilitate an exploration of the underlying factors contributing to learning and adaptive challenges and help determine the effectiveness of support strategies.

Intellectual tests are also instrumental in assessing potential delays in intellectual functioning. In Japan, IQ plays a pivotal role in the process of obtaining a Rehabilitation Certificate. This certificate serves as a gateway for children with an IQ score of approximately 75 or lower to access various government support services. It also plays a significant role in determining the suitability of special-needs education for these individuals.

In clinical practice, a comprehensive evaluation is imperative when diagnosing ASD. This evaluation extends beyond the sole consideration of IQ. It necessitates a holistic assessment that encompasses the content of interviews, behavioral observations, attitudes, and error patterns observed during intelligence tests. Additionally, it entails an examination of problem-solving characteristics and the results of assessments other than traditional intelligence tests.

This comprehensive approach ensures a more nuanced and accurate diagnosis, enabling healthcare professionals to develop tailored intervention strategies for individuals with ASD. It is through this multidimensional assessment that we can better understand the diverse needs and abilities of those on the autism spectrum.

Diagnostic Assessment for Intelligence Quotient

Assessment for IQ for a precise diagnosis of ASD is important in clinical settings. An IQ test is helpful in clarifying the strengths and weaknesses in ASD. ASD often shows scatter among skills, with areas of significant strength and weakness. For example, in some ASD children with no intellectual disability, verbal ability is more developed than processing speed skills. In addition, the diagnosis of ASD poses a substantial challenge, particularly when dealing with adults (Kanai et al., 2012). The difficulties arise in part from the limited recollection of developmental history by primary caregivers during the patient's early childhood, making it challenging to gather accurate information for a differential diagnosis of ASD in adults. Moreover, some adults with ASD may have lost contact with their primary caregivers, leading to potential gaps in understanding their childhood experiences. Consequently, the development of efficient diagnostic indicators is paramount within the clinical context.

In the assessment of intellectual functioning, there exists a myriad of methods. This chapter offers a comprehensive overview of widely employed assessment techniques in Japan.

Preschool Age

[TB Scale-V (Tanaka-Binet Intelligence Scale, Fifth Edition)]

The Tanaka-Binet Intelligence Scale, a modified Binet test by Tanaka, assesses the intelligence and cognitive abilities in individuals from children to adults. The Tanaka-Binet Intelligence Scale is also called the Japanese version of the Stanford-Binet Intelligence Scale (Tanaka, 2003). The Tanaka-Binet Intelligence Scale, Fifth Edition (TB Scale-V) is the current version used in Japan. The TB Scale-V, as well as the Wechsler Intelligence Scale, the most popular standardized intelligence test in Japan, is useful for testing individuals who have limited language abilities. A full IQ is obtained by a mental age over a chronological age ratio. For people under 13 years of age, IQ is calculated based on the chronological age. For people over 14 years of age, TB Scale-V measures deviation IQ for four factors of cognitive abilities ((1) crystallized IQ, (2) fluid IQ, (3) memory, (4) Logic, and rational faculty). The TB Scale-V can be administered in approximately 30 min.

The items of TB Scale-V are shown in Table 1. In TB Scale-V, subjects start with items of an age-equivalent level. When a subject fails a task of the age-equivalent level, he or she is asked to answer tasks of a lower age-equivalent level until he or she passes all tasks of a specific age-equivalent level. Then, he or she is asked to answer tasks of higher age-equivalent levels until he or she fails all tasks of another specific age-equivalent level.

School Age

[WISC-V; Wechsler Intelligence Scale for Children-Fifth Edition]

The Wechsler Intelligence Scale for Children-Fifth Edition (WISC-V), developed by Wechsler, is an individually administered instrument for assessing cognitive ability in children (Wechsler, 2003) from age 6 to 16. The Japanese version of the WISC-V is still under development. The result based on profile of the WISC-V could

Table 1 Examples of items of the Tanaka-Binet Intelligence Scale, Fifth Edition

Age	Items	Age	Items	Age	Items
1	Discrimination: animal pictures (a dog) Body images Stereo composition: building blocks	7	Similarities: two things Comparison numbers Mutilated stories (A)	13	Way: south, north, east, west Code languages
2	Picture vocabulary Small and large concepts Repeating two words	8	Repeating short sentences Forming sentences	Over 14 ages	Abstract words Meaning of proverbs Matrix
3	Comprehension: a lifestyle habit Similarities and differences Memory of designs	9	Memory of figures (A) Enumeration of words		
4	Number concepts: counting (1–3) Memory of orders Opposite analogies	10	Numerical thinking Completing sentences		
5	Drawing a triangle Number concepts: counting (1–10) Concepts of right and left	11	Meaning of words Mutilated stories (B)		
6	Mutilated pictures Naming the days of the weeks Problem situations	12	Classification Memory of figures (A)		

serve as a tool in appropriate treatments and educational guidance. The WISC-V has two formats (traditional paper and pencil and digital version on Q-interactive). Also, the WISC-V is faster and easier to administer than the WISC-IV due to such factors as reduced testing time to obtain a full-scale IQ.

The WISC-V yields a full-scale IQ and five primary index scales ((1) verbal comprehension, (2) visual spatial, (3) fluid reasoning, (4) working memory, (5) processing speed), five ancillary index scales, and three complementary index scales (see Fig. 1). The WISC-V can be completed in approximately 45–60 min.

Adult

[WAIS-IV; Wechsler Adult Intelligence Scale-Fourth Edition]

The Wechsler Adult Intelligence Scale is one of the most widely used behavioral tests to examine cognitive profiles of adults in the world; it has been translated into many languages. Wechsler Adult Intelligence Scale-Fourth Edition (WAIS-IV) is a new version of the Wechsler intelligence test for adults. The Japanese version of WAIS-IV is under development. The purpose of WAIS-IV is for educational planning and the support of job skills. The WAIS-IV has two formats (traditional paper and pencil and web-based on Q-interactive).

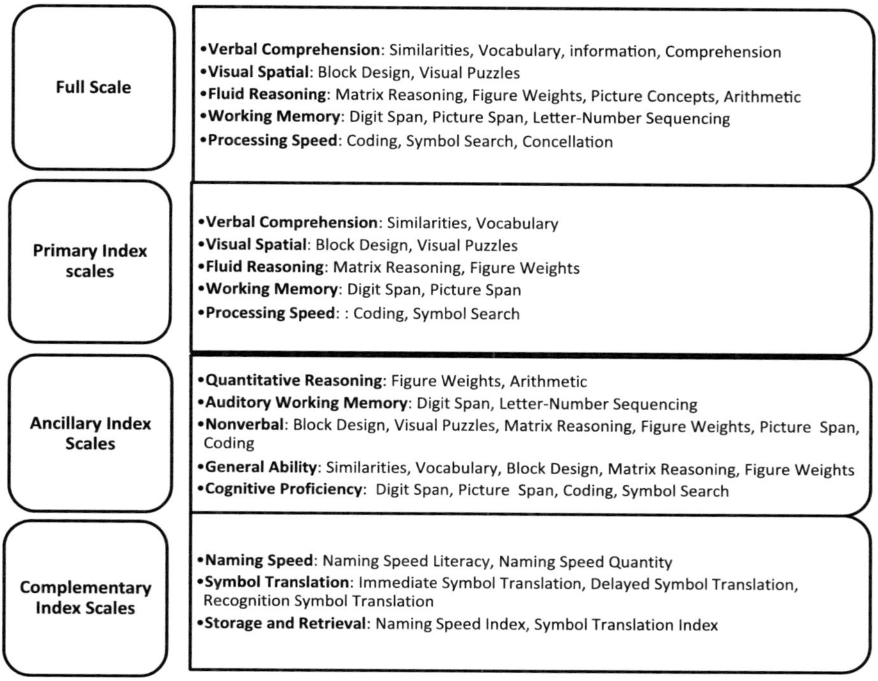

Fig. 1 WISC-V structure

The WAIS-IV has Full IQ [FIQ], four index scales ((1) verbal comprehension, (2) perceptual reasoning, (3) working memory, (4) processing speed) and fifteen subtests (ten subtests and five supplemental subtests) (see Fig. 2).

Studies of Intelligence Quotient for Children with ASD

ASD is a neurodevelopmental condition recognized in early childhood, characterized by persistent social and communication impairments, as well as restricted and stereotyped patterns of interests and behaviors. The developmental level and cognitive functioning of individuals with ASD have emerged as pivotal predictors of outcome (Lai et al., 2014; Volkmar & McPartland, 2016). Prior research has highlighted the association between lower IQ and social, behavioral, and various psychiatric disorders (Edirisooriya et al., 2021; Riccioni et al., 2022).

The Wechsler Intelligence test, available in various translated and standardized versions worldwide, is among the most widely utilized behavioral assessments for examining the cognitive profiles of children and adults. It comprises the Wechsler Adult Intelligence Scale (WAIS; Wechsler, 1939), developed subsequent to

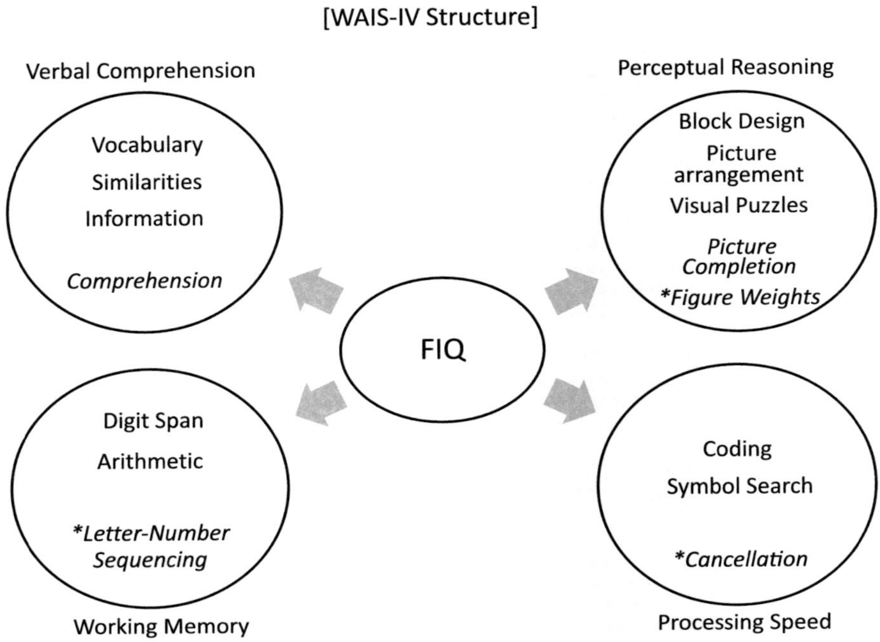

Fig. 2 WAIS-IV structure

the Wechsler Intelligence Scales for Children (WISC; Wechsler, 1949). Analyzing cognitive profiles based on the Wechsler Intelligence test, encompassing Full Intelligence Quotient (FIQ), Verbal Intelligence Quotient (VIQ), Performance Intelligence Quotient (PIQ), as well as index and subtest scores, can be instrumental in the diagnosis of adults with ASD.

The discrepancy between Verbal Intelligence Quotient (VIQ) and Performance Intelligence Quotient (PIQ) is frequently observed in individuals with ASD (Feczko et al., 2018; Joseph et al., 2002), potentially representing a distinctive trait of ASD (Yu et al., 2018). Previous research has indicated that VIQ-PIQ discrepancies are more prevalent in children with ASD compared to typically developing children (TD) (Ankenman et al., 2014; Nowell et al., 2015). These discrepancies manifest as a relatively lower VIQ compared to PIQ in children with ASD (Johnson et al., 2021; Lincoln et al., 1988; Mouga et al., 2016).

Additionally, studies have explored differences in VIQ-PIQ discrepancies between Asperger's and Autism. Some research has reported a VIQ > PIQ profile in certain children with Asperger's (Klin et al., 1995). However, other studies have failed to identify consistent patterns distinguishing Asperger's from Autism (Manjiviona & Prior, 1999; Ozonoff et al., 2000). The inconsistencies in these findings may stem from variations in the criteria used for diagnosing Asperger's (Joseph et al., 2002).

In a previous study, a comparative analysis of Six Subtest Profiles (Similarities, Vocabulary, Comprehension, Block Design, Digit Span, and Coding) based on Intellectual Level was conducted across 34 studies involving children with ASD. The children were categorized into three groups: the lower range (lower range ($IQ \leq$ ~85), borderline range (IQ = 86~100), higher range (IQ > 100)).

Among the four studies in the lower range groups, scores for Similarities, Vocabulary, and Comprehension were notably low, with Comprehension scores creating a prominent trough. Block Design scores were considerably high, forming a peak, while Digit Span and Coding scores were relatively lower. This pattern exhibited classic "islets of ability" profiles. In contrast, among the remaining thirty-two groups, some displayed high Block Design scores and low Comprehension scores. Higher IQ was associated with relatively higher language proficiency, indicating a distinct pattern from the typical profiles (Takayanagi et al., 2022).

In the present study, I conducted a comparative analysis of the scores of the Six Subtest Profiles within the three groups as outlined in Takayanagi's research. The lower range groups exhibited troughs in Comprehension scores and peaks in Block Design scores (Mean IQ score, 71.5: Similarities, M = 5.5; Vocabulary, 4.3; Comprehension, 3.0; Block Design, 9.9; Digit Span, 6.3; and Coding, 5.5). The borderline range groups showed a more moderate "islets of ability" profile compared to the lower range groups, with Coding scores indicating the lowest performance (IQ, 95.0: Similarities, 10.3; Vocabulary, 9.3; Comprehension, 7.7; Block Design, 10.7; Digit Span, 9.2; and Coding, 7.4).

The higher range group exhibited higher Similarities and Vocabulary scores than Block Design scores, while Coding scores were lower than Comprehension scores, suggesting a different pattern from the classic "islets of ability" profiles (IQ, 107.1: Similarities, 12.6; Vocabulary, 12.3; Comprehension, 10.1; Block Design, 11.8; Digit Span, 10.5; and Coding, 8.0). Therefore, children with lower IQs tended to have relatively more typical "islets of ability" profiles, whereas children with higher IQs displayed enhanced verbal ability but lower processing speed.

Studies of Intelligence Quotient for Adults with ASD

While several studies have delineated the cognitive profiles of children with ASD using WISC, relatively little is known about the cognitive distinctions of adults with ASD, who do not exhibit intellectual disability, as assessed by the WAIS. In our investigation, we delved into the cognitive profiles of adults with ASD who had no intellectual disabilities ($IQ \geq 70$), employing WAIS-III (Kanai et al., 2012, 2017). On the other hand, adults with ASD demonstrated an IQ split characterized by higher Verbal Intelligence Quotient (VIQ) and lower Performance Intelligence Quotient (PIQ) (Ghaziuddin & Mountain-Kimchi, 2004; Kanai et al., 2012; Kosaka et al., 2010). This finding underscores the prevalence of superior verbal skills relative to nonverbal skills in adults with ASD (Woodbury-Smith & Volkmar, 2009).

In the context of cognitive characteristics of adults with ASD having an IQ score > 70 (mean IQ level, 101.7) assessed using WAIS-III, the Six Subtest Profiles did not align with the typical "islets of ability" profile. ASD adults exhibited scores for Similarities (mean = 11.7), Vocabulary (12.4), and Comprehension (11.5) that surpassed those for Block Design (9.2). The Coding subtest (7.6) was consistently the lowest among the Six Subtest Profiles (Kanai et al., 2017), aligning with our earlier findings (Kanai et al., 2012). This pattern may be associated with visuomotor coordination and cognitive flexibility challenges (Hedvall et al., 2013; Manjiviona & Prior, 1995; Noterdaeme et al., 2010; Takayanagi et al., 2022).

To facilitate a comparison between the IQs of children and adults, we contrasted the mean scores of the Six Subtest Profiles in both borderline and higher range groups of children with ASD with those of adults. Notably, Comprehension was higher in adults with ASD than in children, while Block Design was lower in adults with ASD. Coding also remained the lowest among the Six Subtest Profiles in both groups (children, IQ, 101.0: Similarities, 11.4; Vocabulary, 10.8; Comprehension, 8.9; Block Design, 11.2; Digit Span, 9.8; and Coding, 7.7). Our study, encompassing both children and adults with ASD, indicates that while characteristics such as superior visual spatial and verbal abilities and challenges related to visuomotor coordination and cognitive flexibility are present in children, they may acquire the knowledge necessary to comprehend social common sense, which pertains to items in the Comprehension subtest, owing to their high level of verbal ability as they mature. Further studies with larger participant samples drawn from the general population are required to gain deeper insights into the cognitive profiles of adults with ASD.

Relationship Between Intellectual Development and Cognitive Functioning in Persons with Autism Spectrum Disorders and Intellectual Disability

Essential Questions and Research Directions

Research on ASD is one of the most widely funded areas in many parts of the world. Advances in fundamental research in neurological science (e.g., brain circuits and dynamic processes in individual brain development, functional connectivity), genetics, epigenetics, gene–environment interactions, and environmental risk factors all aim to interpret the causes of autistic symptoms and find connections to other causes that occur with non-autistic symptoms. Social information processing, lack of a theory of the mind, neurocognitive function, intellectual attribution bias, under-connectivity in neural systems, unconventional sensory information processing, level changes in motivation, and social attention are the most researched diagnostic domains of ASD (Happe, 1994; Scheuffgen et al., 2000; Williamson & Jakobson, 2014; Yirmiya et al., 1996).

Presently, ASD and ID are the most common (approximately 3–5%) developmental disorders in the human population. Many of the new research methods on ASD and ID seek to isolate specific brain circuits that could cause disrupted brain functions related to social and cognitive impairment in neurodevelopment. The presence or absence of ID is considered one of the most critical factors affecting developmentally related outcomes in individuals with ASD (Henninger & Taylor, 2013; Howlin et al., 2004). It is a widely accepted view that ID co-occurs in approximately two-thirds of persons with ASD (Thomas et al., 2014). ASD and ID are both complex and multi-factorial neurodevelopmental disorders with high heritability, and they share overlapping risk factors (Betancur et al., 2009). The development and recent advances in etiology, functional brain scanning (fMRI), and developmental neuroscience all show the importance of early social experiences for cognitive development and intellectual/developmental functioning (Amaral et al., 2008).

The relationship between environmental influences and intellectual/cognitive development includes socioeconomic status, including the quality of the home environment (early developmental environment), and various environmental risk factors (specific and indirect) like an absent father, maternal anxiety, and mental health, parents' education, knowledge of early childhood development, parental attitude, and level of positive parent–child interaction, etc. (Landry et al., 2001; Sameroff, 2005; Seifer, 2001). Hartup (1986) assumes a two-way relationship between social interactions and children's cognitive development, i.e., not only the quality of the interaction affects development, but also the child's level of development affects the kind of interactions s/he will receive.

Significant limitations in intellectual functioning and adaptive behavior characterize ID. ID might occur as an isolated developmental disability problem or be accompanied by impairment in sensory processing development, epileptic seizures, and behavioral disturbances. During childhood (before the age of 18 years), adaptive behavior and intellectual functioning strongly contribute to the development of conceptual, social, and practical adaptive skills (Schalock, 2011). Recent research results show that ID in ASD might emerge as a consequence of severe social-communication deficits on the experience-dependent mechanism underlying various neuro-cognitive developments. The study results of Vivanti et al. (2013) suggest that ASD symptom severity contributes to the extent to which environmental input is required to support typical brain development. This study states that the risk of developing ID increases as the number and severity of ASD social-communicative impairments increase (Vivanti et al., 2013).

Two main conceptual frameworks relate to the nature of ASD-ID/ID-ASD association. One is the so-called "co-morbid condition theory," which states that ID is a co-morbid condition that occurs over and above the ASD symptoms (Matson & Williams, 2014; Matson et al., 2011). The "co-morbid condition" explanation emphasizes the unrelated causality and etiology. Thus, the co-morbid condition and symptoms are conceptually distinct from the principal diagnosis.

The second concept is the so-called "distinct additional theory" that suggests the aetiological relationship between ASD and ID. Some researchers think that there are common aetiological factors that could cause ASD and could cause ID (Waterhouse,

2013). Waterhouse (2013) states that the aetiological background of ASD is too broad to be sure of anything. She uses a metaphoric "illusive butterfly" to explain that 30 years of tremendous research could not give any "certain" answer to the aetiological concept of ASD, and every "new door" that science opens provides us with access to another that needs to be opened.

Developmental theory-dominated clinical neuropsychology research emphasizes that the early neurocognitive development of the human brain is experience-dependent by nature (Karmiloff-Smith et al., 2002). Therefore, unbalanced and insufficient early social experiences could cause an inadequate cognition of self- and peer awareness by proxy and adversely impact cognitive brain functioning (Makinodan et al., 2012). Many of the recent ASD- and ID-related studies focus on the best possible early detection and early intervention to be able to provide (e.g., design, develop, arrange, modify) the necessary social and physical environment for psychosocial and cognitive development for children at high risk of developmental delay or disability (Toth, 2010). Structured early intervention programs and development therapies could make a difference in sensory processing, sensorimotor development, and speech-language abilities (Gernsbacher et al., 2008). Developmental delay and impairment in the communication and speech domain could be the secondary results of the ID and ASD symptoms (Dziuk et al., 2007). Suppose a child during the early "sensitive developmental period" does not have or cannot respond well to early sensory and social inputs from the closed physical and social environment. In that case, he or she will not be able to demonstrate adequate adaptive responses and will show signs of either ID, ASD, or both (Klin et al., 2014; Travers et al., 2015; Ventola et al., 2014). Researchers of experience-dependent neurocognitive development emphasize that, in the case mentioned above, ID is not a co-morbid condition but the ultimate result of inefficient functional brain development. In this case, the severe ASD symptoms could be found responsible for the developmental delay of intellectual development and cognitive functions. This does not mean that ASD could necessarily cause ID, but it emphasizes the fact that severe ASD symptoms cause an at-risk situation for intellectual developmental delay (Gotham et al., 2012; Grossmann & Johnson, 2007).

Interrelation Between Intellectual Functioning and Autism Spectrum Disorders

ASD core symptoms appear in the social communication and interaction domain of development and atypical patterns of behavior (restricted and repetitive) and interest (Wilkins & Matson, 2009). Symptoms of ID are usually grouped into two main diagnostic categories. The first is called intellectual functioning. It includes delayed cognitive information processing and altered development of basic intellectual skills, abilities, and virtues. The second is called adaptive functioning. It includes conceptual skills for learning (e.g., language, literacy, mathematics), social skills (interpersonal relationships), and practical skills related to self-care, health, and safety. Many researchers have questioned the presence of ID in the case of children with ASD for several reasons (Kraijer, 2000; Matson et al., 2013). One of these reasons is the reliability or unreliability of intelligence scales used to assess the IQ of children with ASD. Certain limitations make testing difficult for a child with ASD. Scheuffgen et al. (2000) state that a child with ASD might not be able to complete intellectual measurement tests. For instance, if a child with ASD has moderate or severe speech and language difficulty, the child may not be able to respond to interview questions (Scheuffgen et al., 2000).

Another difficulty is that, in most cases, the diagnosis of ASD symptoms in children with ID is based on clinical criteria validated for populations with average intelligence, thus compromising the diagnostic accuracy of ASD criteria (Javaloyes, 2006). Specific verbal subtests show low performance, while others, like block design, show superior performance results (Shah & Frith, 1993). A person with ASD could have one or a set of unique abilities called savant skills. These are areas of surprising talent in otherwise low-functioning individuals. The estimated prevalence of savant abilities in autism is 10%, whereas the prevalence in the non-autistic population is less than one percentile. The most common forms of savant abilities involve mathematical calculations, extraordinary memory, musical abilities (with perfect pitch and excellent musical memory), and other artistic abilities (e.g., drawing, painting, singing, and playing an instrument). A mathematical ability that many autistic individuals display is calendar memory. At the same time, others can multiply and divide large numbers without writing them down and can also calculate prime numbers in their heads in only seconds (Frith, 1993).

Research on ASD and ID co-morbid features concludes that the severity of ASD symptoms should be independent and separately measured from the severity of cognitive functioning and intellectual abilities. A longitudinal study with 345 participants documented that ID is a distinguishable part of the whole disability feature in children with severe ASD symptoms but less in cases with mild ASD symptom representation; thus, cognitive functioning and ASD symptom severity are not entirely independent features (Gotham et al., 2012). Another study by Vivanti et al. (2013) targeted this latest hypothesis by developing an intervention program to improve ASD symptoms. Vivanti and colleagues predicted that children with severe ASD symptoms are likely to have lower intellectual ability. Therefore, if these children receive a targeted therapy program for their ASD symptoms, they should have improved results in intellectual skill development as well. They based their intervention on recent results in developmental neuroscience that support the "experience-dependent" nature of early brain development (Kuhl, 2007). Positive changes in intellectual functioning could be gained from early behavioral interventions, even if the original aim was to weaken core ASD symptoms. Early appearance of social-communication difficulties in children with ASD could result in sensory processing differences or disorders and cause an unintentional neuropsychological "block" against receiving essential inputs from the closed environment, thus negatively affecting cognitive skill development (Schoen et al., 2009). These results suggest the possible interdependent relation between ASD and ID (Vivanti et al., 2013). The above-mentioned sensory processing issues or differences can affect one or several senses (vision, hearing, touch, smell, taste, proprioception, the vestibular system, and interoception). When these issues cause developmental differences, it is called Sensory Processing Difficulties or Disorders (SPD) (Miller et al., 2007). It is a condition that has an etiological connection to how the central nervous system receives messages (stimuli input) from sensory receptors, interprets impulses, and responds appropriately with adequate behavior. SPD occurs when a sensory signal is not correctly detected on the reception level or later in the nervous system; thus, it cannot respond correctly. These responses could cause the person to inadequately process sensory information, either over-respond when the sensory stimuli are overwhelming or under-respond when stimuli cause weak responses or none—with little or no reaction. SPDs are commonly observed in individuals with ASD, leading to atypical responses to sensory stimuli. SPDs refer to how individuals receive, process, and respond to sensory information from the environment. People with SPDs may be hypersensitive (over-reactive) or hyposensitive (under-reactive) to sensory input, or they may experience fragmented or distorted perceptions. These differences can make it difficult for individuals with SPDs to filter out irrelevant sensory information and integrate sensory information from different sources (Miller et al., 2021). SPD could cause difficulty organizing sensory information and making an appropriate response. Thus, it could cause discomfort, stress, extreme responses, restlessness, inadequate balance, and deficient motor coordination. Sensory processing issues are often first recognized during the early childhood period—mainly during the toddler years, usually one to three years of age—when caregivers notice unusual or aversive behavioral reactions to a stimulus (light, sound, movement, touch, tight- or irritating garments, etc.). These sensory dysregulation issues are challenging to deal with, especially during early childhood, but they might get better with sufficient environmental control and neurological maturation; however, in many cases, these issues will stay with the person during their entire life, possibly in a partly controlled way, by learning coping strategies while receiving social skill training and different other therapies. Since 2013, the SPDs have been linked to ASD by their inclusion in the Fifth Edition of the DSM-5 diagnostic criteria.

Nevertheless, SPDs were NOT included in the DSM-5 as distinctive disorders. In contrast, Sensory Processing and Sensory-Based Movement Disorders in infants and young children were already included in the revised version of "DC:0–3™" Diagnostic Classification of Mental Health and Developmental Disorders of Infancy and Early Childhood (DC:0–3R, 2005). Stanley Greenspan and Serena Weider chaired the Task Force at Zero to Three in 1994 and 2005 (Greenspan & Weider, 2008). The new "DC:0–5™" was released in 2016, and then the updated DC:0–5™ Version 2.0 was released in 2021. The new version keeps up with the tradition. It captures new findings relevant to diagnosis and addresses issues in the earliest years by identifying and describing disorders not addressed in other classification systems like the DSM-5. The Diagnostic Classification of Mental Health and Developmental Disorders

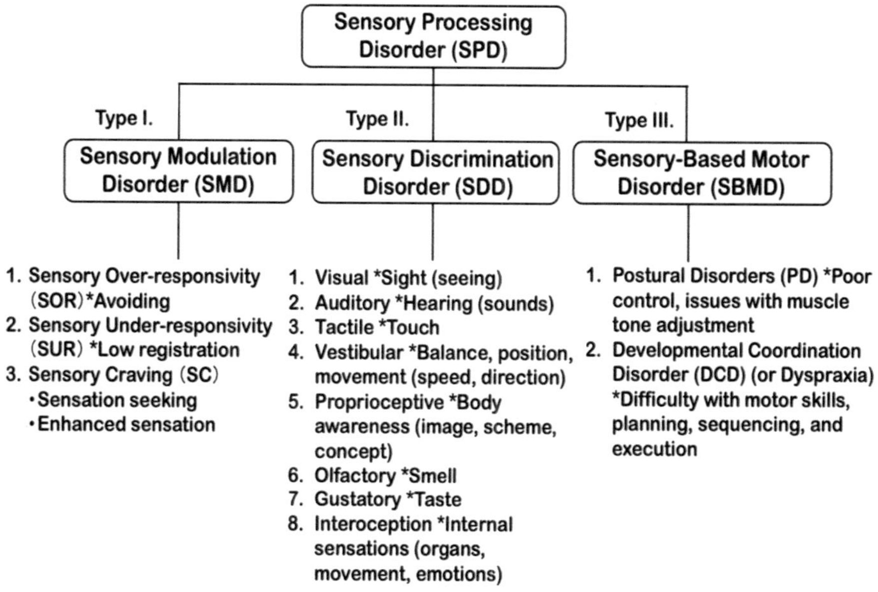

Fig. 3 Subtypes of sensory processing disorder as an umbrella term for identified sensory-based neurological conditions (Modified version based on Miller et al., 2007)

of Infancy and Early Childhood, with an open mind and after careful investigations, points to practical intervention approaches because a child's brain makes one million neural connections per second during the first years of infants and toddlers. For example, sensory pathways during the development of hearing, language, and other higher cognitive functions peak by the first three years of a child's life, while emotionally nourishing relationships establish the foundation of health and well-being. This early social environment is full of human connections (experiences and relationships with parents and siblings directly influence the development of the nervous system, social and emotional self-regulation, and cognitive skills (Fig. 3).

Genetic and Epigenetic Causality Research on Autism Spectrum Disorders and Intellectual Disability

Neurodevelopmental disorders like ASD, ID, and Attention Deficit Hyperactivity Disorder (ADHD) are complex traits that are influenced by more than one factor (genetic or environmental); multiple genetic determinants interact in the context of poorly understood environmental factors to give rise to clinically diverse phenotypes. Research results from genetic, epigenetic, and environmental studies seek to identify candidate genes that could cause ASD, ID, and ADHD and contribute to the understanding of these conditions from the comparative pathobiological viewpoint (Ben-David & Shifman, 2012; Betancur et al., 2009; Kou et al., 2012). These molecular- and cellular-based results could contribute to possible therapeutic approaches in the future. From the genetic standpoint, ASD and ID are likely to be related on the molecular and biochemical levels. The genetic approach sees the causal factors of ASD and ID as both similar and, in many ways, very different.

On the one hand, an estimated 70% of diagnosed ASD individuals have some level of ID as well. In contrast, the others have dysfunctions in speech-language and communication and difficulties in cognitive and social behavioral areas. On the other hand, at least 10–15% of persons with ID diagnosis have autistic tendencies or identified ASD symptoms (Mefford et al., 2012). Recent results from various genetic studies reported that no single gene could be significantly associated with ASD, and there is a high possibility that gene mutation and hundreds of gene variants might be responsible for causing the ASD condition (Anney et al., 2012; Liu et al., 2013). A large number of these gene variants and mutations could be associated with either ASD or ID, while some (e.g., SHANK1, SHANK2, NRXN1) are found to be associated with both conditions (Berkel et al., 2010; Sato et al., 2012). Kou et al. (2012) used systems biology and a combined network approach to predict candidate genes for ASD and ID. Their results showed that ASD and ID share common pathways that could perturb (i.e., alter the regular state or path of) an overlapping synaptic regulatory sub-network (Kou et al., 2012).

During last ten years, significant progress has been made in identifying rare variants of major effect in both ASD and ID; however, it is still challenging to find the best possible explanation for the underlying molecular mechanism of high-risk family traits and rare inherited mutations (Srivastava & Schwartz, 2014). As a result of extensive worldwide genetic research related to specific genetic causes, science has identified many individually rare genes that could be associated with a high risk for ASD, and some of them extensively overlap with genes for ID. A particular genetic etiology can currently be identified in about 15% of patients with ASD (van Bokhoven, 2011). Presently, ongoing studies estimate that in the future, 60–80% of ASD-ID genes and "loci" (position of a gene or mutation on a chromosome) remain to be discovered, and hundreds of genes would be identified to be causally associated with these conditions (Topper et al., 2011). The California Autism Twins Study (CATS) reported research results on 192 identical and fraternal twin pairs. The research study reported a concordance rate of 77% for male monozygotic twins and 50% for female identical twins. The rates among fraternal twins were 31% (male) and 36% (female) (Hallmayer et al., 2011).

Although the high correlation between autism and genetic factors has been long established, the exact genetic background of ASD remains unclear. Some new findings were mere chance associations reported by studies because they looked significant at the time. There is a regular line of new studies reporting on possible associations between recently identified genetic conditions and ASD. Zafeiriou et al. (2013) reported ASD as a heterogeneous group of neurodevelopmental disabilities with various etiologies but with a heritability estimate of more than 90% (Zafeiriou et al., 2007, 2013). Their study concludes that it is essential to identify ASD in patients with genetic syndromes in order to ensure correct management, future therapeutic approaches, and appropriate educational placement. Findings from the study of genetic syndromes are incorporated into the ongoing research on autism etiology and pathogenesis. Different syndromes converge upon common biological backgrounds (such as disrupted molecular pathways and brain circuitries), which probably account for their co-morbidity with ASD (Zafeiriou et al., 2013).

Some well-known syndromes and conditions could cause ID and ASD as well. It is estimated that these syndromes account for more than 10% of ASD cases. These syndromes include Fragile X syndrome, Down syndrome, Prader–Willi syndrome, Williams syndrome, Angelman syndrome, Duchenne syndrome, etc. This chapter gives a short research summary on the first three concerning ID and ASD.

Fragile X syndrome is an inherited genetic disease that causes ID and could cause developmental disabilities as well. Fragile X syndrome is found in about 1 in every 4000 males and about 1 in every 8000 females. Fragile X syndrome is the most common hereditary source of ID in men. People with Fragile X syndrome may show a combination of the following signs as children and throughout life: anxiety (general or social), ASD-like symptoms (e.g., social problems, such as not making eye contact, disliking being touched, trouble understanding body language), ADHD-like symptoms (e.g., impulsiveness, attention problems, hyperactivity), epileptic seizures and sleeping disorders. Nowadays, fragile X syndrome is recognized as the most common identifiable genetic cause of ID and ASD, with many overlapping phenotypic features (Yu & Berry-Kravis, 2014).

Another well-known syndrome that could cause ID and sometimes ASD co-morbidity is Down syndrome. There has been an increase in the number of children with Down syndrome who are being diagnosed as having ASD as well (Gray et al., 2011; Starr et al., 2005). These children with Down syndrome and identified autistic tendencies or ASD are referred to as having a so-called "dual diagnosis," which means that these two are coexisting conditions. There have also been some survey studies in Europe (UK and Sweden) and the USA suggesting that about 5–10% of children with Down syndrome could have been diagnosed with co-morbid ASD (Kent et al., 1999; Rasmussen et al., 2001). Some of the researchers in the field are worried about a tendency to over-diagnose ASD in children with Down syndrome, so it is essential to say that a vast majority of individuals with Down syndrome show no evidence of ASD (Howlin et al., 1995; Starr et al., 2005).

Prader–Willi syndrome is a rare genetic condition caused by an error in one or more genes. The responsible genes are not yet identified, but research shows that most likely the problem lies in a particular region of chromosome 15 (e.g., missing, doubled from the maternal and none from the paternal side, or defective paternal chromosome) (Dimitropoulos et al., 2013). It presents several physical, intellectual, and behavioral problems. A key symptom of Prader–Willi syndrome is the constant sense of hunger (hyperphagia) that usually begins at the age of two and is caused by the dysfunction of the hypothalamus, which controls hunger and thirst. Children with Prader–Willi syndrome often show mild to moderate impairment in intellectual functioning (e.g., thinking, reasoning, problem-solving). Even those without significant ID have some learning disabilities. Infants with Prader–Willi syndrome have poor muscle tone (e.g., hypotonic muscles, poor sucking reflex), lack of eye coordination (strabismus), and poor responsiveness or reaction to various stimuli. During early childhood, the person with Prader–Willi syndrome feels constant hyperphagia and usually has trouble with weight control (Bohm et al., 2015). Children with Prader–Willi syndrome have underdeveloped sex organs (hypogonadism), delayed motor development, speech-language disorder (e.g., delayed language development: dysarthria), sleep disorder, abnormal curvature of the spine (scoliosis), endocrine problems (e.g., hypothyroidism, growth hormone deficiency, central adrenal insufficiency) and high pain tolerance that makes it very difficult to identify injury or illness. They also have various social and behavioral problems (e.g., sharp temper, rigidity, repetitive and obsessive–compulsive behavior, and aggressiveness toward themselves and others) (Lo et al., 2013).

Several studies investigated the co-morbidity of Prader–Willi syndrome with ASD. The study of Descheemaeker et al. (2006) investigated 59 individuals with Prader–Willi syndrome and 59 controls with non-specific ID. They were matched for levels of intelligence (IQ), age, and gender. Results of this study showed prominent autistic-like behavioral phenotypes in most individuals with Prader–Willi syndrome (Descheemaeker et al., 2006). Results revealed that even if a person with Prader–Willi syndrome had a higher level of intelligence, s/he still developed autistic behavioral tendencies. Descheemaeker et al. suggest reconsidering the classic symptomatology of persons with Prader–Willi syndrome to a broader ASD symptomatology.

Recently, Dimitropoulos et al. (2013) compared social functioning in Prader-Willi syndrome to individuals with ASD using the Social Responsiveness Scale (SRS) and the Social Competence Inventory (SCI). This study aims to measure if there is an increased risk of social and behavioral deficits in people with the maternally derived uniparental disomy (mUPD) subtype of Prader–Willi syndrome in comparison to those with 15q11-13 paternal deletion (DEL) type by comparing them to a group of individuals with ASD. The study results showed similar scores across most SRS domains in the ASD and mUPD subtype groups. All groups showed great difficulty with the SCI scores, even though the DEL subtype group had the highest score on prosocial behavior that promotes positive social interaction (e.g., helpfulness, generosity, empathy, social understanding, cooperating, handling of conflict). These findings suggest further characterization of social behavior in Prader–Willi syndrome to understand better genes' contributions in the DEL subtype to ASD susceptibility (Dimitropoulos et al., 2013).

Other X-linked disorders cause ID and, in many cases, epilepsies as well. These are less common than the fragile X syndrome but have been scientifically proven to cause ID. There are few known examples of X-linked mutations that cause ID, for instance, the Coffin–Lowry syndrome (mutations in ribosomal protein S6 kinase: RSK2) and the Borjeson–Forssman–Lehmann syndrome. These are still under study to find out whether they could cause ASD. Introduced a preliminary result on a small subset of patients with Coffin–Lowry syndrome who have also presented with autism or transient autistic behavior.

In summary, some single specific genes can be associated with ASD. However, it seems that the current genetic research and study groups support the idea of polygenic inheritance, meaning that multiple genes are likely to be involved and predispose an individual to develop ASD symptoms (The Simons VIP Consortium, 2012). However, contemporary results and conclusions of these genetic studies still need to be completed and have limited explanations; thus, they cannot be applied to clinical diagnosis yet.

Synaptic Plasticity and Cognitive Disorders

The human central nervous system processes and transmits information in the form of nerve impulses (electrical signals) through its specialized brain cells (neurons). The human brain has a trillion (10^{12}) neurons, and these vast numbers of nerve cells connect with adhesive junctions called synapses. The human synaptic system comprises a quadrillion (10^{15}) synapses. Synapses are highly specialized for mediating communication between neurons in the nervous system (Ho et al., 2011). Cell-based communication through synapses involves the release of chemical information substances (neurotransmitters) from the presynaptic terminals at the end of the nerve fiber by the arrival of an electrical nerve impulse (i.e., action potential). The information carried by the neurotransmitter diffuses across the synapse (transsynaptic interaction) to another nerve fiber. Synapses are morphologically highly dynamic and can be subjected to rapid structural changes in response to stimuli (Missler et al., 2012). Synaptic plasticity is the ability to change structurally as a functional reaction to a particular impulse. This activity-dependent adaptability (dendritic morphogenesis and synaptogenesis) gives the human brain the strength to learn; in other words, synaptic plasticity represents the cellular basis of memory and learning.

Regulated synaptic connectivity and elimination of synapses are critical for learning, memory, and behavioral function in the developing brain. Changes in the synaptic structure can lead to immense changes in information processing. Recent evidence from various studies suggests that this adaptable function of neural plasticity is disrupted in many neurodevelopmental disorders (i.e., ASD, ID, ADHD). As a result of this, intellectual and behavioral functions are strongly affected (Durand et al., 2012; Tsai et al., 2012; Valnegri et al., 2012). The dysfunction of synapse plasticity and dendrite formation is a significant developmental factor of intellectual and behavioral functions in persons with ASD and ID (Hutsler & Zhang, 2010). Tsai et al. (2012) concluded in their study that multiple ASD- and ID-associated genes are involved in the previously mentioned activity-dependent adaptability and synapse elimination process, which elaborates the accuracy of neuronal circuit formation. Dendritic morphogenesis and synaptogenesis are essential neural activities that affect the neural development of a person with ASD (Ebert & Greenberg, 2013; Gilman et al., 2011).

Environmental Aetiology Research on Autism Spectrum Disorders and Intellectual Disability

Other than genetic causes, there is an active interest in various primary environmental causative factors that could also be strongly related (directly or indirectly) to ASD and ID.

In a complete sense, human evolution and, in a narrow sense, child development have been the subjects of genetic and environmental research since the early 1960s. In 1960, Zazzo (Les Jumeaux, le Couple et la Personne) suggested that genetic effects tend to be erased by environmental influences, especially in twins. In addition to genetic heritability, common factors such as the shared prenatal environment might play a role in the formation of ASD. Therefore, to understand and interpret early childhood development, it is necessary to consider information on genetic or hereditary research and environmental and mental changes. Environmental chemicals with hormone-like activity can disrupt the programming of endocrine signaling pathways during development. These so-called "environmental hormones" could result in adverse effects. Recent reports link exposure to environmental endocrine-disrupting chemicals during development with adverse health consequences. Recent research attempts to connect environmental changes with the rapid increase in ASD prevalence, and especially to the potential involvement of toxins in our environment (Grabrucker, 2012). Specific environmental factors might act as risk factors triggering the development of autistic tendencies with limited cognitive functions. Some studies link children's early brain development changes to their mothers' exposure to hormone-disrupting environmental chemicals. However, a few of these studies have explicitly looked at whether they contribute to ASD or ID. Scientists suspect that hormones play a role in ASD and AIDS because boys are four times more likely than girls to be diagnosed, and several hormones are known to control brain development and psychosocial behavior. Thus, the role of environmental factors in ASD-ID etiology is an essential area of research (Grandgeorge et al., 2009).

One of the most important environmental risk factors is the exposure to toxins. Other essential factors include maternal nutrition, tobacco, alcohol, and other drugs, infection during pregnancy and prematurity, as well as parental age at conception. These factors are under continuous study to find a concrete relation to ASD-ID symptomatology.

Frequent and Varied Co-morbid Conditions with Autism Spectrum Disorders and Intellectual Disability

ASD and ID as neurodevelopmental disorders are associated with various comorbidities, such as attention problems, externalizing behaviors such as aggression, affective disorders, and sensory processing difficulties (Dunn, 2007). Neurological comorbidities are motor disorders or developmental motor impairment, epilepsy, and sleeping dysfunction. These co-morbidities also have a significant impact on cognitive functioning and social behavior (Dowell et al., 2009; Dziuk et al., 2007; Goldman et al., 2009; Mandelbaum et al., 2006; Van Waelvelde et al., 2010).

Perception (senses) and movement (body) are present in early childhood experiences. However, these very complex experiences are simultaneously mediated through movement-action and other sensory systems and constitute, for example, the basis of spatial awareness, comprehension, and learning. Correspondingly, self-regulation has both emotional and cognitive dimensions, and according to the National Academies of Sciences, Engineering, and Medicine (2015), it is considered part of executive functioning, socio-emotional competence, and learning competencies. In other words, emotional and cognitive self-regulation are essential for children to utilize their learning competencies. In addition to the persistent deficits in the areas of social communication and interaction and the restricted, repetitive patterns of behavior, interests, or activities as diagnostic criteria for children with ASD, there are measurable sensorimotor difficulties, repetitive motor movements, and atypical reactivity to sensory input (Baranek, 2002). Studies have shown that atypical reactivity to sensory input (problems with sensory modulation and discrimination) could cause difficulties in motor planning and execution (sensory-based motor disorder), and that could account for difficulties in the development of social and communication skills, furthermore, for reduced social attention in early development (Hannant et al., 2016; Kadlaskar et al., 2023; Patil & Kaple, 2023). In other words, motor skill development supports cognitive, speech-language communication, and sensory development. Sensorimotor development combines receiving sensory input and giving a movement (behavioral) response (motor output). It is estimated that at least 80 out of 100 people with ASD have poorer motor coordination skills than their neurotypical peers (Fournier et al., 2010). Difficulties with motor coordination that affect a range of movement activities, including planning, gross-motor development (roll, sit, crawl, gate movement, balance, walk, run, jump, kick, climb, skip, etc.), and fine motor skills (reaching-grasping, eye-hand coordination, finger movements, and dexterity, etc.) could be present from infancy or toddler years until adulthood (Gowen & Hamilton, 2013; Lloyd et al., 2013).

Children with ASD usually experience developmental disorders in one or more areas of development, mainly in the area of sensory perception (processing, discrimination), the area of cognitive skills (attention, memory, problem-solving, following instructions, logical reasoning, and learning, etc.), the area of both gross- and fine motor skills (movement coordination, motor planning, motor control, etc.), the speech-language and communication area (using and understanding language, difficulty speaking words, understanding others, etc.), and the area of social and emotional skills (understanding social cues, expressing feelings, showing adequate emotional reactions, dealing with changes to a routine, etc.) (Schaaf et al., 2014). Typically developing children could also experience a developmental delay, which usually manifests in slower development of specific skills and delayed developmental milestones in two or three areas; however, those can be corrected with general early intervention and supported practical training because they develop specific skills slower than their peers. In the case of ASD and other developmental disabilities, problems of the above-mentioned developmental skills are not only delayed by a time factor (slower development), but those are usually lifelong conditions with the need for continuous support in skill development. Persons with ASD have atypical cognitive deficits (impaired social cognition, atypical perception, disruption in information processing, executive dysfunction, etc.). Thus, these problems are more in the category of developmental disorders rather than developmental delays.

Motor function is essential for broader aspects of development like language, social interaction, and learning. Motor disorders include delayed movement development and deficits in different motor functions. Motor deficits include dyspraxia (difficulty in activities requiring coordinated and skilled movement like writing), motor coordination disorder or developmental coordination disorder (DCD), stereotypic movement disorder (SMD), and gait problems (walking-related abnormalities) (Bodison, 2015; Fournier et al., 2010; Miller et al., 2021). SMD is a repetitive, nonfunctional involuntary motor behavior (e.g., unintentional hand waving or self-injurious behavior like head banging or hand biting) that significantly interferes with normal daily life activities and could result in bodily injuries. Individuals with ASD and ID are at higher risk for SMD. Altogether, movement and motor dysfunction are developmental issues that facilitate earlier diagnosis of ASD and ID during early childhood, particularly in infants and young children (Dziuk et al., 2007).

The importance of a developmental therapy-based sensorimotor program like Sensory Integration Therapy for children with ASD in small group sessions as a therapeutic environment is its self-assertive motivational factor (Miller et al., 2007; Schoen et al., 2019). At the same time, the activity happens together with peers, and the personal behavior through the movement of the individual becomes part of the group dynamics, giving the individual impetus. The participants give each other a model to imitate, which works like peer reinforcement while learning to cooperate. Group members reinforce each other's behavior and start cooperating upon their similar behavioral traits, thus accepting that they are not alone, which might help them develop adaptive behavioral features (Bhat, 2020).

The risk of epilepsy in persons with ASD is linked to lower IQ, with peaks of incidence occurring at preschool age and adolescence. Between 18% and 29% of children with ASD are affected, and any seizure type can occur (Cass et al., 2006). Relationships between autistic traits, epilepsy, and cognitive functioning remain poorly understood. Although in recent studies, the relationship between ASD and epilepsy has been extensively recognized, the underlying mechanism is still unclear. Research data shows that ASD and epilepsy co-occur in about 30% of all cases in either group. However, there is no classic epilepsy syndrome associated with ASD, though it is well documented that ID itself presents a higher specific risk factor for epilepsy (Tuchman et al., 2010; Turk et al., 2009; van Eeghen et al., 2013). The study of Tuchman et al. (2010) summarizes that investigators suggest that the most common reason for the co-occurrence of ASD and epilepsy is that the same brain pathology causes both disorders. The second reason could be an epileptic process during early development that interferes with the developing function of distinct brain networks, leading to the ASD phenotype. The third reason could come from the idea that the coexistence of both ASD and epilepsy aetiologically is a focal or multifocal process affecting structures common to both ASD and epilepsy, such as the limbic system.

Results from various research studies show that it is very likely that multiple biological and genetic substrates could lead to ASD-epilepsy phenotypes. Most study results conclude that there is no single unifying ASD-epilepsy phenotype. On the other hand, it is crucial to understand potential commonalities in subgroups of children with an ASD-epilepsy phenotype. In the near future, the research-based understanding of such phenomena should help us to understand the pathophysiology of both ASD and epilepsy. Now, the research question that needs to be addressed is whether some specific causes or genes differ in individuals with both ASD and epilepsy versus those with either disorder alone (Tuchman et al., 2010).

Finally, sleeping disorder is one of the high-risk co-morbidities in persons with developmental disorders (e.g., ASD, ID, ADHD). The development and maintenance of sleep are controlled by melatonin. Melatonin is a hormone secreted by the brain's pineal (or endocrine) gland (epiphysis cerebri) behind the third ventricle). It works as a "body clock," turned on during hours of darkness and switched off at dawn by the light of day. Melatonin helps the person to sleep and regulates the sleep cycle (called circadian rhythm). Typical symptoms of sleeping dysfunction are prolonged awakening time, sleep fatigue, lack of energy, and lapses in memory and concentration (Grabrucker, 2012; Maski et al., 2011). Some of the studies suggest that anxiety and SPDs, two well-known co-morbid conditions for ASD, might be related to the high-risk co-morbidity for sleeping problems. The most common problems include prolonged sleep latency, bedtime resistance, sleep onset delay, reduced sleep duration, decreased sleep efficacy, sleep anxiety, and night awakening (Hollway & Aman, 2011). Bruni et al. (2015) reported a study on melatonin use for children with sleep disturbances. The study states that melatonin decreases sleep onset latency and increases total sleep time but does not decrease night awakenings.

Recent studies collected data on the sleeping dysfunction of children with ASD from parents related to their daily rhythm and everyday life difficulties. The data show that typically developing children experience an average of 25–40% disrupted sleep cycle, while 40–80% of children with ASD experience a sleep problem (Reynolds & Malow, 2011). Sleeping is a critical factor for early development in children. Sleeping has multiple related functions, and it significantly contributes to brain growth, enhanced memory functions, cognition, and energy conservation. Therefore, insufficient sleep could cause deficits in all of these areas for every child, but especially for those with a developmental disability. Studies on sleep problems in children with ASD show that insufficient sleep accelerates the severity of ASD symptoms (e.g., repetitive behavior, emotional dysregulation, self-injurious behavior, social and communication difficulties).

There is evidence that shows a significant relationship between sleeping dysfunction and problematic daytime behavior. The study of Cohen et al. (2014) proposed that profiling the sleep problems of children with ASD on the nature of their sleep disruption could provide significant data for further research. This profiling system on sleep disturbances could reveal important details and new insight better to understand the behavioral profiles of persons with ASD. On the other hand, analysis of behavior profiles of children with ASD might help to understand sleep problems and contribute to the design of better intervention strategies to manage these symptoms.

Neurophysiological Basis of Intellectual Function in People with Autism Spectrum Disorder

Concept of "Intelligence" and Its Neurophysiological Basis

People with autism spectrum disorder (ASD) show atypicalities in several domains of cognitive and perceptual functions. Diversity in behavioral phenotypes is a characteristic of ASD (Masi et al., 2017). Moreover, ASD as a whole includes patients with heterogeneous patterns of intellectual abilities (Billeiter & Froiland, 2023). As the types of support and intervention requests differ greatly depending on the level of intelligence (Lorenc et al., 2018; Reichow et al., 2013), a precise and objective assessment of intellectual ability is essential in clinical practice.

The term "intelligence" is notoriously hard to define. There is a general consensus regarding the multidimensionality of intelligence, and many intelligence assessment tools have been developed to evaluate multiple aspects of intellectual ability. For example, in the widely used Wechsler Intelligence Scale for Children (WISC) and Wechsler Adult Intelligence Scale (WAIS), the full intelligence quotient (IQ) can be decomposed into verbal and performance IQ (Wechsler, 1991, 1997), whereas the Kaufman Assessment Battery for Children (K-ABC 2; Kaufman & Kaufman, 2013) has its roots in the theoretical framework of fluid and crystallized intelligence (Cattell, 1963).

Psychologists have accumulated abundant information about various aspects of cognitive functions by using existing test-batteries, thus succeeding, to some extent, in characterizing "cognitive profile" of people with ASD. People with ASD show visuospatial performance, as measured by intelligence assessment tools, that is comparable or superior to typically developed (TD) people (Dawson et al., 2007; Takayanagi et al., 2022). Within ASD population, subgroups exhibit different pattern of cognitive performance (Nader et al., 2015). Thus, the assessment of intelligence is useful not only in characterizing the patterns of cognitive function but also in quantifying the heterogeneity among people with ASD.

The Research Domain Criteria (RDoC) framework of psychiatric research (Cuthbert & Insel, 2013) proposes to re-conceptualize psychiatric conditions within multidimensional space defined by constructs such as reward responsiveness, cognitive control, and working memory. Each construct expresses itself as a behavioral phenotype and is derived from genetic and neural morphology or function. Thus, under the RDoC framework, researchers search for the aetiology of psychiatric disorders, not at the level of the currently accepted nosology, but empirically defined cognitive and perceptual functions that can be quantified by rigorous scientific procedures.

Information obtained from the intelligence scale can be useful in refining the dimensional constructs advocated by the RDoC framework. As stated above, many assessment tools have been designed to quantify the multiple dimensions of intellectual ability. Moreover, the intelligence scale was not tailored to any specific population. Instead, widely used instruments are designed such that they are applicable to as wide a population as possible across sex and medical history (Doi et al., 2022; Sumiyoshi et al., 2022). This feature is useful for directly comparing the behavioral phenotypes of psychiatric conditions within an identical dimensional space.

Behavioral assessments of cognitive and perceptual functions are not sufficient to gain an in-depth understanding of intellectual functions in people with ASD. This is partly because knowledge about intellectual ability in TD individuals or those with other conditions cannot be extrapolated simply to ASD. Let's assume that patients with conditions A and B shared similar symptoms. In such cases, it is often concluded that the symptoms are derived from identical biological causes. However, this assumption should be subjected to empirical testing, as it is equally possible that the symptoms are derived from distinct biological causes in conditions A and B (Flagel et al., 2016). In the latter case, the surface similarity in symptoms at the behavioral level is incidental and cannot be substantiated at the biological level. Moreover, even when TD individuals and people with ASD are matched for intellectual ability, the biological mechanisms underlying intellectual function may differ between these two groups.

Thus, investigating the neurophysiological basis of each dimension of intelligence provides valuable information for characterizing cognitive function in people with ASD and understanding the biological basis of this condition. This chapter aims to provide a qualitative review of the existing findings on the neurophysiological correlates of intellectual function in people with ASD.

Neurophysiological Correlates of Intelligence in TD People

Numerous studies have investigated the association between intelligence and brain function and morphology. Electroencephalography (EEG) has been a useful tool for noninvasive brain function measurements for over a century. Its application has led to several seminal discoveries related to human neurophysiological functions. EEG oscillations are considered to be generated by cortical cell populations. After preprocessing, continuous EEG data were decomposed into frequency components. The amplitude and phase of each frequency component were calculated in the frequency domain (Zhang et al., 2023). The amplitude or power of each frequency component and its association with intelligence has been intensively studied in the TD population. These studies revealed correlation between EEG spectral power and intelligence level (Lui et al., 2008; Marosi et al., 1999; Schmid et al., 2002).

Reflecting the multidimensionality of intelligence, the activation pattern of the global neural network, rather than the local neural region, is considered the basis of intellectual ability. In multichannel EEG measurements, time-series EEG data are recorded from distributed scalp regions. Based on multi-channel EEG data, the coherence of the EEG time series across paired electrode sites is estimated as a measure of the network structure. There are multiple methodologies to compute the coherence between EEG time series; many studies have used the cross-correlation coefficient and phase-lag coherence at each frequency band (Zhang et al., 2023).

Multiple indices of activation patterns in local neural regions and global neural networks can be extracted from the EEG data. To address the high dimensionality of EEG data, several studies (Thatcher et al., 2005, 2016) have used multivariate analyses to identify EEG indices that are predictive of intelligence in the TD population. One illustrative study (Thatcher et al., 2005) constructed a linear discriminant classifier to distinguish high-intelligence TD individuals from those with low intelligence. Importantly, the features included measures of both the activation of the local cortical region and global activation of the neural network; the former included the power of the frequency component at each frequency band (delta, theta, alpha, and gamma), and the latter included cross-channel coherence and phase lag indices between pairwise channels. The linear discriminant classifier showed acceptable performance in the prediction of intelligence. The researchers obtained two key findings by analyzing the resultant classifier. First, band power and coherence were positively correlated with intelligence in all the frequency ranges tested. Second, there was a difference in the pattern of relationship between absolute phase lag and intelligence. In the anterior scalp regions surrounding the frontal cortex, phase lag in the delta and beta frequency bands negatively correlated with intelligence, whereas the sign of the correlation was reversed in the posterior regions.

Using EEG, researchers can measure neural activation data with a high temporal resolution on the order of milliseconds. However, the spatial resolution of the EEG data is severely degraded because of volume conduction (Luck, 2014). The electrical activity generated in the neuron population in one focal region spreads widely on the scalp surface, making it difficult for researchers to infer the spatial location of the focal electrical activity generator. Magnetic resonance imaging (MRI) complements this caveat of EEG by providing high-resolution images of neural activation and brain structures on the order of millimeters. The high spatial resolution of MRI enables researchers to quantify the morphological indices of brain structures such as gray matter volume or density, cortical thickness, and white matter microstructure. One line of research links morphological features to intelligence. For example, many studies have found correlations between gray matter volume in the frontal and parietal cortices and intelligence (Flashman et al., 1997; Narr et al., 2007; Rushton & Ankney, 2009). Another line of research has investigated the association between the activation patterns of neural networks and intelligence (Dubois et al., 2018). Since the discovery of resting activation (Raichle et al., 2001), large amounts of data have accumulated regarding the activation of the default mode network (DMN). Through human connectome projects, large amounts of resting-state functional MRI (fMRI) data were made public, together with behavioral indices, which gave researchers the opportunity to observe the association between functional connectivity among neural regions and intelligence. One study (de Souza et al., 2023) directly compared the utilities of morphometric features and network activation as intelligence predictors.

This study first decomposed neural network activation into independent components (ICs) and constructed regressors with regularization terms that predicted general IQ. The predictors included ICs reflective of functional connectivity and the morphometric features of cortical thickness and surface area. The results revealed a larger contribution of functional connectivity to intelligent prediction. Detailed observations revealed that the ICs related to functional connectivity in the DMS, salience network, and ventral-stream network were particularly informative.

Neurophysiological Correlates of Intelligence in People with ASD

The association between neural activation patterns and intelligence in patients with ASD is understudied. Children with ASD often present with co-morbidity epilepsy. The excitatory-inhibition (E-I) theory of ASD (Rubenstein & Merzenich, 2003) claims that one cause of ASD is an imbalance of cortical excitation and inhibition, which in turn is attributable to the dysregulation of GABAergic and glutaminergic neuromodulation. From the perspective of the E-I theory, the frequent co-morbidity of epilepsy in ASD can be explained by the excessive excitation of widespread cortical regions. Co-morbidity of epilepsy is reported to be more prevalent in people with ASD who have severer cognitive disabilities than high-functioning ones (Zarakoviti et al., 2023). Thus, there may be a link between intellectual ability and an imbalance in cortical excitability. This possibility was explored in a multisite EEG study (Orekhova et al., 2007) that revealed a positive correlation in boys with ASD between developmental delay measured by intelligence assessment tools and the spectral power of gamma frequency at the mid-posterior electrode sites. A later study (Orekhova et al., 2008) measured an event-related potential component of P50 to quantify the efficiency of sensory gating—the ability to suppress sensory stimuli—in the auditory cortex of children with ASD, with and without intellectual disability. Children with ASD and normal intellectual ability showed comparable levels of sensory gating to TD children. However, sensory gating was less efficient in children with ASD with intellectual disability than in the other two groups, that is children with ASD without intellectual disability and TD children. Furthermore, there is a negative correlation between the efficiency of sensory gating and EEG gamma power in children with ASD. Together, these findings from EEG studies support the view that intellectual disability in children with ASD is linked to excessive excitability, or dysregulation of excitability, in cortical regions.

Magnetic encephalography (MEG) quantifies neural activation by measuring the phasic fluctuations in the magnetic field induced by electrical activation generated in the brain. In the power spectrum of the MEG/EEG data, the power of the high-frequency aperiodic activity shows decreased power compared to relatively low-frequency range, which relationship can be captured by scale-free 1/f characteristics in spectral power (Lendner et al., 2020). The aperiodic activity is not necessarily relevant to ongoing cognitive and perceptual operations. Hence, individuals with dysregulated cortical excitation show a flatter 1/f slope of spectral power within high-frequency range. Researchers (Manyukhina et al., 2022) collected MEG data from children with ASD, with and without intellectual disabilities, and computed 1/f slope in the high-frequency range in the source space. The main finding was a flatter 1/f slope in children with ASD with intellectual disability than those without intellectual disability, linking excessive cortical activation to intellectual disability in children with ASD.

Limited fMRI studies are available on the neural correlates of intelligence in people with ASD. Several recent studies have adopted a network approach and compared the functional connectivity predictive of IQ between people with ASD and TD patients. One study (Pua et al., 2018) found increased functional connectivity in neural networks related to fluid intelligence in patients with ASD compared with TD controls matched for fluid intelligence. Importantly, this tendency was more prominent in younger individuals with ASD than in older people, indicating a developmental change in the neural basis of intellectual ability. Another study (Dryburgh et al., 2020) that recruited an adolescent population reported that the summary value of functional connectivity showed a stronger correlation with full and verbal IQ in TD individuals than in people with ASD. These findings indicate that distinct neural networks contribute to intelligence in TD individuals and people with ASD.

Early Neurophysiological Function and Later Intellectual Development in Children with ASD

In recent years, an increasing number of studies have indicated that the risk of ASD can be predicted using behavioral and neuropsychological measures collected during infancy (Bosl et al., 2018; Tanner & Dounavi, 2021). These studies show that children with ASD show atypical patterns of behavior and neural responses well before the formal diagnosis of ASD during toddlerhood. For example, a seminal study by Elsabbagh et al. (2012) reported atypical ERP responses to eye stimuli in children with familial risk of ASD who were later diagnosed with ASD 6–10-months after birth. Thus, the search for the early signs of ASD is an active area of investigation.

Regarding early predictors of the later development of intellectual ability, one recent study (Jones et al., 2020) measured the percent change in frontal theta power, a potential indicator of information learning or encoding, while 12-month-old were viewing naturalistic videos. The sample included infants with familial risk of ASD. The researchers tracked the cognitive development of children longitudinally and investigated whether frontal theta power changes predict cognitive ability at later developmental stages. They reported a positive correlation between the percent change in frontal theta power at 12 months and verbal skills at 36 months. Interestingly, this relationship was the strongest in at-risk infants who were later diagnosed with ASD. The number of children with ASD in this study was relatively small;

however, considering that this line of research is still at a nascent stage, this observation warrants further investigation into the early indicators of later intellectual development in children with ASD.

Conclusion and Future Directions

There is a wealth of studies on the neural correlates of intelligence in TD people at various developmental stages. However, the number of empirical studies on the neural basis of intellectual ability in patients with ASD is relatively small. Previous EEG/MEG studies have suggested that intellectual disability in children with ASD is attributable to the dysregulation of excitatory-inhibitory modulation of cortical activation (Manyukhina et al., 2022; Orekhova et al., 2007, 2008). Analysis of functional connectivity raised the possibility that differential patterns of functional networks contribute to intellectual ability in people with and without ASD (Dryburgh et al., 2020; Pua et al., 2018). However, the detailed results of MRI studies are not necessarily convergent, and interpretations vary widely in the literature. Promising results have been reported regarding the early signs of intellectual ability (Jones et al., 2020), but the number of relevant studies is disproportionally small.

Overall, given the dearth of empirical studies on the relevant topics, little can be said about the neurophysiological basis of intellectual ability in people with ASD. Therefore, attention should be paid to the following points in future investigations: First, the multidimensional nature of intelligence is rarely considered in analyses of the association between brain function and morphology and intellectual ability in ASD. For example, four cognitive indices—verbal comprehension, perceptual organization, working speed, and processing speed—can be obtained using the WAIS (Wechsler, 1991, 1997). However, few studies on people with ASD investigated the neural basis of each type of cognitive index. Second, most studies have compared the neural correlates of intellectual ability only between people with ASD and TD individuals, and transdiagnostic comparisons are lacking. Thus, it is not clear at this point whether the existing findings are specific to ASD or whether similar observations can be made for other neurodevelopmental conditions, such as ADHD. Third, most studies have measured neural activation in the resting state. However, a recent study (Sripada et al., 2020) recruiting TD adults indicated that the association between intelligence and neural activation becomes clearer when a cognitive load is imposed on them. Thus, the association between intelligence and neural function should be tested under diverse conditions or environments in people with ASD. From this perspective, the neural activation during sleep is of particular interest. Several studies have reported a correlation between sleep stage-specific EEG patterns and IQ in TD children and adults (Fogel & Smith, 2011). According to one study (Tessier et al., 2015), the density of sleep spindles during sleep stage 2 was negatively correlated with verbal IQ in TD children and those with ASD. However, this correlation was observed in the frontal electrode in TD individuals and in the central electrode sites in people with ASD, providing further support for the view that intellectual ability is linked to different neural regions between TD individuals and people with ASD.

Research on the neural underpinnings of intelligence in people with ASD is a burgeoning field. Investigating the neurophysiological basis of intellectual ability can contribute to the elucidation of the cause of endophenotypes in ASD and is also important from the standpoint of clinical practice because this knowledge is valuable in planning interventions and support strategies for people with ASD with varying levels of intellectual abilities. However, considerable efforts are required to establish a reliable and comprehensive understanding.

References

Amaral, D. G., Schumann, C. M., & Nordahl, C. W. (2008). Neuroanatomy of autism. *Trends in Neurosciences, 31*(3), 137–145.

Ankenman, K., Elgin, J., Sullivan, K., Vincent, L., & Bernier, R. (2014). Nonverbal and verbal cognitive discrepancy profiles in autism spectrum disorders: Influence of age and gender. *American Journal on Intellectual and Developmental Disabilities, 119*(1), 84–99. https://doi.org/10.1352/1944-7558-119.1.84

Anney, R., Klei, L., Pinto, D., Almeida, J., Bacchelli, E., Baird, G., & Devlin, B. (2012). Individual common variants exert weak effects on the risk for autism spectrum disorders. *Human Molecular Genetics, 21*(21), 4781–4792.

Baranek, G. T. (2002). Efficacy of sensory and motor interventions for children with autism. *Journal of Autism and Developmental Disorders, 32*(5), 397–422.

Bhat, A. N. (2020). Is motor impairment in autism spectrum disorder distinct from developmental coordination disorder? A report from the SPARK study. *Physical Therapy, 100*(4) 633–644.

Ben-David, E., & Shifman, S. (2012). Networks of neuronal genes affected by common and rare variants in autism spectrum disorders. *PLoS Genetics, 8*(3), e1002556.

Berkel, S., Marshall, C. R., Weiss, B., Howe, J., Roeth, R., Moog, U., & Rappold, G. A. (2010). Mutations in the SHANK2 synaptic scaffolding gene in autism spectrum disorder and mental retardation. *Nature Genetics, 42*(6), 489–491.

Betancur, C., Sakurai, T., & Buxbaum, J. D. (2009). The emerging role of synaptic cell-adhesion pathways in the pathogenesis of autism spectrum disorders. *Trends in Neurosciences, 32*(7), 402–412.

Billeiter, K. B., & Froiland, J. M. (2023). Diversity of intelligence is the norm within the autism spectrum: Full scale intelligence scores among children with ASD. *Child Psychiatry & Human Development, 54*(4), 1094–1101.

Bodison, S. C. (2015). Developmental dyspraxia and the play skills of children with autism. *The American Journal of Occupational Therapy, 69*(5), 6905185060. https://doi.org/10.5014/ajot.2015.017954

Bohm, B., Ritzen, E. M., & Lindgren, A. C. (2015). Growth hormone treatment improves vitality and behavioural issues in children with Prader-Willi syndrome. *Acta Paediatrica, 104*(1), 59–67.

Bosl, W. J., Tager-Flusberg, H., & Nelson, C. A. (2018). EEG Analytics for early detection of autism spectrum disorder: A data-driven approach. *Scientific Reports, 8*, 6828.

Bruni, O., Alonso-Alconada, D., Besag, F., Biran, V., Braam, W., Cortese, S., & Moavero, R. (2015). Current role of melatonin in pediatric neurology: Clinical recommendations. *European Journal of Paediatric Neurology, 19*(2), 122–133.

Cass, H., Sekara, D., & Baird, G. (2006). Medical investigation of children with autistic spectrum disorders. *Child: Care, Health and Development, 32*(5), 521–533.

Cattell, R. B. (1963). Theory of fluid and crystallized intelligence: A critical experiment. *Journal of Educational Psychology., 54*, 1–22.
Cohen, S., Conduit, R., Lockley, S. W., Rajaratnam, S. M., & Cornish, K. M. (2014). The relationship between sleep and behavior in autism spectrum disorder (ASD): A review. *Journal of Neurodevelopmental Disorders, 6*(1), 44.
Cuthbert, B. N., & Insel, T. R. (2013). Toward the future of psychiatric diagnosis: The seven pillars of RDoC. *BMC Medicine, 11*, 126.
Dawson, M., Soulières, I., Gernsbacher, M. A., & Mottron, L. (2007). The level and nature of autistic intelligence. *Psychol Science, 18*(8), 657–662.
Descheemaeker, M. J., Govers, V., Vermeulen, P., & Fryns, J. P. (2006). Pervasive developmental disorders in Prader-Willi syndrome: The Leuven experience in 59 subjects and controls. *American Journal of Medical Genetics, 140*(11), 1136–1142.
de Souza, E. A., Silva, S. A., Vieira, B. H., & Garrido Salmon, C. E. (2023). fMRI functional connectivity is a better predictor of general intelligence than cortical morphometric features and ICA parcellation order affects predictive performance. *Intelligence, 97*, 101727.
Dimitropoulos, A., Ho, A., & Feldman, B. (2013). Social responsiveness and competence in Prader-Willi syndrome: Direct comparison to autism spectrum disorder. *Journal of Autism and Developmental Disorders, 43*(1), 103–113.
Doi, H., Kanai, C., & Ohta, H. (2022). Transdiagnostic and sex differences in cognitive profiles of autism spectrum disorder and attention-deficit/hyperactivity disorder. *Autism Research, 15*(6), 1130–1141.
Dowell, L. R., Mahone, E. M., & Mostofsky, S. H. (2009). Associations of postural knowledge and basic motor skill with dyspraxia in autism: Implication for abnormalities in distributed connectivity and motor learning. *Neuropsychology, 23*(5), 563–570.
Dryburgh, E., McKenna, S., & Rekik, I. (2020). Predicting full-scale and verbal intelligence scores from functional connectomic data in individuals with autism spectrum disorder. *Brain Imaging and Behavior, 14*(5), 1769–1778.
Dubois, J., Galdi, P., Paul, L. K., & Adolphs, R. (2018). A distributed brain network predicts general intelligence from resting-state human neuroimaging data. *Philosophical Transactions of the Royal Society, B: Biological Sciences, 373*(1756), 20170284.
Dunn, W. (2007). Supporting children to participate successfully in everyday life by using sensory processing knowledge. *Infant and Young Children, 20*(2), 84–101.
Durand, C. M., Perroy, J., Loll, F., Perrais, D., Fagni, L., Bourgeron, T., & Sans, N. (2012). SHANK3 mutations identified in autism lead to modification of dendritic spine morphology via an actin-dependent mechanism. *Molecular Psychiatry, 17*(1), 71–84.
Dziuk, M. A., Gidley Larson, J. C., Apostu, A., Mahone, E. M., Denckla, M. B., & Mostofsky, S. H. (2007). Dyspraxia in autism: Association with motor, social, and communicative deficits. *Developmental Medicine and Child Neurology, 49*(10), 734–739.
Ebert, D. H., & Greenberg, M. E. (2013). Activity-dependent neuronal signaling and an autism spectrum disorder. *Nature, 493*(7432), 327–337.
Edirisooriya, M., Dykiert, D., & Auyeung, B. (2021). IQ and internalising symptoms in adolescents with ASD. *Journal of Autism and Developmental Disorders, 51*(11), 3887–3907. https://doi.org/10.1007/s10803-020-04810-y
Elsabbagh, M., Mercure, E., Hudry, K., Chandler, S., Pasco, G., Charman, T., Pickles, A., Baron-Cohen, S., Bolton, P., Johnson, M. H., & BASIS Team. (2012). Infant neural sensitivity to dynamic eye gaze is associated with later emerging autism. *Current Biology: CB, 22*(4), 338–342.
Feczko, E., Balba, N. M., Miranda-Dominguez, O., Cordova, M., Karalunas, S. L., Irwin, L., Demeter, D. V., Hill, A. P., Langhorst, B. H., Grieser Painter, J., Van Santen, J., Fombonne, E. J., Nigg, J. T., & Fair, D. A. (2018). Subtyping cognitive profiles in Autism Spectrum Disorder using a Functional Random Forest algorithm. *NeuroImage, 172*, 674–688. https://doi.org/10.1016/j.neuroimage.2017.12.044
Flagel, S. B., Pine, D. S., Ahmari, S. E., First, M. B., Friston, K. J., Mathys, C., Redish, A. D., Schmack, K., Smoller, J. W., & Thapar, A. (2016). A novel framework for improving psychiatric

diagnostic nosology. In A. Redish & J. A. Gordon (Eds.), *Computational psychiatry: New perspectives on mental illness* (pp. 169–199). MIT Press.

Flashman, L. A., Andreasen, N. C., Flaum, M., & Swayze, V. W. (1997). Intelligence and regional brain volumes in normal controls. *Intelligence, 25*(3), 149–160.

Fogel, S. M., & Smith, C. T. (2011). The function of the sleep spindle: A physiological index of intelligence and a mechanism for sleep-dependent memory consolidation. *Neuroscience and Biobehavioral Reviews, 35*, 1154–1165.

Fournier, K. A., Hass, C. J., Naik, S. K., Lodha, N., & Cauraugh, J. H. (2010). Motor coordination in autism spectrum disorders: A synthesis and meta-analysis. *Journal of Autism and Developmental Disorders, 40*(10), 1227–1240.

Frith, U. (1993). Autism. *Scientific American, 268*(6), 108–114.

Gernsbacher, M. A., Sauer, E. A., Geye, H. M., Schweigert, E. K., & Hill Goldsmith, H. (2008). Infant and toddler oral- and manual-motor skills predict later speech fluency in autism. *Journal of Child Psychology and Psychiatry, 49*(1), 43–50.

Ghaziuddin, M., & Mountain-Kimchi, K. (2004). Defining the intellectual profile of Asperger Syndrome: Comparison with high-functioning autism. *Journal of Autism and Developmental Disorders, 34*(3), 279–284. https://doi.org/10.1023/b:jadd.0000029550.19098.77

Gilman, S. R., Iossifov, I., Levy, D., Ronemus, M., Wigler, M., & Vitkup, D. (2011). Rare de novo variants associated with autism implicate an extensive functional network of genes involved in the formation and function of synapses. *Neuron, 70*(5), 898–907.

Goldman, S., Wang, C., Salgado, M. W., Greene, P. E., Kim, M., & Rapin, I. (2009). Motor stereotypies in children with autism and other developmental disorders. *Developmental Medicine and Child Neurology, 51*(1), 30–38.

Gotham, K., Pickles, A., & Lord, C. (2012). Trajectories of autism severity in children using standardized ADOS scores. *Pediatrics, 130*(5), e1278-1284.

Gowen, E., & Hamilton, A. (2013). Motor abilities in autism: A review using a computational context. *Journal of Autism and Developmental Disorders, 43*(2), 323–344.

Grabrucker, A. M. (2012). Environmental factors in autism. *Front Psychiatry, 3*, 118.

Grandgeorge, M., Hausberger, M., Tordjman, S., Deleau, M., Lazartigues, A., & Lemonnier, E. (2009). Environmental factors influence language development in children with autism spectrum disorders. *PLoS ONE, 4*(4), e4683.

Gray, L., Ansell, P., Baird, G., & Parr, J. R. (2011). The continuing challenge of diagnosing autism spectrum disorder in children with Down syndrome. *Child: Care, Health and Development, 37*(4), 459–461.

Greenspan, S. I., & Weider, S. (2008). The interdisciplinary council on developmental and learning disorders diagnostic manual for infants and young children—An overview. *Journal of the Canadian Academy of Child and Adolescent Psychiatry, 17*(2), 76–89.

Grossmann, T., & Johnson, M. H. (2007). The development of the social brain in human infancy. *European Journal of Neuroscience, 25*(4), 909–919.

Hallmayer, J., Cleveland, S., Torres, A., Phillips, J., Cohen, B., Torigoe, T., & Risch, N. (2011). Genetic heritability and shared environmental factors among twin pairs with autism. *Archives of General Psychiatry, 68*(11), 1095–1102.

Hannant, P., Tavassoli, T., & Cassidy, S. (2016). The role of sensorimotor difficulties in autism spectrum conditions. *Frontiers in Neurology, 7*(124), 1–11. https://doi.org/10.3389/fneur.2016.00124

Happe, F. G. (1994). Wechsler IQ profile and theory of mind in autism: A research note. *Journal of Child Psychology and Psychiatry, 35*(8), 1461–1471.

Hartup, W. W. (1986). Relationships and their significance in cognitive development. In R. A. Hinde, A. Perret-Clermont, & J. Stevenson-Hinde (Eds.), *Social relationships and cognitive development* (pp. 66–82). Oxford University Press.

Hedvall, Å., Fernell, E., Holm, A., Åsberg Johnels, J., Gillberg, C., & Billstedt, E. (2013). Autism, processing speed, and adaptive functioning in preschool children. *The Scientific World Journal, 2013*, 158263. https://doi.org/10.1155/2013/158263

Henninger, N. A., & Taylor, J. L. (2013). Outcomes in adults with autism spectrum disorders: A historical perspective. *Autism, 17*(1), 103–116.

Ho, V. M., Lee, J. A., & Martin, K. C. (2011). The cell biology of synaptic plasticity. *Science, 334*(6056), 623–628.

Hollway, J. A., & Aman, M. G. (2011). Sleep correlates of pervasive developmental disorders: A review of the literature. *Research in Developmental Disabilities, 32*(5), 1399–1421.

Howlin, P., Goode, S., Hutton, J., & Rutter, M. (2004). Adult outcome for children with autism. *Journal of Child Psychology and Psychiatry, 45*(2), 212–229.

Howlin, P., Wing, L., & Gould, J. (1995). The recognition of autism in children with Down syndrome—Implications for intervention and some speculations about pathology. *Developmental Medicine and Child Neurology, 37*(5), 406–414.

Hutsler, J. J., & Zhang, H. (2010). Increased dendritic spine densities on cortical projection neurons in autism spectrum disorders. *Brain Research, 1309*, 83–94.

Javaloyes, M. A. (2006). The need for reviewing international diagnostic categories in pervasive developmental disorders. *Autism, 10*(5), 525.

Johnson, C. N., Ramphal, B., Koe, E., Raudales, A., Goldsmith, J., & Margolis, A. E. (2021). Cognitive correlates of autism spectrum disorder symptoms. *Autism Research, 14*(11), 2405–2411. https://doi.org/10.1002/aur.2577

Jones, E. J. H., Goodwin, A., Orekhova, E., et al. (2020). Infant EEG theta modulation predicts childhood intelligence. *Scientific Reports, 10*, 11232.

Joseph, R. M., Tager-Flusberg, H., & Lord, C. (2002). Cognitive profiles and social-communicative functioning in children with autism spectrum disorder. *Journal of Child Psychology and Psychiatry, 43*(6), 807–821. https://doi.org/10.1111/1469-7610.00092

Kadlaskar, G., Mao, P. H., Iosif, A. M., Amaral, D., Wu Nordahl, C., & Miller, M. (2023). Patterns of sensory processing in young children with autism: Differences in autism characteristics, adaptive skills, and attentional problems. *Autism, 27*(3), 723–736.

Kanai, C., Hashimoto, R., Itahashi, T., Tani, M., Yamada, T., Ota, H., Iwanami, A., & Kato, N. (2017). Cognitive profiles of adults with high-functioning autism spectrum disorder and those with attention-deficit/hyperactivity disorder based on the WAIS-III. *Research in Developmental Disabilities, 61*, 108–115. https://doi.org/10.1016/j.ridd.2016.12.008

Kanai, C., Tani, M., Hashimoto, R., Yamada, T., Ota, H., Watanabe, H., Iwanami, A., & Kato, N. (2012). Cognitive profiles of adults with Asperger's disorder, high-functioning autism, and pervasive developmental disorder not otherwise specified based on the WAIS-III. *Research in Autism Spectrum Disorders, 6*(1), 58–64. https://doi.org/10.1016/j.rasd.2011.09.004

Karmiloff-Smith, A., Scerif, G., & Thomas, M. (2002). Different approaches to relating genotype to phenotype in developmental disorders. *Developmental Psychobiology, 40*(3), 311–322.

Kaufman, A. S., & Kaufman N. L. (2013). *Kaufman assessment battery for children* (2nd ed.). NCS Pearson, Inc.

Kent, L., Evans, J., Paul, M., & Sharp, M. (1999). Comorbidity of autistic spectrum disorders in children with Down syndrome. *Developmental Medicine and Child Neurology, 41*(3), 153–158.

Klin, A., Shultz, S., & Jones, W. (2014). Social visual engagement in infants and toddlers with autism: Early developmental transitions and a model of pathogenesis. *Neuroscience & Biobehavioral Reviews, 50*, 189–203.

Klin, A., Volkmar, F. R., Sparrow, S. S., Cicchetti, D. V., & Rourke, B. P. (1995). Validity and neuropsychological characterization of Asperger syndrome: Convergence with nonverbal learning disabilities syndrome. *Journal of Child Psychology and Psychiatry, 36*(7), 1127–1140. https://doi.org/10.1111/j.1469-7610.1995.tb01361

Kosaka, H., Omori, M., Munesue, T., Ishitobi, M., Matsumura, Y., Takahashi, T., Narita, K., Murata, T., Saito, D. N., Uchiyama, H., Morita, T., Kikuchi, M., Mizukami, K., Okazawa, H., Sadato, N., & Wada, Y. (2010). Smaller insula and inferior frontal volumes in young adults with pervasive developmental disorders. *Neuroimage, 50*(4), 1357–1363. https://doi.org/10.1016/j.neuroimage.2010.01.085

Kou, Y., Betancur, C., Xu, H., Buxbaum, J. D., & Ma'ayan, A. (2012). Network- and attribute-based classifiers can prioritize genes and pathways for autism spectrum disorders and intellectual disability. *American Journal of Medical Genetics Part C: Seminars in Medical Genetics, 160C*(2), 130–142.

Kraijer, D. (2000). Review of adaptive behavior studies in mentally retarded persons with autism/pervasive developmental disorder. *Journal of Autism and Developmental Disorders, 30*(1), 39–47.

Kuhl, P. K. (2007). Is speech learning 'gated' by the social brain? *Developmental Science, 10*(1), 110–120.

Lai, M. C., Lombardo, M. V., & Baron-Cohen, S. (2014). Autism. *Lancet, 383*(9920), 896–910. https://doi.org/10.1016/s0140-6736(13)61539-1

Landry, S. H., Smith, K. E., Swank, P. R., Assel, M. A., & Vellet, S. (2001). Does early responsive parenting have a special importance for children's development, or is consistency across early childhood necessary? *Developmental Psychology, 37*(3), 387–403.

Lendner, J. D., Helfrich, R. F., Mander, B. A., Romundstad, L., Lin, J. J., Walker, M. P., Larsson, P. G., & Knight, R. T. (2020). An electrophysiological marker of arousal level in humans. *eLife, 9*, e55092

Lincoln, A. J., Courchesne, E., Kilman, B. A., Elmasian, R., & Allen, M. (1988). A study of intellectual abilities in high-functioning people with autism. *Journal of Autism and Developmental Disorders, 18*(4), 505–524. https://doi.org/10.1007/bf02211870

Liu, L., Sabo, A., Neale, B. M., Nagaswamy, U., Stevens, C., Lim, E., & Roeder, K. (2013). Analysis of rare, exonic variation amongst subjects with autism spectrum disorders and population controls. *PLoS Genetics, 9*(4), e1003443.

Lloyd, M., MacDonald, M., & Lord, C. (2013). Motor skills of toddlers with autism spectrum disorders. *Autism, 17*(2), 133–146.

Lo, S. T., Siemensma, E., Collin, P., & Hokken-Koelega, A. (2013). Impaired theory of mind and symptoms of Autism Spectrum Disorder in children with Prader-Willi syndrome. *Research in Developmental Disabilities, 34*(9), 2764–2773.

Lorenc, T., Rodgers, M., Marshall, D., Melton, H., Rees, R., Wright, K., & Sowden, A. (2018). Support for adults with autism spectrum disorder without intellectual impairment: Systematic review. *Autism, 22*(6), 654–668.

Luck, S. J. (2014). *An introduction to the event-related potential technique* (2nd ed.). MIT Press.

Lui, T., Shi, J., Zhao, D., & Yang, J. (2008). The relationship between EEG Band power, cognitive processing and intelligence in school aged children. *Psychology Science Quarterly, 50*, 259–268.

Makinodan, M., Rosen, K. M., Ito, S., & Corfas, G. (2012). A critical period for social experience-dependent oligodendrocyte maturation and myelination. *Science, 337*(6100), 1357–1360.

Mandelbaum, D. E., Stevens, M., Rosenberg, E., Wiznitzer, M., Steinschneider, M., Filipek, P., & Rapin, I. (2006). Sensorimotor performance in school-age children with autism, developmental language disorder, or low IQ. *Developmental Medicine and Child Neurology, 48*, 33–39.

Manjiviona, J., & Prior, M. (1995). Comparison of asperger syndrome and high-functioning autistic children on a test of motor impairment. *Journal of Autism and Developmental Disorders, 25*(1), 23–39. https://doi.org/10.1007/bf02178165

Manjiviona, J., & Prior, M. (1999). Neuropsychological profiles of children with Asperger syndrome and autism. *Autism, 3*, 327–356.

Manyukhina, V. O., Prokofyev, A. O., Galuta, I. A., Goiaeva, D. E., Obukhova, T. S., Schneiderman, J. F., Altukhov, D. I., Stroganova, T. A., & Orekhova, E. V. (2022). Globally elevated excitation-inhibition ratio in children with autism spectrum disorder and below-average intelligence. *Molcular Autism, 13*(1), 20. https://doi.org/10.1186/s13229-022-00498-2. PMID: 35550191; PMCID: PMC9102291.

Marosi, E., Rodríguez, H., Harmony, T., Yañez, G., Rodrìguez, M., Bernal, J., Fernàndez, T., Silva, J., Reyes, A., & Guerrero, V. (1999). Broad band spectral EEG parameters correlated with different IQ measurements. *International Journal of Neuroscience, 97*(1–2), 17–27.

Maski, K. P., Jeste, S. S., & Spence, S. J. (2011). Common neurological co-morbidities in autism spectrum disorders. *Current Opinion in Pediatrics, 23*(6), 609–615.
Masi, A., DeMayo, M. M., Glozier, N., & Guastella, A. J. (2017). An overview of autism spectrum disorder, heterogeneity and treatment options. *Neuroscience Bulletin, 33*(2), 183–193.
Matson, J. L., Dempsey, T., LoVullo, S. V., Fodstad, J. C., Knight, C., Sevin, J. A., & Sharp, B. (2013). The moderating effects of intellectual development on core symptoms of autism and PDD-NOS in toddlers and infants. *Research in Developmental Disabilities, 34*(1), 573–578.
Matson, J. L., Kozlowski, A. M., Worley, J. A., Shoemaker, M. E., Sipes, M., & Horovitz, M. (2011). What is the evidence for environmental causes of challenging behaviors in persons with intellectual disabilities and autism spectrum disorders? *Research in Developmental Disabilities, 32*(2), 693–698.
Matson, J. L., & Williams, L. W. (2014). The making of a field: The development of comorbid psychopathology research for persons with intellectual disabilities and autism. *Research in Developmental Disabilities, 35*(1), 234–238.
Mefford, H. C., Batshaw, M. L., & Hoffman, E. P. (2012). Genomics, intellectual disability, and autism. *The New England Journal of Medicine, 366*(8), 733–743.
Miller, L. J., Anzalone, M. E., Lane, S. J., Cermak, S. A., & Osten, E. T. (2007). Concept evolution in sensory integration: A proposed nosology for diagnosis. *American Journal of Occupational Therapy, 61*(2), 135–140.
Miller, H. L., Sherrod, G. M., Mauk, J. E., Fears, N. E., Hynan, L. S., & Tamplain, P. M. (2021). Shared features or co-occurrence? Evaluating symptoms of developmental coordination disorder in children and adolescents with autism spectrum disorder. *Journal of Autism and Developmental Disorders, 51*(10), 3443–3455.
Missler, M., Sudhof, T. C., & Biederer, T. (2012). Synaptic cell adhesion. *Cold Spring Harbor Perspectives in Biology, 4*(4), a005694.
Mouga, S., Café, C., Almeida, J., Marques, C., Duque, F., & Oliveira, G. (2016). Intellectual profiles in the autism spectrum and other neurodevelopmental disorders. *Journal of Autism and Developmental Disorders, 46*(9), 2940–2955. https://doi.org/10.1007/s10803-016-2838-x
Nader, A. M., Jelenic, P., & Soulières, I. (2015). Discrepancy between WISC-III and WISC-IV cognitive profile in autism spectrum: What does it reveal about autistic cognition? *PLoS ONE, 10*(12), e0144645.
Narr, K. L., Woods, R. P., Thompson, P. M., Szeszko, P., Robinson, D., Dimtcheva, T., Gurbani, M., Toga, A. W., & Bilder, R. M. (2007). Relationships between IQ and regional cortical gray matter thickness in healthy adults. *Cerebral Cortex, 17*(9), 2163–2171.
National Academies of Sciences, Engineering, and Medicine. (2015). Child development and early learning. In *Transforming the workforce for children birth through age 8: A unifying foundation* (Chapter 4, pp. 85–86). The National Academies Press.
Noterdaeme, M., Wriedt, E., & Höhne, C. (2010). Asperger's syndrome and high-functioning autism: Language, motor and cognitive profiles. *European Child & Adolescent Psychiatry, 19*(6), 475–481. https://doi.org/10.1007/s00787-009-0057-0
Nowell, K. P., Schanding, G. T., Jr., Kanne, S. M., & Goin-Kochel, R. P. (2015). Cognitive profiles in youth with autism spectrum disorder: An investigation of base rate discrepancies using the differential ability scales-second edition. *Journal of Autism and Developmental Disorders, 45*(7), 1978–1988. https://doi.org/10.1007/s10803-014-2356-7
Orekhova, E. V., Stroganova, T. A., Nygren, G., Tsetlin, M. M., Posikera, I. N., Gillberg, C., & Elam, M. (2007). Excess of high frequency electroencephalogram oscillations in boys with autism. *Biological Psychiatry, 62*(9), 1022–1029.
Orekhova, E. V., Stroganova, T. A., Prokofyev, A. O., Nygren, G., Gillberg, C., & Elam, M. (2008). Sensory gating in young children with autism: Relation to age, IQ, and EEG gamma oscillations. *Neuroscience Letters, 434*(2), 218–223.
Ozonoff, S., South, M., & Miller, J. (2000). DSM-IV defined Asperger disorder: Cognitive, behavioral, and early history differentiation from high-functioning autism. *Autism, 4*, 29–46.

Patil, O., & Kaple, M. (2023). Sensory processing differences in individuals with autism spectrum disorder: A narrative review of underlying mechanisms and sensory-based interventions. *Cureus, 15*(10), e48020. https://doi.org/10.7759/cureus.48020

Pua, E. P. K., Malpas, C. B., Bowden, S. C., & Seal, M. L. (2018). Different brain networks underlying intelligence in autism spectrum disorders. *Human Brain Mapping, 39*(8), 3253–3262.

Raichle, M. E., et al. (2001). A default mode of brain function. *Proceedings of the National Academy of Sciences of the United States of America, 98*, 676–682.

Rasmussen, P., Borjesson, O., Wentz, E., & Gillberg, C. (2001). Autistic disorders in down syndrome: Background factors and clinical correlates. *Developmental Medicine and Child Neurology, 43*(11), 750–754.

Reichow, B., Servili, C., Yasamy, M. T., Barbui, C., & Saxena, S. (2013). Non-specialist psychosocial interventions for children and adolescents with intellectual disability or lower-functioning autism spectrum disorders: A systematic review. *PLoS Medicine, 10*(12), e1001572.

Reynolds, A. M., & Malow, B. A. (2011). Sleep and autism spectrum disorders. *Pediatric Clinics of North America, 58*(3), 685–698.

Riccioni, A., Siracusano, M., Arturi, L., Marcovecchio, C., Postorino, V., Gialloreti, L. E., & Mazzone, L. (2022). Developmental and intelligence quotient in autism: A brief report on the possible long-term relation. *Behavioral Sciences, 12*(9). https://doi.org/10.3390/bs12090304

Rubenstein, J. L. R., & Merzenich, M. M. (2003). Model of autism: Increased ratio of excitation/inhibition in key neural systems. *Genes Brain & Behavior, 2*, 255–267.

Rushton, J. P., & Ankney, C. D. (2009). Whole brain size and general mental ability: A review. *International Journal of Neuroscience, 119*(5), 692–732.

Sameroff, A. J. (2005). The science of infancy: Academic, social, and political agendas. *Infancy, 7*(3), 219–242.

Sato, D., Lionel, A. C., Leblond, C. S., Prasad, A., Pinto, D., Walker, S., & Scherer, S. W. (2012). SHANK1 deletions in males with Autism Spectrum Disorder. *The American Journal of Human Genetics, 90*(5), 879–887.

Schaaf, R. C., Benevides, T., Mailloux Z. Faller, P., Hunt, J., van Hooydonk, E., Freeman, R., Leiby, B., Sednecki, J., & Kelly, D. (2014). An intervention for sensory difficulties in children with autism: A randomized trial. *Journal of Autism and Developmental Disorders, 44*(7), 1493–1506.

Schalock, R. L. (2011). The evolving understanding of the construct of intellectual disability. *Journal of Intellectual and Developmental Disability, 36*(4), 223–233.

Scheuffgen, K., Happe, F., Anderson, M., & Frith, U. (2000). High "intelligence," low "IQ"? Speed of processing and measured IQ in children with autism. *Development and Psychopathology, 12*(1), 83–90.

Schmid, R. G., Tirsch, W. S., & Scherb, H. (2002). Correlation between spectral EEG parameters and intelligence test variables in school-age children. *Clinical Neurophysiology, 113*(10), 1647–1656.

Schoen, S. A., Lane, S. J., Mailloux, Z., May-Benson, T., Parham, L. D., Smith Roley, S., & Schaaf, R. C. (2019). A systematic review of Ayres sensory integration intervention for children with autism. *Autism Research, 12*(1), 6–19.

Schoen, S. A., Miller, L. J., Brett-Green, B. A., & Nielsen, D. M. (2009). Physiological and behavioral differences in sensory processing: A comparison of children with autism spectrum disorder and sensory modulation disorder. *Frontiers in Integrative Neuroscience, 3*, 29.

Seifer, R. (2001). Socioeconomic status, multiple risks, and development of intelligence. In R. J. Sternberg & E. L. Grigorenko (Eds.), *Environmental effects on cognitive abilities* (pp. 59–81). Lawrence, Erlbaum Associates Inc.

Shah, A., & Frith, U. (1993). Why do autistic individuals show superior performance on the block design task? *Journal of Child Psychology and Psychiatry, 34*(8), 1351–1364.

Sripada, C., Angstadt, M., Rutherford, S., Taxali, A., & Shedden, K. (2020). Toward a "treadmill test" for cognition: Improved prediction of general cognitive ability from the task activated brain. *Hum Brain Mapping, 41*(12), 3186–3197.

Srivastava, A. K., & Schwartz, C. E. (2014). Intellectual disability and autism spectrum disorders: Causal genes and molecular mechanisms. *Neuroscience & Biobehavioral Reviews, 46*(Pt 2), 161–174.

Starr, E. M., Berument, S. K., Tomlins, M., Papanikolaou, K., & Rutter, M. (2005). Brief report: Autism in individuals with Down syndrome. *Journal of Autism and Developmental Disorders, 35*(5), 665–673.

Sumiyoshi, C., Ohi, K., Fujino, H., Yamamori, H., Fujimoto, M., Yasuda, Y., Uno, Y., Takahashi, J., Morita, K., Katsuki, A., Yamamoto, M., Okahisa, Y., Sata, A., Katsumoto, E., Koeda, M., Hirano, Y., Nakataki, M., Matsumoto, J., Miura, K., … Hashimoto, R. (2022). Transdiagnostic comparisons of intellectual abilities and work outcome in patients with mental disorders: Multicentre study. *British Journal of Psychiatry Open, 8*(4), e98.

Takayanagi, M., Kawasaki, Y., Shinomiya, M., Hiroshi, H., Okada, S., Ino, T., Sakai, K., Murakami, K., Ishida, R., Mizuno, K., & Niwa, S. I. (2022). Review of cognitive characteristics of autism spectrum disorder using performance on six subtests on four versions of the Wechsler intelligence scale for children. *Journal of Autism and Developmental Disorders, 52*(1), 240–253.

Tanaka Institute for Educational Research. (2003). *Tanaka Binet Chinou Kensa V* [Tanaka-Binet Intelligence Scale V]. Taken Publishing (in Japanese).

Tanner, A., & Dounavi, K. (2021). The emergence of autism symptoms prior to 18 months of age: A systematic literature review. *Journal of Autism and Developmental Disorders, 51*, 973–993.

Tessier, S., Lambert, A., Chicoine, M., Scherzer, P., Soulières, I., & Godbout, R. (2015). Intelligence measures and stage 2 sleep in typically-developing and autistic children. *International Journal of Psychophysiology, 97*(1), 58–65.

Thatcher, R. W., North, D., & Biver, C. (2005). EEG and intelligence: Relations between EEG coherence, EEG phase delay and power. *Clinical Neurophysiology, 116*(9), 2129–2141.

Thatcher, R. W., Palmero-Soler, E., North, D. M., & Biver, C. J. (2016). Intelligence and EEG measures of information flow: Efficiency and homeostatic neuroplasticity. *Scientific Reports, 6*, 38890.

The Simons VIP Consortium. (2012). Simons Variation in Individuals Project (Simons VIP): A genetics-first approach to studying autism spectrum and related neurodevelopmental disorders. *Neuron, 80*(6), 1063–1067 (Correspondence: Spiro, J. E., & Chung, W. K.).

Thomas, N., Singh, A., Sankaran, S., Russell, P. S., Tsheringla, S., Viswanathan, S. A., & Nair, M. K. (2014). ICD-10 and alternative diagnostic criteria for childhood autism among children with intellectual disability. *Indian Journal of Pediatrics, 81*(Suppl. 2), 173–178.

Topper, S., Ober, C., & Das, S. (2011). Exome sequencing and the genetics of intellectual disability. *Clinical Genetics, 80*(2), 117–126.

Toth, G. (2010). Early intervention theories and practice—A comprehensive historical overview of foundations and approaches in early childhood care and education. *Journal of Education and Child Studies, 2*(1), 1–20.

Travers, B. G., Kana, R. K., Klinger, L. G., Klein, C. L., & Klinger, M. R. (2015). Motor learning in individuals with autism spectrum disorder: Activation in superior parietal lobule related to learning and repetitive behaviors. *Autism Research, 8*(1), 38–51.

Tsai, N. P., Wilkerson, J. R., Guo, W., Maksimova, M. A., DeMartino, G. N., Cowan, C. W., & Huber, K. M. (2012). Multiple autism-linked genes mediate synapse elimination via proteasomal degradation of a synaptic scaffold PSD-95. *Cell, 151*(7), 1581–1594.

Tuchman, R., Alessandri, M., & Cuccaro, M. (2010). Autism spectrum disorders and epilepsy: Moving towards a comprehensive approach to treatment. *Brain and Development, 32*(9), 719–730.

Turk, J., Bax, M., Williams, C., Amin, P., Eriksson, M., & Gillberg, C. (2009). Autism spectrum disorder in children with and without epilepsy: Impact on social functioning and communication. *Acta Paediatrica, 98*(4), 675–681.

Valnegri, P., Sala, C., & Passafaro, M. (2012). Synaptic dysfunction and intellectual disability. *Advances in Experimental Medicine and Biology, 970*, 433–449.

van Bokhoven, H. (2011). Genetic and epigenetic networks in intellectual disabilities. *Annual Review of Genetics, 45*, 81–104.

van Eeghen, A. M., Pulsifer, M. B., Merker, V. L., Neumeyer, A. M., van Eeghen, E. E., Thibert, R. L., & Thiele, E. A. (2013). Understanding relationships between autism, intelligence, and epilepsy: A cross-disorder approach. *Developmental Medicine & Child Neurology, 55*(2), 146–153.

Van Waelvelde, H., Oostra, A., Dewitte, G., Van Den Broeck, C., & Jongmans, M. J. (2010). Stability of motor problems in young children with or at risk of autism spectrum disorders, ADHD, and or developmental coordination disorder. *Developmental Medicine and Child Neurology, 52*(8), e174-178.

Ventola, P., Saulnier, C. A., Steinberg, E., Chawarska, K., & Klin, A. (2014). Early-emerging social adaptive skills in toddlers with autism spectrum disorders: An item analysis. *Journal of Autism and Developmental Disorders, 44*(2), 283–293.

Vivanti, G., Barbaro, J., Hudry, K., Dissanayake, C., & Prior, M. (2013). Intellectual development in autism spectrum disorders: New insights from longitudinal studies. *Frontiers in Human Neuroscience, 7*, 354.

Volkmar, F. R., & McPartland, J. C. (2016). Moving beyond a categorical diagnosis of autism. *Lancet Neurology, 15*(3), 237–238. https://doi.org/10.1016/s1474-4422(15)00299-9

Waterhouse, L. (2013). *Rethinking autism—Variation and complexity*. Academic Press, Elsevier.

Wechsler, D. (2003). *Wechsler Intelligence Scale for Children edition (WISC-IV)*. Psychological Corporation.

Wechsler, D. (1997). *Wechsler Adult Intelligence Scale—Third Edition* (WAIS-III) [Database record]. APA PsycTests.

Wechsler, D. (1991). *The Wechsler intelligence scale for children—Third edition*. The Psychological Corporation.

Wechsler, D. (1949). *Wechsler intelligence scale for children: Manual*. The Psychological Corp.

Wechsler, D. (1939). *The measurement of adult intelligence*. Williams & Wilkins.

Wilkins, J., & Matson, J. L. (2009). A comparison of social skills profiles in intellectually disabled adults with and without ASD. *Behavior Modification, 33*(2), 143–155.

Williamson, K. E., & Jakobson, L. S. (2014). Social perception in children born at very low birthweight and its relationship with social/behavioral outcomes. *Journal of Child Psychology and Psychiatry, 55*(9), 990–998.

Woodbury-Smith, M. R., & Volkmar, F. R. (2009). Asperger syndrome. *European Child & Adolescent Psychiatry, 18*(1), 2–11. https://doi.org/10.1007/s00787-008-0701-0

Yirmiya, N., Solomonica-Levi, D., Shulman, C., & Pilowsky, T. (1996). Theory of mind abilities in individuals with autism, Down syndrome, and mental retardation of unknown etiology: The role of age and intelligence. *Journal of Child Psychology and Psychiatry, 37*(8), 1003–1014.

Yu, T. Y., Chou, W., Chow, J. C., Lin, C. H., Tung, L. C., & Chen, K. L. (2018). IQ discrepancy differentiates levels of fine motor skills and their relationship in children with autism spectrum disorders. *Neuropsychiatric Disease and Treatment, 14*, 597–605. https://doi.org/10.2147/ndt.S153102

Yu, T. W., & Berry-Kravis, E. (2014). Autism and Fragile X syndrome. *Seminars in Neurology, 34*(3), 258–265.

Zafeiriou, D. I., Ververi, A., & Vargiami, E. (2007). Childhood autism and associated comorbidities. *Brain and Development, 29*(5), 257–272.

Zafeiriou, D. I., Ververi, A., Dafoulis, V., Kalyva, E., & Vargiami, E. (2013). Autism spectrum disorders: The quest for genetic syndromes. *American Journal of Medical Genetics, Part B, 162B*, 327–366.

Zarakoviti, E., Shafran, R., Skuse, D., McTague, A., Batura, N., Palmer, T., Dalrymple, E., Bennett, S. D., & Reilly, C. (2023). Factor associated with the occurrence of epilepsy in autism: A systematic review. *Journal of Autism and Developmental Disorders, 53*(10), 3873–3890.

Zhang, H., Zhou, Q. Q., Chen, H., Hu, X. Q., Li, W. G., Bai, Y., Han, J. X., Wang, Y., Liang, Z. H., Chen, D., Cong, F. Y., Yan, J. Q., & Li, X. L. (2023). The applied principles of EEG analysis methods in neuroscience and clinical neurology. *Military Medical Research, 10*(1), 67.
Zazzo, R. (1960). *Les jumeaux, le couple et la personne* [Twins, the couple, and the person] (2 Vols.). Presses Universitaires de France.

Executive Functions in Autism

Adam W. McCrimmon, Erica M. Makarenko, Abdullah S. Bernier, Sydney Dickner, and Madison Waller

Abstract This chapter provides a comprehensive exploration of executive functioning in individuals on the autism spectrum. It begins by defining executive functioning (EF) and examining its theoretical factor structure, highlighting its role in inhibition, working memory, and cognitive flexibility. The chapter then outlines the typical developmental trajectory of EF in neurotypical individuals, and the relation of EF to cognitive abilities, and approaches to measurement of EF before transitioning to a discussion of EF in autistic individuals. We describe how these differences influence and interact with core diagnostic behaviours of autism. The chapter also reviews neuroimaging studies that investigate the neural underpinnings of EF in autism, shedding light on areas of brain activity that may contribute to observed EF differences. We highlight the connection between EF and support needs of those on the autism spectrum and describe current intervention approaches aimed at improving EF in autistic individuals. The chapter concludes by summarizing key insights and suggesting directions for future research and intervention strategies to better support autistic individuals in managing EF differences.

Keywords Executive Function · Autism · Cognition · Cognitive development

Researchers and clinicians have striven to understand the core and secondary impairments observed in individuals diagnosed with autism[1] (spectrum disorder). The Executive Function (EF; Ozonoff et al., 1991) theory has been studied comprehensively to aid in these efforts. The primary focus of this work has been to understand and describe EF abilities in autistic individuals, and to link those abilities to diagnostic behaviours demonstrated by autistic individuals. The purpose of this chapter is to

[1] In alignment with current perspectives on language and labelling, and to respect the recommendations and views of self-advocates, the terms "autistic", "autism" or "on the autism spectrum" will be used throughout this chapter when referring to the diagnosis and individuals in receipt of it (Kapp et al., 2013; Kenny et al., 2016).

A. W. McCrimmon (✉) · E. M. Makarenko · A. S. Bernier · S. Dickner · M. Waller
Werklund School of Education, University of Calgary, Calgary, AB, Canada
e-mail: awmccrim@ucalgary.ca

J. L. Matson (ed.), *Assessment and Diagnosis in Autism*, Autism and Child Psychopathology Series, https://doi.org/10.1007/978-3-032-11802-8_10

review information pertaining to EF in individuals on the autism spectrum. We begin with an overview of EF and its relation to neuropsychological functioning. Common approaches to measurement/evaluation of EF are described. Subsequently, neurotypical development of EF is reviewed and compared to EF development in autistic people. EF abilities its relation to the social and behavioural differences often seen in autistic individuals is also presented. Additional research regarding EF and neural structures in autistic individuals is then reviewed. The chapter ends with a discussion of intervention strategies for EF in autism, implications of the findings of EF in autism, and future research opportunities.

Executive Functions

The term *Executive Functions* was introduced in relation to the work of Luria (1966), who proposed a cognitive system in charge of intentionality and formulation of thoughts and actions, identification of goal-appropriate cognitive routines, and evaluation of outcomes of tasks leveraging these abilities. This area of mental functioning is predominantly regulated by the prefrontal cortex, though that region is not solely responsible for these cognitive processes (Diamond, 2020). As such, this area of the brain is thought to act primarily as a *control centre* to mediate these cognitive functions with connections extending to other brain regions (Miller & Cohen, 2001).

Baddeley and Hitch (1974) were the first to describe EF as a *central executive*, further defined by Lezak (1983) to include a central process that controls how human behaviour is expressed. According to Diamond (2013), EFs are a coordinated set of mental processes that are engaged when one attends, concentrates, inhibits prepotent responses, or shifts to a different cognitive state. While concrete definitions have varied over time, a compelling and comprehensive definition has been put forth by Jurado and Rosselli (2007):

> In a constantly changing environment, executive abilities allow us to shift our mind set quickly and adapt to diverse situations while at the same time inhibiting inappropriate behaviors. They enable us to create a plan, initiate its execution, and persevere on the task at hand until its completion. Executive functions mediate the ability to organize our thoughts in a goal directed way and are therefore essential for success in school and work situations, as well as everyday living. (p. 214)

EF was historically seen to exist as a unitary construct; however, more recent work indicates that the factor structure evolves with an individual's maturation and neural development (Laureys et al., 2022). Specifically, EF abilities in younger children are reported to fit best under a unitary factor model whereas adolescents' abilities better fit under a multi-factor model. The exact nature of the multi-factor model is inconsistent; however, most findings support a tripartite structure in which various EF tasks/abilities are seen to exemplify three core domains: inhibition (IN), working memory (WM), and cognitive flexibility (CF; Diamond, 2013; Friedman et al., 2016; Miyake et al., 2000). There is moderate evidence for a fourth factor in the form of planning (Miyake & Friedman, 2012); however, debate continues as to whether this is a separate factor, a component of WM (Cirino et al., 2018), or part of IN (Lehto et al., 2003). Evidence for the differentiation of EF abilities into the three factors comes from research indicating high correlation among tasks that engage the same aspect of EF and low correlations between EF tasks seen to be based upon divergent EF abilities (e.g., Miyake et al., 2000); however, there is little evidence that EF abilities exist and can be used by people independently of one another. That is, people's everyday use of EF abilities typically involves a simultaneous combination of IN, WM, and/or CF to plan, execute, and evaluate goal-directed behaviour.

Inhibition

IN is the ability to control a response that will not support goal attainment and instead activate an appropriate alternative (Diamond, 2020). In essence, it is one's ability to control their thoughts, behaviours, or emotions such that automatic instances of these are overridden to obtain an intended goal. IN can be conceptualized as either simple, where a prepotent response must be resisted, or complex, where an arbitrary rule must be held in mind to hold back a response in favour of an alternate one. An example of simple inhibition would be withholding an automatic response to scratch an itch, or to cross the street as one last car speeds through the intersection even if the walk sign has already turned on. A more complex example may be resisting the desire to make a large purchase to instead review one's finances and consult with a significant other before doing so. Inhibitory ability has been postulated as foundational to both the development and function of EF as it underlies the regulation of emotion, cognition, and behaviour (Miyake et al., 2000; Nigg, 2000). Barkley (1997) strongly defines accurate performance among all areas of EF as relying upon a basis of behavioural IN ability. Thus, it remains an important focus for study in childhood and adolescence due to the importance of inhibitory development (and ability) and its underlying importance to EF development in general.

Working Memory

WM is the ability to hold information in one's mind while either mentally manipulating it or while experiencing circumstances of distraction (Diamond, 2020). For example, WM would be engaged when conducting mental calculations or mentally reorganizing information. This ability is distinguished from short-term memory by the processes by which information is maintained or manipulated as well as neural structures involved in each (Gathercole et al., 2004). WM is further differentiated by the modality of information to be maintained and/or manipulated (verbal versus nonverbal; Diamond, 2013). Other research has provided information on a subprocess of WM termed *updating*, which refers to the important cognitive process of not just maintaining information in WM, but choosing what information enters and leaves WM due to the limited capacity it has.

Cognitive Flexibility

CF, also referred to as mental flexibility, is the ability to perceive events in a different manner, respond in unique ways, and/or to switch between different mindsets (Diamond, 2013). For example, there are different social expectations for how an individual should act in a shopping mall versus during a church service, and switching appropriately between these sets is optimal to participating in each situation. CF is also important during conversational exchanges, or any situation in which topics or ideas may switch rapidly and one must show adaptability. For example, an individual must shift their mindset during an argument with a peer to account for the other person's perspective to find a solution to the issue at hand.

Hot Versus Cold EF

EFs have also been conceptualized as either *hot* or *cold* to understand them more clearly (Salehinejad et al., 2021). Hot EF skills are typically demonstrated in emotionally arousing situations that occur in our daily lives. Alternately, cold EF skills tend to be demonstrated in relation to academic or problem-solving situations. Cold EF is more similar to the types of tasks psychologists administer to measure EF as part of a psychoeducational assessment whereas hot EF tends to be a more emotionally driven process that is typically measured using rating scales (Metcalfe & Mischel, 1999). Salehinejad and colleagues (2021) postulate that specific EFs can be situated under these cold and hot EF domains; examples of hot EF include emotion regulation, reward processing, delayed gratification, risky decision-making, and social cognition. Cold EF includes inhibition, working memory, cognitive flexibility, problem solving, attentional control, and multitasking (Salehinejad et al., 2021).

Development of EF

Despite the prior notion that frontal lobes are relatively inactive during early childhood, neuroimaging studies have shown that the frontal lobes begin activation at approximately six months of age (Chugani et al., 1987; Jurado & Rosselli, 2007). The frontal lobes, the anterior cingulate cortex (ACC), and the prefrontal cortex (PFC) continue to mature through late adolescence and up to early adulthood through neurological processes like myelination, synaptic pruning, and synaptic growth (Arain et al., 2013; Casey et al., 2006; Spear, 2013). Considering that most EF processes occur in the PFC and the ACC, the developmental trajectory for EF and these brain regions are one and the same. However, although the stages of childhood are associated with EF maturity (e.g., an infant's stimulus-based reactions; preschoolers' ability to think of the past, plan for the future, and begin making complex decisions), significant specialized plasticity occurs during adolescence, an identified critical period for further EF development (Garon et al., 2008; Larsen & Luna, 2018; Tervo-Clemmens et al., 2023). This is because at this stage, the brain has more capacity to engage in higher order cognitive processes that require more complex functions, resulting in more EF activity than in previous stages (Larsen & Luna, 2018). In general, EF ability appears to develop sequentially early on following PFC maturity, with specific growth periods identified between birth to 2 years and 7 to 9 years; EF development then shifts to a cañonical trajectory, significantly growing at 10 to 15 years, before stabilizing to adult-ability levels at 18 to 20 years, with trajectories varying for every child (Anderson et al., 2001a, 2001b, 2002; Tervo-Clemmens et al., 2023).

Regarding the development and differentiation of early EF abilities, researchers continue to debate whether control processes (i.e., IN, WM, and CF) are fully separable early in development. Some argue that since the assessment of EF in young children requires language, visual-spatial abilities, memory, and motor skills, all of which are still in the early stages of development, they are likely to influence assessment outcomes (Wiebe et al., 2011). Earlier EF models that use statistical modelling, like confirmatory factor analyses, have indicated that a single-factor EF model best describes EF abilities. This trend appeared to exist especially for children between 3–6 years old, where no improvement in statistical models was seen when separate IN, WM, or CF components are added (Hughes et al., 2010; Wiebe et al., 2008). However, more recent approaches describe EF component frameworks to be both unitary and diverse, suggesting IN, WM, and CF can be measured separately in later development like preschool years (Garon et al., 2008; Miyake et al., 2000).

EF develops through infancy and childhood, with critical maturation present in adolescence and young adulthood. IN is the first EF observed in children's behaviour, with CF significantly improving later in childhood and adolescence, and WM continuing to strengthen into late adolescence and early adulthood. Researchers including Diamond (2013) and Best and Miller (2010) suggest that these differing trajectories of development are in support of the diversified EF framework, whereby EF components are measured separately in later development. Notably, EF abilities obtain varying developmental patterns, with some acting as a necessary foundation for others, and certain components not achieving full maturity until early adulthood (Best & Miller, 2010; Diamond, 2013; Luna et al., 2015). It is important to mention that contextual factors including environmental stress or enrichment can significantly alter such trajectories of EF development. Nevertheless, the following description outlines the typical developmental course of IN, WM, and CF.

Inhibition

Infants can demonstrate basic IN ability like delaying the urge to eat a treat, showing rapid gains observed through early childhood (Amso & Johnson, 2005; Garon et al., 2008). By one year of age, babies can inhibit an over-learned response, with the largest gains in IN ability observed in children between 6–9 years (Brocki & Bohlin, 2004; Klenberg et al., 2001). Similar to the differential development of EF abilities, IN components tend to mature at varying rates, with more simplistic components laying the ground for the development of subsequent complex ones that continue to be refined through adolescence and into adulthood (Best & Miller, 2010).

Working Memory

Simple memory function like holding information in the phonological loop (e.g., remembering a five-digit verification code for a password) is present during the preschool years. More complex WM ability involving mental manipulation of items, such as being able to recite given digits in reverse order, begins to develop at around six years of age (Garon et al., 2008; Gathercole et al., 2004). However, like other growth patterns, WM matures nonlinearly, with most rapid growth occurring during childhood (ages 3–10), followed by a period of brief accelerated growth in youth 13–16 years (Ahmed et al., 2022). Researchers theorize that WM abilities improve as the capacity to hold and manipulate items, also known as WM capacity, improves (Reynolds et al., 2022). In general, WM ability develops into adolescence and adulthood, likely due to cognitive and neural maturation.

Cognitive Flexibility

Miyake and colleagues (2000) point out that IN is essential for shifting between mental sets, as a new set must be the focus of attention and the previous one inhibited. Moreover, WM abilities are also required to switch between sets of mental rules (Best & Miller, 2010). Considering the need of other EF abilities for CF performance, CF follows the same trajectory as other EFs and improves with age. The ability to shift between two simple response sets is apparent at around 3–4 years of age (Anderson et al., 2002; Hughes, 1998), though children at this stage still make errors and often perseverate on an initial rule/response set (Buttelmann & Karbach, 2017). As children reach 7–9 years of age, they begin to show the ability to maintain and shift between multiple mental sets, with the ability levelling off at approximately 15 years of age (Huizinga et al., 2006; Karbach & Kray, 2007), and continuing to mature throughout adolescence (Anderson et al., 2002; Davidson et al., 2006; Zelazo & Frye, 1998).

Relation to Cognition

Cognitive intelligence (IQ) is difficult to define; it generally refers to "the aggregate or global capacity of the individual to act purposefully, to think rationally, and to deal effectively with his environment" (Wechsler, 1944). This construct is most often used in reference to standardized testing where an individual is compared to age-related peers to determine an individual's cognitive strengths and/or areas of weakness.

Research findings have consistently noted that, although EF and IQ are related (e.g., Brydges et al., 2012), they represent unique cognitive constructs (Duggan & Garcia-Barrera, 2015). Intelligence has been defined in various ways over the decades that it has been researched and studied; the most comprehensive model of human cognitive abilities is the Cattell-Horn-Carroll (CHC) model (McGrew, 2009) that provides evidence of a factor structure consisting of two main constructs (crystallized and fluid intelligence) and additional factors representing different information processing abilities. Research investigating the correlations between EF and cognitive test scores reflecting the CHC model (Floyd et al., 2010) has shown a strong relation between EF task performance and overall cognitive ability. At the same time, findings indicate that EF is not equivalent to general cognitive ability, nor does EF task performance explain cognitive task performance entirely (Floyd et al., 2010; Crinella & Yu, 2000). Indeed, research findings have shown that the relation between IQ and EF is positive, though not strong enough to indicate substantial overlap (Ardila et al., 2000; Arffa, 2007). Further, EF is more strongly correlated to individual cognitive ability factors reflected in CHC theory (rather than to overall cognitive ability), suggesting that EF is not overly related to general intelligence (Floyd et al., 2010).

Another line of research investigating the relation between EF and cognitive ability assumes that a strong overlap between these two constructs would mean that individuals who present with impairments in one would also present with impairments in the other. Findings from this work indicate that many individuals, such as those with attention-deficit/hyperactivity disorder (ADHD), can present with strong cognitive abilities yet demonstrate EF impairments (Antshel et al., 2010; Craig et al., 2016).

In general, a positive relation exists between EF and cognitive ability in that tasks of EF typically require a baseline level of cognitive ability and vice-versa. Indeed, common sense dictates that problems cannot be solved without EF; however, the relation between these two constructs is far from direct. EF is just one information processing component necessary for problem solving, and correlations between cognition and EF measures tend to be small to moderate, suggesting that many factors other than EF influence an individual's cognitive ability. As succinctly pointed out by Duncan et al. (1995) "frontal patients have impaired 'planning', 'problem solving', etc. but preserved 'intelligence'" (p. 262).

Measurement of EF

The relevance of EF to children and adolescents has long been a topic of debate (Toplak et al., 2013). This discussion has centred primarily around questions of the theoretical factor structure of the construct (i.e., is EF appropriately conceptualized as IN, WM, and CF; Miyake et al., 2000), the development of EF from infancy through to adolescence (i.e., is the theoretical factor structure stable throughout development; Willoughby et al., 2010), and effective measurement processes (i.e., how can we appropriately measure EF abilities in children of various ages; Willoughby et al., 2011). Regarding the latter, clinical practice and empirical literature indicates that EFs are generally measured through two approaches: Task or performance-based measures and/or rating scales (Toplak et al., 2013).

Task-based approaches typically employ the use of standardized measures designed to isolate and examine a specific EF ability and are typically considered measures of cold EF skills. Some common measures used in childhood and adolescence are the Delis-Kaplan Executive Function System (DKEFS; Delis et al., 2001), the NEPSY-II (Korkman et al., 2007), and the Wisconsin Card Sorting Task (WCST; Heaton et al., 1993). Tasks are typically selected based upon the EF domain that they are purported to evaluate, and performance is judged based on accuracy and/or speed of response in comparison to a norm-referenced group.

In contrast, rating scales require an informant (often a parent and/or a teacher) to judge the child's challenges with common behaviours that require EF and are typically considered measures of hot EF skills. The most common measures in this domain are the Behavior Rating Inventory of Executive Function, Second Edition (BRIEF2; Gioia et al., 2015) and the Comprehensive Executive Function Inventory (CEFI; Naglieri & Goldstein, 2013). Raters are asked to indicate the frequency with which a child demonstrates various specified important behaviours related to or mediated by EF abilities. Scores are then compared to a norm-referenced comparison group to provide an ecologically valid representation of a child's competence with EF abilities as the individual being reported on is not directed or instructed to engage in behaviours.

Despite the use of these two forms of EF measurement, research indicates that they do not assess EF in a cohesive manner (Toplak et al., 2013). Indeed, these two formats correlate poorly (rs ≈ 0.2) and so it has been proposed that they likely measure different aspects of EF, with task-based measures evaluating cognitive aspects of the construct (e.g., cold EF), and rating scales measuring behavioural implementation of EF abilities (e.g., hot EF). This position is supported by research that indicates that individuals who demonstrate EF impairment on rating scales (i.e., behavioural impairment) are often capable of adequate performance on task-based measures (Gioia et al., 2008). In general, clinicians and researchers are advised that task-based and ratings scales are not interchangeable and can provide important and unique information about an individual's EF abilities (Biederman et al., 2008).

Executive Function in Autism

Research advancements regarding the interplay between EF and autism have extended beyond the proposition that the invariance of autism-related behaviours and rigidity could be explained as a primary impairment in executive control (Hughes & Russell, 1993; Ozonoff et al., 1991; Pellicano, 2012) to include broad and heterogenous impairments in areas such as social cognition, mental health, lifelong functioning, and disability (Demetriou et al., 2019). Certainly, autism is heterogeneous; however, so too are the EF impairments seen in those on the autism spectrum (Demetriou et al., 2019). Despite this heterogeneity, EF difficulties have consistently been demonstrated across the lifespan of those on the spectrum (Brady et al., 2017; Demetriou et al., 2018; Fossum et al., 2021; Geurts et al., 2014b; Leung et al., 2014; Wang et al., 2017).

As suggested by Demetriou and colleagues (2019), recent research on EF and autism has illuminated a potential common underlying pathway that influences the culmination of impairment. There has been a shift away from measuring discrete EF domains with neuropsychological testing to ecologically valid measurement tools (e.g., rating scales) to understand the level of functional impact in everyday life (Demetriou et al., 2018, 2019; Kenworthy et al., 2009). As such, EF has recently been proposed as a biomarker for autism due to correlations between neuropsychological, cognitive, and behavioural domains of EF impairments (e.g., WM, CF, IN) and autism symptom severity (Demetriou et al., 2019; Van Eylen et al., 2015). Other studies, however, indicate heterogeneity in EF skills across the lifespan, with certain EF strengths among autistic individuals (e.g., St. John et al., 2021). This heterogeneity is reduced when utilizing ecologically valid measurement tools since the artificial nature of task-based measurement reduces reliability in predicting performance in real-life situations (St. John et al., 2021).

Despite contention surrounding the attribution of these impairments, it is important to consider specific EF impairments for those on the autism spectrum. A meta-analysis from Lai and colleagues (2017) reported that autistic individuals perform below typically developing matched controls on common EF measures of CF (WCST, Trail Making Test), IN (Opposite Word subtest of the TEA-Ch, the Stroop Task), verbal WM (Digit Span, Sentence Repetition), spatial WM (Spatial Working Memory task of the CANTAB; Rey Complex Figure Test), planning (NEPSY Tower Task/D-KEFS Tower of London, Stocking of Cambridge task of the CANTAB), and generativity (ideational fluency of the Use of Common Objects task). Some tasks showed less impairment when compared to allistic (non-autistic) peers, such as the extradimensional stage of the IED task on the CANTAB (Lai et al., 2017). According to this meta-analysis and despite all EF domains being impaired, verbal WM, spatial WM, flexibility, and generativity were considered core EF impairments among autistic individuals that were consistently evident despite co-occurring ADHD (Lai et al., 2017).

A more recent review reported mixed findings regarding the level of impairment experienced by autistic individuals in particular EF domains (St. John et al., 2021).

The differences in findings may be due to contextual factors, such as task demands (e.g., more structure leads to less impairment), co-occurring conditions (e.g., ADHD contributes to poorer IN performance), and social expectations (e.g., better decision-making as a feature of less social pressures; St. John et al., 2021). This view is further supported by research that aimed to eliminate the *task impurity problem*. According to this perspective, the findings indicate that autistic individuals exhibit EF impairments in prepotent response inhibition, CF, and WM (Van Eylen et al., 2015; White, 2013); however, difficulties with generativity and planning were observed only during open-ended tasks, suggesting that the impairment in inferring implicit information, which is inherent to autism, may confound EF measurement (Van Eylen et al., 2015; White, 2013). Certainly, EF impairments are varied and exist along a continuum as not all EF domains are consistently affected among autistic individuals (e.g., Demetriou et al., 2018; Johnston et al., 2019).

EF impairments have impacts on the functioning of autistic individuals across multiple domains of functioning. Reduced CF may manifest as perseverative responses and difficulty shifting focus from external objects to internal perspectives, leading to challenges in social interactions and maintaining conversations with changing topics (Pellicano, 2012). Further, given that autistic individuals tend to have verbal and/or communicative challenges, EF tasks that are language-laden tend to suggest greater impairment (Lai et al., 2017). EF skills are associated with social functioning and certain metacognitive executive processes (e.g., initiation, WM, planning, organization, and self-monitoring) are uniquely affected in autism; reduced skills in these areas indicate higher autism-related social-communicative behaviours (Leung et al., 2016). Generally, EF challenges impact independent living, academic success, and quality of life (Demetriou et al., 2018; St. John et al., 2021). Poorer EF performance has been linked to increased social difficulties and repetitive behaviours (Van Eylen et al., 2015). To mitigate these challenges, accommodations such as adjusting contextual factors (e.g., structure, time, prompting) may enhance functioning for autistic individuals (St. John et al., 2021).

Given that the presence of co-occurring conditions is more common than not among autistic individuals (e.g., Lai et al., 2019), it is important to consider the role of additional diagnoses in EF. Despite some research finding core EF impairments in autism (Demetriou et al., 2019), other research indicates that features of EF are not tied to specific diagnoses and are shared transdiagnostically (Cordova et al., 2020). In fact, EF impairments may be considered a transdiagnostic indicator of atypical development and, thus, neurodevelopmental conditions (Zelazo, 2020). There are certain subgroups among autistic and ADHD individuals characterized by certain EF profiles rather than diagnostic class, indicating shared neurocognitive challenges despite heterogeneity between and within these populations (Cordova et al., 2020).

Further, although proponents of the executive dysfunction theory of autism continue to exist, there have been negative research findings that have cast doubt on that hypothesis as a primary problem in autism as it cannot explain all autistic symptomatology (Griffith et al., 1999; Yerys et al., 2007). As such, researchers have suggested that we must shift away from the idea that there is a single framework that explains the causality of autism, and instead focus on the underlying causes that encompass multiple atypicalities (Happé et al., 2006). Although autistic individuals show greater impairment in certain EF skills (e.g., CF), these skills do not distinctly differentiate between diagnoses as there are shared impairments across neurodevelopmental conditions, such as ADHD (Margari et al., 2016). Typically, the presence of co-occurring conditions is characterized by more severe EF impairments (Benallie et al., 2021). While EF deficits are correlated with symptom severity, they are not the sole contributor to associated symptoms (Cordova et al., 2020). This correlation is further complicated in adulthood wherein EF impairments were not found to be associated with behavioural indicators of an autism profile (Johnston et al., 2019). Therefore, regardless of whether EF is considered a primary cause of autistic symptomatology or not, EF impairments are likely to place an autistic individual at risk for a poorer developmental outcome (Pellicano, 2012).

The challenge within the literature is to move from research that focuses on attributing symptomatology to executive dysfunction and instead incorporating a developmental perspective (Geurts et al., 2014a) to better understand causality. For instance, the level of impairment and maturation pattern for WM, IN, and CF were tracked from childhood to young adulthood in a recent longitudinal study (Fossum et al., 2021). Using neuropsychological tests, the results indicated significant delays in EF at baseline. Despite a similar maturation pattern as typically developing participants, the EF impairments for autistic individuals were considerable and persisted across time. There has also been research that has postulated positive developmental outcomes for certain EF domains. It is suggested that the planning capacity of autistic children improved at a faster rate than that of neurotypical children (Pellicano, 2010). These findings suggest that at least certain EF impairments in autism might decline over time (Geurts et al., 2014b). This proposition is supported by research which found that autistic young adults generally meet normative expectations on neuropsychological measures of EF (Brady et al., 2017). However, there are many studies that indicate executive dysfunction remains present in adulthood (Fossum et al., 2021; Geurts & Vissers, 2012; Johnston et al., 2019), thus providing an atypical course of EF development in autism over time. The variability in developmental trajectory for distinct EFs across peak developmental periods "may be contributing to some of the heterogeneity observed in EF performance" among autistic individuals (Demetriou et al., 2019, p. 8). Therefore, it is essential that future research focus on how and when EF develops in autistic individuals, with a specific focus on EF impairments and how they evolve among such a heterogeneous population.

Relation to Restricted and/or Repetitive Behaviours

Challenges with CF are commonly and consistently reported in autism (Lage et al., 2023). This impairment to shift one's cognitive mindset has been associated with the restricted and/or repetitive behaviour (RRB) diagnostic criterion of autism (Faja & Darling, 2019). This connection makes intuitive sense as an inability to flexibly shift from one topic/context to another can be seen to manifest in behaviours such as insistence on sameness and perseverative interests present in many individuals on the spectrum (APA, 2022). Other studies (Lopez et al., 2005; South et al., 2007) have reported links between repetitive behaviours as evaluated on comprehensive autism diagnostic measures such as the ADOS-2 (Lord et al., 2012) and ADI-R (Le Couter et al., 1989).

In addition to CF, other core EFs have been investigated in relation to RRBs. Early work by Turner (1997) found significant correlations between both IN and CF performance with repetitive behaviours. Lopez and colleagues (2005) reported that IN, WM, and CF were negatively correlated to repetitive behaviour. Subsequently, Kenworthy and colleagues (2009) found a strong link between EF and repetitive behaviours in their sample.

More recently, meta-analytical work has reported moderate associations between RRBs and both IN and CF based on both task-based and parental report of autistic children's EF abilities (Iverson & Lewis, 2021). Based on these findings from nearly 3000 participants, Iverson and Lewis suggested that the connection between EF and RRBs, although likely bi-directional, is worthy of continued study to enhance our understanding of causal factors and additional associations related to these constructs.

Relation to Social-Communication Deficits

Regarding social communication, EF impairments are seen to underlie one's control of their behaviour in social contexts (IN), shifting social behaviour or conversational topics depending on the circumstance and situational demands (CF), and holding social information in mind while processing the ever-changing features of social interactions to form appropriate responses (WM; Landa & Goldberg, 2005). Despite this intuitive connection, much less research has focused on links between EF impairments and the social-communication diagnostic domain of autism in comparison to the RRB domain.

Very early work identified that impairments in CF were related to autistic children's difficulties with joint attention, which is the natural tendency to follow the gaze of a social partner that is significantly important in social interaction, communication, and social development (McEvoy et al., 1993). Subsequent research has yielded inconsistent findings with some researchers indicating that EF is related to social and communicative behaviours in autism (Gilotty et al., 2002; Joseph & Tager–Flusberg, 2004; Kenworthy et al., 2009) and others reporting no relation (Bishop & Norbury, 2005a, 2005b). A more recent study comparing autistic children and adolescents to an allistic control group indicated that while IN and CF were related to social functioning in both participant groups, some aspects of EF (WM, planning) predicted social functioning in the autistic sample but not the comparison group (Leung et al., 2016). Overall, the connection between EF and social ability remains tenuous and in need for further investigation.

EF Imaging and Brain Studies in Autism

There is significant evidence linking frontal lobe abnormalities with executive dysfunction in autistic children. Researchers have demonstrated that autistic individuals often exhibit atypical connectivity between the frontal lobe and other brain regions (Doyle-Thomas et al., 2015; Reiter et al., 2019). For example, using fMRI, Juster and colleagues (2020) found reduced connectivity between the frontal cortex and parietal regions in children on the spectrum, which are crucial for integrative functions hypothesized to underlie difficulties in social cognition and executive functions commonly seen in autism. Similarly, Doyle-Thomas and colleagues (2015) found that autistic individuals showed inconsistent connectivity between the posterior cingulate cortex and Default Mode Network areas of the brain, suggesting that the presence of neural atypicalities may impact the development of socio-cognitive abilities in autistic children.

It has also been proposed that autistic symptomatology may be associated with atypical myelination patterns (Galvez-Contreras et al., 2020; Kleinhans et al., 2012). Using diffusion tensor imaging (DTI), Travers et al. (2020) examined white matter integrity in autistic children and reported abnormalities in white matter tracts, specifically in the prefrontal cortex. Impaired myelination could disrupt signal transmission across neural networks, which may lead to difficulty processing social information, a hallmark of autism symptomology. Additional studies have also observed atypical myelination in infants who were later diagnosed with autism (Wolff et al., 2019). These myelination deficits were correlated with atypical social responsiveness, which supports the premise that atypical myelination is related to autism symptom development.

Researchers also suggest that atypical frontal lobe activity and structure itself may be involved in autism (Gilbert et al., 2008; Ha et al., 2015). Han and colleagues (2022) found that autistic children showed significantly weaker prefrontal functional connectivity than neurotypical individuals on tasks requiring speeded processing and accuracy on a novel problem-solving task. This suggests that the structure of the frontal lobe is related to EF in autism. Relatedly, Sokolowski and colleagues (2020) observed reduced activation in the dorsolateral prefrontal cortex (DLPFC) during inhibitory control tasks in children on the spectrum, suggesting that lower activation in this area may underlie difficulties with inhibitory control, emphasizing the role of frontal lobe abnormalities in executive dysfunction in an autism population.

Finally, other research suggests the findings of atypical or delayed postnatal maturation of the frontal lobes in autism (Chomiak et al., 2010; Trutzer et al., 2019). This viewpoint posits that the failure of the frontal lobe to follow a typical maturation pattern leads to long-term consequences in development, reflected in the abnormal development of other connected systems and thus increased expression of autism symptomology (Chomiak et al., 2010).

Results from studies of neurotypical individuals indicate that many brain regions are required for the coordination of EF such as the prefrontal cortex and its connection to the basal ganglia, anterior cingulate cortex, and others (Menon & D'Esposito,

2022; Zink et al., 2021). Generally, ongoing evidence supports the importance of the frontal lobes as the primary location for EF-related activity and coordination in the brain with connections projecting to many other areas (Menon & D'Esposito, 2022). Brain imaging has found both structural and functional differences in frontal lobe functioning in autistic individuals (Taylor et al., 2014). A recent review of neuroimaging in autism by May and Kana (2020) concluded that different brain functioning is observed when autistic individuals are compared to an allistic comparison group during most EF tasks used.

In regard to IN, Voorhies and colleagues (2018) observed differences between autistic children and a comparison group, with the autistic participants showing significantly greater functional connectivity of the right inferior frontal junction with the posterior cingulate gyrus, and left and right frontal poles, demonstrating the differential patterns of brain function when inhibiting responses. Kana et al. (2007) observed similar results in their sample of autistic participants. Despite similar performance to allistic controls on a go/no-go task, the autistic group had poor functional connectivity in fronto-striatial brain regions (Kana et al., 2007). The inconsistency of specific brain areas, and increased versus decreased activation, may be the result of study composition (e.g., age, diagnoses, tasks used, sample size, etc.). Nevertheless, studies support altered brain function during IN tasks and the likelihood of increased effort required for typical cognitive and behavioural IN for autistic individuals.

As WM is proposed to be important for social processing such as facial and emotional expressions (Gambarota & Sessa, 2019), there has been some attention given to brain functioning during WM tasks among autistic individuals. In general, neuroimaging has revealed that a fronto-parietal network is the primary location for WM function in neurotypical individuals (Sala-Llonch et al., 2015). In a meta-analysis of phonological and visuospatial WM tasks comparing autistic individuals and controls, Habib and colleagues (2019) found that WM scores were significantly lower for individuals on the spectrum in both the visuospatial and phonological domains, suggesting impairment in both accuracy and error recognition in both domains for autism. Urbain and colleagues (2015) used magnetoencephalography in children on the spectrum and matched controls during an n-back WM task to examine differences in functional brain activity. Their results showed that autistic children demonstrated reduced activation in the right hippocampus and the cingulate gyrus compared with the controls, who showed greater activation in the left DLPFC and insulae (Urbain et al., 2015). They also reported reduced activity in the ACC, which was correlated with symptom severity in autistic children (Urbain et al., 2015).

Few studies have focused on isolating CF in relation to brain function. Using a set-shifting paradigm adopted from developmental cognitive neuroscience literature involving flexible switching between stimulus categories, Dirks and colleagues (2020) demonstrated that autistic participants showed similar behavioural performance to controls. However, parallel to other neuroimaging research during EF tasks, underlying brain function was different (Dirks et al., 2020). Autistic individuals showed greater activation of the parahippocampal gyrus during performance on trials requiring switching, suggesting that those on the spectrum may leverage memory-based neural systems more so than allistic peers when CF is required (Dirks et al., 2020). In a meta-analysis of CF in autistic individuals, Lage and colleagues (2023) examined 59 studies with an age range of 4 through 85 years. Their results showed that autistic individuals had greater difficulties with CF, with perseverative errors obtaining the largest effect size (Lage et al., 2023); however, this profile is characterised by substantial heterogeneity, particularly in terms of results across the lifespan. This supports the notion that CF, and possibly EF broadly, may improve over time for autistic individuals.

In summary, research supports both structural and functional differences in how autistic individuals demonstrate EF during traditional measures. Primary activity differences between autistic individuals compared with control peers have been observed in the prefrontal cortex, parts of the corpus collosum, fronto-striatial, and fronto-parietal regions (Zhang et al., 2020). Though more research is needed to understand the importance of these findings, there is consensus that the observed differences reflect inefficient brain function and increased effort required for autistic individuals to execute typical EF tasks and behaviours.

EF and Support Needs

As it relates to EF and autism-related behaviours more generally, literature in the recent decade has shifted to the prospects of autism research and support needs for autistic individuals. More specifically, there has been a focus on developing recommendations that are conducive to the long-term benefits of autistic individuals into adulthood, including enhanced quality of life in the areas of autonomy, community participation, and well-being (Lord et al., 2022). Although "no single treatment for autism exists" (Lord et al., 2022, p. 291) owed to the "substantial clinical, biological, and aetiological heterogeneity of autism" (Lai et al., 2020, p. 445), the focus of this section will be EF-related support needs for autism. Importantly, however, the *DSM-5-TR* severity metrics for autism are determined by the level of support individuals require, which highlights the importance of a nuanced understanding of need based on individual profiles (APA, 2022). Therefore, acknowledging the diverse and complex needs of autistic people, community collaboration, systemic change, and the importance of evidence-based interventions are crucial (Lord et al., 2022). In fact, Lai and colleagues (2020) indicated a "framework for the care and support of autistic people across the lifespan" (p. 435) that includes aims of maximizing potential, minimizing barriers, and optimising the person-environment fit.

Further, the type of support autistic individuals require changes with time. Indeed, as autistic individuals develop from the preschool age (where the family's role is of utmost importance) to school-age and adolescence (where the school environment becomes more significant), their need for community support tends to increase in adulthood (Lai et al., 2020; Lord et al., 2022). Nested within this transformation is the need for a multi-disciplinary approach with varied and changing relative significance regarding the roles of professionals, caregivers, community members, systems, and school personnel (see Lai et al., 2020). Still, however, the general trend of support needs of autistic individuals remains or gradually increases while support availability decreases as individuals transition toward adulthood (Bishop-Fitzpatrick et al., 2014; Turcotte et al., 2016).

Generally, although EF difficulties are not a diagnostic feature of autism, attending to the support needs of autistic individuals is important to both bolster quality of life and reduce the negative impacts that EF struggles can have on everyday life (Desideri et al., 2020; de Vries & Geurts, 2015; Fletcher-Watson & Happé, 2019; Wallace et al., 2016). Given the impact of EF on adaptive functioning, autistic individuals typically require support with independence, social functioning, and adaptive communication (Tsermentseli et al., 2018). Further, the play, language, and academic outcomes of autistic children are, in part, predicted by their EF (Faja et al., 2016; Friedman & Sterling, 2019; Pellicano et al., 2017). There are both individual teaching and environmental accommodation or compensatory strategies to support EF difficulties in autistic individuals (Dawson & Guare, 2018). One such compensatory strategy includes assistive technologies for cognition (ATC) that are used for certain EF domains, which include a metacognitive component (e.g., self-monitoring); however, there is a dearth of research regarding the use of ATC, which should be further investigated (Desideri et al., 2020). Given differences in support and cognitive development across the lifespan (Lai et al., 2020; Lord et al., 2022), it is important to consider individual needs of autistic children, adolescents, and adults.

Among children and adolescents, there are practical EF difficulties that permeate both the home and school environment which impact academic and adaptive outcomes, and these tend to increase with age (Tschida & Yerys, 2022). Certainly, the functional impact of these EF impairments highlights the support needs of autistic youth across settings, especially as it pertains to shifting abilities (Tschida & Yerys, 2022), planning, CF, and WM (Kenny et al., 2024). One qualitative study examining EF difficulties for autistic youth highlighted that EF skills varied greatly depending on the context, particularly in unpredictable, demanding, and emotionally charged situations, and this variability may be linked to broader differences in how they process information (Kenny et al., 2024). In schools, the implementation of school-based strategies via Individualized Education Programs (IEPs) to address support needs of autistic youth is mediated by certain factors such as communication between school staff, staff expertise, home-school relationship, and technology use (Duncan et al., 2023). However, primary EF challenges are seldom addressed through IEPs despite these challenges permeating many domains of impairment (e.g., academic success, peer interaction, emotion regulation) among autistic youth (Duncan et al., 2023). As autistic youth develop and tasks become more complex requiring planning, organizing, and prioritising, they report heightened difficulty with executing EF-related tasks (Kenny et al., 2024). Parents expressed concerns regarding a tension between their role as external sources of executive control and providing their children enough opportunities to develop autonomy; a tension mirrored in the youth's apprehension about future demands, highlighting the need for collaborative efforts to reconcile this balance (Kenny et al., 2024). Further, as youth transition toward adulthood, there is a need for schools to support EF skills to enhance functioning in areas such as independence, increased responsibility, employment, and/or post-secondary education

(Pugliese et al., 2024). Indeed, EF skills can help autistic individuals transitioning to adulthood identify their support needs and "self-determine their lives" (Shogren et al., 2021, p. 297).

Like childhood and adolescence, autistic adults require supports to bolster their academic success in post-secondary due to the EF challenges that they experience (Stark & Lindo, 2022). Traditional accommodations in post-secondary (e.g., time extensions) tend to not address EF difficulties and, thus, autistic individuals experience persistent challenges (Anderson et al., 2017; Barnhill, 2014). Certainly, autistic adults require non-academic supports (e.g., skill-based training, mentorship, group therapy, academic strategists) to bolster development of EF skills, such as time-management, organization, CF, WM, and IN (Stark & Lindo, 2022). As autistic adults obtain employment, their reported EF challenges impact both their "self-perceived social and employment functioning" (Woolard et al., 2021, p. 2129). According to these researchers, promoting EF skills in the form of specific interventions or training programmes would optimize autistic adults' employment and social outcomes and, thus, is an area of support need (Woolard et al., 2021).

Overall, EF development has been linked to quality of life and other positive long-term outcomes (Demetriou et al., 2018; Lord et al., 2022; St. John et al., 2021). Further, several studies have identified difficulties in daily life, academic settings, social functioning, and employment, which indicates that EF challenges persist across developmental stages. Despite varying severity metrics for autism and the need for personalized approaches based on individual profiles (APA, 2022), there remains a need for addressing the supports required by autistic individuals for their EF-related challenges. Certainly, given the impact of EF on the everyday life of autistic individuals, the literature contends that support needs for EF across the lifespan is crucial.

Intervention for EF in Autism

To date, there are limited EF interventions specifically designed for individuals on the spectrum. However, there are several interventions that target anxiety and social skills within this population using a cognitive behavioural therapy (CBT) approach (Dawson & Burner, 2011), which also appear to target EF skills (e.g., problem solving; Bauminger, 2002; Stichter et al., 2012). However, these are not considered EF interventions per say. Promisingly, a recently developed EF intervention designed for autistic children, *Unstuck and On Target* (UOT), has shown promising results (Kenworthy et al., 2014). UOT is an intervention that can be implemented in both school and home environments and that targets EF skills such as flexibility, goal setting, and planning. UOT is a cognitive behavioural programme consisting of self-regulation scripts, scaffolding, and visual/verbal cueing. Using a randomized controlled effectiveness trial, Kenworthy and colleagues (2014) found support for the effectiveness of the UOT intervention among autistic children. Specifically, students on the spectrum showed significantly more improvements in problem solving, flexibility, planning/organization, rule following, and transitions, than a comparison group who received a social skills intervention. Nevertheless, these researchers indicated that more studies are required to address questions regarding the ability to streamline this lengthy intervention, as well as examining other components of the intervention (e.g., features of interventionists that affect outcomes, etc.). Overall, there are a variety of books and resources available that address EF development among children and adolescents; however, more research is needed that focuses specifically on EF interventions for individuals on the spectrum.

The remainder of this section describes a variety of strategies that exist to improve EF abilities among children and adolescents in both home and school settings, which are not specific to autism. At home, parenting practices such as scaffolding and structured discipline have been found to support EF development. Scaffolding consists of parents providing support, while also instilling independence in their children to help them reach their goals. Structured discipline, on the other hand, refers to the practice of maintaining consistency with respect to reward and punishment, to ensure that children are reinforced for good behaviour and receive consequences for negative behaviour (Hughes & Ensor, 2009; Rhoades et al., 2011). Although no known formal interventions have been developed, early EF difficulties among preschoolers may be improved by identifying maladaptive parenting practices, and by implementing consistent discipline, scaffolding, and modeling to support the development of EF abilities (Anderson & Reidy, 2012).

Regular aerobic activity has been found to improve EF and prefrontal cortex activity among children and adults (Chaddock et al., 2011; Hillman et al., 2008). Among children in particular, intervention outcomes have been small but significant, suggesting that children between the ages of 7–12 years may show improvements in WM and CF after taking part in fitness training for a few days per week for 60–120 min (Davis et al., 2011; Kamijo et al., 2011). Furthermore, studies have found that martial arts training improves WM and CF, likely because of the behavioural monitoring components of this sport. Importantly, these improvements have been shown to transfer to classroom conduct and remain significant, even when controlling for the aerobic aspects of martial arts (Lakes & Hoyt, 2004). Also, the effects of mindfulness training have shown promise with respect to improving EF abilities. In a study of 7- to 9-year-olds practising mindfulness techniques (e.g., meditation, body awareness, attention regulation), parents and teachers rated significant improvements among child participants' EF due to mindfulness practices (Flook et al., 2010).

Within the classroom setting, teachers may target EF development via specific curriculum add-ons or the use of individualized strategies. Three examples of curricula shown to improve EF include *Tools of the Mind* (TOOLS; Bodrova & Leong, 2007), *Promoting Alternative Thinking Strategies* (PATHS; Kusche & Greenberg, 1994), and the *EF Curriculum Series* (Boseday et al., 2010). Moreover, there are a vast number of individual strategies that can be used in the classroom to accommodate student differences in EF abilities (Winters et al., 2015). For example, to target IN, teachers can place visual cues on desks (e.g., "stop and think!"), use nonverbal cues (e.g., raised hand, finger to nose), or establish sounds with individual students as a cue. Additionally, students who struggle with IN (e.g., blurting out answers) may benefit from universal classroom strategies such as having all students use small white boards to write down their answers to show the teacher. Moreover, students who struggle with CF may have trouble transitioning to different activities (e.g., gym to math). Teachers can assist these students by making classroom routines and activities clear and accessible in advance (e.g., visual schedules) as well as with reminders or warnings throughout the day (e.g., "In 10 min, when this timer goes off, it is time to put our books away"). If students struggle to switch between rule sets (e.g., in math), the use of visual reminders and charts can be useful to accommodate such challenges. Additionally, teachers can help students with WM impairments by breaking complex tasks down into smaller steps, and reminding students to write down steps (e.g., display math work, plan out writing in advance using graphic organizers, take notes while reading to ensure comprehension, etc.). Generally, to support WM, teachers can reduce the amount of information that a student must hold in their mind, which can be done without compromising the overall complexity of the task (Winters et al., 2015).

Finally, computerized training has been explored in both school and home settings as a possible method for improving a variety of EF abilities. The appeal of computerized training is not surprising given the increasing prevalence of technology paired with demands on classroom teachers, such as large class sizes (Otero et al., 2014). The primary focus of computerized training programmes, such as *CogMed*, has been to improve working memory and general attention. Using repeated practice and reinforcement, these programmes aim to produce structural brain changes to improve WM capacity (Klingberg et al., 2005). This modality is an attractive approach to improve EF, especially due to the possibility of delivering interventions in a group setting as well as the reduction of human error in implementation (Otero et al., 2014). Despite the fact that WM has been shown to improve as a result of computerized training (Bergman-Nutley et al., 2011; Wong et al., 2014), a meta-analysis by Melby-Lervag and Hulme (2013) indicated that there appears to be little generalization to other areas of cognitive or academic performance using computerized training (despite improving IN and WM on the tasks used to teach the skills). Nevertheless, due to the appeal of computerized training and its ease of use and availability (e.g., tablets, phones, computers, etc.), research in this area continues to develop.

Implications of Research Findings and Future Directions

Researchers have emphasized differences in neurological structure, function, and the development of EF in autistic individuals. While more investigation is necessary to understand how and when EF development occurs in those on the spectrum, researchers currently hold that such differences among autistic individuals require increased effort to execute typical EF tasks and behaviours. Further, it is important to recognize that EF differences are quite heterogenous among autistic individuals; the type of EF ability and severity of impairment varies across those on the spectrum; as such, EF impairment cannot be defined as a primary feature of autism symptomology. Nonetheless, EF clearly plays a significant role in social communication abilities, RRBs, and important life skills needed for autonomous living.

To advance the field, researchers must identify which individuals on the autism spectrum experience EF impairments, and which do not. This differentiation is critical for determining the most effective EF interventions and tailoring them to individual needs (Geurts et al., 2014a). Although few interventions are explicitly designed for autistic individuals, many indirectly address EF development and execution. Additionally, there are numerous books, resources, and strategies available to support EF development in children more broadly. However, further research is necessary to focus specifically on EF interventions for autistic individuals. This includes assessing the applicability and effectiveness of EF-specific strategies originally developed for allistic populations. Continued development of tools like UOT will be vital in enhancing intervention effectiveness and identifying any additional components that contribute to positive outcomes.

In summary, our understanding of EF in autism has significantly advanced over the past two decades, but further research is needed to explore EF in autism comprehensively across the lifespan. While there is considerable variability in developmental outcomes among autistic individuals, emerging empirical evidence is beginning to shed light on the underlying causes of this condition and its variability (Pellicano, 2012). Initially, the executive dysfunction hypothesis was proposed as a primary explanation for autism; however, it fails to account for the diverse range of autism symptomatology (Yerys et al., 2007). As a result, researchers have shifted away from viewing EF as the sole underlying cause of autism and are instead working toward a deeper understanding of EF development and progression in autistic individuals. Addressing this complex issue will require thorough investigation, likely through longitudinal studies, to evaluate the impact of EF on functional outcomes in autistic children. Insights gained may also hold relevance for children with other developmental disabilities and those who are typically developing.

References

Ahmed, S. F., Ellis, A., Ward, K. P., Chaku, N., & Davis-Kean, P. E. (2022). Working memory development from early childhood to adolescence using two nationally representative samples. *Developmental Psychology, 58*(10), 1962–1973. https://doi.org/10.1037/dev0001396

American Psychiatric Association. (2022). *Diagnostic and statistical manual of mental disorders* (5th ed., Text Rev.). https://doi.org/10.1176/appi.books.9780890425787

Amso, D., & Johnson, S. P. (2005). Selection and inhibition in infancy: Evidence from the spatial negative priming paradigm. *Cognition, 95*(2), B27–B36. https://doi.org/10.1016/j.cognition.2004.08.006

Anderson, A. H., Stephenson, J., & Carter, M. (2017). A systematic literature review of the experiences and supports of students with autism spectrum disorder in post-secondary education. *Research in Autism Spectrum Disorders, 39*, 33–53. https://doi.org/10.1016/j.rasd.2017.04.002

Anderson, P. J., & Reidy, N. (2012). Assessing executive function in preschoolers. *Neuropsychological Review, 22*, 345–360. https://doi.org/10.1007/s11065-012-9220-3

Anderson, V., Anderson, P., Northam, E., Jacobs, R., & Catroppa, C. (2001a). Development of executive functions through late childhood and adolescence in an Australian sample. *Developmental Neuropsychology, 20*(1), 385–406. https://doi.org/10.1207/S15326942DN2001_5
Anderson, V., Northam, E., Hendy, J., & Wrenall, J. (2001b). *Developmental neuropsychology: A clinical approach.* Psychology Press.
Anderson, V., Levin, H. S., & Jacobs, R. (2002). Executive functions after frontal lobe injury: A developmental perspective. In D. T. Stuss & R. T. Knight (Eds.), *Principles of frontal lobe function* (pp. 504–527). Oxford University Press.
Antshel, K. M., Faraone, S. V., Maglione, K., Doyle, A. E., Fried, R., Seidman, L. J., & Biederman, J. (2010). Executive functioning in high-IQ adults with ADHD. *Psychological Medicine, 40*(11), 1909–1918. https://doi.org/10.1017/S0033291709992273
Arain, M., Haque, M., Johal, L., Mathur, P., Nel, W., Rais, A., Sandhu, R., & Sharma, S. (2013). Maturation of the adolescent brain. *Neuropsychiatric Disease and Treatment, 9*, 449–461. https://doi.org/10.2147/NDT.S39776
Ardila, A., Pineda, D., & Rosselli, M. (2000). Correlation between intelligence test scores and executive function measures. *Archives of Clinical Neuropsychology, 15*(1), 31–36. https://doi.org/10.1016/S0887-6177(98)00159-0
Arffa, S. (2007). The relationship of intelligence to executive function and non-executive function measures in a sample of average, above average, and gifted youth. *Archives of Clinical Neuropsychology, 22*, 969–978. https://doi.org/10.1016/j.acn.2007.08.001
Baddeley, A., & Hitch, G. (1974). Working memory. In G. H. Bower (Ed.), *Recent advances in learning and motivation* (Vol. 8). Academic.
Barkley, R. A. (1997). Behavioral inhibition, sustained attention, and executive functions: Constructing a unifying theory of ADHD. *Psychological Bulletin, 121*, 65–94. https://doi.org/10.1037/0033-2909.121.1.65
Barnhill, G. P. (2014). Supporting students with Asperger Syndrome on college campuses. *Focus on Autism and Other Developmental Disabilities, 31*(1), 3–15. https://doi.org/10.1177/1088357614523121
Bauminger, N. (2002). The facilitation of social-emotional understanding and social interaction in high-functioning children with autism: Intervention outcomes. *Journal of Autism and Developmental Disorders, 32*, 283–298. https://doi.org/10.1023/A:1016378718278
Benallie, K. J., McClain, M. B., Bakner, K. E., Roanhorse, T., & Ha, J. (2021). Executive functioning in children with ASD + ADHD and ASD + ID: A systematic review. *Research in Autism Spectrum Disorders, 86*, Article 101807. https://doi.org/10.1016/j.rasd.2021.101807
Bergman-Nutley, S., Soderqvist, S., Bryde, S., Thorell, L. B., Humpreys, K., & Klingberg, T. (2011). Gains in fluid intelligence after training nonverbal reasoning in 4 year old children: A controlled, randomized study. *Developmental Science, 14*, 591–601. https://doi.org/10.1111/j.1467-7687.2010.01022.x
Best, J. R., & Miller, P. H. (2010). A developmental perspective on executive function. *Child Development, 81*(6), 1641–1660. https://doi.org/10.1111/j.1467-8624.2010.01499.x
Biederman, J., Petty, C. R., Fried, R., Black, S., Faneuil, A., Doyle, A. E., & Faraone, S. V. (2008). Discordance between psychometric testing and questionnaire-based definitions of executive function deficits in individuals with ADHD. *Journal of Attention Disorders, 12*, 92–102. https://doi.org/10.1177/1087054707305111
Bishop, D. V. M., & Norbury, C. F. (2005a). Executive functions in children with communication impairments, in relation to autistic symptomology. 1. Generativity. *Autism, 9*, 9–27. https://doi.org/10.1177/1362361305049027
Bishop, D. V. M., & Norbury, C. F. (2005b). Executive functions in children with communication impairments, in relation to autistic symptomology. 2. Response inhibition. *Autism, 9*, 29–43. https://doi.org/10.1177/1362361305049028
Bishop-Fitzpatrick, L., Minshew, N. J., & Eack, S. M. (2014). A systematic review of psychosocial interventions for adults with autism spectrum disorders. *Adolescents and Adults with Autism Spectrum Disorders, 315–327*. https://doi.org/10.1007/978-1-4939-0506-5_16

Bodrova, E., & Leong, D. J. (2007). *Tools of the mind: The Vygotskian approach to early childhood education.* Merrill/Prentice Hall.
Boseday, G., Gidaspow, J., Minton, S., & Smith, M. E. (2010). *Executive functions curriculum notebook series.* Rush University Medical Center Press.
Brady, D. I., Saklofske, D. H., Schwean, V. L., Montgomery, J. M., Thorne, K. J., & McCrimmon, A. W. (2017). Executive functions in young adults with autism spectrum disorder. *Focus on Autism and Other Developmental Disabilities, 32*(1), 31–43. https://doi.org/10.1177/1088357615609306
Brocki, K. C., & Bohlin, G. (2004). Executive functions in children aged 6 to 13: A dimensional and developmental study. *Developmental Neuropsychology, 26*, 571–593. https://doi.org/10.1207/s15326942dn2602_3
Brydges, C. R., Reid, C. L., Fox, A. M., & Anderson, M. (2012). A unitary executive function predicts intelligence in children. *Intelligence, 40*(5), 458–469. https://doi.org/10.1016/j.intell.2012.05.006
Buttelmann, F., & Karbach, J. (2017). Development and plasticity of cognitive flexibility in early and middle childhood. *Frontiers in Psychology, 8*, 1040. https://doi.org/10.3389/fpsyg.2017.01040
Casey, B. J., Amso, D., & Davidson, M. C. (2006). Learning about learning and development with modern imaging technology. In Y. Manukata & M. H. Johnson (Eds.), *Process of change in brain and cognitive development: Attention and performance XXI* (Vol. 21, pp. 513–533). Oxford University Press.
Chaddock, L., Pontifex, M. B., Hillman, C. H., & Kramer, A. F. (2011). A Review of the relation of aerobic fitness and physical activity to brain structure and function in children. *Journal of the International Neuropsychological Society, 17*(6), 975–985. https://doi.org/10.1017/S1355617711000567
Chomiak, T., Karnik, V., Block, E., & Hu, B. (2010). Altering the trajectory of early postnatal cortical development can lead to structural and behavioural features of autism. *BMC Neuroscience, 11*, 1–10.
Chugani, H. T., Phelps, M. E., & Mazziotta, J. C. (1987). Positron emission tomography study of human brain functional development. *Annals of Neurology, 22*, 287–297. https://doi.org/10.1002/ana.410220408
Cordova, M., Shada, K., Demeter, D. V., Doyle, O., Miranda-Dominguez, O., Perrone, A., Schifsky, E., Graham, A., Fombonne, E., Langhorst, B., Nigg, J., Fair, D. A., & Feczko, E. (2020). Heterogeneity of executive function revealed by a functional random forest approach across ADHD and ASD. *NeuroImage: Clinical, 26*, 102245. https://doi.org/10.1016/j.nicl.2020.102245
Cirino, P. T., Ahmed, Y., Miciak, J., Taylor, W. P., Gerst, E. H., & Barnes, M. A. (2018). A framework for executive function in the late elementary years. *Neuropsychology, 32*(2), 176. https://doi.org/10.1037/NEU0000427
Craig, F., Margari, F., Legrottaglie, A. R., Palumbi, R., de Giambattista, C., & Margari, L. (2016). A review of executive function deficits in autism spectrum disorder and attention-deficit/hyperactivity disorder. *Neuropsychiatric Disease and Treatment, 12*, 1191–1202. https://doi.org/10.2147/NDT.S104620
Crinella, F., & Yu, J. (2000). Brain mechanisms and intelligence. Psychometric g and executive function. *Intelligence, 27*(4), 299–327. https://doi.org/10.1016/S0160-2896(99)00021-5
Davis, C. L., Tomporowski, P. D., McDowell, J. E., Austin, B. P., Miller, P. H., Yanasak, N. E., et al. (2011). Exercise improves executive function and achievement and alters brain activation in overweight children: A randomized, controlled trial. *Health Psychology, 30*(1), 91–98. https://doi.org/10.1037/a0021766
Davidson, M. C., Amso, D., Anderson, L. C., & Diamond, A. (2006). Development of cognitive control and executive functions from 4 to 13 years: Evidence from manipulations of memory, inhibition, and task switching. *Neuropsychologia, 44*(11), 2037–2078. https://doi.org/10.1016/j.neuropsychologia.2006.02.006

Dawson, G., & Burner, K. (2011). Behavioral interventions in children and adolescents with autism spectrum disorder: A review of recent findings. *Current Opinion in Pediatrics, 23*, 616–620. https://doi.org/10.1097/MOP.0b013e32834cf082
Dawson, P., & Guare, R. (2018). *Executive skills in children and adolescents: A practical guide to assessment and Intervention.* Guilford Press.
Delis, D. C., Kaplan, E., & Kramer, J. H. (2001). *Delis-Kaplan Executive Function System (D-KEFS).* The Psychological Corporation.
Demetriou, E. A., DeMayo, M. M., & Guastella, A. J. (2019). Executive function in autism spectrum disorder: History, theoretical models, empirical findings, and potential as an endophenotype. *Frontiers in Psychiatry, 10.* https://doi.org/10.3389/fpsyt.2019.00753
Demetriou, E. A., Lampit, A., Quintana, D. S., Naismith, S. L., Song, Y. J., Pye, J. E., Hickie, I., & Guastella, A. J. (2018). Autism spectrum disorders: A meta-analysis of executive function. *Molecular Psychiatry, 23*(5), 1198–1204. https://doi.org/10.1038/mp.2017.75
Desideri, L., Di Santantonio, A., Varrucciu, N., Bonsi, I., & Di Sarro, R. (2020). Assistive technology for cognition to support executive functions in autism: A scoping review. *Advances in Neurodevelopmental Disorders, 4*(4), 330–343. https://doi.org/10.1007/s41252-020-00163-w
de Vries, M., & Geurts, H. (2015). Influence of autism traits and executive functioning on quality of life in children with an autism spectrum disorder. *Journal of Autism and Developmental Disorders, 45*(9), 2734–2743. https://doi.org/10.1007/s10803-015-2438-1
Diamond, A. (2013). Executive functions. *Annual Review of Psychology, 64*, 135. https://doi.org/10.1146/ANNUREV-PSYCH-113011-143750
Diamond, A. (2020). Executive functions. In *Handbook of clinical neurology* (Vol. 173, pp. 225–240). Elsevier B.V. https://doi.org/10.1016/B978-0-444-64150-2.00020-4
Dirks, B., Romero, C., Voorhies, W., Kupis, L., Nomi, J. S., Dajani, D. R., & Uddin, L. Q. (2020). Neural responses to a putative set-shifting task in children with autism spectrum disorder. *Autism Research, 13*(9), 1501–1515. https://doi.org/10.1002/aur.2347
Doyle-Thomas, K. A., Lee, W., Foster, N. E., Tryfon, A., Ouimet, T., Hyde, K. L., & NeuroDevNet ASD Imaging Group. (2015). Atypical functional brain connectivity during rest in autism spectrum disorders. *Annals of Neurology, 77*(5), 866–876.
Duggan, E. C., & Garcia-Barrera, M. A. (2015). Executive functioning and intelligence. In S. Goldstein, D. Princiotta, & J. A. Naglieri (Eds.), *Handbook of intelligence: Evolutionary theory, historical perspective, and current concepts* (pp. 435–458). Springer.
Duncan, A., Risley, S., Combs, A., Lacey, H. M., Hamik, E., Fershtman, C., Kneeskern, E., Patel, M., Crosby, L., Hood, A. M., Zoromski, A. K., & Tamm, L. (2023). School challenges and services related to executive functioning for fully included middle schoolers with autism. *Focus on Autism and Other Developmental Disabilities, 38*(2), 90–100. https://doi.org/10.1177/10883576221110167
Duncan, J., Burgess, P., & Emslie, H. (1995). Fluid intelligence after frontal lobe lesions. *Neuropsychologia, 33*(3), 261–268. https://doi.org/10.1016/0028-3932(94)00124-8
Faja, S., & Darling, L. N. (2019). Variation in restricted and repetitive behaviors and interests relates to inhibitory control and shifting in children with autism spectrum disorder. *Autism, 23*(5), 1262–1272. https://doi.org/10.1177/1362361318804192
Faja, S., Dawson, G., Sullivan, K., Meltzoff, A. N., Estes, A., & Bernier, R. (2016). Executive function predicts the development of play skills for verbal preschoolers with autism spectrum disorders. *Autism Research, 9*(12), 1274–1284. https://doi.org/10.1002/aur.1608
Fletcher-Watson, S., & Happé, F. (2019). *Autism: A new introduction to psychological theory and current debate.* Routledge.
Flook, L., Smalley, S. L., Kitil, M. J., Galla, B. M., Kaiser-Greenland, S., Locke, J., et al. (2010). Effects of mindfulness awareness practices on executive functions in elementary school children. *Journal of Applied School Psychology, 26*, 70–95. https://doi.org/10.1080/15377900903379125

Floyd, R. G., Bergeron, R., Hamilton, G., & Parra, G. R. (2010). How do executive functions fit with the Cattell–Horn–Carroll model? Some evidence from a joint factor analysis of the Delis-Kaplan executive function system and the Woodcock-Johnson III tests of cognitive abilities. *Psychology in the Schools, 47*(7), 721–738. https://doi.org/10.1002/pits.20500

Fossum, I. N., Andersen, P. N., Øie, M. G., & Skogli, E. W. (2021). Development of executive functioning from childhood to young adulthood in autism spectrum disorder and attention-deficit/hyperactivity disorder: A 10-year longitudinal study. *Neuropsychology, 35*(8), 809–821. https://doi.org/10.1037/neu0000768

Friedman, L., & Sterling, A. (2019). A review of language, executive function, and intervention in autism spectrum disorder. *Seminars in Speech and Language, 40*(04), 291–304. https://doi.org/10.1055/s-0039-1692964

Friedman, N. P., Miyake, A., Altamirano, L. J., Corley, R. P., Young, S. E., Rhea, S. A., & Hewitt, J. K. (2016). Stability and change in executive function abilities from late adolescence to early adulthood: A longitudinal twin study. *Developmental Psychology, 52*(2), 326–340. https://doi.org/10.1037/dev0000075

Galvez-Contreras, A. Y., Zarate-Lopez, D., Torres-Chavez, A. L., & Gonzalez-Perez, O. (2020). Role of oligodendrocytes and myelin in the pathophysiology of autism spectrum disorder. *Brain Sciences, 10*(12), 951–968. https://doi.org/10.3390/brainsci10120951

Gambarota, F., & Sessa, P. (2019). Visual working memory for faces and facial expressions as a useful "tool" for understanding social and affective cognition. *Frontiers in Psychology, 10*(2392), 1–7. https://doi.org/10.3389/fpsyg.2019.02392

Garon, N., Bryson, S. E., & Smith, I. M. (2008). Executive function in preschoolers: A review using an integrative framework. *Psychological Bulletin, 134*, 31–60. https://doi.org/10.1037/0033-2909.134.1.31

Gathercole, S. E., Pickering, S. J., Ambridge, B., & Wearing, H. (2004). The structure of working memory from 4 to 15 years of age. *Developmental Psychology, 40*, 177–190. https://doi.org/10.1037/0012-1649.40.2.177

Geurts, H. M., de Vries, M., & Sanne, F. W. M. (2014a). Executive functioning theory and autism. In S. Goldstein & J. A. Naglieri (Eds.), *Handbook of executive functioning* (pp. 121–141). Springer.

Geurts, H. M., van den Bergh, S. F., & Ruzzano, L. (2014b). Prepotent response inhibition and interference control in autism spectrum disorders: Two meta-analyses. *Autism Research, 7*(4), 407–420. https://doi.org/10.1002/aur.1369

Geurts, H. M., & Vissers, M. E. (2012). Elderly with autism: Executive functions and memory. *Journal of Autism and Developmental Disorders, 42*(5), 665–675. https://doi.org/10.1007/s10803-011-1291-0

Gilbert, S. J., Bird, G., Brindley, R., Frith, C. D., & Burgess, P. W. (2008). Atypical recruitment of medial prefrontal cortex in autism spectrum disorders: An FMRI study of two executive function tasks. *Neuropsychologia, 46*(9), 2281–2291.

Gilotty, L., Kenworthy, L., Sirian, L., Black, D. O., & Wagner, A. E. (2002). Adaptive skills and executive function in autism spectrum disorders. *Child Neuropsychology, 8*(4), 241–248. https://doi.org/10.1076/chin.8.4.241.13504

Gioia G. A., Isquith P. K., Guy S. C., Kenworthy L. (2015). *Behavior Rating Inventory of Executive Function®, Second Edition (BRIEF®2)*. PAR Inc.

Gioia, G. A., Isquith, P. K., & Kenealy, L. E. (2008). Assessment of behavioral aspects of executive function. In V. Anderson, R. Jacobs, & P. J. Anderson (Eds.), *Executive functions and the frontal lobes: A lifespan perspective* (pp. 179–202). Psychology Press.

Griffith, E. M., Pennington, B. F., Wehner, E. A., & Rogers, S. J. (1999). Executive functions in young children with autism. *Child Development, 70*(4), 817–832. https://doi.org/10.1111/1467-8624.00059

Ha, S., Sohn, I. J., Kim, N., Sim, H. J., & Cheon, K. A. (2015). Characteristics of brains in autism spectrum disorder: Structure, function and connectivity across the lifespan. *Experimental Neurobiology, 24*(4), 273–284. https://doi.org/10.5607/en.2015.24.4.273

Habib, A., Harris, L., Pollick, F., & Melville, C. (2019). A meta-analysis of working memory in individuals with autism spectrum disorders. *PLoS ONE, 14*(4), Article e0216198.

Han, Y. M., Chan, M. C., Chan, M. M., Yeung, M. K., & Chan, A. S. (2022). Effects of working memory load on frontal connectivity in children with autism spectrum disorder: A FNIRS study. *Scientific Reports, 12*(1), 1522. https://doi.org/10.1038/s41598-022-05432-3

Happé, F., Ronald, A., & Plomin, R. (2006). Time to give up on a single explanation for autism. *Nature Neuroscience, 9*(10), 1218–1220. https://doi.org/10.1038/nn1770

Heaton, R. K., Chelune, G. J., Talley, J. L., Kay, G. G., & Curtis, G. (1993). *Wisconsin Card Sorting Test (WCST) manual—Revised and expanded.* Psychological Assessment Resources, Odessa, FL.

Hillman, C. H., Erickson, K. I., & Kramer, A. F. (2008). Be smart, exercise your heart: Exercise effects on brain and cognition. *Nature Reviews Neuroscience, 9*(1), 58–65. https://doi.org/10.1038/nrn2298

Hughes, C. (1998). Executive function in preschoolers: Links with theory of mind and verbal ability. *British Journal of Developmental Psychology, 16*, 233–253. https://doi.org/10.1111/j.2044-835X.1998.tb00921.x

Hughes, C., & Russell, J. (1993). Autistic children's difficulty with mental disengagement from an object: Its implications for theories of autism. *Developmental Psychology, 29*(3), 498. https://doi.org/10.1037/0012-1649.29.3.498

Hughes, C., Ensor, R., Wilson, A., & Graham, A. (2010). Tracking executive function across the transition to school: A latent variable approach. *Developmental Neuropsychology, 35*(1), 20–36. https://doi.org/10.1080/87565640903325691

Hughes, C. H., & Ensor, R. A. (2009). How do families help or hinder the emergence of early executive function? *New Directions in Child and Adolescent Development, 2009*, 35–50. https://doi.org/10.1002/cd.234

Huizinga, M., Dolan, C. V., & Van der Molen, M. W. (2006). Age-related change in executive function: Developmental trends and a latent variable analysis. *Neuropsychologia, 44*, 2017–2036. https://doi.org/10.1016/j.neuropsychologia.2006.01.010

Iversen, R. K., & Lewis, C. (2021). Executive function skills are linked to restricted and repetitive behaviors: Three correlational meta analyses. *Autism Research, 14*(6), 1163–1185. https://doi.org/10.1002/aur.2468

Johnston, K., Murray, K., Spain, D., Walker, I., & Russell, A. (2019). Executive function: Cognition and behaviour in adults with Autism Spectrum Disorders (ASD). *Journal of Autism and Developmental Disorders, 49*(10), 4181–4192. https://doi.org/10.1007/s10803-019-04133-7

Joseph, R. M., & Tager-Flusberg, H. (2004). The relationship of theory of mind and executive functions to symptom type and severity in children with autism. *Development and Psychopathology, 16*, 137–155. https://doi.org/10.1017/S095457940404444X

Jurado, M. B., & Rosselli, M. (2007). The elusive nature of executive functions: A review of our current understanding. *Neuropsychology Review, 17*, 213–233. https://doi.org/10.1007/s11065-007-9040-z

Juster, R., Rosenthal, M., Goorin, A., & Carpenter, K. (2020). Frontal-parietal connectivity and its role in executive dysfunction in autism spectrum disorder: A resting-state fMRI study. *Journal of Neurodevelopmental Disorders, 12*(3), 445–460.

Kamijo, K., Pnontifex, M. B., O'Leary, K. C., Scudder, M. R., Wu, C. T., Castelli, D. M., et al. (2011). The effects of an afterschool physical activity program on working memory in preadolescent children. *Developmental Science, 14*(5), 1046–1058. https://doi.org/10.1111/j.1467-7687.2011.01054.x

Kana, R. K., Keller, T. A., Minshew, N. J., & Just, M. A. (2007). Inhibitory control in high-functioning autism: Decreased activation and underconnectivity in inhibition networks. *Biological Psychiatry, 62*(3), 198–206. https://doi.org/10.1016/j.biopsych.2006.08.004

Kapp, S. K., Gillespie-Lynch, K., Sherman, L. E., & Hutman, T. (2013). Deficit, difference, or both? Autism and neurodiversity. *Developmental Psychology, 49*(1), 59–71. https://doi.org/10.1037/A0028353

Karbach, J., & Kray, J. (2007). Developmental changes in switching between mental task sets: The influence of verbal labeling in childhood. *Journal of Cognition and Development, 8*(2), 205–236. https://doi.org/10.1080/15248370701202430

Kenny, L., Hattersley, C., Molins, B., Buckley, C., Povey, C., & Pellicano, E. (2016). Which terms should be used to describe autism? Perspectives from the UK autism community. *Autism, 20*(4), 442–462. https://doi.org/10.1177/1362361315588200

Kenny, L., Remington, A., & Pellicano, E. (2024). Everyday executive function issues from the perspectives of autistic adolescents and their parents: Theoretical and empirical implications. *Autism, 28*(9), 2204–2217. https://doi.org/10.1177/13623613231224093

Kenworthy, L., Anthony, L. G., Naiman, D. Q., Cannon, L., Wills, M. C., et al. (2014). Randomized controlled effectiveness trial of executive function intervention for children on the autism spectrum. *Journal of Child Psychology and Psychiatry, 55*(4), 374–383. https://doi.org/10.1111/jcpp.12161

Kenworthy, L., Black, D. O., Harrison, B., Della Rosa, A., & Wallace, G. L. (2009). Are executive control functions related to autism symptoms in high-functioning children? *Child Neuropsychology, 15*(5), 425–440. https://doi.org/10.1080/09297040802646983

Kleinhans, N. M., Pauley, G., Richards, T., Neuhaus, E., Martin, N., Corrigan, N. M., & Dager, S. R. (2012). Age-related abnormalities in white matter microstructure in autism spectrum disorders. *Brain Research, 1479*, 1–16. https://doi.org/10.1016/j.brainres.2012.07.056

Klenberg, L., Korkman, M., & Lahti-Nuutila, P. (2001). Differential development of attention and executive functions in 3- to 12-year-old Finnish children. *Developmental Neuropsychology, 20*, 407–428. https://doi.org/10.1207/S15326942DN2001_6

Klingberg, T., Fernell, E., Olesen, P. J., Johnson, M., Gustafsson, P., Dahlström, K., & Westerberg, H. (2005). Computerized training of working memory in children with ADHD-a randomized, controlled trial. *Journal of the American Academy of Child & Adolescent Psychiatry, 44*(2), 177–186. https://doi.org/10.1097/00004583-200502000-00010

Korkman, M., Kirk, U., & Kemp, S. (2007). *NEPSY-II: Clinical and interpretive manual.* Pearson.

Kusche, C. A., & Greenberg, M. T. (1994). *The PATHS curriculum.* Developmental Research and Programs.

Lage, C., Smith, E. S., & Lawson, R. P. (2023). A Meta-analysis of cognitive flexibility in autism spectrum disorder. *Neuroscience & Biobehavioral Reviews, 157*, Article 105511. https://doi.org/10.1016/j.neubiorev.2023.105511

Lai, C. L., Lau, Z., Lui, S. S., Lok, E., Tam, V., Chan, Q., Cheng, K. M., Lam, S. M., & Cheung, E. F. (2017). Meta-analysis of neuropsychological measures of executive functioning in children and adolescents with high-functioning autism spectrum disorder. *Autism Research, 10*(5), 911–939. https://doi.org/10.1002/aur.1723

Lai, M.-C., Anagnostou, E., Wiznitzer, M., Allison, C., & Baron-Cohen, S. (2020). Evidence-based support for autistic people across the lifespan: Maximising potential, minimising barriers, and optimising the person–environment fit. *The Lancet Neurology, 19*(5), 434–451. https://doi.org/10.1016/s1474-4422(20)30034-x

Lai, M.-C., Kassee, C., Besney, R., Bonato, S., Hull, L., Mandy, W., Szatmari, P., & Ameis, S. H. (2019). Prevalence of co-occurring mental health diagnoses in the autism population: A systematic review and meta-analysis. *The Lancet Psychiatry, 6*(10), 819–829. https://doi.org/10.1016/s2215-0366(19)30289-5

Lakes, K. D., & Hoyt, W. T. (2004). Promoting self-regulation through school based martial arts training. *Applied Developmental Psychology, 25*, 283–302. https://doi.org/10.1016/j.appdev.2004.04.002

Landa, R. J., & Goldberg, M. C. (2005). Language, social, and executive functions in high functioning autism: A continuum of performance. *Journal of Autism and Developmental Disorders, 35*(5), 557–573. https://doi.org/10.1007/s10803-005-0001-1

Larsen, B., & Luna, B. (2018). Adolescence as a neurobiological critical period for the development of higher-order cognition. *Neuroscience and Biobehavioral Reviews, 94*, 179–195. https://doi.org/10.1016/j.neubiorev.2018.09.005

Laureys, F., De Waelle, S., Barendse, M. T., Lenoir, M., & Deconinck, F. J. A. (2022). The factor structure of executive function in childhood and adolescence. *Intelligence, 90*. https://doi.org/10.1016/j.intell.2021.101600
Le Couter, A., Rutter, M., Lord, C., Rios, P., Robertson, S., Holdgrafer, M., et al. (1989). Autism diagnostic interview: A standardized investigator-based instrument. *Journal of Autism and Developmental Disorders, 19*, 363–387. https://doi.org/10.1007/BF02212936
Lehto, J. E., Juujärvi, P., Kooistra, L., & Pulkkinen, L. (2003). Dimensions of executive functioning: Evidence from children. *British Journal of Developmental Psychology, 21*(1), 59–80. https://doi.org/10.1348/026151003321164627
Leung, R. C., Vogan, V. M., Powell, T. L., Anagnostou, E., & Taylor, M. J. (2016). The role of executive functions in social impairment in autism spectrum disorder. *Child Neuropsychology, 22*(3), 336–344. https://doi.org/10.1080/09297049.2015.1005066
Lezak, M. D. (1983). *Neuropsychological assessment* (2nd ed.). Oxford University Press.
Lord, C., Charman, T., Havdahl, A., Carbone, P., Anagnostou, E., Boyd, B., Carr, T., de Vries, P. J., Dissanayake, C., Divan, G., Freitag, C. M., Gotelli, M. M., Kasari, C., Knapp, M., Mundy, P., Plank, A., Scahill, L., Servili, C., Shattuck, P., & McCauley, J. B. (2022). The Lancet Commission on the future of care and clinical research in autism. *The Lancet, 399*(10321), 271–334. https://doi.org/10.1016/s0140-6736(21)01541-5
Lord, C., Rutter, M., DiLavore, P. C., Risi, S., Gotham, K., & Bishop, S. (2012). *Autism diagnostic observation schedule* (2nd ed.). Western Psychological Services.
Lopez, B. R., Linoln, A. J., Ozonoff, S., & Lai, Z. (2005). Examining the relationship between executive functions and restricted, repetitive symptoms of autistic disorder. *Journal of Autism and Developmental Disorders, 35*, 445–460. https://doi.org/10.1007/s10803-005-5035-x
Luna, B., Marek, S., Larsen, B., Tervo-Clemmens, B., & Chahal, R. (2015). An integrative model of the maturation of cognitive control. *Annual Review of Neuroscience, 38*, 151–170. https://doi.org/10.1146/annurev-neuro-071714-034054
Luria, A. (1966). *Higher cortical functions in man*. Basic Books Inc.
Margari, L., Craig, F., Margari, F., Legrottaglie, A., Palumbi, R., & De Giambattista, C. (2016). A review of executive function deficits in autism spectrum disorder and attention-deficit/hyperactivity disorder. *Neuropsychiatric Disease and Treatment, 1191*. https://doi.org/10.2147/ndt.s104620
May, K. E., & Kana, R. K. (2020). Frontoparietal network in executive functioning in autism spectrum disorder. *Autism Research, 13*(10), 1762–1777. https://doi.org/10.1002/aur.2403
McEvoy, R. E., Rogers, S. J., & Pennington, B. F. (1993). Executive function and social communication deficits in young autistic children. *Journal of Child Psychology and Psychiatry, 34*(4), 563–578. https://doi.org/10.1111/j.1469-7610.1993.tb01036.x
McGrew, K. S. (2009). CHC theory and the human cognitive abilities project: Standing on the shoulders of the giants of psychometric intelligence research. *Intelligence, 37*, 1–10. https://doi.org/10.1016/j.intell.2008.08.004
Melby-Lervag, M., & Hulme, C. (2013). Is working memory training effective? A meta-analytic review. *Developmental Psychology, 49*, 270–291. https://doi.org/10.1037/a0028228
Menon, V., & D'Esposito, M. (2022). The role of PFC networks in cognitive control and executive function. *Neuropsychopharmacology, 47*(1), 90–103. https://doi.org/10.1038/s41386-021-01152-w
Metcalfe, J., & Mischel, W. (1999). A hot/cool-system analysis of delay of gratification: Dynamics of willpower. *Psychological Review, 106*, 3–19. https://doi.org/10.1037/0033-295X.106.1
Miller, E., & Cohen, J. (2001). An integrative theory of prefrontal cortex function. *Annual Review of Neuroscience, 24*(1), 167–202. https://doi.org/10.1146/annurev.neuro.24.1.167
Miyake, A., & Friedman, N. P. (2012). The nature and organization of individual differences in executive functions four general conclusions. *Current Directions in Psychological Science, 21*(1), 8–14. https://doi.org/10.1177/0963721411429458
Miyake, A., Friedman, N. P., Emerson, M. J., Witzki, A. H., Howerter, A., & Wager, T. D. (2000). The unity and diversity of executive functions and their contributions to complex "frontal lobe"

tasks: A latent variable analysis. *Cognitive Psychology, 41*, 49–100. https://doi.org/10.1006/cogp.1999.0734
Naglieri, J. A., & Goldstein, S. (2013). *Comprehensive executive function inventory*. Multi-Health Systems Inc.
Nigg, J. T. (2000). On inhibition/disinhibition in developmental psychopathology: Views from cognitive and personality psychology and a working inhibition taxonomy. *Psychological Bulletin, 126*, 220–246. https://doi.org/10.1037/0033-2909.126.2.220
Otero, T. M., Barker, L. A., & Naglieri, J. A. (2014). Executive function treatment and intervention in schools. *Applied Neuropsychology: Child, 3*(3), 205–214. https://doi.org/10.1080/21622965.2014.897903
Ozonoff, S., Pennington, B. F., & Rogers, S. J. (1991). Executive function deficits in high-functioning autistic individuals: Relationship to theory of mind. *Journal of Child Psychology and Psychiatry, 32*(7), 1081–1105. https://doi.org/10.1111/j.1469-7610.1991.tb00351.x
Pellicano, E. (2010). The development of core cognitive skills in autism: A 3-year prospective study. *Child Development, 81*(5), 1400–1416. https://doi.org/10.1111/j.1467-8624.2010.01481.x
Pellicano, E. (2012). The development of executive function in autism. Autism research and treatment, 2012: Article ID 146132. https://doi.org/10.1155/2012/146132
Pellicano, E., Kenny, L., Brede, J., Klaric, E., Lichwa, H., & McMillin, R. (2017). Executive function predicts school readiness in autistic and typical preschool children. *Cognitive Development, 43*, 1–13. https://doi.org/10.1016/j.cogdev.2017.02.003
Pugliese, C. E., Werner, M. A., Alexander, K. C., Cannon, L., Strang, J. F., Caplan, R., Klinger, L., Mandell, D., Dieckhaus, M., Handsman, R., Kenworthy, L., & Anthony, L. G. (2024). Development of a high school-based executive function intervention for transition-age autistic youth: Leveraging multi-level community partnerships. *School Mental Health, 16*(3), 862–878. https://doi.org/10.1007/s12310-024-09661-x
Reiter, M. A., Mash, L. E., Linke, A. C., Fong, C. H., Fishman, I., & Müller, R. A. (2019). Distinct patterns of atypical functional connectivity in lower-functioning autism. *Biological Psychiatry: Cognitive Neuroscience and Neuroimaging, 4*(3), 251–259.
Reynolds, M. R., Niileksela, C. R., Gignac, G. E., & Sevillano, C. N. (2022). Working memory capacity development through childhood: A longitudinal analysis. *Developmental Psychology, 58*(7), 1254–1263. https://doi.org/10.1037/dev0001360
Rhoades, B. L., Greenberg, M. T., Lanza, S. T., & Blair, C. (2011). Demographic and familial predictors of early executive function development: Contribution of a person-centered perspective. *Journal of Experimental Child Psychology, 108*(3), 638–662. https://doi.org/10.1016/j.jecp.2010.08.004
Sala-Llonch, R., Palacios, E. M., Junqué, C., Bargalló, N., & Vendrell, P. (2015). Functional networks and structural connectivity of visuospatial and visuoperceptual working memory. *Frontiers in Human Neuroscience, 9*(340), 1–9. https://doi.org/10.3389/fnhum.2015.00340
Salehinejad, M. A., Ghanavati, E., Rashid, M. H. A., & Nitsche, M. A. (2021). Hot and cold executive functions in the brain: A prefrontal-cingular network. *Brain and Neurosciences Advances, 5*, 1–9. https://doi.org/10.1177/23982128211007769
Shogren, K. A., Mosconi, M. W., Raley, S. K., Dean, E. E., Edwards, B., Wallisch, A., Boyd, B., & Kiblen, J. C. (2021). Advancing the personalization of assessment and intervention in autistic adolescents and young adults by targeting self-determination and executive processes. *Autism in Adulthood, 3*(4), 289–299. https://doi.org/10.1089/aut.2021.0010
Sokolowski, H. M., Lewandowski, E., & Sabbagh, M. A. (2020). Frontal lobe hypoactivation during inhibition tasks in children with autism spectrum disorder. *Cognitive, Affective, & Behavioral Neuroscience, 20*(3), 560–572.
South, M., Ozonoff, S., & McMahon, W. M. (2007). The relationship between executive functioning, central coherence, and repetitive behaviors in the high-functioning autism spectrum. *Autism, 11*, 437–451. https://doi.org/10.1177/1362361307079606
Spear, L. P. (2013). Adolescent neurodevelopment. *The Journal of Adolescent Health: Society for Adolescent Medicine, 52*(2 Suppl 2), S7–S13. https://doi.org/10.1016/j.jadohealth.2012.05.006

Stark, M. D., & Lindo, E. J. (2022). Executive functioning supports for college students with an autism spectrum disorder. *Review Journal of Autism and Developmental Disorders, 10*(4), 604–614. https://doi.org/10.1007/s40489-022-00311-z

Stichter, J. P., O'Connor, K. V., Herzog, M. J., Lierheimer, K., & McGhee, S. D. (2012). Social competence intervention for elementary students with Aspergers syndrome and high functioning autism. *Journal of Autism and Developmental Disorders, 42*, 354–366.

St. John, T., Woods, S., Bode, T., Ritter, C., & Estes, A. (2021). A review of executive functioning challenges and strengths in autistic adults. *The Clinical Neuropsychologist, 36*(5), 1116–1147. https://doi.org/10.1080/13854046.2021.1971767

Taylor, M. J., Doesburg, S. M., & Pang, E. W. (2014). Neuromagnetic vistas into typical and atypical development of frontal lobe functions. *Frontiers in Human Neuroscience, 8*(453), 1–12. https://doi.org/10.3389/fnhum.2014.00453

Tervo-Clemmens, B., Calabro, F. J., Parr, A. C., Fedor, J., Foran, W., & Luna, B. (2023). A canonical trajectory of executive function maturation from adolescence to adulthood. *Nature Communications, 14*(1). https://doi.org/10.1038/s41467-023-42540-8

Toplak, M. E., West, R. F., & Stanovich, K. E. (2013). Practitioner review: Do performance-based measures and ratings of executive function assess the same construct? *Journal of Child Psychology and Psychiatry, 54*(2), 131–143. https://doi.org/10.1111/jcpp.12001

Travers, B. G., Ennis, C., & Alexander, A. L. (2020). Altered myelination in autism spectrum disorder and its impact on connectivity: A diffusion imaging study. *Brain Connectivity, 10*(5), 323–334.

Trutzer, I. M., García-Cabezas, M. Á., & Zikopoulos, B. (2019). Postnatal development and maturation of layer 1 in the lateral prefrontal cortex and its disruption in autism. *Acta Neuropathologica Communications, 7*, 1–23.

Tschida, J. E., & Yerys, B. E. (2022). Real-world executive functioning for autistic children in school and home settings. *Autism, 26*(5), 1095–1107. https://doi.org/10.1177/13623613211041189

Tsermentseli, S., Tabares, J. F., & Kouklari, E. C. (2018). The role of every-day executive function in social impairment and adaptive skills in autism spectrum disorder with intellectual disability. *Research in Autism Spectrum Disorders, 53*, 1–6. https://doi.org/10.1016/j.rasd.2018.05.006

Turcotte, P., Mathew, M., Shea, L. L., Brusilovskiy, E., & Nonnemacher, S. L. (2016). Service needs across the lifespan for individuals with autism. *Journal of Autism and Developmental Disorders, 46*(7), 2480–2489. https://doi.org/10.1007/s10803-016-2787-4

Turner, M. A. (1997). Towards an executive dysfunction account of repetitive behaviour in autism. In J. Russel (Ed.), *Autism as an executive disorder* (pp. 57–100). Oxford University Press.

Urbain, C. M., Pang, E. W., & Taylor, M. J. (2015). Atypical spatiotemporal signatures of working memory brain processes in autism. *Translational Psychiatry, 5*(8), e617–e617. https://doi.org/10.1038/tp.2015.107

Van Eylen, L., Boets, B., Steyaert, J., Wagemans, J., & Noens, I. (2015). Executive functioning in autism spectrum disorders: Influence of task and sample characteristics and relation to symptom severity. *European Child & Adolescent Psychiatry, 24*(11), 1399–1417. https://doi.org/10.1007/s00787-015-0689-1

Voorhies, W., Dajani, D. R., Vij, S. G., Shankar, S., Turan, T. O., & Uddin, L. Q. (2018). Aberrant functional connectivity of inhibitory control networks in children with autism spectrum disorder. *Autism Research, 11*(11), 1468–1478. https://doi.org/10.1002/aur.2014

Wallace, G. L., Yerys, B. E., Peng, C., Dlugi, E., Anthony, L. G., & Kenworthy, L. (2016). Assessment and treatment of executive function impairments in autism spectrum disorder: An update. *International Review of Research in Developmental Disabilities, 85–122*. https://doi.org/10.1016/bs.irrdd.2016.07.004

Wang, Y., Zhang, Y., Liu, L., Cui, J., Wang, J., Shum, D. H., van Amelsvoort, T., & Chan, R. C. (2017). A meta-analysis of working memory impairments in autism spectrum disorders. *Neuropsychology Review, 27*(1), 46–61. https://doi.org/10.1007/s11065-016-9336-y

Wechsler, D. (1944). *The measurement of adult intelligence*. Williams & Wilkins.

White, S. J. (2013). The triple I hypothesis: Taking another('s) perspective on executive dysfunction in autism. *Journal of Autism and Developmental Disorders, 43*(1), 114–121. https://doi.org/10.1007/s10803-012-1550-8

Wiebe, S. A., Espy, K. A., & Charek, D. (2008). Using confirmatory factor analysis to understand executive control in preschool children: 1. Latent structure. *Developmental Psychology, 44*(2), 575–587. https://doi.org/10.1037/0012-1649.44.2.575

Wiebe, S. A., Sheffield, T., Nelson, J. M., Clark, C. A. C., Chevalier, N., & Espy, K. A. (2011). The structure of executive function in 3-year-olds. *Journal of Experimental Child Psychology, 108*(3), 436–587. https://doi.org/10.1016/j.jecp.2010.08.008

Willoughby, M. T., Blair, C. B., Wirth, R. J., & Greenberg, M. (2010). The measurement of executive function at age 3 years: Psychometric properties and criterion validity of a new battery of tasks. *Psychological Assessment, 22*(2), 306–317. https://doi.org/10.1037/a0018708

Willoughby, M. T., Wirth, R. J., & Blair, C. B. (2011). Contributions of modern measurement theory to measuring executive function in early childhood: An empirical demonstration. *Journal of Experimental Child Psychology, 108*(3), 414–435. https://doi.org/10.1016/j.jecp.2010.04.007

Winters, K., Altomare, A., Colp, M., & Matchullis, R. (2015). Classroom strategies for students with special needs. In J. Andrews & J. L. Lupart (Eds.), *Diversity education: Understanding and addressing student diversity* (pp. 601–620). Nelson Education.

Wolff, J. J., Gerig, G., & Piven, J. (2019). Delayed myelination and its relationship to social and cognitive development in autism: Evidence from a longitudinal study of infants at risk. *Translational Psychiatry, 9*(1), 234–246. https://doi.org/10.1016/j.jaac.2020.07.910

Wong, A. S., He, M. Y., & Chan, R. W. (2014). Effectiveness of computerized working training program in Chinese community settings for children with poor working memory. *Journal of Attention Disorders, 18*(4), 318–330. https://doi.org/10.1177/1087054712471427

Woolard, A., Stratton, E., Demetriou, E. A., Boulton, K. A., Pellicano, E., Glozier, N., Gibbs, V., Rogerson, N., Quinn, P., Hickie, I. B., & Guastella, A. J. (2021). Perceptions of social and work functioning are related to social anxiety and executive function in autistic adults. *Autism, 25*(7), 2124–2134. https://doi.org/10.1177/13623613211013664

Yerys, B. E., Hepburn, S. L., Pennington, B. F., & Rogers, S. J. (2007). Executive function in preschoolers with autism: Evidence consistent with a secondary deficit. *Journal of Autism and Developmental Disorders, 37*(6), 1068–1079. https://doi.org/10.1007/s10803-006-0250-7

Zelazo, P. D. (2020). Executive function and psychopathology: A neurodevelopmental perspective. *Annual Review of Clinical Psychology, 16*(1), 431–454. https://doi.org/10.1146/annurev-clinpsy-072319-024242

Zelazo, P. D., & Frye, D. (1998). Cognitive complexity and control: The development of executive function in childhood. *Current Directions in Psychological Science, 7*, 121–126. https://doi.org/10.1111/1467-8721.ep10774761

Zhang, Z., Peng, P., & Zhang, D. (2020). Executive function in high-functioning autism spectrum disorder: A meta-analysis of fMRI studies. *Journal of Autism and Developmental Disorders, 50*, 4022–4038. https://doi.org/10.1007/s10803-020-04461-z

Zink, N., Lenartowicz, A., & Markett, S. (2021). A new era for executive function research: On the transition from centralized to distributed executive functioning. *Neuroscience & Biobehavioral Reviews, 124*, 235–244.

Forensic Mental Health Assessments for Individuals with Autism Spectrum Disorder

A. J. McConnell, Lindsay Lewandowski, Michael Mayo, and Bob Stinson

Abstract This chapter provides an overview of the interaction between individuals with autism spectrum disorder and the legal system, highlighting the need for professionals to utilize a neurodevelopmental framework when completing a forensic mental health assessment for this population. Common types of forensic mental health assessments requested by courts and attorneys are described. Specifically, assessments focusing on psycholegal issues related to competency to stand trial, criminal responsibility/the insanity defense, risk assessment, and guardianship are addressed. Given the lack of specific training and best practices available for assessing individuals with autism spectrum disorder in forensic contexts, ethical considerations and strategies for completing a forensic mental health assessment are provided.

Keywords Autism spectrum disorder · Forensic psychology · Competency to stand trial · Guardianship · Criminal responsibility · Forensic mental health assessment · Testimony

The interaction between individuals with Autism Spectrum Disorder (ASD) and the legal system is increasing, raising concerns among judges and attorneys regarding these individuals' diagnosis of ASD and how it impacts their functional capabilities relevant to psycholegal issues and court proceedings. Debate exists regarding the exact prevalence rates of individuals diagnosed with ASD being charged with a crime or encountering other legal issues related to court involvement. Some studies

A. J. McConnell (✉)
Alvis, Inc., Columbus, OH, US
e-mail: allen.mcconnell@alvis180.org

L. Lewandowski
Littleton, Colorado, US

M. Mayo
Capella University, Westerville, OH, US

B. Stinson
Forum Ohio, LLC, Columbus, OH, US

J. L. Matson (ed.), *Assessment and Diagnosis in Autism*, Autism and Child Psychopathology Series, https://doi.org/10.1007/978-3-032-11802-8_11

suggest individuals with ASD are similar or less likely to be involved with the legal system compared to the general population (King & Murphy, 2014; Lindsay et al., 2014), while others contend they are overrepresented (Collins et al., 2023; Loureiro et al., 2018). Additionally, it is posited that individuals with ASD are more likely to interact with law enforcement than the general population (Browning & Caulfield, 2011; Lindsay et al., 2014; Rainer & Linksey, 2020). Research indicates that at least 20% of individuals with ASD have had contact with the police or legal system by the age of 22 years old (Rainer & Linksey, 2020; Rava et al., 2017). It is therefore a strong likelihood that forensic mental health professionals working in the forensic domain will be asked to complete a forensic mental health assessment (FMHA) on an individual with ASD.

Given the increasing frequency of requests for forensic mental health professionals to assess individuals with ASD for legal matters, it is imperative that FMHAs adhere to ethical guidelines and emphasize the relevant functional capacities that may be impacted by virtue of the individual's diagnosis. However, there is a dearth of training, research, and attention from researchers and practitioners regarding best practices for assessing and evaluating this population in forensic settings. Consequently, there are few forensic mental health professionals who specialize in both FMHAs and neurodevelopmental disorders (Brown, 2017). From an ethical standpoint, mental health professionals must possess sufficient experience working with individuals with ASD to conduct a thorough and precise assessment (American Psychological Association [APA], 2017). To cultivate competency in this area, this chapter aims to provide information on ASD characteristics pertinent to common forensic assessments requested by courts and attorneys, and strategies for conducting effective FMHAs.

Prevalence of Individuals with ASD Involved in Criminal Cases

When reviewing literature that concentrates on ASD it is first important to take note of how the researchers are demarcating their subject groups. While there are consistent characteristics of ASD across various forms of literature, there are great variations in how it is distinguished. Some researchers design subject groups based on historical ASD diagnoses, while others utilize ASD characteristics alone. Some articles define ASD groups by qualifications for developmental disabilities, and others center on types of services that subjects receive. These differences in how various researchers define ASD and utilize criteria to create subject groups can contribute to inconsistent data findings and disparities in implications that are drawn. Whenever reviewing literature about ASD populations, it is important to ensure special attention is given to how the researcher(s) define their subject groups, and how that may or may not relate to a particular case.

Additionally, it is important to highlight the multi-faceted nature of the ASD diagnosis itself. Although an ASD diagnosis is characterized by 3 symptoms of social communication deficits and 2 to 4 symptoms of restricted and repetitive behaviors with a developmental onset, individuals with a diagnosis of ASD can vary greatly in their presentations. For example, they may have an accompanying intellectual impairment or language impairment, and their symptoms are categorized by assigning one of three levels of severity for each symptom category. Forensic mental health professionals are encouraged to recognize that these diagnostic distinctions will alter a variety of factors related to a particular case, including the applicability of relevant literature and data.

Furthermore, there have been a remarkable number of individuals with ASD who went undiagnosed until their adult years. How forensic mental health professionals and researchers have understood and conceptualized ASD has changed drastically over the last 10 years. Original prevalence rates were thought to be 1 in 100, but more recent literature has highlighted prevalence rates as high as 1 in 59 (Baio, 2018; Railey et al., 2020). In 2022, the CDC calculated the rate of ASD in children between the ages of four years and eight years to be 1 in 31 (Shaw et al., 2022). This is likely not only due to the major shift in diagnostic criteria that was released with the fifth edition of the Diagnostic and Statistical Manual of Mental Disorders (DSM-5, American Psychiatric Association, 2013), but also to our understanding of how ASD can manifest. Historically, only individuals with the most overt and glaring symptoms of ASD were diagnosed. Rigidity was seen solely as strong adherence to routines, and stereotyped behaviors centered on rapid and rhythmic body movements. Lack of eye contact, delayed verbal developmental milestones, and lack of friendships were also key indicators. What mental health professionals now know, however, is that rigidity in thought processes, difficulty with transitions, black-and-white rule following and problem solving, restricted interests that lead to expertise, and trouble with perspective taking are more subtle but clear indicators of ASD. For many adults, ASD has gone undiagnosed due to the more covert nature of their symptoms. Rather than being seen through the lens of neurodivergence, these individuals have been viewed as rigid, unsympathetic, egocentric, and even grandiose at times. Monologuing, dominating conversations, and failing to read social cues may have been incorrectly discerned as undesirable personality traits, rather than a manifestation of social communication deficits. Understanding how ASD can manifest in adults without intellectual or language impairments, who have average to above average functioning, is key. Within the legal system, forensic mental health professionals are likely to encounter adolescents and adults who were not identified as neurodivergent in childhood. Thus, becoming more familiar with how ASD can present in these populations will be an important part of a clinician's work.

Criminal Involvement in Individuals with ASD

There are great inconsistencies in the literature surrounding the prevalence of ASD in juvenile and criminal justice systems. Cheely et al. (2012) conducted a study on youth diagnosed with ASD and found that out of 609 people between the ages of 12 and 18 years old, 5% were charged with offenses. Similarly, Yu et al. (2021) found that about 3% of individuals diagnosed with ASD have been charged with at least one offense by the time they reach adulthood. There are, however, some common themes across research. King and Murphy (2014) undertook a systematic review of people with ASD and their involvement in the criminal justice system. The review focused on two types of research studies: those that reviewed findings of individuals with ASD already in the criminal justice system, and those that reviewed criminal justice involvement within the ASD population. Only papers that included a DSM-IV-TR or ICD-10 diagnosis were included. They concluded that individuals who were diagnosed with ASD were neither over nor underrepresented in the criminal justice system. Despite this, they noted a wide range of results in their review, namely, prevalence of ASD in offender populations was as low as 3% and as high as 27%. When assessing rates of offending behavior in individuals who are diagnosed with ASD, prevalence again varied greatly, with some articles citing a 2.74% prevalence rate and others citing a rate as high as 48% for individuals who self-reported offending behavior. All of these rates exceed the 1% diagnostic prevalence rate cited in the article, which suggests some level of disproportionality.

King and Murphy (2014) further noted inconsistent results when researchers tried to assess the prevalence of different types of offending behavior. Again, these results varied greatly. Some articles showed little difference in types of offenses, whereas others showed increased rates of sexual crimes, arson, and school disturbances. Some literature reported higher rates of violent conduct and threatening behaviors, but only when assessing those with ASD in psychiatric facilities, suggesting the setting and context may contribute to the elevated rates and not the ASD diagnosis itself. Overall, the authors argued that sample bias and poor methodology were the primary reasons for these discrepancies across research results. They noted that inclusion criteria, type of criminal justice setting, comorbid diagnoses, and comparison groups were a few of the factors that influenced results.

Several years after the King and Murphy article was released, a number of updated studies and reviews were conducted to expand upon the original data that was published in 2014. In 2020, Railey et al. (2020) published a scoping, rather than systematic, literature review of 55 articles centered on individuals with ASD and their involvement in the criminal justice system. The article broadened their definition of what they considered to be "involvement" in the system, to include perpetrators, victims, those involved in domestic disputes or elopements, and witnesses. Railey et al. (2020) not only again noted the wide range in ASD and criminal justice prevalence rates, but they also explored literature in the following categories: characteristics and profiles of people with ASD in the criminal justice system; autism community experiences with and perceptions of the criminal justice system; interviewing individuals with ASD within the criminal justice system; and professionals' knowledge, experiences, and training related to ASD. They concluded that, while proportions vary, interactions between ASD and the criminal justice system are not uncommon. They reasoned that more training is needed to support individuals who are involved in these proceedings.

In 2023, Collins et al. distributed another systematic review in an attempt to update the data published in 2014 by King and Murphy. The authors reviewed 47 papers all published after 2013, using the same inclusion criteria as King and Murphy. The authors continued to highlight the challenges in cross comparing literature based on differences in methodology and subject groups. For example, Collins et al. (2023) noted that prevalence of ASD in the criminal justice system varied from 0.2% (in a sample of offenders across several detainment facilities) to as high as 62.8% (when surveying a juvenile court ordered sexual offender program), suggesting that perhaps juvenile sexual offenses may be a particular area of interest in the population. When examining criminal justice involvement in the ASD community, rates varied from 0.7% to 5%.

Furthermore, types of offenses included arson, property crime, sexual offending, drug offenses, traffic incidents, stalking, fraud, theft, and robbery, but rates differed between studies, as did the prevalence of comorbid diagnoses (Collins et al., 2023). Additional risk factors highlighted among ASD offenders included being male, single, not having children, presence of birth defects, childhood behavioral difficulties, low educational achievement, history of aggression, offending/antisocial behavior, sexually inappropriate behavior, substance use, and victimization. They noted that few studies used comparisons to explore unique characteristics or similarities, but one finding did highlight difficulties in understanding and following trial processes and proceedings. This is particularly relevant for forensic mental health professionals conducting competency to stand trial evaluations. The authors also underlined a dearth of information regarding female offenders. Again, the range in diagnostic methodologies and biased samples were cited as an area of concern in determining the rates.

Across the literature, there is consistent variability in rates that explore the relationship between criminal justice involvement and individuals who are diagnosed with ASD. What is clear, and what these authors find important to highlight, however, is that individuals with ASD are represented to some extent in the juvenile and criminal justice systems and, thus, it is important that professionals be aware of how to identify neurodivergent populations, as well as how their symptoms may factor into their offending behaviors and the relevance of their symptom presentation as it relates to various forensic mental health assessments.

Clinical Frameworks for Explaining Offending Behaviors Related to ASD

In addition to being aware of what is noted in the literature about ASD and criminal justice involvement, it is important for forensic mental health professionals to be familiar with the clinical symptoms of ASD, and ways in which they may contribute to offending behaviors and impact on FMHAs.

As discussed in Howlin (2004), King and Murphy (2014) suggested four factors of ASD that may relate to an individual's offending behaviors, including the following: (1) their increased social naiveté may leave people with an ASD open to manipulation by others; (2) a disruption of routines, or over-rigid adherence to rules, might lead people with ASD to become aggressive; (3) a lack of understanding of social situations (and poor negotiating skills) might lead people with an ASD to become aggressive; and (4) an obsessional interest might lead someone to commit an offense in the pursuit of that interest, perhaps exacerbated by a failure to recognize the implications of their behavior. Here, we elaborate upon this framework, and provide examples of how this may manifest in forensic assessment practice.

ASD is characterized by social communication deficits. This may manifest as trouble with social reciprocity, difficulty expressing oneself, lack of shared conversations, trouble understanding social norms, or flattened nonverbal expressions. This can cause a host of difficulties for individuals with ASD that may be relevant to their legal system involvement. These individuals may appear affectively unemotional in response to distressing situations or altercations. They are likely to have more difficulty navigating challenging social situations or seeking support. Some individuals with ASD experience "autistic meltdowns," in which they are unable to express themselves verbally altogether during times of distress, which would create complications when interacting with law enforcement personnel or others in a courtroom. Perhaps most noteworthy, individuals with ASD have trouble reading, interpreting, and responding to social cues. They are less likely to be aware of how their behaviors impact those around them. This may lead to a misperception of someone's intentions, an experience of overly negative or argumentative attitudes, or trouble with conflict resolution. On the opposite end of the spectrum, an individual with ASD may also be more likely to be exploited, due to their difficulty in reading the intentions of others. This is particularly concerning for those with ASD who have an accompanying intellectual or language impairment.

This is pivotal as it relates to dating and sexual relationships. Individuals with ASD may be more likely to misinterpret cues for consent. Oftentimes, neurotypical individuals correctly perceive body language associated with consent (e.g., strong eye contact, smiling, moving one's body closer to another, nodding their head yes). Nonverbal cues signaling nonconsent (e.g., turning away, covering up one's body, frowning, crossing one's legs) will be far more difficult for an individual with ASD to read and accurately translate. Even verbal cues that an individual is uncomfortable, such as hinting that they want to transition conversation topics or activities, will not be as blatant to an individual with ASD. This can lead to a variety of charges related to unwanted physical touch or sexual contact that stemmed from a miscue during the social interaction.

Theory of mind (ToM), or the ability to attribute mental states to others, is another important concept to be aware of when working with individuals who are diagnosed with ASD. ToM includes the ability to identify the thoughts and feelings in others based on situations and/or the facial expressions of others. Individuals with ASD often have deficits in TOM because they play a role in social communication, resulting in a real or perceived lack of empathy (Baron-Cohen, 2000). Individuals with ASD generally think more logically and factually instead of thinking with emotions. Taken a step further, people with ASD who lack ToM may also struggle with implementing empathetic behaviors.

Empathy has two main components: cognitive empathy, or the ability to understand the perspectives of others; and affective empathy, the ability to feel someone else's emotions. In order to properly demonstrate cognitive empathy, a person would need to mentally put themselves in the shoes of another person in order to better understand that person's thoughts and emotions. Similar to cognitive empathy, affective empathy involves the ability to mirror others' emotions and to accurately recognize what someone else might be feeling. In order to successfully demonstrate empathy, a connection needs to be made between the recognition of an affective state of another and valuing their feelings and perspective. While individuals with ASD are not inherently unempathetic, and they do often experience regret, remorse, and a sense of understanding, their deficits in recognizing social norms and understanding emotion in others may lead to challenges within the realm of empathy. Many times, once an individual can concretely recognize why an individual may feel or respond in a certain way, their empathetic response shifts.

Stemming beyond social communication differences, restricted and repetitive behaviors can also yield problematic behaviors that may result in legal system involvement. In addition to the propensity for direct and blunted communication, individuals with ASD can be rigid and unyielding in their beliefs, opinions, and actions. This may lead to behaviors that feel argumentative or verbally aggressive. Demands to follow rules that they do not agree with may result in noncompliance with authority or violations of legal expectations, and it may be more difficult for an individual with ASD to recognize the wrongfulness of "hands-off" crimes, such as those involving child pornography.

Special interests present another domain in which legal charges may arise. While some individuals experience restricted interests that are typical in topic but unusual in their intensity, others have topics of interest that are inherently unique. For example, individuals with ASD may have special interests surrounding sexual topics such as child pornography, masturbation, voyeurism, or exhibitionism. They may also have fascinations with individual people or places that lead to violations of personal space, boundaries, or contact. Special interests can even manifest in crimes related to theft.

Another deficit that can exist in ASD is one that relates to central coherence (i.e., gestalt formation), or the ability to integrate numerous details into a bigger picture. In the context of ASD, this could also be referred to as weak central coherence. Common characteristics of weak central coherence typically involve concrete, literal thinking; social challenges that involve missing out on subtle cues and emotional overtones; and excelling in detail-oriented tasks, but struggling with the integration of information to better understand context. In other words, weak central coherence may lead to struggles with understanding social nuances and integrating both verbal and nonverbal cues in order to appropriately understand the context of social interactions.

The deficits that may occur in ToM, weak central coherence, and the core symptoms of ASD may help explain the function of offending behavior in someone with ASD. For example, misunderstanding social cues, such as misinterpreting facial expressions to be unfriendly, paired with restricted interests that are violent may result in aggressive behaviors (Brewer et al., 2023). Being able to identify these deficits and how they relate to the referral issue in a FMHA is an important skill for forensic mental health professionals to develop.

Developmental Considerations

While the research above focuses primarily on the criminal justice system, those working within the juvenile justice arena should also be aware of this literature and the ASD clinical framework. Interestingly, despite the fact that ASD is a neurodevelopmental disorder (i.e., symptom onset in early childhood), there appears to be far less research overall on the ASD population and their involvement in the juvenile justice system, as opposed to in the adult criminal justice system. Some literature adjacently addresses the topic. For example, Slaughter et al. (2019) discussed school discipline and criminal behavior in juvenile justice involved youth with ASD. In their article, they briefly noted the dearth of research around juvenile justice involvement rates, and summarized that the few articles that have been published range from 1.3 to 18.2%. External to the studies explored there, little research has addressed juvenile justice ASD prevalence, or highlighted the unique needs of the population.

What is perhaps more important to consider, are the clinical and environmental contexts that differ for youth when compared to adult populations. When working within the juvenile justice system, the same clinical framework explored in the section above applies, but the circumstances of how those symptoms may manifest will differ. Thus, forensic mental health professionals might see cases that relate to school truancy or altercations with peers. For instance, forensic mental health professionals may be conducting school threat assessments, and need to consider how ASD may impact the juvenile's presentation. A clinician may consider if social isolation, trouble with reciprocity, or special interests may factor into the juvenile being flagged for a threat assessment. Forensic mental health professionals may be examining group youth activity in which a juvenile was manipulated or exploited, and not able to read the social cues that led up to the incident, a key element to consider in mitigation. Additionally, Collins et al. (2023) highlighted literature suggesting that in a juvenile court ordered sexual offender program as many as 62.8% of the group was diagnosed with ASD. Awareness of how social cues factor into budding sexual development, interests, and interactions should also be considered in the context of juvenile FMHAs.

Types of FMHAs

Forensic mental health professionals may be asked to complete a FMHA for the court or by attorneys for a variety of reasons. This section will focus on some of the most often requested types of FMHAs. Specifically, we will focus on assessments for competency to stand trial, criminal responsibility/insanity, risk assessments, and guardianship. It should also be noted that the remainder of this chapter focuses primarily on psycholegal issues relevant to laws and statutes in the United States. We recommend reviewing (Freckelton et al., 2021) for additional information on evaluations or topics relevant to international law.

Competency to Stand Trial

Competency to stand trial has to do with one's present mental capacity (note: *Competence to proceed* or *adjudicative competence* is sometimes the language used to describe this legal issue). In the landmark case of *Dusky v. United States* (1960), the United States Supreme Court held that a defendant is competent when he has "sufficient present ability to consult with his lawyer with a reasonable degree of rational understanding—and [when] he has a rational as well as factual understanding of the proceedings against him." Someone who is not competent to stand trial cannot proceed to trial or be sentenced (*Pate v. Robinson*, 1966).

Competency to stand trial evaluations are the most commonly requested forensic psychological evaluations by courts (Zapf & Roesch, 2009). Forensic mental health professionals are called upon to assess individuals' functional capacities as it relates to competence to stand trial. These functional capacities can include all of the following: appraisal of available legal defenses, unmanageable behavior, appraisal of the likely outcome, capacity to disclose to one's attorney, ability to testify relevantly, ability to cope with stress, understanding the role of participants in the courtroom, understanding of the charges, understanding of court procedures, appreciation of the seriousness of the charges, appraisal of the range and nature of possible penalties, capacity to assist one's attorney in planning a legal strategy, and capacity to realistically challenge prosecution witnesses (McGarry, 1965). Thus, decision-making abilities, the reliability of information provided, flexibility in thinking, emotional regulation, abstract thinking, social and communication skills, and other factors related to ASD are implicated in competency to stand trial evaluations. A comprehensive forensic evaluation that focuses on the relevant psycholegal issue of competency to stand trial will include a clinical interview, mental status examination, review of the legal discovery and other collateral records, and possibly psychological testing. Table 1 provides topics that may be reviewed as part of a competency to stand trial evaluation.

It is standard practice during a FMHA to provide an opinion to the referral source on whether the individual has a mental illness or mental defect that interferes with

Table 1 Examples of topical areas and questions to assess and explain in forensic evaluation reports

Competency to stand trial	
Understanding the nature and objective of the court proceedings	Capability to assist in defense
Description of legal charges Range and nature of possible penalties Appraisal of available legal options Plea Options Pros and Cons of a plea bargain Ability to identify courtroom participants (e.g., judge, defense attorney, prosecutor, jury) Ability to describe the roles of courtroom participants Alternatives to the use of a jury	Quality of relating to an attorney Capacity to disclose available pertinent facts Capacity to help plan and/or discuss a legal strategy A defendant's motivation for a favorable outcome Capacity to comprehend instructions, challenge witnesses, and testify Stress tolerance
Criminal responsibility	
The presence of a severe mental disease or mental defect at the time of the act charged An analysis of whether the behavior at the time of the act charged is consistent with a severe mental disease or defect The individual's motivation and motives at the time of the act charged. Is the act charged explained by typical criminal motives? The presence or absence of a ruse Exploration on whether drugs or alcohol were involved at the time of the act charged Post-offense behavior (e.g., How did the individual respond to being arrested? What behaviors did the individual have immediately following the act charged?) Past and present knowledge that the alleged criminal behavior is wrong, and when and how the defendant acquired that knowledge	
Guardianship	
Identification of the individual's mental illness, mental impairment, neurodevelopmental disorder, neurocognitive disorder, or other condition(s) Impairment in mental status at the time of the evaluation List of medications and identification of any signs of physical and/or mental impairments caused by the medications Deficits in adaptive behavior Capability to make decisions concerning medical treatments, living arrangements, diet, and finances Any indications of abuse, neglect, or exploitation of the individual Other special characteristics of the individual that should be considered	

their competency to stand trial. The presence of a diagnosis, such as ASD, alone does not indicate that a person is incompetent to stand trial (Mayes, 2003). Rather, it is their functional deficits at the time related to their diagnosis that may interfere with their competency to stand trial. Therefore, it is important for forensic mental health professionals to have the necessary expertise in evaluating individuals with ASD so that they can describe to the fact finder and referral source the individual's capabilities and limitations.

It is common for individuals with more severe impairments to be found incompetent to stand trial when compared to individuals with minimal impairments. For example, a comprehensive meta-analysis (Pirelli et al., 2011) found that defendants diagnosed with a psychotic disorder were approximately eight times more likely to be deemed incompetent compared to those without such a diagnosis. This finding that a person with a more severe disorder is more likely to be found incompetent to stand trial holds true for individuals with ASD, too. Individuals with ASD have been found to have a poorer understanding of courtroom procedures compared to individuals not diagnosed with ASD (Brewer et al., 2016). Characteristics of ASD may also interfere with an individual with ASD being able to assist in their defense. For instance, deficits in ToM and central coherence may result in an individual with ASD becoming preoccupied with certain aspects of the case or specific legal terminology while ignoring the "big picture." An individual with ASD's rigid beliefs and preoccupations may also relate to them irrationally rejecting legal advice or not fully assisting their attorney in planning a legal defense.

Furthermore, Allely (2022) noted that characteristics of ASD may be misinterpreted or viewed in a negative manner by evaluators, courtroom personnel, and jurors. Specifically, Allely noted that difficulties with memory, lack of emotional expression, unusual ways of speaking, inappropriate behaviors, difficulty with establishing or maintaining eye contact, impaired social communication and interaction, echolalia or repetitive vocalizations, difficulties with unstructured environments (e.g., a courtroom), or unusual body movements can be viewed in a negative manner. Mahoney et al. (2021) also indicated that problems with receptive and expressive language, working memory, intellectual or reasoning impairments, emotional regulation, sensory processing problems, and deficits in executive functioning may impact an individual with ASD's competency to stand trial. It is common for individuals with ASD to mask their deficits, which could result in the defense team working with the individual with ASD not recognizing the individual's true limitations. Forensic mental health professionals, therefore, can play a vital role in helping to educate the court and others about ASD, how deficits related to ASD impact the psycholegal issue, and best practices for interacting with the individual.

Individuals with ASD may be referred to competency restoration services if they are not competent to stand trial. Competency restoration services can be provided in an outpatient or inpatient setting; however, the United States ruled in *Jackson v. Indiana* (1972) that a defendant cannot be confined for more than a reasonable period of time needed to determine if they are capable of regaining competency in the future. Thus, individuals cannot be held for an indefinite amount of time for competency restoration. A "reasonable period of time" for competency restoration may differ depending on the legal jurisdiction in which the case is being held.

The rate of defendants referred for an evaluation that have been found incompetent to stand trial is 27.5% though the amount of individuals being referred for competency evaluations and restoration services is rising (Murrie et al., 2023). An exact number of individuals with ASD being referred for a competency to stand trial evaluation or restoration services is not currently known. The majority of research related to competency to stand trial on neurodevelopmental disorders has focused on individuals with Intellectual Developmental Disorder (IDD). For example, Tsargis et al. (2015) examined demographic characteristics of 315 adult offenders with neurodevelopmental disorders in an urban environment in northern Ohio. Competency to stand trial was not raised as a legal issue in every case; however, it was found that 16% were found incompetent to stand trial—unrestorable and an additional 16% had their cases dismissed. The remaining individuals were sentenced to prison (21.4%) or up to 60 months of community control/probation (43%). Research on individuals with IDD participating in competency restoration found that 61% attained competency after participating in a competency restoration program specifically designed for individuals with IDD (Wall & Christopher, 2012). Other studies have found that there are high rates of competency restoration (81 to 90%) in individuals with no or mild cognitive impairment, whereas individuals with IDD were less likely to attain competency (Pirelli & Zapf, 2020; Staats et al., 2021; Wood, 2025).

There is no standardized or evidence-based curriculum available for competency restoration services for individuals with ASD. Individuals with ASD who are ordered to undergo competency restoration services in an inpatient setting or correctional facility are typically placed in competency restoration programming with other defendants. This may include individual and group restoration sessions in which the individual is frequently being assessed and reevaluated to determine if they have been restored. We recommend that professionals providing competency restoration services to individuals with ASD utilize other evidence-based curriculums, such as the UCLA PEERS program (Laugeson et al., 2012), to assist individuals with ASD in learning and practicing social skills and other skills that are relevant to understanding courtroom proceedings and assisting in their defense. This may include lessons on conversational skills, exchanging information, appropriate use of humor, cognitive flexibility, handling disagreements, adjusting to change, and expected courtroom behavior. The Slater Method is another curriculum that could be considered for individuals with ASD who have a co-occurring diagnosis of an IDD. The Slater Method is a five-module program that has been found to be helpful in restoring individuals with IDD to competency (Wall & Christopher, 2012). It reviews topics aimed to help the individual understand their charges, plea options, potential consequences of each plea option, courtroom personnel, courtroom proceedings, plea bargaining, communicating with the attorney, giving testimony, tolerating the stress of the proceedings, and other skills needed to assist in their defense. More research on using the Slater method and other competency restoration curriculums with individuals with ASD is needed.

Criminal responsibility/the Insanity Defense

Two principles must be present in order for a person to be held responsible for a crime. First, a person must have actually committed the physical element of the offense in question (*Actus Reus*, meaning the commission or omission that comprises an element of an offense), and the individual must have the requisite mental state (i.e., *Mens Rea*), such as acting intentionally, knowingly, recklessly, or negligently. In other words, the individual must have committed the offense with a particular mental state or intent (sometimes referred to as a "guilty mind"). Individuals with a mental disease or defect, however, may engage in criminal conduct without meeting the principle of having the requisite Mens Rea. The insanity defense and other forms of a (in)capacity defense are used to address the concept of Mens Rea. Therefore, individuals may be referred for an evaluation to help determine if pursuing the insanity defense is an appropriate legal strategy. The insanity defense is the most controversial issue in criminal law (Melton et al., 2018). Common misperceptions of the insanity defense include that a large number of defendants use the defense, most individuals using this defense are successful, individuals are released upon acquittal, and the individual is still dangerous even after release (Melton et al., 2018). In reality, the plea of not guilty by reason of insanity (NGRI) is rarely used and is estimated to be raised in less than 0.5% of felony cases. It is estimated the defense is successful in only 25% of the cases in which the NGRI plea is rarely raised, and individuals found NGRI may spend a longer time involuntarily hospitalized or confined compared to individuals that otherwise would have been convicted and sentenced (Melton et al., 2018).

"Insanity" or NGRI is an affirmative legal defense—an excuse from punishment under the criminal law. It is an assertion that the person committed the offense or offenses charged, but should not be held responsible. The first conception of insanity was the "Wild Beast Test." Under the Wild Beast Test, one would not be held criminally responsible if they were "totally deprived of [their] understanding and memory, and doth not know what [they are] doing, no more…than a brute, or a wild beast" (Rex v. Arnold, 1724). Since then, four formulations of insanity have been used in the United States that focus on a cognitive and/or volitional test (Yu, 2021):

1. A person is insane if, due to a mental disease or defect, they did not know or appreciate the nature of what they were doing (the first prong of the *M'Naghten* rule, see M'Naghten's Case, 1843, a cognitive test).
2. A person is insane if, due to a mental disease or defect, they did not know or appreciate that what they were doing was wrong, even though they knew or appreciated the nature of what they were doing (the second prong of the M'Naghten rule, a cognitive test).
3. A person is insane if, due to a mental disease or defect, they were suffering from an irresistible and uncontrollable impulse, and thus, substantially lacked the capacity to control their actions (known as the "irresistible impulse test," a volitional test).
4. A person is insane if what they were doing, a culpable act, was the result or product of a mental disease or defect (known as the *Durham* rule, or the "product" test; see Durham v. United States, 1954).

The Insanity Defense Reform Act of 1984, enacted by Congress in response to John Hinckley's attempted assassination of then-President Ronald Reagan and subsequently adopted in most states, uses a form of the M'Naghten rule and thus is a cognitive test. It emphasizes that at the time of the offense charged, as a result of mental disease or defect, the person was unable to appreciate the nature and quality or the wrongfulness of their conduct. This is the standard of the insanity defense that is used in all federal cases in the United States. Notably, the Supreme Court of the

United States has rejected the notion that the states must adopt one of these tests (*Kahler v. Kansas*, 2020). Therefore, forensic mental health professionals should be aware of how their local jurisdiction statutorily defines insanity when completing criminal responsibility evaluations for non-federal cases. Kansas, Utah, Montana, and Idaho are four states that do not recognize an insanity defense but may allow individuals to argue they lacked intent and to present evidence regarding mitigating factors.

A FMHA to determine if an individual meets criteria for the Insanity defense differs from other types of evaluations because it is not focusing on an individual's current presentation. Rather, this type of FMHA is analyzing past behavior and actions at the time of the offense being charged. Key components of this type of FMHA include data collection, a current mental status examination, and a review of collateral information. Data collection involves collecting historical background information on the individual, such as their developmental history, legal history, and course of mental health treatment. This may be conducted through a record review, clinical interview, or interviewing of collateral sources. A clinical interview in which the evaluator obtains the individual's account of what happened before and after the offense charged is also needed; however, individuals charged with a crime may not always be forthcoming or they may provide inconsistencies (Packer, 2009). During the process of completing a mental status examination, evaluators also need to assess if the individual's current mental state is consistent or inconsistent with the behavior around the time of the offense being charged. It is always possible that an individual's mental health symptomatology has improved or deteriorated since the time of the accused offense. A review of offense-related information is essential as police reports, video or audio recordings of the offense, and third-party collateral interviews (e.g., family, co-worker, direct care staff) may provide additional insight into the person's mental state at the time of the offense being charged. We caution the use of psychological testing in criminal responsibility evaluations because most tests do not relate directly to the legal issue (see Packer, 2009). Any testing completed will portray the individual's mental state at the time of the evaluation and, therefore, may not be representative of how the individual was functioning at the time of the offense they are accused of. In interpreting the data collected, it is important to consider conflicting data, develop hypotheses, and determine which hypothesis best fits the data (Packer, 2009). We provided examples of areas and questions to assess in criminal responsibility evaluations in Table 1.

In general, forensic mental health professionals conclude that an individual meets criteria for the insanity defense less than 15% of the time (Melton et al., 2018). If a person is found NGRI, they may be confined for treatment if the individual has a mental illness and poses a danger to themselves or others (*Jones v. United States*, 1983). In addition to or in lieu of an NGRI evaluation, evaluators may sometimes be requested by the individual's legal counsel to provide a sentencing mitigation report. This allows the individual's defense team to present mitigating factors related to a person's mental illness (including information related to the person's neurodevelopmental disorder), treatment recommendations, and other factors that should be taken into consideration during sentencing.

Legal arguments using the insanity defense are difficult to prove in individuals with ASD (Crehan et al., 2021). Cea (2014) argues that present standards for the Insanity defense in the United States are inadequate for individuals with ASD because individuals with ASD may commit a crime due to a lack of knowledge (which aligns with the cognitive test), whereas other individuals with ASD may commit a crime due to a lack of control related to rigid beliefs, repetitive or stereotyped behaviors, sensory concerns, or other clinical features of ASD (which aligns with a volitional test). Cea (2014) also critiques the use of terms in insanity defense laws, such as "severe" or "substantial" in regards to describing a mental disease or mental defect or the ability to appreciate the wrongfulness of an action. Current standards and terminology may be disadvantageous to individuals with ASD that present as higher functioning because they may appear to court personnel and the jury as not presenting with functional deficits related to the insanity defense as statutorily defined (Cea, 2014). Thus, this may limit the use of the insanity defense by individuals with ASD. This stresses the importance of forensic mental health professionals conducting a FMHA on an individual with ASD to consider the individual's insight into their behavior, understanding of social norms or understanding of explicit rules of what not to do, sensory responses and repetitive behaviors that may be misinterpreted, and/or intellectual functioning when considering if the insanity defense is appropriate (Crehan et al., 2021; Mahoney et al., 2021).

Risk Assessments

Drawing on the available literature, Douglas and colleagues (2013) defined risk assessment "as the process of gathering information about people in a way that is consistent with and guided by the best available scientific and professional knowledge to understand their potential for engaging in violence in the future and to determine what should be done to prevent them from doing so." It has been argued by some that mental health professionals, individually and as a group, cannot predict with an acceptable degree of reliability that a particular person will commit other crimes in the future and, thus, represent a danger to the community (American Psychiatric Association, 1982). However, the Supreme Court of the United States rejected this position (Barefoot v. Estelle, 1983). Indeed, as the Court held in a prior case, "[P]rediction of future criminal conduct is an essential element in many of the decisions rendered throughout our criminal justice system," including for example, whether to admit a defendant to bail, what sentence to impose, and whether to grant parole (*Jurek v. Texas*, 1976). As such, forensic mental health professionals are routinely called upon to render opinions on future risk.

The process of completing risk assessments has evolved over time. Douglas et al. (2013) summarized the various approaches to risk assessments. Broadly speaking, there are discretionary approaches and nondiscretionary approaches. Discretionary approaches include at least three types: (1) unaided clinical judgment which, while perhaps the most common method, is not an empirical approach and lacks validity and reliability as it relies solely on intuition and so-called "clinical judgment"; (2) an anamnestic approach, which focuses on personal and situational factors associated with past violence, which adds some structure, but still lacks empiricism; and (3) structured professional judgment (SPJ), a guided clinical approach where decision-making is guided by the scientific and professional literature, which contributes to valid and reliable decisions. Nondiscretionary approaches come in at least two types: (1) actuarial use of psychological tests (e.g., the Hare Psychopathy Checklist; Hare, 2003), which use cutoff scores but are limited by relying on a single test that is typically inferior to other approaches; and (2) actuarial risk assessment instruments (ARAIs), used solely to predict the future, where items are chosen rationally or empirically and then weighted and combined to reach a decision about the likelihood of violence over some period of time. While a complete literature review of the strengths and weaknesses of each approach is beyond the scope of this chapter, we agree with Douglas et al. and others who have argued or demonstrated that the SPJ approach is structured, evidence-based, valid, and reliable; and, thus, superior to other approaches (Douglas & Kropp, 2002; Hart et al., 2007; Singh et al., 2011; Viljoen et al., 2010; Webster et al., 1997).

Assessing individuals with ASD, however, provides unique challenges, and while the field of risk assessment has enjoyed evolution, particularly in the past 50 years, that process is in its infancy when it comes to assessing the unique factors specific to individuals with ASD.

Individuals with ASD, social difficulties, or other neurodevelopmental and psychiatric disorders are viewed as being responsible for many acts of violence (Schwartz, 2023; White et al., 2017), which may prompt referral sources to request a risk assessment when concerns of violence arise. Prevalence of violence in individuals with ASD is unclear with some studies suggesting that as low as 1.5% and as high as 67% of individuals with ASD are violent. For example, Allely et al. (2017) examined 73 lone shooter cases from 1982 to 2014 and found that six of the individuals (8%) were diagnosed with ASD with another 16 individuals (21%) exhibiting traits associated with ASD. In a study of 157 youth that participated in a threat assessment between 1998 to 2019, over half (51.6%) received special education services, with many of the individuals being diagnosed with ASD, Attention-Deficit/Hyperactivity Disorder (ADHD), depression, anxiety, and/or a learning disability (Weisbrot et al., 2023). A verbal threat was made by 80% of the students and 29.3% students brought a weapon to school. Consequently, placement in a therapeutic school setting or psychiatric hospitalization was more likely to be recommended by evaluators if the youth had a prior history of violence (or threats of violence) and symptoms related to ASD, mood disorders, paranoia, and/or other behaviors associated with a conduct disorder. Other risk management strategies can include referrals to psychiatry for medication management, psychotherapy, case management, and/or linkage to social service agencies.

A limitation to risk assessment measures is that they don't explain the function of behavior; therefore, an examination of the link between ASD characteristics and concerning behavior should be utilized by evaluators. Common factors related to increased risk of violence or other offending behaviors in individuals with ASD have included deficits in ToM, social naivety and vulnerability to manipulation by others, disruption of routine or rigid rules followed by the individual, misinterpretation of social situations or social norms, emotional dysregulation, impaired moral reasoning, and preoccupation or obsessional interests that can become deviant or results in the individual not recognizing the consequences of their behavior (Howlin, 2004; Lerner et al., 2012; Matthews & Bell, 2020). Other risk factors may include a prior history of violence, substance abuse, being male, a diagnosis of a comorbid psychiatric disorder, parental criminal history, parental mental health history, and a delayed diagnosis of ASD (Heeramun et al., 2017; Murphy, 2022).

Risk assessment and management strategies for individuals with ASD have received some scholarly attention; however, it is still necessary to recognize the dearth of research pertaining to specific assessment tools applicable to this population. The bulk of the literature on individuals with ASD has focused on the use of risk assessment measures of violence but not measures assessing the risk for recidivism of sexual offending. For instance, the HCR-20 is a structured professional judgment tool used for assessing risk of violence in adults. The presence of a "major mental illness" is a risk factor on the HCR-20 and ASD and other neurodevelopmental disorders are included in this category. Although specific characteristics related to ASD may not be risk factors captured by the HCR-20, the diagnosis of ASD is considered a "major mental illness." Murphy (2013) used the HCR-20 to assess violence in 20 individuals with ASD admitted to a high security psychiatric facility. These individuals were assigned into high versus low violence groups based on whether their offense was related to an act of violence that led to severe injury compared to offenses in which minimal injury or no direct harm to the victim occurred. There were no significant group differences on the number of items on the HCR-20 that were present, but three historical factors (relationship instability, early maladjustment, diagnosis of a personality disorder), one clinical item (lack of insight), and one risk item (vulnerability to future stress) were frequently present. It was also noted that individuals in the high violence group were more likely to exhibit verbal difficulties, particularly in word knowledge and abstract verbal reasoning, compared to individuals in the low violence group. More interestingly, Murphy also concluded that the use of the HCR-20 was of minimal use to case formulation and development of risk management strategies. Another study examined the use of the Psychopathy Checklist Short Version (PCL:SV) in adults with ASD in a psychiatric facility and found that the PCL:SV was correlated with the HCR-20 (Maguire et al., 2025). Specifically, higher scores on the PCL:SV, which suggests a higher degree of antisocial traits and psychopathy in individuals, were associated with more items on the HCR-20, poorer treatment progress, and a longer length of stay in the hospital.

The Structured Assessment of Violence Risk in Youth (SAVRY; Borum et al., 2002), an SPJ instrument, is commonly employed in the evaluation of violence risk among adolescents aged–18 years. There are no published studies on the use of the SAVRY in youth with ASD specifically, but Adamson, Dixon, and McLean (2011) report that there is some evidence that it is a strong predictor of violence in youth with neurodevelopmental disorders in general. ASD is not a risk factor included in the SAVRY; however, the SAVRY is designed to allow evaluators to include additional historical, social and contextual, individual/clinical, and protective factors that are noteworthy. Thus, the diagnosis of ASD, or characteristics and behaviors related to ASD, can be considered when relevant. In addition, already established risk factors on the SAVRY, such as poor school performance, peer rejection, stress and poor coping, risk taking and impulsivity, lack of personal/social support, low empathy/ remorse, and anger management problems may be relevant risk factors to further explore when using the SAVRY to assess adolescents with ASD.

Given the limited research on risk assessment measures for individuals with ASD, current best practices for risk assessment in individuals with ASD include consideration of the same risk factors and use of standardized risk assessment measures designed for the general population (Matthews & Bell, 2020). This recommendation has the caveat that conceptualization of risk includes considerations of ASD related characteristics, such as deficits in theory of mind, social communication, emotional regulation, and executive functioning, that help give a possible explanation of the individual's behavior related to risk (Matthews & Bell, 2020). This aligns with recommendations provided by Shine and Cooper-Evans (2016) to confirm the diagnosis of ASD and identification of specific ASD characteristics prior to completing risk assessment measures. Additionally, Shine and Cooper-Evans advise to conduct a functional behavioral analysis to discern antecedents and consequences associated with the individual's potential for engaging in future violent or offending behaviors. This analysis can then assist forensic mental health professionals in accurately scoring assessment measures based on the presence and relevance related to the individual's risk.

Guardianship

Guardianship constitutes a legal process wherein the state designates a family member, attorney, or an organization to act as a decision-maker for an individual who has been adjudicated as lacking the capacity for independent decision-making. It is based on the principle of *parens patriae* or "parent of the state," which allows the state to intervene or protect those who are unable to protect or care for themselves (Jameson et al., 2015; Melton et al., 2018). Fell (1994, as cited in Bloom, 2015, p. 960) states, "A person is not made the subject of a guardianship because he transgressed social standards in a manner that presents a danger to others, but because, through illness or other disability, he lacked the present ability to make decisions necessary to carry on life affairs. The court acts in a protective role, like a parent, to assure control and management of the subject's affairs while the subject is not competent to do so." In order for a person to be appointed a guardian, a petition to the court that the person is incompetent in their decision-making capabilities or are unable to care for or protect themselves must be made by any concerned person (Melton et al., 2018). If a guardianship hearing is scheduled, the court will hear evidence and, if warranted, appoint a person or organization as guardian of the individual.

Legal definitions for what constitutes a person in need of a guardian varies by jurisdiction. There are also various forms of guardianship. A general or plenary guardianship refers to a person or organization being appointed control over the person and their estate. Thus, the guardian is responsible for decision-making and controlling the person's finances and other assets. Limited or specific guardianships are used in some jurisdictions, which allow the guardian to only have authority over certain parts of the individual, such as only the person or only the estate. This type of guardianship is rarely used in most jurisdictions (Bloom, 2015; Jameson et al., 2015; Melton et al., 2018). Almost all jurisdictions encourage those petitioning the court to consider less restrictive alternatives to guardianship before legal guardianship is pursued (Ferguson et al., 2025). Less restrictive alternatives may include developing an advance directive, appointing a representative payee to manage the individual's finances or estate, or utilizing a supported decision-making model. A supported decision-making model allows individuals to still maintain control over their life but gives them access to an advocate or consultant that can give them information and advice to aid them with their decision-making (Jameson et al., 2015).

Although the pursuit of a legal guardian is justified under certain circumstances, there are also several critiques to pursuing guardianship for an individual. Barnes (2003) examined 566 guardianship cases and found that most hearings lasted less than 15 min, the individual presumably in need of a guardian was not present in 66% of the hearings, counsel representing the individual was not always present, the FMHA lacked details, and the expert completing the FMHA that recommended guardianship was rarely in attendance at the hearing. This brings into question whether the court has fully examined the individual's strengths and weaknesses in relation to their ability to make decisions and manage their estate. Other critiques of the guardianship process is that most courts rarely monitor appointed guardians and their ability to assist the individual, most courts do not track the number of active guardians, and individuals can still be exploited by their appointed guardian or others (Melton et al., 2018).

Bloom (2015) also noted that the focus on plenary guardianship over limited guardianship is concerning, particularly for individuals with ASD. Most courts prefer plenary guardianship because they believe that there is a "downward trend" in which the individual, most often an older adult, will continue to deteriorate over time and, thus, the role of a guardianship will continue to be necessary in order to make important decisions for the individual to receive appropriate treatment and care (Bloom, 2015). However, individuals with ASD do not necessarily follow the "downward trend" but have the potential to learn new skills and increase their functional independence over time. Furthermore, courts may prefer plenary guardianship because they are more familiar with this model, believe that considering a limited guardianship will take more time and be less cost effective, and experience difficulty with identifying how a limited guardianship can meet the specific needs of the individual (Bloom, 2015).

As an individual with ASD turns 18 and becomes a legal adult, parents and caregivers may become concerned regarding the individual's capacity to live independently, avoid becoming a victim of exploitation, and personal and healthcare decision-making abilities. Adults with ASD may struggle making treatment decisions, maintaining employment, living independently, managing finances, or completing other daily living activities such as shopping or maintaining personal hygiene. Deficits related to cognition, socialization, and communication are common reasons that guardianship may be pursued for individuals with ASD (Bloom, 2015; Ferguson et al., 2025). Farley et al. (2018) reported that 75 (44%) out of 169 adults with ASD were appointed a legal guardian, with the majority of the individuals with ASD also being diagnosed with IDD. Similarly, Ferguson et al. (2025) reported that 69 out of 114 adults with ASD had a legal guardian. Adults with a legal guardian had significantly lower verbal and nonverbal IQ scores, higher scores on the Autism Diagnostic Observation Schedule (ADOS; Lord et al., 2012), and lower scores on the communication and socialization domains of the Vineland Adaptive Behavior Scale (Sparrow et al., 2016) compared to adults without a guardian.

However, it should also be mentioned that there could be consequences to the mental health of an individual with ASD if guardianship is pursued. In general, losing the ability to make one's own decisions can interfere with physical and mental health and limit one's ability to use adaptive coping skills (Melton et al., 2018). In individuals with ASD and other disabilities, the appointment of a guardian can also limit the person's opportunity to engage in self-determination, reduce opportunities to integrate into the community, and decrease overall quality of life (Jameson et al., 2015). This stresses the importance of forensic mental health professionals recommending the need for a guardian only when no other justifiable alternatives are available in individuals with ASD.

Guardianship evaluations typically consist of a clinical interview, mental status examination, psychological testing, and reliance on information from collateral sources. Psychological testing can be useful to help establish the individual's diagnoses, current symptomatology, and adaptive behavior abilities. Melton et al. (2018) recommend that evaluators completing guardianship evaluations focus more on the range of functional and adaptive behavior abilities of the individual rather than solely on the diagnoses or symptoms that are present. It is important to specifically outline what the individual can do independently versus what assistance the individual may need from a guardian because there are various functional impairments that may be present in an individual with ASD. When determining if a guardian should be recommended, the forensic mental health professional should also consider whether less restrictive alternatives are available that can alleviate the individual's functional and adaptive deficits. In other words, it is important to determine if support staff or an advocate can help the individual complete a task or make a decision without the need for a legal guardian to be appointed. The evaluator's report to the court should provide information on the pros and cons of each alternative considered as well as the justification for their clinical opinion on whether a guardian or other alternative is being recommended. Common areas of a guardianship evaluation are outlined in Table 1.

Strategies for Completing a FMHA

Developing Competency in Conducting a FMHA

Forensic mental health professionals should have the appropriate level of competence to evaluate an individual with ASD. The American Psychological Association's (APA) *Ethical Principles of Psychologists and Code of Conduct* recommends psychologists "provide services… with populations and in areas only within the boundaries of their competence based on their education, training, supervised experience, consultation, study, or professional experience" (APA, 2017, see Ethical Standard 2.01 (a)). This includes individuals with disabilities (APA, 2017; see Ethical Standard 2.01 (b)). Similarly, APA's *Speciality Guidelines for Forensic Psychology* state that "forensic practitioners strive to understand how factors associated with age, gender, gender identity, race, ethnicity, culture, national origin, religion, sexual orientation, disability, language, socioeconomic status, or other relevant individual and cultural differences may affect and be related to the basis for people's contact and involvement with the legal system" (2013, p. 10). If evaluators do not believe they have the competence necessary to complete an evaluation, it is recommended that they "make an appropriate referral if indicated, or gain the necessary training, experience, consultation, or supervision necessary to gain competency" (APA, 2013, p. 10; see also APA, 2017, Ethical Standard 2.01(b)).

Gaining competency in working with individuals with ASD can be a lengthy process because it takes time to become updated on best practices for ASD assessments, understanding differential diagnoses, and identifying characteristics of ASD that may be overlooked by general practitioners. Furthermore, individuals with ASD have differing presentations and no two individuals are alike. Forensic mental health professionals need to assess their level of competency in working with individuals with ASD prior to accepting a referral to complete a forensic psychological evaluation. Consulting with non-forensic professionals that work with ASD, attending training, reading relevant research and other sources, and obtaining supervision are a start to begin building competency. Table 2 provides some recommended reading and trainings related to ASD that will help forensic mental health professionals begin to develop competency in working with this population.

Strategies to Modify an Interview with the Individual with ASD

Completing a FMHA with an individual with ASD also poses unique challenges. Some individuals with ASD may have limitations in their ability to read, write, or comprehend common legal terms. Even when cognitive functioning (i.e., intelligence) is not of concern, deficits in abstract thinking and a limited vocabulary are also common. When interacting with the legal system, individuals with ASD may not fully appreciate the serious nature of participating in an evaluation. At times,

Table 2 Resources to help develop competency in evaluating individuals with ASD

Organizations providing professional and educational resources		
Agency	Website	Description
The arc: national center for criminal justice and disability	https://www.thearc.org/nccjd	Online trainings, publications, videos, and other resources on forensic issues for individuals with developmental disabilities is provided
American association on intellectual and developmental disabilities	http://aaidd.org	Information on policies, research, effective practices, and additional educational resources for working with individuals with developmental disabilities is provided
UCLA Program for the Education and Enrichment of Relational Skills (PEERS)	https://www.semel.ucla.edu/peers	The PEERS program is an evidence-based curriculum that focuses on teaching adults with ASD basic social skills
Autism Society of America	https://www.autismsociety.org	The Autism Society of America website provides education and information on advocacy, community programming and other resources related to ASD
Association for science and autism treatment	https://www.asatonline.org	Information on research and evidence-based treatments for professionals is provided. This includes recommendations related to ethics, transitioning from adolescence to adulthood, intervention, and other guidance for practitioners
Recommended readings		
Book title	Author	Year published
Autism spectrum disorder in the criminal justice system: a guide to understanding suspects, defendants and offenders with Autism	Clare S. Allely	2022
Working with autistic people in the criminal justice and forensic mental health systems: a handbook for practitioners	Edited by Nichola Tyler and Anne Sheeran	2022
What science tells us about autism spectrum disorder	Raphael A. Bernier, Geraldine Dawson, and Joel T. Nigg	2020

(continued)

Table 2 (continued)

Organizations providing professional and educational resources		
Agency	Website	Description
Handbook of autism spectrum disorder and the law	Edited by Fred R. Volkmar, Rachel Loftin, Alexander Westphal, and Marc Woodbury-Smith	2021
Landmark cases in forensic psychiatry (2nd Ed.)	Edited by Merrill Rotter, Jeremy Colley, and Heather Ellis Cucolo	2019
Forensic mental health assessment in criminal contexts: key concepts and cases	Noah K. Kaufman, Shane S. Bush, Nicole R. Schneider, and Scotia J. Hicks	2022
Psychological evaluations for the courts: a handbook for mental health professionals and lawyers	Gary B. Melton, John Petrila, Norman G. Poythress, Christopher Slobogin, Randy K. Otto, Douglas Mossman, and Lois O. Condie	2018
Trainings and other media		
Title	Website	Description
Concept at Palo Alto University	https://concept.paloaltou.edu/	Concept provides several webinars focusing on autism and the law as well as completing competency, criminal responsibility, and threat assessments on individuals with ASD
University of New Mexico: Law and Mental Health Series	https://hsc.unm.edu/medicine/departments/psychiatry/divisions/forensic-services/	This weekly didactic series focuses on a range of topics related to forensic psychology and psychiatry. There are some available trainings related to conducting evaluations on individuals with ASD and other neurodevelopmental disorders
Autastic	https://www.autastic.com/asd-friendly-podcasts	Autastic provides a variety of podcasts and other media that provides information on ASD

they may not fully respond to questions or they may limit the amount of details they provide in their verbal responses. Individuals with ASD may also become preoccupied with certain topics related to their restricted interests, which may be viewed by others as a deflection strategy. Individuals with ASD also tend to exhibit deficits in emotional expression, empathy, and understanding the perspective of others. Thus, a lack of experience and competency in working with individuals with ASD may result in a forensic mental health professional misinterpreting the individual's behaviors and responses as the individual being disinterested in participating in the evaluation, not cooperating or putting forth good effort, or presenting themselves as arrogant or narcissistic (Mattison & Allely, 2022).

Individuals with ASD are known in some cases to be overly compliant, suggestible, eager to please, and avoidant of conflict and confrontation (Mattison & Allely, 2022). In contrast, some individuals with ASD may present as rigid and confrontational. They may also attempt to mask their true deficits and be over accommodating to others, particularly individuals in positions of authority (Criminal Justice Advocacy Program, 2014). These factors are a barrier to a forensic mental health professional trying to inquire about an individual's knowledge of a topic or other strengths and weaknesses of the individual. Forensic mental health professionals should be sensitive to an individual's nonverbal cues and tendency to become overly compliant or guarded with disclosing details. Prior to interviewing the individual with ASD, it may be helpful to obtain information about the individual's adaptive strengths and weaknesses from previous records, caregivers, treatment providers, and other collateral sources to obtain an accurate perspective for the relevant factors of the individual's disorder that is related to the context and purpose of the evaluation. Forensic mental health professionals should also frequently check-in with the individual to assess the individual's comprehension of topics that are being discussed. Having individuals with ASD use terms that they are comfortable with as well as having them restate concepts in their own words is encouraged.

At the onset of the evaluation, it is helpful to provide individuals with ASD a thorough explanation of the purpose of the FMHA, the limits of confidentiality, and expectations of their role and participation in the FMHA. Using literal language that provides explicit instructions and guidelines is recommended. When interviewing the individual, using a variety of question formats can be useful to gauge the individual's level of comprehension and understanding. Wood (2025) proposed using a combination of formats during FMHA with individuals with IDD that include an open-ended format, multiple-choice format, forced-choice format (e.g., true/false or yes/no questions), or recognition questions where respondents select responses from a list of items. A similar approach can also be utilized with individuals with ASD. Other recommendations for interviewing an individual with ASD include providing extra time to build rapport and establish trust, extra time for individuals to process a question and provide a response, use of visual aides and cuing, do not assume prior knowledge of a topic, plan questions in advance, avoid multi-part questions, use simple terminology, be concise and avoid unnecessary wording, and phrase questions in a non-leading manner (Mattison & Allely, 2022).

Establishing ASD as a Diagnosis

The primary purpose of FMHA is to address the psycholegal issue that prompted the evaluation referral. However, a valuable aspect of the role of a forensic mental health professional is to determine if the individual officially meets diagnostic criteria for ASD. Unfortunately, many individuals with ASD who have been charged with a crime have not been properly diagnosed (Mayes, 2003). For example, Hofvander et al. (2019) examined 249 violent offenders with and without ASD. Only 19% of the violent offenders with ASD were officially diagnosed with ASD prior to becoming involved with the legal system. In fact, over 73% of the individuals that were not previously diagnosed with ASD were instead diagnosed with Attention-Deficit / Hyperactivity Disorder (ADHD). This suggests that many forensic mental health professionals may be diagnosing an individual with ASD for the first time or may be working with an individual who has been diagnosed with a different disorder that may or may not be an accurate representation of their symptoms and behavior.

The "gold standard" and best practices for establishing an ASD diagnosis has been the use of multidisciplinary teams that use the ADOS-2 (Lord et al., 2012) and/or Autism Diagnostic Interview-Revised (ADI-R; Lord et al., 1994) as part of their assessment battery. However, utilizing a multidisciplinary team for a FMHA is not always cost or time effective as many courts give evaluators strict timeframes to complete the FMHA, whereas a referral to a multidisciplinary team can result in an individual being placed on a lengthy waiting list. Furthermore, there has been recent criticisms suggesting that we rethink best practices and the "gold standard" approach in diagnosing ASD. (Kaufman, 2022). Specifically, Kaufman argues that more testing that focuses on core components of the neurodevelopmental disorder, such as working memory, processing speed, personality, attention, and executive functioning is needed rather than relying on two "gold standard" tests. Forensic mental health professionals should also consider that the ADOS-2 can produce a high number of false positives, particularly among individuals diagnosed with more severe psychiatric conditions (Maddox et al., 2017). Therefore, an ADOS-2 score above the recommended cutoff does not necessarily indicate that the person meets criteria for ASD, but rather that they may exhibit difficulties in social communication and behavior that coincide with their psychiatric diagnosis. Overall, the use of additional testing to help establish a diagnosis of ASD provides more data points for the evaluator to consider and formulate an opinion on whether the individual meets criteria for ASD and what specific strengths and weaknesses the individual may possess. Evaluators should keep in mind that some jurisdictions and courts may prefer the inclusion of the ADOS-2 and/or ADI-R as part of a FMHA because these tests are still considered the "gold standard." Therefore, we recommend that evaluators administer the ADOS-2 and/or ADI-R as part of their assessment battery when (1) previous clinical evaluations that utilized an ADOS-2 and/or ADI-R are not available to review and include as a collateral source in the evaluator's current evaluation report, (2) the individual has not been previously diagnosed with ASD, or (3) the referral source or court has either requested or preferred to have these tests completed given their reputation as the "gold standard" for diagnosing ASD.

The Use of Psychological Testing in FMHAs

There are benefits and limitations of using psychological testing in FMHAs. One of the primary benefits for using psychological testing is that it can provide a sense of scientific reasoning and objectivity to the opinions that are provided (Melton et al., 2018), which is typically viewed positively and a boost to an evaluator's credibility by judges (Brannon et al., 2025). Limitations to including psychological testing is that information that addresses the referral question can be obtained via alternative methods, administration time for psychological testing can increase the cost of the FMHA, and some evaluators may select tests without rationale—they administer the test just because it is part of their standard battery regardless of the referral question (Melton et al., 2018). Thus, tests should be carefully selected and administered, particularly when there are no alternative methods available to directly assess a construct related to the psycholegal issue.

When selecting which testing measures to administer, evaluators need to be cognizant of the Federal Rules of Evidence (2020) and relevant legal cases related to the admission of evidence. There are numerous federal rules of evidence that cover various forms of evidence. The federal rules emphasize that evidence presented to the court needs to be relevant and assist in determining if a fact is more or less probable that it would be without the evidence (Rule 401); evidence can be excluded if it is prejudicial, confusing, misleading, causes delay, or wastes time (Rule 403); evidence needs to be "reasonably relied upon" by professionals in the field (Rule 703); and hearsay is often not admissible (Rule 802). Two relevant legal cases that evaluators should also reference are Frye v. U.S (1923) and Daubert v. Merrell Dow Pharmaceuticals (1993). The outcome of Frye v. U.S. (1923) indicated that evidence presented to the court "must be sufficiently established to have gained general acceptance in the particular field." In Daubert v. Merrell Dow Pharmaceuticals (1993), it was argued that the Frye test had been superseded by the Federal Rules of Evidence and was no longer the appropriate standard for admitting scientific evidence into court. The U.S. Supreme Court provided guidelines for judges to consider when determining the appropriateness of evidence: "(1) Are the methods and/or rationale scientifically valid? (2) Has the theory been subject to peer review or publication? (3) Can or has the theory been tested? (4) What is the theory's or technique's known or potential error rate? (5) Are there standards that relate to the technique? (6) Is there widespread acceptance of the technique in the scientific community?" (Rotter et al., 2019, p. 44).

In line with the Federal Rules of Evidence and landmark cases related to FMHAs, Melton et al. (2018) identified several factors for forensic mental health professionals to consider in using psychological testing measures as part of a forensic evaluation. Specifically, evaluators need to first determine if the test directly answers the specific construct or psycholegal issue based on the purpose of the evaluation. Additionally, evaluators are recommended to select tests that are commercially available, have a user's manual, possess an adequate level of reliability and validity, and have been peer reviewed. Furthermore, it is important that evaluators have the necessary qualifications to use the test. For example, evaluators attempting to identify whether a person has ASD should have the necessary training and competency to administer assessments that help establish whether ASD is present, such as the ADOS-2, ADI-R, or the Monteiro Interview Guidelines for Diagnosing the Autism Spectrum—Second Edition (MIGDAS-2; Monteiro & Stegall, 2018). An evaluator should also have similar competency in the ability to use forensic assessment instruments (FAIs).

Three categories of testing measures can be present in a forensic psychological evaluation: clinical assessment instruments (CAIs), forensic related instruments (FRIs), and FAIs (Heilbrun et al., 2002; Melton et al., 2018). CAIs primarily focus on diagnosis, treatment, and other clinical factors. Examples of CAIs may include the ADOS-2, Behavior Assessment System for Children—Third Edition (BASC-3; Reynolds & Kamphaus, 2015), or the Vineland Adaptive Behavior Scale—Third Edition (Vineland-3; Sparrow et al., 2016). In comparison, FRIs are similar to CAIs but emphasize constructs more relevant to the legal issue, such as a person's response style or risk for violence or sexual offending. The use of CAIs and FRIs may or may not aid an evaluator in directly answering a psycholegal question posed by the court; therefore, these instruments should only be used when necessary. FAIs, however, are measures specifically designed to help evaluators assess a specific legal standard and the capacities that an individual must possess to meet that legal standard (Heilbrun et al., 2002).

Unfortunately, many of the FAIs used by forensic psychologists have not been normed on individuals with ASD. For example, Melton et al. (2018) suggests including a measure of response style to determine if an individual is malingering or feigning psychiatric symptoms or knowledge of a psycholegal topic. However, there are currently no specific measures designed to assess response style or malingering in individuals with ASD and measures developed for the general population may not always be an appropriate selection. Faccini and Burke (2021) suggest that the use of general measures assessing response style in the general population should not be used on individuals with ASD because these measures "assume knowledge of social or communication constructs" (p. 440) and may be difficult for individuals with ASD with language deficits to fully comprehend. Given the complexities of ASD, more research is needed to determine which FAIs are appropriate to use with individuals with ASD. Table 3 provides a description of some of the FAIs and FRIs developed for the general population and their appropriateness of use for individuals with ASD. We advise that forensic mental health professionals develop a rationale for the use of psychological testing measures that are selected as part of the battery that aligns with the Federal Rules of Evidence, landmark cases, and guidelines suggested by Melton et al. (2018). Developing a rationale for test selection can be useful if called to testify in court.

Report Writing

Producing a well written evaluation report to the court is important because it gives the court a good first impression of the evaluator's expertise, outlines evidence that

Table 3 Description of select forensic assessment instruments (FAIs) and forensic relevant instruments (FRIs) and their appropriateness of use for individuals with ASD

Competency to stand trial		
Test	Description of test and appropriateness for individuals with ASD	Select peer-reviewed research references focusing specifically on ASD
Competence assessment for standing trial for defendants with intellectual disabilities (CAST*ID)	The CAST*ID is a standardized instrument used to assess competency to stand trial in individuals with IDD (Everington & Luckasson, 1992). It consists of three scales, measuring (1) Understanding of Basic Legal Concepts, (2) Skills to Assist in Defense, and (3) Understanding of Case Events. The CAST*ID consists of a number of multiple-choice and open-ended questions that utilize simple language. The CAST*ID was the first validated competency to stand trial instrument for individuals with IDD. It is appropriate for individuals with ASD that have intellectual deficits. There are norms in the user's manual for individuals from the general population without an ID, and theoretically can be used for all populations	None available
Evaluation of competence to stand trial—revised (ECST-R)	The ECST-R is a semi-structured interview designed to assess psycholegal questions related to the legal standard for competency to stand trial as outlined in Dusky v. United States (Rogers et al., 2003). It includes four scales related to competency to stand trial: Factual Understanding of the Courtroom Proceedings, Rational Understanding of the Courtroom Proceedings, Consult with Counsel, and Overall Rational Ability. There is also an Atypical Presentation scale that screens for feigned psychotic and nonpsychotic symptoms as well as other signs that an individual is feigning incompetency to stand trial. The ECST-R has not been validated in individuals with an IQ below 60. We caution the use of the ECST-R in individuals with ASD with intellectual deficits	None available

(continued)

Table 3 (continued)

Competency to stand trial		
Test	Description of test and appropriateness for individuals with ASD	Select peer-reviewed research references focusing specifically on ASD
MacArthur Competence Assessment Tool—Criminal Adjudication (MacCAT-CA)	The MacCAT-CA is a structured interview used to assess a defendant's understanding, reasoning, and appreciation as related to their competence to stand trial (Poythress et al., 1999). The understanding and reasoning domains focus on a brief vignette involving an altercation between two individuals that escalates and results in a legal situation. The appreciation domain focuses on the defendant's own legal case, such as the likelihood of being treated fairly or their ability to assist in their defense. The MacCAT-CA is not validated for individuals with IDD. The MacCAT-CA also involves some level of abstract thinking, which may be difficult for individuals with ASD, but is helpful to assess their ability to understand abstract concepts in a trial situation. We caution the use of the MacCAT-CA in individuals with ASD and do not recommend it for individuals with intellectual deficits	None available
Response style		
Test	Description	Select ASD references
Inventory of Legal Knowledge (ILK)	The ILK (Musick & Otto, 2010) is a 61 item true/false measure designed to detect feigning regarding the lack of legal knowledge during competency to stand trial evaluations. No specific research studies are available for the ASD population. Other research cautions the use of this measure with individuals with IDD because it can lead to a mislabel of feigning. We also caution the use of this measure for individuals with ASD with intellectual deficits	None available

(continued)

Table 3 (continued)

Competency to stand trial		
Test	Description of test and appropriateness for individuals with ASD	Select peer-reviewed research references focusing specifically on ASD
Structured interview of reported symptoms—version 2 (SIRS-2)	The SIRS-2 is a structured interview designed to detect feigning of psychiatric symptoms (Rogers et al., 2010). It includes scales that assess the feigning of rare symptoms, symptom combinations, improbable or absurd symptoms, over endorsement of symptoms, and other indicators of feigned symptomatology. Results provide a qualitative description of the individual's response style, which may include an honest response style, indeterminate response style, probably feigning, or definitely feigning. Although there is no peer-reviewed research on using the SIRS-2 on individuals with ASD, it may be helpful in situations in which an evaluator suspects that an individual with ASD may be feigning other psychiatric difficulties	None available
Test of Memory Malingering (TOMM)	The TOMM is a 50-item visual recognition test used to distinguish between feigned memory deficits and true memory impairments (Tombaugh, 1996). Two trials are administered and a retention trial is optional. The TOMM has been used in individuals with a variety of clinical presentations (i.e., traumatic brain injury, intellectual disability, head injuries, dementia, neurocognitive disorders, etc.); however, use of the cutoff scores in the manual may need to be modified depending on the individual's diagnostic presentation. We caution the use of the TOMM in individuals with ASD that may also have intellectual deficits	Loughan & Pema (2014) Moss (2013)
Validity Indicator Profile (VIP)	The VIP is a general assessment of response style that is helpful to distinguish between valid and invalid responding to intellectual or neurocognitive testing (Frederick, 1997). It includes both a verbal and nonverbal subtest. According to the manual, it is not recommended to use the VIP on individuals with a documented IDD or neurocognitive disorder. We do not recommend this test for individuals with ASD that have intellectual deficits, and caution the use for individuals with ASD without IDD	None available

(continued)

Table 3 (continued)

Competency to stand trial		
Test	Description of test and appropriateness for individuals with ASD	Select peer-reviewed research references focusing specifically on ASD
Risk assessment		
Test	Description	Select ASD references
Assessment of risk and manageability of individuals with developmental and intellectual limitations who offend—sexually (ARMIDILO-S)	The ARMIDILO-S is a measure specifically designed for individuals with borderline intellectual functioning or mild intellectual impairment who have offended sexually or have displayed sexually inappropriate behavior (Boer et al., 2012). The ARMIDILO-S does include a process for examining dynamic risk factors in the individual and considers the impact of the living environment and the relationship the individual has with family, support staff, and others. In general, the ARMIDILO-S has not been researched extensively; therefore more studies are needed to provide psychometric data. There are no specific studies available on the ASD population. We caution the use of the ARMIDILO-S, particularly given the limited research and that it may not meet the Daubert standard that the legal system requires for evidence used in a forensic evaluation	Matthews and Bell (2020)
Child Pornography Offender Risk Tool (CPORT)	The CPORT is a risk assessment tool used to predict recidivism in adult males with a conviction of an offense related to CASM (Eke et al., 2018). In general, the actual use of the CPORT recidivism probabilities are not recommended until there are further validation studies. However, there are six risk categories that can help evaluators obtain information on an individual's recidivism risk. There have been no specific studies on using the CPORT in individuals with ASD; however, given the increasing number of cases of individuals with ASD being charged with offenses related to CASM, the CPORT may be helpful to provide some information on risk for recidivism. Caution should still be used when using the CPORT	Allely and Dubin (2018)

(continued)

Table 3 (continued)

Competency to stand trial		
Test	Description of test and appropriateness for individuals with ASD	Select peer-reviewed research references focusing specifically on ASD
Historical clinical and risk management scale (HCR-20)	The HCR-20 is used to assess the risk of violence in adults between 18 to 65 years old (Douglas et al., 2013). It focuses on 10 historical risk factors related to violence history and psychosocial adjustment, five dynamic risk factors related to current symptoms and functioning, and five risk management factors focusing on potential future concerns for the individual's mental health and psychosocial adjustment. The HCR-20 appears to be an appropriate risk assessment tool based on the limited studies available	Girardi et al. (2019) Matthews and Bell (2020) Murphy (2013) Murphy (2022) Shine and Cooper-Evans (2016)
Sex Offender Risk Appraisal Guide (SORAG)	The SORAG is an actuarial risk assessment measure that focuses on 14 static items that assess an individual's risk of sexual recidivism, including non-contract sexual offenses, in adult men who have committed at least one previous sexual offense (Quinsey et al., 2006). Similar to the VRAG, the SORAG has been studied on individuals with IDD but there are no specific studies on ASD. We recommend the SORAG be used with caution in individuals with ASD	None Available
Static-99 revised/static-2002	The Static-99R (Phenix et al., 2017) and Static-2002 (Phenix et al., 2008) are actuarial risk assessment instruments used to assess risk of sexual reoffending in adult males who have been charged or convicted of at least one sexual offense against a child or an adult. It is not designed for use with individuals that have only been charged or convicted of possession or distribution of child sexual abuse material. According to the users' manual, the original normative samples for the Static-99R and Static-2002 contained individuals with developmental delays and, therefore, is appropriate to use with this population	None available

(continued)

Table 3 (continued)

Competency to stand trial		
Test	Description of test and appropriateness for individuals with ASD	Select peer-reviewed research references focusing specifically on ASD
Structured Assessment of Violence Risk in Youth (SAVRY)	The SAVRY is an assessment guide that assists forensic mental health professionals in utilizing a structured clinical judgment approach regarding a juvenile's risk of future violence (Borum et al., 2002). It contains 10 static risk factors pertaining to past behavior, six dynamic items pertaining to social and contextual factors in a juvenile's environment, and eight items assessing current behavior and other clinical concerns. Six protective factors are also provided. Limited research is available specifically for youth with ASD	Adamson et al. (2011) Sinclair et al. (2013)
Violence Risk Appraisal Guide (VRAG)	The VRAG is an actuarial risk assessment tool that primarily focuses on 12 static items that assess the long-term likelihood of violent or sexually violent reoffending in adult males (Quinsey et al., 2006). Examples of items contained in the VRAG include substance abuse problems, criminal history, age at index offense, and psychopathy. It has been studied on individuals with IDD but there are no specific studies on ASD. We recommend the VRAG be used with caution in individuals with ASD	Matthews and Bell (2020)
Other measures		
Test	Description	Select ASD references
Gudjonsson Suggestibility Scales (GSS)/ Gudjonsson Compliance Scale (GCS)	The GSS (Gudjonsson, 1997) is a tool focusing on an individual's level of suggestibility in response to leading questions and negative feedback. It can be used to assess how an individual may respond during police interrogation. There is also a separate Gudjonsson Compliance Scale (Gudjonsson, 1989) that can be completed by the individual or a collateral source (e.g., caregiver, guardian) and provides data on how compliant an individual is in a variety of situations. There are a few research studies showing that individuals with ASD have comparable scores on the GSS to a non-ASD sample; however, individuals with ASD may be more compliant (i.e., score higher on the GCS) than individuals without ASD. We believe the GSS and GCS are appropriate for individuals with ASD but still caution the use given the limited studies available	Maras and Bowler (2012) North et al. (2008)

(continued)

Table 3 (continued)

Competency to stand trial		
Test	Description of test and appropriateness for individuals with ASD	Select peer-reviewed research references focusing specifically on ASD
Multiphasic Sexual Inventory—Second Edition (MSI-II)	The MSI-II (Nichols & Molinder, 2010) is a self-report measure that assesses different psychosexual topics in an individual engaging in sexually inappropriate behavior or charged with a sex-related offense. Although there is no research specifically on individuals with ASD, our communication with the publisher has indicated that the MSI-II is appropriate to use in individuals with ASD. We still caution the use of the MSI-II in individuals with ASD until there is additional research available	None Available
Psychopathy Checklist Screening Version (PCL:SV)	The PCL:SV (Hart et al., 1995) is a brief measure assessing psychopathy. It is a shorter version of the Psychopathy Checklist-Revised (PCL-R). The PCL:SV is a strong predictor of violence in psychiatric inpatient units. There is evidence that it predicts future violence among adults with ID. Cautioned use for individuals with ASD due to limited research available	Maguire et al. (2025) Matthews and Bell (2020)
Risk-Sophistication-Treatment Inventory (RSTI)	The RSTI (Salekin, 2004) is a semi-structured interview and rating scale that is used by forensic mental health professionals to assess the functioning of juvenile offenders age 9 to 18 years, in three important areas: (1) risk for dangerousness (2) sophistication-maturity, and (3) treatment amenability. We recommend that forensic mental health professionals using the RSTI use a neurodevelopmental framework when conceptualizing the results	None available
Socio-Sexual Knowledge and Attitudes Assessment Tool—Revised (SKAAT-R)	The SKAAT-R measures sexual knowledge and attitudes in individuals with developmental disabilities that are 15 years old and older (Griffiths & Lunsky, 2003). Subtests focus on anatomy, a person's knowledge of men's and women's bodies, intimacy, pregnancy, childbirth, childrearing, birth control and sexually transmitted diseases, and healthy socio-sexual boundaries. The SKAAT-R is not a predictive or diagnostic tool but can be used to assess sexual knowledge. The normative sample consisted of 276 adolescents and adults with developmental disabilities. Specific information on individuals with ASD was not included in the manual. Given the SKAAT-R's focus on developmental disabilities, it is likely an appropriate measure for individuals with ASD. An updated version of the SKAAT-R is currently going through field research testing	None available

the court can use when making a legal decision, and can be used to defend the evaluator's opinion and conclusions if the evaluator is called to testify in court. There are common errors that evaluators should avoid when writing the report. These may include having missing or inadequate data, failure to use multiple sources and methods when conducting the evaluation, having insufficient logic or lacking a detailed explanation for opinions and conclusions, a lack of clarity or organization of the report, or problems with the clinical interview and/or mental status examination, such as having inconsistent information or missing parts/sections (Dicataldo et al., 2020). Similarly, Grisso (2010) described 10 common errors in the reports of 36 candidates that applied for certification with the American Board of Forensic Psychology. The 10 errors included providing opinions without sufficient explanation (56% of the reports), the purpose of the forensic evaluation was not clearly stated (53%), poor organization of the report (36%), providing irrelevant data or opinions (31%), failure to describe or consider alternative opinions (30%), using inadequate data (28%), placing the summary of data and interpretations of the data in the same section of the report (26%), over-reliance on a single source of data (22%), language problems (e.g., use of psychojargon or biased phrases), and using tests improperly (15%). We have already highlighted in earlier sections some strategies that evaluators can use to avoid these common errors.

When writing the report, evaluators should keep in mind that the report is a legal document that is intended for a legal audience. The goal is to educate the reader and, ultimately, the fact finder—whether it be the judge, a magistrate, or jury—about ASD and how it relates to the legal issue. The appropriate use of terminology can bring a sense of significance and importance to the report. The use of jargon should be limited. Evaluators should appropriately balance professional standards with layman's terminology when writing the report. We recommend avoiding using terms, such as mild or high functioning, because it may be misinterpreted by the audience. For example, describing an individual as "mildly autistic" or a "high functioning" individual, while also arguing that they are incompetent to stand trial may bring a sense of confusion to the reader who believes that the individual only has minimal deficits because of the terminology that was used. A general rule is to not use terms that are outdated (e.g., Pervasive Developmental Disorder—Not Otherwise Specified, Asperger's Syndrome) but rather use official terminology described in the current edition of the DSM, DM-ID, or ICD classification system.

It should also be noted that the FMHA report significantly differs from the type of report produced by a clinical practitioner in a clinical setting. Clinical evaluations primarily rely on self-report and information that the client presents is often assumed to be reliable. FMHAs, in contrast, minimally rely on self-report measures but instead rely on the combination of all data points including the individual's self-report, testing, and collateral sources of data, such as police reports, collateral interviews, and historical records. It is important to include a detailed list of all information considered in the FMHA report and a section of the report devoted to providing a summary of collateral interviews, historical records, and other information derived from collateral sources. All opinions and conclusions provided in the report should be based on multiple data points and not on a single source of data.

In summary, a well written FMHA report should include the purpose of the evaluation, be organized in a coherent manner, educate the reader about ASD, describe how the characteristics and behaviors of the individual with ASD are related to the legal issue, include relevant testing that is appropriate to address the diagnosis of ASD and the legal issue, utilize multiple data points to support the opinions and conclusions contained within the report, and balance professional standards with layman's terminology.

Providing Testimony

Expert testimony based on the FMHA report may be requested. Evaluators need to be aware of the rules of evidence (and hence the rules of testimony) for the jurisdiction in which they are called to testify (see "Report Writing" section of this chapter for examples of the Federal Rules of Evidence and relevant case law). The U.S. Supreme Court has ruled that psychologists can testify as expert witnesses in relation to mental health issues (see Jenkins v. United States, 1962). However, it is still common for judges and jurors to be skeptical of information provided by an expert witness (Allely & Cooper, 2017; Edens et al., 2012; Fradella et al., 2002). Experts in mental health may sometimes be viewed as a "hired gun" for the defense or prosecution, lack neutralization, and/or using "junk science" or be "charlatans" (Edens et al., 2012; Fradella et al., 2002, p. 443).

Testifying in court can be anxiety provoking and is one reason why experts in ASD often choose not to conduct FMHAs. At the beginning of providing testimony, the expert will be expected to present their credentials, including relevant education and experience, in order for the court to determine if the evaluator is deemed an expert witness. This is known as the voir dire process. Evaluators should be prepared to discuss anything presented on their curriculum vitae during this process. Once appointed as an expert, the focus of testimony is on content found within the FMHA report. The testimony should be based on science and, thus, experts should be proficient in both practice and scientific knowledge regarding the subject matter (Heilbrun et al., 2008). Effective testimony is based on the content of the report and the "style" in which the testimony is delivered (Heilbrun et al., 2008). Boccaccini et al. (2016) also note that effective testimony is based on the expert being viewed as credible, the expert's ability to provide clarity in the information presented, the clinical knowledge demonstrated by the expert, and certainty in responses provided by the expert. Table 4 provides additional strategies to help professionals prepare for testimony, provide effective testimony, and improve upon their skills for future testimony.

Table 4 Strategies on providing effective testimony (Boccaccini et al., 2016; Brodsky, 1999; Heilbrun et al., 2008; Melton et al., 2018)

Preparing to testify
• Know the case • Review the written report several times leading up to the hearing • Consult with legal counsel to help prepare a list of questions that will be asked during the direct examination and potential areas of the report that will be targeted during cross examination • Dress professionally • Consider preparing a testimony outline • Arrive to the courtroom early to become aware of your surroundings and to give you additional time to review the report and testimony outline • Bring copies of your CV and an unmarked copy of your report • Know that anything that is taken to the witness stand when testifying could be entered into evidence • Anticipate attacks to your credibility and weaknesses in the report • Practice relaxation or mindfulness techniques prior to testifying to help reduce anxiety • Overprepare • Know details of the case and timeline of events related to the report • Practice answering questions out loud before arriving to court
Providing testimony
• Tell the truth • Only answer the question that is asked. Only respond with a Yes/No response if a Yes/No question is asked • It is better to say "I don't know" than to take a guess • Avoid jargon or overusing abbreviations without explaining what the abbreviation means first. Provide an explanation of test results, diagnoses, and other facts in terms that the judge or jury can understand • Explain the core features of Autism and give examples that the client exhibits to support the diagnosis • Do not become defensive during cross examination • Be confident but do not present as being overconfident or narcissistic • Avoid unclear or confusing responses • Pay attention to nonverbal communication (overuse of gestures, smiling, or other facial expressions)
Strategies to improve skills
• Participate in mock trials • Videotape the mock trial if possible • Observe others by watching colleagues testify in court and/or reviewing available videos of experts providing. Videos of trials can be found on social media platforms and YouTube • Ask for feedback from attorneys after the hearing • Review books related to providing expert testimony

Conclusion

This chapter has provided a broad overview of the challenges in understanding the prevalence of ASD within the legal system, highlighted features of ASD that may contribute to offending behavior or referral for a FMHA, and described common types of FMHAs that may be requested by a court or attorney. Strategies for establishing a diagnosis, modifying an interview, selecting appropriate testing instruments and measures, producing a well written report, and providing effective testimony was discussed. With standards for conducting a FMHA for individuals with ASD still being in its infancy, there is a need for additional research and establishment of best practices in conducting FMHAs for this population. Many of the FRIs and FAIs used by forensic mental health professionals have not been researched or normed on individuals with ASD. Therefore, forensic mental health professionals that complete a FMHA need to be aware of the complexities of these types of assessments because experience and competency in diagnostic procedures and case conceptualization from a neurodevelopmental perspective is necessary in addition to the ability to assess psycholegal matters relevant to a specific legal issue. Providing courts and others involved in the legal system information on how characteristics of the individual with ASD is related to a legal matter is a valuable resource that forensic mental health professionals competent in this area can provide.

References

Adamson, L., McLean, A., & Sher, M. (2011). Risk assessment in adolescents with developmental disabilities. In *Forensic issues in adolescents with developmental disabilities* (pp. 142–154). Jessica Kingsley Publishers.

Allely, C. S. (2022). *Autism spectrum disorder in the criminal justice system: A guide to understanding suspects, defendants and offenders with autism.* Routledge.

Allely, C. S., & Cooper, P. (2017). Jurors' and judges' evaluation of defendants with autism and the impact on sentencing: A systematic Preferred Reporting Items for Systematic Reviews and Meta-Analyses (PRISMA) review of autism spectrum disorder in the courtroom. *Journal of Law and Medicine, 25*(1), 105–123.

Allely, C. S., & Dubin, L. (2018). The contributory role of autism symptomatology in child pornography offending: Why there is an urgent need for empirical research in this area. *Journal of Intellectual Disabilities and Offending Behaviour, 9*(4), 129–152.

Allely, C. S., Wilson, P., Minnis, H., Thompson, L., Yaksic, E., & Gilberg, C. (2017). Violence is rare in autism: When it does occur, is it sometimes extreme? *The Journal of Psychology, 151*, 49–68.

American Psychiatric Association. (1982). Brief for the American Psychiatric Association as Amicus Curiae, *Barefoot v. Estelle*, 463 U.S. 880, 1983.

American Psychiatric Association. (2013). *Diagnostic and statistical manual of mental disorders* (5th ed.). Author.

American Psychological Association. (2013). Specialty guidelines for forensic psychology. *American Psychologist, 68*(1), 7–19. https://doi.org/10.1037/a0029889

American Psychological Association. (2017). *Ethical principles of psychologists and code of conduct* (2002, amended effective June 1, 2010, and January 1, 2017). https://www.apa.org/ethics/code.

Baio, J. (2018). Prevalence of autism spectrum disorder among children aged 8 years—autism and developmental disabilities monitoring network, 11 sites, United States, 2014. *MMWR. Surveillance Summaries, 67*.

Barefoot v. Estelle. (1983). 463 U.S. 880.

Barnes, A. (2003). The liberty and property of elders: Guardianship and will contests as the same claim. *Elder Law Journal, 11*(1), 9–10.

Baron-Cohen, S. (2000). Theory of mind and autism: A review. *International Review of Research in Mental Retardation, 23*, 169–184.
Bloom, M. E. (2015). Asperger's disorder, high-functioning autism, and guardianship in Ohio. *Akron Law Review, 42*(3), 955–1002.
Boccaccini, M. T., Kwartner, P. P., & Harris, P. B. (2016). Testifying in court: Evidence-based recommendations for expert-witness testimony. In R. Jackson & R. Roesch (Eds.), *International perspective on forensic mental health. Learning forensic assessment: Research and practice* (pp. 506–520). Routledge/Taylor & Francis Group.
Boer, D. P., Haaven, J., Lambrick, F., Lindsay, W. R., McVilly, K. R., Sakdalan, J., & Frize, M. (2012). Assessment of risk and manageability for individuals with developmental and intellectual limitations who offend-sexually (ARMIDILO-S). *Unpublished manuscript*.
Borum, R., Bartel, P., & Forth, A. (2002). Manual for the Structured Assessment of Violence Risk in Youth (SAVRY) University of South Florida. *Tampa, FL, USA*.
Brannon, M., Speiser, M. A., Singhal, A., Scherer, E. A., & Perillo, A. (2025, May 6). *Judicial perspectives of the strengths and weaknesses of forensic mental health assessments and testimony* [Webinar]. The University of New Mexico Health Sciences: Division of Forensic Behavioral Sciences - Law and Mental Health. https://www.youtube.com/watch?v=DgYZx5LlrzE
Brewer, N., Lucas, C. A., Alliyza, L., & Young, R. L. (2023). Detecting dodgy behavior: The role of autism, autistic traits, and theory of mind. *Autism, 27*(4), 1026–1035. https://doi.org/10.1177/1362361125564
Brewer, R. J., Davies, G. M., & Blackwood, N. J. (2016). Fitness to plead: The impact of autism spectrum disorder. *Journal of Forensic Psychology Practice, 16*(3), 182–197.
Brodsky, S. L. (1999). *The expert witness: More maxims and guidelines for testifying in court*. American Psychological Association.
Brown, J. (2017). Autism Spectrum Disorder (ASD) and competency to stand trial (CST): A need for greater understanding and further research. *Forensic Scholars Today, 3*(1), Article 1.
Browning, A., & Caulfield, L. (2011). The prevalence and treatment of people with Asperger's Syndrome in the criminal justice system. *Criminology & Criminal Justice, 11*(2), 165–180.
Cea, C. N. (2014). Autism and the criminal defendant. *St. John's Law Review, 88*(2), 495–530.
Cheely, C. A., Carpenter, L. A., Letourneau, E. J., Nicholas, J. S., Charles, J., & King, L. B. (2012). The prevalence of youth with autism spectrum disorders in the criminal justice system. *Journal of Autism and Developmental Disorders, 42*(9), 1856–1862. https://doi.org/10.1007/s10803=01101427-2
Collins, J., Horton, K., Gale-St. Ives, E., Murphy, G., & Barnoux, M. (2023). A systematic review of autistic people and the criminal justice system: An update of king and murphy (2014). *Journal of Autism and Developmental Disorders, 53,* 3151–3179.
Crehan, E. T., & Ury, F. S., et al. (2021). Legal defense in criminal cases. In F. R. Volkmar (Ed.), *Handbook of autism spectrum disorder and the law* (pp. 127–143). Springer.
Criminal Justice Advocacy Program. (2014). *Individual with intellectual and developmental disabilities who become involved in the criminal justice system: A guide for attorneys*. Author.
Daubert v. Merrell Dow Pharmaceuticals. (1993). 509 U.S. 579.
DiCataldo, F., Serafinski, R. L., Beam, D. C., & Grisso, T. (2020). Feedback on forensic mental health assessments in a juvenile court clinic certification program. *Juvenile and Family Court Journal, 71*(4), 35–51. https://doi.org/10.1111/jfcj.12386
Douglas, K. S., Hart, S. D., Webster, C. D., & Belfrage, H. (2013). *HCR-20V3: Assessing risk for violence: User guide*. Mental Health, Law, and Policy Institute, Simon Fraser University.
Douglas, K. S., & Kropp, P. R. (2002). A prevention-based paradigm for violence risk assessment: Clinical and research applications. *Criminal Justice and Behavior, 29*(5), 617–658.
Durham v. United States. (1954). 214 F.2d 862, 874-75 (D.C. Cir. 1954).
Dusky v. United States. (1960). 362, U.S. 402.
Edens, J. F., Smith, S. T., Magyar, M. S., Mullen, K., Pitta, A., & Petrila, J. (2012). "Hired guns","charlatans", and their "voodoo psychobabble": Case law references to various forms of perceived bias among mental health expert witnesses. *Psychological Services, 9*(3), 259.

Eke, A. W., Helmus, L. M., & Seto, M. C. (2018). *Scoring guide for the Child Pornography Offender Risk Tool (CPORT): Version 2.* Unpublished manual.

Everington, C.T., & Luckasson, R. (1992). Competence assessment for standing trial for defendants with mental retardation (CAST*MR) test manual. International Diagnostic Systems, Inc.

Faccini, L., & Burke, C. (2021). Psychological assessment of Autism spectrum disorder and the law. In *Handbook of autism spectrum disorder and the law* (pp. 439–451). Springer.

Farley, M., Cottle, K. J., Bilder, D., Viskochil, J., Coon, H., & McMahon, W. (2018). Mid-life social outcomes for a population-based sample of adults with ASD. *Autism Research, 11*(1), 142–152.

Federal Rules of Evidence. (2020). In United States Code Annotated, West Publishing. Retrieved from https://www.uscourts.gov/sites/default/files/federal_rules_of_evidence_-_december_2020_0.pdf

Fell, N. (1994). Guardianship and the elderly oversight not overlooked. *The University of Toledo Law Review, 25*, 189.

Ferguson, E. F., Clarke, E. B., Schisterman, N., & Lord, C. (2025). Family experiences with supplemental social security income and legal guardianship for autistic adults: A mixed-methods study. *Research in Autism Spectrum Disorders, 119*, Article 102522. https://doi.org/10.1016/j.rasd.2024.102522

Fradella, H. F., Fogarty, A., & O'Neill, L. (2002). The impact of Daubert on the admissibility of behavioral science testimony. *Pepperdine Law Review, 30*(3), 403–444.

Freckelton, I., et al. (2021). Expert evidence about autism spectrum disorder. In F. R. Volkmar (Ed.), *Handbook of autism spectrum disorder and the law* (pp. 39–69). Springer.

Frederick, R. I. (1997). *Validity indicator profile manual.* NCS Assessments.

Frye v. U.S. (1923). 293 F. 1013.

Girardi, A., Hancock-Johnson, E., Thomas, C., & Wallang, P. M. (2019). Assessing the risk of inpatient violence in autism spectrum disorder. *Journal of the American Academy of Psychiatry and the Law, 47*(4), 427–436.

Griffiths, D. M., & Lunsky, Y. (2003). *Socio-sexual knowledge and attitudes assessment – Revised manual.* Stoelting Co.

Grisso, T. (2010). Guidance for improving forensic reports: A review of common errors. Open access. *Journal of Forensic Psychology, 2*, 102–115.

Gudjonsson, G. H. (1989). Compliance in an interrogation situation: A new scale. *Personality and Individual Differences, 10*, 535–540.

Gudjonsson, G. H. (1997). *The Gudjonsson suggestibility scales manual.* Psychology Press.

Hare, R. D. (2003). The hare psychopathy checklist–Revised (2nd ed.). Multi-Health Systems.

Hart, S. D., Cox, D. N., & Hare, R. D. (1995). *Hare psychopathy checklist: Screening version (PCL: SV).* Multi-Health Systems.

Hart, S. D., Michie, C., & Cooke, D. J. (2007). Precision of actuarial risk assessment instruments: Evaluating the "margins of error" of group versus individual predictions of violence.

Heeramun, R., Magnusson, C., Gumpert, C. H., Granath, S., Lundberg, M., Dalman, C., & Rai, D. (2017). Autism and convictions for violent crimes: Population-based cohort study in Sweden. *Journal of the American Academy of Child & Adolescent Psychiatry, 56*(6), 491–497.

Heilbrun, K., Grisso, T., & Goldstein, A. (2008). *Foundations of forensic mental health assessment.* Oxford University Press.

Heilbrun, K., Rogers, R., & Otto, R. K. (2002). Forensic assessment: Current status and future directions. *Taking Psychology and Law Into the Twenty-First Century*, 119–146.

Hofvander, B., Bering, S., Tärnhäll, A., Wallinius, M., & Billstedt, E. (2019). Few differences in the externalizing and criminal history of young violent offenders with and without autism spectrum disorders. *Frontiers in Psychiatry, 10*, 911.

Howlin, P. (2004). *Autism: Preparing for adulthood* (2nd ed.). Routledge.

Jackson v. Indiana. (1972). 406 U.S. 715.

Jameson, J. M., Riesen, T., Polychronis, S., Trader, B., Mizner, S., Martinis, J., & Hoyle, D. (2015). Guardianship and the potential of supported decision making with individuals with disabilities. *Research and Practice for Persons with Severe Disabilities, 40*(1), 36–51.

Jenkins v. United States. (1962). 307 F.2d 637 (D.C. Cir. 1962).
Jones v. United States. (1983). 463 U.S. 354.
Jurek v. Texas. (1976). 428 U.S. 262.
Kahler v. Kansas. (2020). 140 S. Ct. 1021, 1025-26.
Kaufman, N. K. (2022). Rethinking "gold standards" and "best practices" in the assessment of autism. *Applied Neuropsychology: Child, 11*(3), 529–540.
King, C., & Murphy, G. H. (2014). A systematic review of people with autism spectrum disorder and the criminal justice system. *Journal of Autism and Developmental Disorders, 44*(11), 2717–2733.
Laugeson, E. A., Frankel, F., Gantman, A., Dillon, A. R., & Mogil, C. (2012). Evidence-based social skills training for adolescents with autism spectrum disorders: The UCLA PEERS program. *Journal of Autism and Developmental Disorders, 42*, 1025–1036.
Lerner, M. D., Haque, O. S., Northrup, E. C., et al. (2012). Emerging perspectives on adolescents and young adults with high- functioning autism spectrum disorders, violence, and criminal law. *The Journal of the American Academy of Psychiatry and the Law, 40*(2), 177–190.
Lindsay, W. R., Carson, D., O'Brien, G., Holland, A. J., Taylor, J. L., Wheeler, J. R., & Steptoe, L. (2014). A comparison of referrals with and without autism spectrum disorder to forensic intellectual disability services. *Psychiatry, Psychology and Law, 21*(6), 947–954. https://doi.org/10.1080/13218719.2014.918081
Lord, C., Rutter, M., & Le Couteur, A. (1994). Autism diagnostic interview-revised: A revised version of a diagnostic interview for caregivers of individuals with possible pervasive developmental disorders. *Journal of Autism and Developmental Disorders, 24*(5), 659–685. https://doi.org/10.1007/BF02172145
Lord, C., Rutter, M., DiLavore, P. C., Risi, S., Gotham, K., & Bishop, S. (2012). *Autism diagnostic observation schedule* (2nd ed., ADOS-2). Western Psychological Services.
Loughan, A. R., & Perna, R. (2014). Performance and specificity rates in the Test of Memory Malingering: An investigation into pediatric clinical populations. *Applied Neuropsychology: Child, 3*(1), 26–30.
Loureiro, D., Machado, A., Silva, T., Veigas, T., Ramalheira, C., & Cerejeira, J. (2018). Higher autistic traits among criminals, but no link to psychopathy: Findings from a high-security prison in Portugal. *Journal of Autism and Developmental Disorders, 48*(9), 3010–3020. https://doi.org/10.1007/s10803-018-3576-z.
McGarry, A. L. (1965). Competency for trial and due process via the state hospital. *American Journal of Psychiatry, 122*, 623–631.
M'Naghten's Case. (1843). 10 CI. & Fin. 200.
Maddox, B. B., Brodkin, E. S., Calkins, M. E., Shea, K., Mullan, K., Hostager, J., Mandell, D., & Miller, J. S. (2017). The accuracy of the ADOS-2 in identifying autism among adults with complex psychiatric conditions. *Journal of Autism and Developmental Disorders, 47*, 2703–2709. https://doi.org/10.1007/s10803-017-3188-z
Matthews, M., & Bell, E. (2020). Assessment of risk of violent offending for adults with intellectual disability and/or autism spectrum disorder. *The Wiley Handbook of What Works in Violence Risk Management: Theory, Research and Practice*, 349–366.
Maguire, K., Barnoux, M., Collins, J., Melvin, C. L., Inkson, I., Alexander, R. T.,... & Langdon, P. E. (2025). The factor structure and validity of the psychopathy checklist-short version when used with autistic psychiatric inpatients. *Autism Research, 18*(3), 614–631.
Mahoney, M. J., et al. (2021). Defending men with autism accused of online sexual offenses. In F. R. Volkmar (Ed.), *Handbook of autism spectrum disorder and the law* (pp. 269–306). Springer.
Maras, K. L., & Bowler, D. M. (2012). Brief report: Suggestibility, compliance and psychological traits in high-functioning adults with autism spectrum disorder. *Research in Autism Spectrum Disorders, 6*(3), 1168–1175.
Mattison, M., & Allely, C. (2022). Questioning autistic people: Police and courts. In *Working with autistic people in the criminal justice and forensic mental health systems* (pp. 55–66). Routledge.

Mayes, T. (2003). Persons with autism and criminal justice: Core concepts and leading cases. *Journal of Positive Behavioral Interventions, 5*(2), 92–100.

Melton, G. B., Petrila, J., Poythress, N. G., Slobogin, C., Otto, R. K., Mossman, D., & Condie, L. O. (2018). *Psychological evaluations for the courts: A handbook for mental health professionals and lawyers* (4th ed.). The Guilford Press.

Monteiro, M. J., & Stegall, S. (2018). *Monteiro interview guidelines for diagnosing the autism spectrum* (2nd ed.). Western Psychological Services.

Moss, R. A. (2013). Neuropsychological evaluation in an adolescent with cerebellar hypoplasia diagnosed with Asperger's Syndrome. *Neurocase, 19*(1), 85–89.

Murphy, D. (2013). Risk assessment of offenders with an autism spectrum disorder. *Journal of Intellectual Disabilities and Offending Behaviour, 4*(2), 33–41. https://doi.org/10.1108/JJDOB-02-2013-0004

Murphy, D. (2022). Risk assessment with autistic people. In *Working with autistic people in the criminal justice and forensic mental health systems* (pp. 105–116). Routledge.

Murrie, D. C., Gowensmith, W. N., Kois, L. E., & Packer, I. K. (2023). Evaluations of competence to stand trial are evolving amid a national "competency crisis." *Behavioral Sciences & the Law, 41*(5), 310–325.

Musick, J., & Otto, R. (2010). *The inventory of legal knowledge.* Psychological Assessment Resources.

Nichols, H. R., & Molinder, I. (2010). *Multiphasic sex inventory - Second edition.* Available at https://www.nicholsandmolinder.com/sex-offender-assessment-msi-ii.php

North, A. S., Russell, A. J., & Gudjonsson, G. H. (2008). High functioning autism spectrum disorders: An investigation of psychological vulnerabilities during interrogative interview. *The Journal of Forensic Psychiatry and Psychology, 19*(3), 323–334. https://doi.org/10.1080/14789940701871521

Packer, I. K. (2009). *Evaluation of criminal responsibility.* Oxford University Press.

Pate v. Robinson. (1966). 383, U.S. 375.

Phenix, A., Doren, D., Helmus, L., Hanson, R. K., & Thornton, D. (2008). *Coding rules for Static-2002.* Retrieved from https://saarna.org/static-2002r/

Phenix, A., Fernandez, Y., Harris, A. J., Helmus, M., Hanson, R. K., & Thornton, D. (2017). *Static-99R coding rules, revised-2016.* Public Safety Canada.

Pirelli, G., Gottdiener, W. H., & Zapf, P. A. (2011). A meta-analytic review of competency to stand trial research. *Psychology, Public Policy, and Law, 17*(1), 1–53.

Pirelli, G., & Zapf, P. A. (2020). An attempted meta-analysis of the competency restoration research: Important findings for future directions. *Journal of Forensic Psychology Research and Practice, 20*(2), 134–162.

Poythress, N., Nicholson, R., Otto, R., et al. (1999). *The MacArthur competence assessment tool - Criminal adjudication: Professional manual.* Psychological Assessment Resources.

Quinsey, V. L., Harris, G. T., Rice, M. E., & Cormier, C. A. (2006). *Violent offenders: Appraising and managing risk* (2nd ed.). American Psychological Association.

Railey, K. S., Love, A. M. A., & Campbell, J. M. (2020). A scoping review of autism spectrum disorder and the criminal justice system. *Review Journal of Autism and Developmental Disorders, 35*(10). https://doi.org/10.1177/1088357620922152

Rainer, H., & Linksey, J. P. (2020). Autism and the criminal justice system. *International Journal of Education and Social Science, 7*(6), 2415–1246.

Rava, J., Shattuck, P., Rast, J., & Roux, A. (2017). The prevalence and correlates of involvement in the criminal justice system among youth on the autism spectrum. *Journal of Autism and Developmental Disorders, 47*(2), 340–346.

Rex v. Arnold. (1724). 16 How. St. Tr. 695, 764-65.

Reynolds, C. R., & Kamphaus, R. W. (2015). *Behavior assessment system for children* (3rd ed.). Pearson.

Rogers, R., Sewell, K. W., & Gillard, N. D. (2010). *Structured Interview of Reported Symptoms (SIRS)* (2nd ed.). Psychological Assessment Resources Inc.

Rogers, R., Tillbrook, C. E., & Sewell, K. W. (2003). *Evaluation of competency to stand trial - Revised professional manual*. Psychological Assessment Resources.

Rotter, M., Cucolo, H., & Colley, J. (Eds.). (2019). *Landmark cases in forensic psychiatry* (2nd ed.). Oxford University Press.

Salekin, R. T. (2004). *Risk-sophistication-treatment-inventory (RSTI): A professional manual*. Psychological Assessment Resources.

Schwartz, H. I. (2023). The mind of the mass school shooter. *Journal of American Academy of Psychiatry and Law, 51*, 314–319.

Shaw, K. A., Williams, S., & Patrick, M. E., et al. (2022). Prevalence and early identification of autism spectrum disorder among children aged 4 and 8 years — autism and developmental disabilities monitoring network, 16 Sites, United States, 2022. *MMWR Surveillance Summaries 2025, 74*(No. SS-2), 1–22. https://doi.org/10.15585/mmwr.ss7402a1

Shine, J., & Cooper-Evans, S. (2016). Developing an autism specific framework for forensic case formulation. *Journal of Intellectual Disabilities and Offending Behaviour, 7*(3), 127–139. https://doi.org/10.1106/JIDOB-04-2015-0006

Sinclair, M., Blencowe, A., McCaig, L., & Misch, P. (2013). Neuropsychological findings from a forensic neuropsychology clinic at a South East London tier 4 CAMHS. *Advances in Mental Health and Intellectual Disabilities, 7*(2), 93–107.

Singh, J. P., Grann, M., & Fazel, S. (2011). A comparative study of violence risk assessment tools: A systematic review and meta-regression analysis of 68 studies involving 25,980 participants. *The British Journal of Psychiatry, 190*(2), 162–167.

Slaughter, A. M., Hein, S., Hong, J. D., Mire, S. S., & Grigorenko, E. L. (2019). Criminal behavior and school discipline in juvenile justice-involved youth with Autism. *Journal of Autism and Developmental Disorder, 49*(6), 2268–2280.

Sparrow, S. S., Cicchetti, D. V., & Saulnier, C. A. (2016). *Vineland adaptive behavior scales* (3rd ed.). Pearson Assessments.

Staats, M. L. P., Kivisto, A. J., & Connell, R. E. (2021). The role of cognitive functioning in predicting restoration among criminal defendants committed for inpatient restoration of competence to stand trial. *International Journal of Law and Psychiatry, 74*, Article 101654.

Tombaugh, T. N. (1996). *Test of memory malingering*. Multi-Health Systems Inc.

Viljoen, J. L., McLachlan, K., & Vincent, G. M. (2010). Assessing risk for violence in adolescents. *Aggression and Violent Behavior, 15*(2), 129–142.

Wall, B. W., & Christopher, P. P. (2012). A training program for defendants with intellectual disabilities who are found incompetent to stand trial. *Journal of the American Academy of Psychiatry and the Law Online, 40*(3), 366–373.

Webster, C. D., Douglas, K. S., Eaves, D., & Hart, S. D. (1997). *HCR-20: Assessing risk for violence (Version 2)*.

Weisbrot, D. M., Carlson, G. A., Ettinger, A. B., et al. (2023). Psychiatric characteristics of students who make threats towards others at school. *Journal of American Academy of Child and Adolescent Psychiatry, 62*(7), 764–776.

White, S. G., Meloy, J. R., Mohandie, K., & Kienien, K. (2017). Autism spectrum disorder and violence: Threat assessment issues. *Journal of Threat Assessment and Management, 4*(3), 144–163.

Wood, M. E. (2025, April 1). *The complexity of adjudicative competence evaluations for defendants with intellectual disability: Arguing (again) for distance practices and procedures* [Webinar]. The University of New Mexico Health Sciences: Division of Forensic Behavioral Sciences - Law and Mental Health. https://www.youtube.com/watch?v=DO2Vx2mppW4

Yu, J. (2021). *Without the forbidden fruit. Returning to the wild beast test. Cornell Journal of Law and Public Policy, 30*, 819 at 823. Fn. 12

Yu, Y., Bradley, C. C., Boan, A. D., Charles, J. M., & Carpenter, L. A. (2021). Young adults with autism spectrum disorder and the criminal justice system. *Journal of Autism & Developmental Disorders, 51*(10), 3624–3636. https://doi-org.library.capella.edu/https://doi.org/10.1007/s10803-020-04805-9

Zapf, P. A., & Roesch, R. (2009). *Evaluation of competence to stand trial*. Oxford University Press.

Ethics in Assessment

Johnny L. Matson

Abstract Autism and related neurodevelopmental disorders have become among the most discussed and studied in the field of mental health. Also, there are many controversies about what constitutes autism, whether it should be treated or indeed whether it should be considered an atypical aspect of the human condition. These and other critical issues also are implicated with respect to ethical concerns. This chapter tackles some of these ethical issues. An effort is made to point out differing positions and goals as they apply to the assessment and diagnosis of autism spectrum disorders.

Keywords Autism · Ethics · Assessment · Diagnosis · Goals of assessment · Goals of diagnosis

The field of autism has seen a dramatic rise in attention from clinicians and researchers in the last few decades. This phenomenon has occurred at a grass roots level which has also affected funding, states and federal laws as well as goals and expectations for all stakeholders. Beginning the process of care is the identification and diagnosis of the disorder. Later, methods to track skills to increase and enhance adaptation to their environment are added. Also, assessment geared toward decreasing excesses such as challenging behaviors deficits in social skills and communication are targeted. These and related issues lead to consider how these questions are addressed and how concerns of stake holders and professionals can be achieved to arrive at mutually agreed upon goals.

Informed consent is necessary for clinical care and for research aimed at enhancing services (Neff, 2008). Based on the Nuremberg Cole which emerged in Germany after WW II (1947) and followed by the Medical Association Declaration of Helsinki (1964), then the Belmont report helped codify informed consent as we know it (1979). Several key points emerged from these documents including, as noted, the need for informed consent, the focus on client autonomy and the need to assess

J. L. Matson (✉)
Department of Psychology, Louisiana State University, Baton Rouge, LA, USA
e-mail: johnmatson@aol.com

J. L. Matson (ed.), *Assessment and Diagnosis in Autism*, Autism and Child Psychopathology Series, https://doi.org/10.1007/978-3-032-11802-8_12

potential risks and benefits of assessment and treatment. Neff (2008) stresses that informed consent at its essence is a non-corrosive process between the patient and the clinician. Preferably the consent is provided by the patient. However, for young children, in some cases for the elderly and among persons with severe autism and/or intellectual disability, this goal may not be possible. And, whether the patient or their advocate provides consent, it should occur without the sense of time constraints or other pressures.

Ethical factors with respect to the assessment of autism involve a number of factors. Among the most important is ensuring that methods selected are relevant for each person, and to ensure that the assessment methods used have an evidence base. Thus, the chapter will begin with a brief overview of evidence-based methods, and what targets can be reliably evaluated.

Within the assessment paradigm, issues include diagnosis, the selection of target behaviors for intervention and the evaluation of treatment effectiveness. Also, it has become more apparent with further study that many ancillary skills can be affected by the core symptoms of autism. Additionally, comorbid disorders such as ADHD and anxiety have proven to be common with autism. Having said that, the most frequent co-occurring problem is intellectual disability. Above all these other problems it is the disorder most likely to adversely affect the understanding of information and thus informed consent (Hamilton et al., 2017). Where applicable, using visual and other technical devices (e.g., pictures may be combined with auditory aids) within a person-centered context should be employed. The need for a multimodal approach should be intensify with respect to comorbid disorders added on to the need to assess autism symptoms.

Differential diagnosis is a major aspect of assessment. It has been and continues to be at the center of debate since autism was first defined by Kanner (1944). Autism was once considered to be separate from intellectual disability, but no longer. Rather, considerable overlap exists between autism and intellectual disabilities and has far reaching implications for both assessment and treatment (Matson et al., 2007). Along these same lines are the conceptual issues regarding how to understand how these two conditions interact and affect each other. For example, when both autism and intellectual disability occur together, which one is the primary condition? The answer to this question has important ethical considerations and the decision should be made on a case by case basis with respect to which diagnosis is primary. The guiding principle for which disorder is primary should be based on how best services can be used to develop goals to produce the best quality of life for the person (Matson & Minshawi, 2006). For example, one or the other diagnosis may trigger more available services in a given geographic location. As alluded to, the diagnosis flow from that. All assessments are critical, but no assessment is more important than the initial assessment which produces or does not produce a diagnosis of autism. Particularly in the former case, delivering the news may be difficult (Abrans & Goodman, 1998). Along these same lines, the assessment and reporting of findings to the parent or client (determined by age and cognitive capacities) should be completed in days or at most 2–3 weeks upon the start of this initial assessment (Canadian Psychological Association, 2000). Often, delaying the reporting of results to stakeholders can cause unnecessary anxiety and frustration. This issue should be viewed in the context of professional competence and ethical guidelines.

Assessment, in the broader context, should take several forms. Foremost are standardized checklists. Basic psychometric properties for these checklists should be in place including norms for the age group and culture of the person being evaluated. These points are essential in terms of providing the most accurate information possible, since further action steps would be based on this data. Also, tests that are a best fit for each client based on clinical characteristics such as target behaviors and learning history as well as potential needs that best conceptualize quality of life should be addressed. Unfortunately, the failure to use evidence-based procedures are far too common.

Given the heterogenetic nature of autism, evaluation needs to cover a range of areas of impairment (Gordijn & Have, 2012). Among these are social impairments, linguistic capacities, intellectual functioning, adaptive behavior fine and gross motor skills, and challenging behaviors. Also deserving attention on an individual clinical level is the cause or causes of the specific behavior excesses and deficits and how they are triggered, exacerbated, and maintained (Hens et al., 2019).

For many years the focus in the field was almost exclusively on children, particularly young children. However, researchers and clinicians are now recognizing and emphasizing the lifelong nature of autism. The focus is now also on the transition from school to the adult world as part of this new approach. Preparation for movement into and adapting to adult society has thus, and rightly become a major focus of assessment and treatment (Lee & Carter, 2012). Paramount among these transition topics is vocational training including the evaluation of work-related social behaviors (Barbaro & Shankardass, 2023).

Informed Consent

Informed consent is the cornerstone of the ethics of assessment and also is a legal requirement (Kadam, 2017; Nijhawan et al., 2013). The philosophy behind informed consent dates to the end of WW II. The mistreatment of people by medical professionals in Nazi Germany led to the Nuremberg Code. The notion behind these developments was that the client had the right to know and understand the procedures to be used, and to have the right to participate or reject participation. And, while a form much be completed, perhaps more importantly is the need to ensure that the client clearly understands what is being asked of them (Pallodino, 2002). This goal requires that the participant understand the risks, benefits, time requirements and the tasks to be completed (Wirshing et al., 1998). As a result, there are a number of factors that are important to consider in ensuring that the clients' rights are protected. Achieving this goal can be particularly important for persons with autism, where lack of process can be a problem. These issues are compounded by the fact that young children in particular, have limited vocabulary and conceptual skills.

The purpose of the assessment and how the information will be used and stored should be addressed (Jefford & Moore, 2008). The consent form should avoid professional jargon where possible. And, where jargon is unavoidable, the clinician should check to ensure that the client or where necessary, their guardian, can clearly understand these profession specific terms. Having said that, concerns have been raised that the understanding of the consent form is often quite low (Nishimura et al., 2013). Various methods have been applied to enhance establishing informed consent such as using multimedia and the use of examples for complex terms and concepts. To date the results of these strategies have produced mixed results (Firoy & Emanuel, 2004).

A number of procedures have been evaluated to enhance informed consent such as multimedia methods and steering away from professional jargon as mentioned earlier. Anderson et al. (2017) asked former research participants what they would recommend to improve informed consent. These authors acknowledge the value of technical factors. In addition, they stress the need to ensure that trust is established between the clinicians and the client. They also stress that client confusion can lead to dissatisfaction with the assessment process. Anderson et al. (2017) note that this effect can lead to higher dropout rates by clients.

Lorenzen et al. (2008) describe a very creative approach to improving informed consent. They describe a model in Iowa where hospitals created "health literacy teams." The purpose of these teams was to improve knowledge of health terms and concepts. Members were multidisciplinary and included professionals in risk management, medical education, general education, and students from a community college extension program. They focused on the structure and form of the consent document. Among the most salient recommendations that were made included keeping the form short and the font size of words large. Also, medical and legal jargon has often been used but is infrequently defined. While on the surface this all makes sense, federal, state, and professional mandates can make the task of simplifying the consent form challenging. Often specific concepts and jargon are required, that is often hard for the general public to understand.

It has been pointed out that patient characteristics, especially lower literacy and minority status are impactful for understanding and then providing consent. These points also apply to parents of young children (Sudore et al., 2006). To underscore the importance of proficient presentation of information, and the unique characteristics of clients, these authors point out that 40% to 80% of patients actually have the capacity to consent (persons with low I.Q. and/or dementia who did not understand one or more aspects of the form). Sudore et al. (2006) as have other authors underscore the need to make consent forms less complex, more readable and better designed.

Lentz et al. (2016) stress the importance of the voluntary nature of informed consent. As with all aspects of clinical care, the process can always be improved to lead to clear, accurate information about the specifics of proposed assessment methods and procedures. Generally speaking, both clinicians and stake holders agree that more could be done to achieve these goals.

In the Lentz et al. (2016) study, efforts to improve informed consent involved a literature review where they focused on identifying methods that have been used to evaluate the effectiveness. Also, they identified barriers to changes in informed consent and factors associated with patient satisfaction with the process. The degree to which informed consent can effect whether the client or their advocate chooses to participate in the assessment process was also identified as an important factor.

A second procedure these authors used was interviewing experts. Included were IRB chairs, FDA and NIH medical directors and officers, ethicists, executives from pharmaceutical and medical device executives, clients, advocates, academic medical center professionals, and electronic consent company executives among others. Then, a two-day meeting with 60 other experts from professional organizations, law firms, academic nonprofits, government employees, client representatives, and professionals from health systems were among the individuals who participated.

Findings covered several topics. First, professional staff should administer the informed consent. This approach is typically followed for research studies. However, in clinical practice often clients or advocates are given forms and then are told to read and sign the forms. This latter approach is far more likely to lead to a lack of understanding of the assessment process. Also, the authors underscore that formalized training of staff should occur using a variety of methods. They cite providing didactic information, interactive opportunities and continuing education. It was also stressed that clients and advocates have different learning styles. Those people who will provide informed consent come to the task with different levels of knowledge and experience with the assessment process. The rate at which individuals learn will differ as well. For example, some stakeholders may wish to be provided with a comprehensive overview of proposed tasks, others may prefer a brief summary. Educational and cultural factors may also impact the process. These authors as with others mentioned in this chapter stress using simplified, plain language, limiting the amount of information presented and incorporating pictograms and lists or bullet point as a means of enhancing comprehension (Nishimura et al., 2013).

E-consent has become common and is likely to be used even more frequently in the future given the trend to paperless documentation. With this electronic trend comes new and unique problems. Among these are concerns about security and confidentiality, a lack of established processes, initial development costs, and the need to establish wide acceptance of e-signatures (Lentz et al., 2016).

Specialized Issues for Informed Consent

There is a copious literature on informed consent. Within this context, various specialization issues have been identified and then discussed. A few of these issues will now be briefly reviewed to give the reader an idea of what has been covered.

Proxy consent is, as previously noted, necessary when the person is not cognitively able to provide consent (Graber, 2016). In Graber's paper, criteria for proxy consent are laid out. The first is the right to an open future, which assumes the future possibility of autonomy. The most common example would be a young child. As they age maturation and experience increase the likelihood of making better and more informed decisions. The second is substitute judgment. This approach implies that a legal guardian is required. The best interest standard would be used on the basis of do no harm either physically, mentally or both.

It is also important for the client to be able to recall possible risks and complications of treatment. Sherlock and Brownie (2014) conducted a review on this topic. They found that the ability to remember risk and complications of interventions was low and was particularly problematic in older people. Other characteristics such as intellectual disabilities and autism can also complicate this informed consent process. As in other studies reviewed in this chapter, Sherlock and Broume (2014) stress that remembering critical information on consent forms follows strategies for initial comprehension. Tips include using interactive multimedia plus didactic material that are easy to read and understand.

Another specialized topic involves the application of digital tools (Gesualdo et al., 2012). These authors found that interactive multimedia was the most commonly used digital tool to assist in obtaining informed consent. Noninteractive multimedia was the next most frequently used digital method followed by videos. These authors concluded from their overview of the literature on the topic found that these media and video methods did not negatively impact the consent process. Having said that, more research and/or better multimedia methods are needed.

Also using technology, Welch et al. (2016) developed a process they call tele consent. The clinician or researchers can, using this method, obtain consent remotely. They imbed the informed consent into a telehealth session. The clinician can display the form and then interact with the client in real time while the consent form is completed and e-signed. Given the rapid move to a more paperless society, methods such as tele consent are likely to become more common.

Ethical Issues in Assessment and Diagnosis

There are a number of factors that are driving this development in diagnostic screening for autism. First, awareness of autism and the persistent increases in the numbers of people diagnosed with the disorder has increased the demand for new, more efficient and effective assessment tools. Second, diagnostic substitution where one diagnosis takes the place of another (e.g., autism being diagnosed rather than intellectual disabilities) increased dramatically in the area of neurodevelopmental disorders. No where is this point more applicable than with autism. A third factor is called diagnostic coupling (Graf et al., 2017). These authors use this term to note that often therapies and other services for autism must be accompanied with a specific diagnosis. Finally, these authors note that pediatric screening for autism has become commonplace. These issues have important implications for ethical practices not only in genetic testing, but also with respect to other screening and diagnostic methods.

Ethical issues in establishing an autism diagnosis are commonly observed. The primary problem revolves around the methods and processes used for a given individual, and if the approach used yields an accurate diagnosis. In practice, often reliable and valid methods are not used. Rather, unproven or unreliable approaches are employed. These questionable practices raise ethical red flags.

One such questionable practice is the use of genetic testing. This practice is growing and has "Uncertain scientific validity and limited clinical utility" (Graf et al., 2017). An important ethical issue as these authors point out is that making diagnoses using this method therefore may also be inaccurate. Additional expense and time are likely.

Natri et al. (2023) have also addressed ethical challenges in autism genomics. They note the great potential for genetic research. This potential applies to not just first diagnosis but possibly new preventative methods and innovative treatment as well. The counterbalance to this issue is the push back by many in the autism community. For example, some people believe that efforts to find causes and studies on genetic markers and prenatal screening should not be conducted (Frazier et al., 2018). These opponents also stress the need to have input from the autistic community regarding genomic research. Their position, at least among many, is that there needs to be a move away from identification prevention or treatment and instead focus on well-being, barrier to inclusion in society and societal benefits of diversity. It has been argued further that ethical guidelines should be revised including the review process and methods for development and implementation (Manzini et al., 2021). At a minimum, safeguards should be in place that allow for input by members of the autism community as it applies to individuals who are participants in genetics or any other form of research. Many of these same concerns are noted for clinical treatments as well.

A good development has been researched that surveys attitudes, priorities, and concerns of the autism community. An example of these types of studies is presented by Wagner et al. (2020). They conducted a survey of parent perspectives on various genetic practices for persons with autism. They administered a 16-item questionnaire to 244 parents of children who were 19–135 months of age and who were identified as meeting criteria for autism. Nineteen percent of the parents could accurately identify basic facts about epigenetics despite over 60% having discussed genetic information with a physician. This data clearly shows that additional thinking about how to enhance knowledge and thus informed consent for stakeholders is needed.

It is generally accepted at this point in time that autism is at least in part a genetic condition. Also, there does not appear to be one specific genetic profile. Rather, it appears to be a number of genetic variants that make autism more likely (Kaufmann et al., 2017; Parisi et al., 2015). Because of this state of affairs, informed consent issues may need to be linked to genetic counseling so that the consent can be put into the broader content of autism, or at least in the future as these methods are further developed and refined. Some authors have stressed that counseling of this sort when accompanied by testing that provides molecular confirmation can help parents accept their autism and "acknowledge that it is permanent and beyond the control thus mitigating feelings of guild (Reiff et al., 2015). Along this line of argument, it is stressed that the identification of genetic causes/confirmation of autism can help motivate parents to consider anticipatory and proactive care (Vorstam et al., 2017). It should be underscored again however, that these genetic diagnostic methods are still in the early stage of development. Thus, proponents of genetic testing also stress that in an attempt to do no harm genetic testing and counseling can enhance knowledge about the nature of the condition. This information can lead to better knowledge of disorder specific characteristics and behaviors that are expressed (Oliver et al., 2011). Also, it is stressed that failing to identify or further help gain new information about a condition is an ethical concern in and of itself. Having said that, issues of informed consent and other aspects of identification and treatment with genetic conditions is one of the major points of emphasis with respect to the entire field of ethics and autism.

Another area recently receiving considerable attention with respect to ethical concerns is artificial intelligence. This topic will in all likelihood continue to grow exponentially in the years to come. Fike et al. (2019) discuss ethical issues as it applies to virtual/robotic therapies. As the reader is most likely aware autistic children often gravitate to robotics (Scassellati et al., 2012). These therapies use an artificially intelligent (AI) algorithm which is preprogrammed into the robot. As a result, human therapist input is not needed in real time. This therapy model differs from telehealth where a therapist counsels the client remotely or where the client engages in self-instruction using didactic materials. Example goals of AI therapy include the recognition of emotions, teaching resilience to aid in anxiety reduction, flagging expressions of emotional distress, teaching about various technical terms that constitute autism, various assessments, and treatment and developing skills for handling difficult social interactions. Robots usually are in the shape of small, cute animals. One example is the Kaspar robot application with autistic children to teach social skills and the development of other adaptive skills (Huijnen et al., 2017).

Given the rapid development of AI, robotics and other AI-based technologies are likely to go from an infant field to widespread use rapidly. Fike et al. (2019) point out that these methods may be useful for some difficult to treat populations, for individuals in resource poor environments, or who are in remote situations. Also, some clients may prefer less intense therapies, or assessments and treatments that can be administered in a private setting such as the home. Finally, a robot therapist could be available at all times if used in this manner.

Several ethical issues have also been identified. Much more research is needed on the effectiveness of AI for the assessment and treatment of autism and related issues such as intellectual disabilities and challenging behaviors. In addition to effectiveness, dependability will also be a significant issue. Also, since electronics can be breached by hackers, data security will always be a major concern. Many of the ethical challenges will mirror current issues. However, much of the AI technology will result in the development of new, novel application to insure the ethical utilization of these methods. Guidelines will need to be developed to ensure that clinicians can train and supervise clients using AI technology in an ethical manner.

As mentioned previously, in addition to AI, telehealth is another electronic medium likely to receive considerable attention moving forward. Quigley et al. (2019) provide a discussion of telehealth as it applies to autism. Among the most frequent concerns are efforts to protect confidentiality. Savin et al. (2006) note that typical internet services are not secure enough to safeguard client data. McDuffie et al. (2013) suggest that this problem can be solved by using a virtual private network. Various software programs may also be employed to meet this objective. What is clear is that new innovations will be needed to protect data. Also, as the technology of hackers advances security measures will need to evolve.

A second major issue involves adherence to various laws and guidelines such as HIPPA. For example, the Individuals with Disabilities Act (IDEA, 2004) mandates that functional behavioral assessment be used when applied behavior analysis programs are employed. Similarly, Quigley et al. (2019) note that professional organization codes such as the American Telehealth Association, Telehemental Health Practice Guidelines (2013) and the ethics code for Behavior Analyst Certification Board, 2014) should be studied and used as a model to adhere to various recognized professional standards.

Ethic Factors in Assessment and Treatment

An ethical approach to assessment and treatment implies that goals need to be established to promote independence among people with autism while enhancing happiness. Bahry et al. (2023) list a number of goals that need to be assessed and implemented to achieve the goal of independence of each client. Among these objectives include; (1) having the therapist, practice within the scope of their competence; (2), using effective, data-based interventions; (3) involve clients and other stakeholders; (4) maximum benefits that accrue while doing no harm, and (5) clients should be treated with compassion, dignity, and respect. These authors also stress the importance of a holistic approach to care. This should include effective treatments that are reliability and validity assessed goals. It also means enhancing goals which increase physical, social and academic inclusion. Particularly for persons with the most severe symptoms of autism and/or secondary intellectual disability and/or forms of psychopathology, lifelong intervention may be necessary. The authors cited above also note that ethical goals require highly individualized goals that teach applied skills. Among the results would be to provide well-being and the support of long-term goals which promote happiness. Teaching specific goals requires systematic assessment, using objective means to determine the magnitude and effectiveness of outcomes.

Cox (2012) makes another very important point with respect to ethical issues in autism. Cox (2012) notes that autism has become a multidisciplinary field. Ethical codes from a number of professions including speech, psychology, medicine, applied behavior analysis, special education, and occupational therapy, therefore, should be considered. Cox (2012) noted several common ethical principles including informed consent, confidentiality, beneficence, non-maleficence, respect for autonomy, and justice. It is stressed that these common ethical characteristics should be viewed as common language for professionals. Another issue pertains to professional competence. It is noted that it is necessary for the professional to acquire the necessary knowledge skill set. These abilities apply to technical knowledge and personal interactive skills. This latter category includes developing trust and good faith to ensure the best interests of the client. And, with respect to interdisciplinary issues, ensuring that what needs to be done by an interdisciplinary colleague occurs, ensuring continuity of information as the key to continuity of care and committing to working as a group are needed to present high-quality care. These points help underscore the need to view the person in a comprehensive way.

Bahry et al. (2023) address the issue of treatment evaluation framed in the context of ethical considerations. In this context, the authors underscore the importance of ensuring that it is incumbent on the clinician to prepare the autistic person to live as independent a life as much as possible across the lifespan. Factors that should be assessed include post-secondary education, social and community participation, employment, accessing services, health issues, independent living, and safety. Also, these authors stress that autism symptoms and comorbidities vary widely in terms of strengths and weaknesses as well as severity of symptoms. Intellectual disability is the most common comorbidity and may affect up to 70% of the autism community. Also, intellectual deficits are more predictive of poor outcomes than even the person's autistic symptoms. Bahry et al. (2023) note several ethical considerations regarding the assessment process. Among these are selecting assessments that are scientifically supported and provide for the diverse needs of clients and stakeholders at their disposal. Also, they recommend continually evaluating interventions. Factors to consider when analyzing data include ongoing evaluation to determine if treatment goals are being achieved. These goals should be evaluated and adjustments to the treatment plan and goals should be modified as needed. It is also possible that services provided by other professionals may make the overall treatment plan less effective. Since most individuals received services from multiple professionals at once (e.g., psychology, applied behavior analyses, speech therapy, educators, social workers, pediatricians, neurologists, psychiatrists, and physical therapists) these issues need to be addressed and coordinated with the relevant professionals. Supervisor competence is another issue these author's address. It is stated that the supervisor should only provide training to staff within the scope of competence and training that the professional possesses. (This point seems obvious but in practice it is often not followed.) Additionally, the supervisor should possess the relevant skills and they should continually evaluate and improve their skills.

Bahry et al. (2023) emphasize the importance of selecting and prioritizing what specific skills need to be taught. From an ethical standpoint, they underscore the importance of developing not only behavior reduction assessment and treatment, but also to emphasize skill development that result in better adjustment and independence. This author has seen numerous examples of inconsequential skills being trained while essential skills were not being trained. Given limited training time and resources, this issue is very important. Prioritizing treatment efforts is essential for all clients and for persons with severe autism symptoms and major intellectual deficits. This priority model is especially crucial. Such is the case because of a slower, more limited rate of learning for people with extreme cognitive deficits. It is also stressed that skills selection, assessment and treatment should help enhance quality of life. A client's needs should consider factors such as age, preferences, strengths, physical and psychological challenges and the demands placed on clients, stakeholders and professionals in current and potential future environments.

Miller (2017) also addressed the value of assessment in the monitoring of treatment. The author stresses the need for program evaluation as a means of informing the clinician about treatment effectiveness. Variables that need to be assessed according to the author are related to implementation of treatment, determining the effectiveness of the intervention, how cost effective the program is (many programs for autism involve intensive applied behavior analysis which can be very costly in money, time and commitment) and what is the stakeholder's satisfaction level with care. It is recommended that specific assessments that are both qualitative and quantitative should be used to achieve this goal. Some of the variables that should be addressed include parent knowledge of principles and procedures that make up the program, parent satisfaction and family stressors, what factors led to participant choice and participant satisfaction. Miller (2017) also points out that providers often are not familiar with many of the assessments they should consider using to evaluate treatment. Thus, assessing agency/staff knowledge should, from an ethical perspective, be part of the overall assessment plan. In addition to a needs assessment for the agency, the population served should be evaluated. Among the questions Miller (2017) suggests should be asked are, who is being served, why is the person being served, and what interventions are being provided. It is stressed that service providers need to learn about variations in the service population's culture, language and knowledge about the intervention(s) to be employed.

Conclusions

In this chapter, the focus has been on ethical factors (variables to consider in the assessment of individuals with autism. Assessment goals include diagnosis, establishing goals for intervention and evaluating treatment effectiveness. Needs assessment for caregiver's stakeholders and clients should also be addressed. These goals are a tall order and must be balanced against the possibilities of overwhelming staff or clients, making the assessment to time consuming and/or expensive. Picking a checklist should be followed by prioritizing what methods and procedures can be utilized in a predetermined time period and what people will be included in the process.

Before these assessment goals can be implemented, informed consent needs to be obtained. In this chapter factors to consider during this process have been reviewed. Also, the content and structure of the form itself were covered. It is underscored that avoiding professional jargon, covering the major issues in how the assessment will be conducted establishing what the potential costs and benefits should be included. Also, the client, or their guardian should be aware that they can withdraw consent at any time. Ethical assessment then, is imbedded in all aspects of the evaluation process.

References

Abrams, E. Z., & Goodman, J. F. (1998). Diagnosing developmental problems in children? Parents and professionals negotiate bad news. *Journal of Pediatric Psychology, 23*, 82–98.

American Telemedicine Association, Telemental Health Practice Guidelines Work Group and the ATA Standards and Guidelines committee. (2013). Practice guidelines for video-based online mental health services.

Anderson, E. E., Newman, S. B., & Matthews, A. K. (2017). Improving informed consent: Stakeholders views. *AJOB Empirical Bioethics, 8*, 178–188.

Bahry, S., Gerhardt, P. F., Weiss, M. J., Leaf, J. B., Putan, R. F., & Bondy, A. (2023). The ethics of actually helping people: Targeting skill acquisition goals that promote meaningful outcomes for individuals with autism spectrum disorder. *Behavior Analysis in Practice, 16*, 672–695.

Barbaro, D., & Shankardass, K. (2023). Work-related social skills interventions for individuals with autism spectrum disorder throughout the life course. *Review Journal of Autism and Developmental Disorders, 10*, 699–711.

Belmont Report. (1979). Ethical principles and guidelines for the protection of human subjects of research. National Commission for the Protection of Human Subjects of Biomedical and Behavioral Research. Washington, D.C.

Behavior Analyst Certification Board. (2014). Professional and ethical compliance code for behavior analysts. Retrieved from http://bacb.com/wp-content/uploads/2015/08/150824-compliance-code-enghlish.pdf

Canadian Psychological Association. (2000). *Canadian code of ethics for psychologists*. Author.

Cox, D. J. (2012). From interdisciplinary to integrate care of the child with autism: The essential role for a code of ethics. *Journal of Autism and Developmental Disorders, 42*, 2729–2738.

Fike, A., Henningsen, P., & Buyx, A. (2019). Your robot therapist will see you now: Ethical implications of embodied artifical intelligence in psychiatry, psychology and psychtherapy. *Journal of Medical Internet Research, 21*, 5.

Fiory, J., & Emanuel, E. (2004). Interventions to improve research participants' understanding in informed consent for research: A systematic review. *Journal of the American Medical Association, 292*, 1593–1601.

Frazier, T. W., Dawson, G., Murray, D., Shh, A., Sachs, J. S., & Geiger, A. (2018). Brief report: A survey of autism research priorities across a diverse community of stakeholders. *Journal of Autism and Developmental Disorders, 48*, 3965–3971.

Gesualdo, F., Daverio, M., Palazani, L., Dimitriou, D., Diez-Domingo, J., Fons-Martinez, J., Jackson, S., Vignally, P., Rizzo, C., & Tozzi, A. E. (2012). Digital tool in the informed consent process: A systematic review. *BMC Medical Ethics, 22*, 18. https://doi.org/10.1186/s12910-021-00585-8

Graber, A. (2016). Autism, intellectual disability and a challenge to our understanding of proxy consent. *Medicine, HealthCare and Philosophy, 20*, 229–236.

Gordijn, B., & ten Have, H. (2012). Ethics of autism. *Mental Health Care and Philosophy, 15*, 253–254.

Graf, W. S., Miller, G., Epstein, L. G., & Rapin, I. (2017). The autism "epidemic": Ethical, legal, and social issues in a developmental spectrum disorder. *American Academy of Neurology, 88*, 1–10.

Hamilton, J., Ingham, B., McKinnon, I. Parr, J. R., Tam, L. Y.-G., & LeCouteur, A. (2017). Mental capacity to consent to research? Experiences of consenting adults with intellectual disabilities and autism to research. *British Journal of Learning Disabilities*, 1–8. 10.111/bid.12198

Hens, K., Robeyns, I., & Schaubroeck, K. (2019). The ethics of autism. *Philosophy Compass, 14*, Article e12559.

Huijnen, C. A., Lexis, M. A., Jansens, R., & deWitt, L. P. (2017). How to implement robots in interventions for children with autism? A co-creation study involving people with autism, parents and professionals. *Journal of Autism and Developmental Disorders, 47*, 3079–3096.

Individuals with Disabilities Act (IDEA). (2004). 20 U.S.C. & 1400.

Jefford, M., & Moore, R. (2008). Improvement of informed consent and the quality of consent documents. *Lancet Oncology, 9*, 485–493.
Kadam, R. A. (2017). Informed consent process: A step further towards making it meaningful! *Perspective Clinical Research, 8*, 107–112.
Kanner, L. (1944). Early infantile autism. *Journal of Pediatrics, 25*, 211–217.
Kaufmann, W. E., Kidd, S. A., Andrews, H. F., Budimirovic, D. B., Esler, A., Haas-Givler, B., Stackhouse, T., Riley, C., Peacock, G., Sherman, S. L., Brown, W. T., & Berry-Kravis, E. (2017). Autism spectrum disorder in fragile X syndrome: Cooccurring conditions and current treatment. *Pediatrics, 139*(Supplement 3), S194–S206. https://doi.org/10.1542/peds.2016-1159F
Lee, G. K., & Carter, E. W. (2012). Preparing transition-age students with high-functioning autism spectrum disorders for meaningful work. Psychology in the Schools. https://doi.org/10.1002/pits.21651
Lentz, J., Kennett, M., Perlmutter, J., & Forrest, A. (2016). Paving the way to a more effective informed consent process: Recommendations from the clinical trials transformation initiative. *Contemporary Clinical Trials, 49*, 65–69.
Lorenzen, B., Melby, C. E., & Earles, B. (2008). Using principles of health literacy to enhance the informed consent process. *AORN Journal, 88*, 23–29.
Manzini, A., Jones, E. J. H., Charman, T., Elsabbagh, M., Johnson, M. H., & Singh, I. (2021). Ethical dimensions of translational developmental neuroscience research in autism. *Journal of Child Psychology and Psychiatry, 62*, 1363–1373.
Matson, J. L., & Minshawi, N. F. (2006). Early intervention for autism spectrum disorders: A critical analysis. Oxford, England: Elsevier Science Inc.
Matson, J. L., Nebel-Schwalm, M., & Matson, J. L. (2007). A review of methodological issues in the differential diagnosis of autism spectrum disorders in children. *Research in Autism Spectrum Disorders, 1*, 38–54.
McDuffie, A., Machalicek, W., Oakes, A., Haebig, E., Weismer, S. E., & Abbeduto, L. (2013). Distance video-teleconferencing in early intervention: Pilot study of a naturalistic parent-implemented language intervention. *Topics in Early Childhood Special Education, 33*, 172–185.
Miller, K. L. (2017). The use of evaluation in treatment programs for children with autism. *Behavior Analysis Practice, 10*, 35–44.
Natri, H. M., Chapman, C. R., Heraty, S., Dwyer, P., Walker, N., Kapp, S. K., Dron, H. A., Martinez-Agosto, J. A., Mikkola, L., & Doherty, M. (2023). Ethical challenges in autism genomics: Recommendations for researchers. *Journal of Medical Genetics, 66*(9). https://doi.org/10.1016/ejmg.2023.104810
Neff, M. J. (2008). Informed consent: What is it? Who can give it? How do we improve it? *Respiratory Care, 53*, 1337–1341.
Njjhawan, L. P., Janodia, M. F., Muddukrishna, B. S., Bhat, K. M. Bairy, K. L., Udupa, N., & Musmade, P. B. (2013). Informed consent; Issues and challenges. *Journal of Advanced Pharmaceutical Technology and Research, 4*, 134–140.
Nishimura, A., Carey, J., Erwin, P. J., Tilburt, J. G., Hassan Murad, M., & McCormick, J. B. (2013). Improving understanding in the research informed consent process: A systematic review of 54 interventions tested in randomized control trials. *BMC Medical Ethics, 14*, 28.
Oliver, C., Berg, K., Moss, J., Arron, K., & Burbidge, C. (2011). Delineation of behavioral phenotypes in genetic syndromes: Characteristics of autism spectrum disorder, affect and hyperactivity. *Journal of Autism and Developmental Disorders, 41*(8), 1019–1032. https://doi.org/10.1007/s10803-010-1125-5
Pallodino, M. (2002). Challengers in the informed consent process: Identifying design strategies that enhance communication in adult clinical trials. *Research Practice, 3*, 164–171.
Parisi, L., DiFilippo, T., & Roccella, M. (2015). Behavioral phenotype and autism spectrum disorders in cornelia de lange syndrome. *Mental Illness, 7*(2), 5988. https://doi.org/10.4081/mi.2015.5988

Quigley, S. P., Blevins, P. R., Cox, D. J., Broadhead, M. T., & Kim, S. Y. (2019). An evaluation of explicit ethical statements in telehealth research with individuals with autism spectrum disorder. *Behavior Analysis Research and Practice, 19*, 123–135.

Reiff, M., Giarelli, E., Bernhardt, B. A., Easley, E., Spinner, N. B., Sankar, P. L., & Mulchandani, S. (2015). Parents' perceptions of the usefulness of chromosomal microarray analysis for children with autism spectrum disorders. *Journal of Autism and Developmental Disorders, 45*(100), 3262–3275. https://doi.org/10.1007/s10803-015-2489-3

Savin, D., Garry, M. T., Zuccaro, P., & Novins, D. (2006). Telepsychiatry for treating rural American Indian youth. *Journal of the American Academy of Child an Adolescent Psychiatry, 45*, 484–488.

Scassellati, B., Admoni, H., & Mataric, M. (2012). Robots for use in autism research. *Annual Review of Biomedical Engineering, 14*, 275–294.

Sherlock, A., & Brownie, S. (2014). Patients' recollection and understanding of informed consent: A literature review. *ANX Journal of Surgery, 84*, 207–210.

Sudore, R. L., Landerfeld, C. S., Williams, B. A., Barnes, D. E., Lindquist, K., & Scillinger, D. (2006). Use of a modified informed consent process among vulnerable patients: A descriptive study. *Journal of General Internal Medicine, 21*, 1009.

Vortman, J. A. S., Parr, J. R., Moreno-De-Luca, D., Anney, R. J. L., Nurnberger, J. I., Jr., & Hallmayer, J. F. (2017). Autism genetics: Opportunities and challenges for clinical translation. *Nature Reviews. Genetics, 18*(6), 362–376. https://doi.org/10.1038/nrg.2017.4[doi]

Wagner, K. E., McCormick, J. B., Barns, S., Carney, M., Middleton, F. A., & Hicks, S. D. (2020). Parent perspectives toward genetic and epigenetic testing for autism spectrum disorder. *Journal of Autism and Developmental Disorders, 50*, 3114–3325.

Welch, B. M., Marshall, E., Oanungo, S., Aziz, A., Laken, M., Lenert, L., & Obeid, J. (2016). Teleconsent: A novel approach to obtain informed consent for research. *Contemporary Clinical Trials Communications, 3*, 74–79.

Wirshing, D. A., Wirshing, W. C., Murder, S. R., Liberman, R. P., & Mintz, J. (1998). Informed consent: Assessment of comprehension. *American Journal of Psychiatry, 155*, 1508–1511.

World Medical Association Declaration of Helsinki. (1964). Ethical principles for medical research involving human subjects. (2013). https://doi.org/10.1001/jama.2013.281053

Index

J. L. Matson (ed.), *Assessment and Diagnosis in Autism*, Autism and Child Psychopathology Series, https://doi.org/10.1007/978-3-032-11802-8

MIX
Papier aus verantwortungsvollen Quellen
Paper from responsible sources
FSC® C105338

If you have any concerns about our products,
you can contact us on
ProductSafety@springernature.com

In case Publisher is established outside the EU,
the EU authorized representative is:
Springer Nature Customer Service Center GmbH
Europaplatz 3, 69115 Heidelberg, Germany

Printed by Libri Plureos GmbH
in Hamburg, Germany